The Paths of Pain 1975–2005

Mission Statement of IASP Press®

The International Association for the Study of Pain (IASP) is a nonprofit, inter-disciplinary organization devoted to understanding the mechanisms of pain and improving the care of patients with pain through research, education, and communi-cation. The organization includes scientists and health care professionals dedicated to these goals. The IASP sponsors scientific meetings and publishes newsletters, tech-nical bulletins, the journal *Pain,* and books.

The goal of IASP Press is to provide the IASP membership with timely, high-quality, attractive, low-cost publications relevant to the problem of pain. These publi-cations are also intended to appeal to a wider audience of scientists and clinicians interested in the problem of pain.

The Paths of Pain 1975–2005

Editors

Harold Merskey, DM, FRCP, FRCP(C), FRCPsych
Professor Emeritus of Psychiatry, University of Western Ontario
London, Ontario, Canada

John D. Loeser, MD
Departments of Neurological Surgery and Anesthesiology,
University of Washington, Seattle, Washington, USA

Ronald Dubner, DDS, PhD
Department of Oral and Craniofacial Biological Sciences
Dental School, University of Maryland,
Baltimore, Maryland, USA

Editorial Committee

Jean-Marie Besson, DSc
Sir Michael R. Bond, MD, PhD, DSc, FRSE, FRCS, FRCPsych
Ronald Dubner, DDS, PhD
Ulf Lindblom, MD, DMSc
John D. Loeser, MD
Harold Merskey, DM, FRCP, FRCP(C), FRCPsych
Barry J. Sessle, MDS, PhD, DSC, FRSC
Manfred Zimmermann, Dr-Ing, Dr med

IASP PRESS® • SEATTLE

Library of Congress Cataloging-in-Publication Data

Available from the publisher.

Published by:

IASP Press
International Association for the Study of Pain
909 NE 43rd Street, Suite 306
Seattle, WA 98105-6020 USA
Fax: 206-547-1703
www.iasp-pain.org
www.painbooks.org

Printed in the United States of America

This volume is dedicated to
Louisa E. Jones

The authors and editors are pleased to dedicate this book to Ms. Louisa E. Jones. She is the key person in the development of IASP since its foundation in 1974. She has helped to translate the dream of John J. Bonica into the mature and flourishing association that we celebrate with this volume. Thirty-two years ago, Dr. Bonica organized an international meeting on pain that was held in a former convent in Issaquah, Washington. His administrative assistant for that critical meeting was Louisa Jones. When IASP was fully established, Louisa became its first employee as Executive Secretary. She has guided the development of our association with great skill, integrity, and wisdom. As our Executive Officer, she has played a crucial role in all of our activities. She has chosen to retire following the 2005 Congress, after 32 years of devoted service, and we will miss her greatly. Louisa will always be appreciated by this association, as will her unfailing commitment to its permanent place in science and medicine.

Contents

Contributing Authors

Allan I. Basbaum, PhD *Departments of Anatomy and Physiology and W.M. Keck Foundation Center for Integrative Neuroscience, University of California, San Francisco, California, USA*

Gary J. Bennett, PhD *Department of Anesthesia, Faculty of Dentistry, and Centre for Research on Pain, McGill University, Montreal, Quebec, Canada*

Jean-Marie Besson, DSc *INSERM Unit 161, Ambroise Paré Hospital, Boulogne-Billancourt, France*

Nikolai Bogduk, MD, PhD *Department of Clinical Research, Royal Newcastle Hospital, University of Newcastle, Newcastle, New South Wales, Australia*

Jörgen Boivie, MD *Department of Neurology, University Hospital, Linköping, Sweden*

Michael R. Bond, Kt, MD, PhD, DSc, FRSE, FRCS, FRCPsych *University of Glasgow, Glasgow, United Kingdom*

Rami Burstein, PhD *Departments of Anesthesia and Critical Care, Beth Israel Deaconess Medical Center; Department of Neurobiology and the Program in Neuroscience, Harvard Medical School, Boston, Massachusetts, USA*

M. Catherine Bushnell, PhD *McGill Centre for Research on Pain, Montreal, Quebec, Canada*

James N. Campbell, MD *Department of Neurosurgery and Applied Physics Laboratory, Johns Hopkins University, Baltimore, Maryland, USA*

Fernando Cervero, MD, PhD *Anaesthesia Research Unit, McGill University, Montreal, Quebec, Canada*

Michael J. Cousins, AM, MD, FANZCA, FRCA, FFPMANZCA, FAChPM (RACP) *Pain Management Research Institute, University of Sydney, Royal North Shore Hospital, St Leonards, New South Wales, Australia.*

Anthony H. Dickenson, PhD *Department of Pharmacology, University College London, London, United Kingdom*

Kim E. Dixon, PhD, MBA *Department of Psychiatry and Behavioral Sciences, Duke University Medical Center, Durham, North Carolina, USA*

Andy Dray, PhD *AstraZeneca Research and Development, Montreal, Quebec, Canada*

Ronald Dubner, DDS, PhD *Department of Biomedical Sciences, University of Maryland Dental School, Baltimore, Maryland, USA*

Michael S. Gold, PhD *Department of Biomedical Sciences, Dental School; Program in Neuroscience; and Department of Anatomy and Neurobiology, Medical School, University of Maryland, Baltimore, Maryland, USA*

Richard H. Gracely, PhD *Chronic Pain and Fatigue Research Program, Departments of Internal Medicine, Rheumatology and Neurology, University of Michigan and VA Medical Center, Ann Arbor, Michigan, USA*

David Hanscom, MD *Private Practice in Orthopedics, Seattle, Washington, USA*

Moshe Jakubowsky *Departments of Anesthesia and Critical Care, Beth Israel Deaconess Medical Center; Department of Neurobiology and the Program in Neuroscience, Harvard Medical School, Boston, Massachusetts, USA*

Louisa E. Jones, BS *International Association for the Study of Pain, Seattle, Washington, USA*

Frances J. Keefe, PhD *Department of Psychiatry and Behavioral Sciences, Duke University Medical Center, Durham, North Carolina, USA*

Linda LeResche, ScD *Department of Oral Medicine, University of Washington, Seattle, Washington, USA*

Dan Levy, PhD *Departments of Anesthesia and Critical Care, Beth Israel Deaconess Medical Center; Department of Neurobiology and the Program in Neuroscience, Harvard Medical School, Boston, Massachusetts, USA*

Ulf Lindblom, MD, DMSc *Department of Clinical Neurosciences, Section of Neurology, Karolinska Institute; Gösta Ekman Laboratory for Sensory Research, Department of Psychology, Stockholm University, Stockholm, Sweden*

Bengt Linderoth, MD, PhD *Department of Clinical Neuroscience, Section of Neurosurgery, Karolinska Institute and Karolinska University Hospital, Stockholm, Sweden*

John D. Loeser, MD *Departments of Neurological Surgery and Anesthesiology, University of Washington, Seattle, Washington, USA*

Steven F. Maier, PhD *Department of Psychology and Center for Neuroscience, University of Colorado at Boulder, Boulder, Colorado, USA*

Patricia A. McGrath, PhD *Department of Anesthesia, Divisional Centre of Pain Management and Research, The Hospital for Sick Children; Brain and Behavior Program, Research Institute at The Hospital for Sick Children; and the Department of Anesthesia, The University of Toronto, Toronto, Ontario, Canada*

Marcia L. Meldrum, PhD *John C. Liebeskind History of Pain Collection, Louise M. Darling Biomedical Library, and Department of History, University of California, Los Angeles, California, USA*

Harold Merskey, DM, FRCP, FRCPC, FRCPsych *Professor Emeritus of Psychiatry, University of Western Ontario, London, Ontario, Canada*

Richard A. Meyer, PhD *Department of Neurosurgery and Applied Physics Laboratory, Johns Hopkins University, Baltimore, Maryland, USA*

Björn A. Meyerson, MD, PhD *Department of Clinical Neuroscience, Section of Neurosurgery, Karolinska Institute and Karolinska University Hospital, Stockholm, Sweden*

Jeffrey S. Mogil, PhD *Department of Psychology and Centre for Research on Pain, McGill University, Montreal, Quebec, Canada*

Harvey Moldofsky, MD, FRCPC *Professor Emeritus, Faculty of Medicine, University of Toronto, Toronto, Ontario, Canada*

Dwight E. Moulin, MD, FRCPC *Departments of Oncology and Clinical Neurological Sciences, University of Western Ontario, and London Regional Cancer Centre, London, Ontario, Canada*

Paul M. Murphy, MB, MRCPI, FCARCSI *Pain Management Research Institute, University of Sydney, Royal North Shore Hospital, St Leonards, New South Wales, Australia.*

Michael H. Ossipov, PhD *Department of Pharmacology, University of Arizona Health Sciences Center, Tucson, Arizona, USA*

Frank Porreca, PhD *Department of Pharmacology, University of Arizona Health Sciences Center, Tucson, Arizona, USA*

Rebecca W. Pryor, BA *Department of Psychiatry and Behavioral Sciences, Duke University Medical Center, Durham, North Carolina, USA*

Dean Ricketts, MD *Private Practice in Orthopedics, Bellevue, Washington, USA*

James P. Robinson, MD, PhD *Department of Rehabilitation Medicine, University of Washington, Seattle, Washington, USA*

Barry J. Sessle, MDS, PhD, DSc, FRSC *Faculty of Dentistry, University of Toronto, Toronto, Ontario, Canada*

Michael Von Korff, ScD *Center for Health Studies, Group Health Cooperative, Seattle, Washington, USA*

Gordon Waddell, CBE, DSc, MD, FRCS *Centre for Psychosocial and Disability Research, University of Cardiff, Cardiff, United Kingdom*

Linda R. Watkins, PhD *Department of Psychology and Center for Neuroscience, University of Colorado at Boulder, Boulder, Colorado, USA*

C. Peter N. Watson, MD, FRCPC *University of Toronto, Toronto, Ontario, Canada*

William D. Willis, Jr., MD, PhD *Department of Neuroscience and Cell Biology, University of Texas Medical Branch, Galveston, Texas, USA*

Tony L. Yaksh, PhD *Department of Anesthesiology, University of California, San Diego, California, USA*

Manfred Zimmermann, Dr-Ing, Dr med *Neuroscience and Pain Research Institute, Heidelberg, Germany*

Foreword

This book is published by the International Association for the Study of Pain in celebration of the 30 years from the 1st World Congress of the Association in Florence in 1975 to the 11th World Congress in Sydney in 2005. The earlier formulation of the gate control theory of pain and the foundation and growth of the association generated a revolution involving almost all aspects of the study of pain and an explosive growth of knowledge. This revolution is reflected in the present volume by members of the IASP.

As dissemination of new information on pain is a major part of the goals of IASP, it is a pleasure to present this book to all participants of the 11th World Congress on Pain in Sydney, Australia. This book has only been made possible by a generous unrestricted grant from Pfizer Inc., and their contribution is gratefully acknowledged.

TROELS STAEHELIN JENSEN, MD, PHD
PRESIDENT-ELECT OF IASP

Preface

This volume is a commissioned work. The Council of the International Association for the Study of Pain (IASP) invited a group of editors to produce the volume to celebrate the 11th triennial World Congress on Pain, being held in Sydney 30 years after the 1st World Congress, held in Florence in 1975. This celebration was proposed because the IASP has flourished as an international institution, founded in unique circumstances as described in Chapter 2, evolving with advances in science and health care, and having an enormous influence, much greater than the number of its professional members might suggest.

The association is a professional scientific, medical, and health care body that provides support for research, patient care, and education about pain throughout the world. In its chosen disciplines the IASP has become a beneficial influence in spreading knowledge about pain and encouraging research on pain in all its aspects.

Such a claim should not be made lightly. It deserves or requires validation. We lack the temerity to claim that we have produced such validation in systematic social science and historical studies. That approach requires examination in depth of the state of pain medicine and other pain studies, including all the relevant sciences and clinical topics with their starting points and current end points. But there have been triumphs, as with the focus upon children's pain (Chapter 30), that the association appears to have facilitated. Many other developments support a favorable view of what has happened over the past 30 years.

We can, indeed, point to a number of indices of achievement between 1975 and 2005. First, there is the organization itself with its widespread membership and creation of chapters in 64 countries, only two or three of which had any sort of pain society, much less national chapters, before the start of the IASP. Notably, unlike most professional and scientific international organizations, the IASP was not founded by a group of existing societies from different countries, but came into being as an international body with specific purposes, thanks to the Herculean efforts of one individual, the late Dr. John J. Bonica, in raising the funds and persuading fellow scientists and clinicians to join his campaign.

The widespread international presence is strongly sustained by the success of the association's journal *PAIN*, which, by the usual criteria of early indexing, difficulty of access, number of papers, level of citation among its peers, and widespread recognition of the high standard of its contents, is unquestionably the leading journal in this field. It is also in the forefront among anesthesiology and neuroscience journals. In addition, the publications of IASP Press rank high in the world of medical science on pain.

Other significant advances in knowledge and practice include the establishment of clinical definitions for clinicians that have largely proved acceptable. Thus, the IASP functions as a body that has developed a classification of pain disorders, has provided criteria for education and training in numerous disciplines, and has published valuable appraisals of the state of knowledge, as in the series *Pain: Clinical Updates.*

The aim of this book is to show, within a limited space, how matters stood concerning knowledge of the many fields in which pain is important, in basic science, in clinical knowledge, and in health care, when the IASP started and where matters stand now. One book of the present size cannot adequately accommodate enough individual chapters to exhaustively appraise the changes that have occurred and the influence the IASP may have had in bringing about these changes. But what has happened in those 30 years is exciting in the history of knowledge and the progress of medicine, and to be able to provide a chronicle of those changes is a wonderful opportunity that allows us to display at least a portion of the progress, the arguments and the advances, the efforts and their outcome that we have witnessed in the life of the IASP.

Accordingly, the editors and the editorial committee agreed upon a series of chapters, each of limited length, with some economy of references but precision of report, that would display the evolution of ideas and information for these 30 years. Hard choices had to be made about topics that were left out, which ideally would have better rounded out the accounts now offered. Some of the editors' own favorite themes have been omitted because we strove to give a representative account without hoping unrealistically for an amply comprehensive statement. We offer sympathy to those who feel justice was not done to their particular focus of interest and seek a little sympathy in return for our efforts at self-restraint. The editors also want to acknowledge on behalf of the authors of chapters that many of them were obliged to omit material and references that they clearly took to be important.

The first chapter provides a highly focused historical account from the early modern period to the second half of the 20th century. The second chapter outlines the development, growth, success, and challenges of the IASP. Most other chapters start with an attempt to characterize the state of knowledge in 1975 and then move at varying speeds to the evolution of knowledge and our current situation. As editors we have not thought it practicable to set quotas on what proportion of each chapter should be devoted respectively to past, present, and future. We would like to believe that most readers will find this approach appropriate and interesting. Should we comment more often on how things did develop or where they are going? As we are historians here, we will avoid prediction. The benefit of historical study is well understood to be as a guide for the student to avoid, if possible, repetition of the errors of the past, and not to pretend to be wise enough to prevent new cases of error, which must be frequent in prophecy.

Difficulty in forecasting is particularly strong when it comes not so much to specific remedies as to organizational and social change. The final chapter of this volume looks ahead to see where the developments of knowledge to date may lead the world in biological knowledge and remedies for pain. We will not expand on this comment, but we should note as well the importance of psychological skills, not just in helping to explain pain, nor in curing it, but rather in helping to ease and support the patients and families who suffer through the maze of problems and the prolonged and often intense distress of severe chronic pain. We think it fair to claim that the international movement to help patients with pain, and to better understand the sources and causes of pain, has contributed to the atmosphere of respect for patients' pain, some reduction in the denigration or disparagement of pain, and a better recognition in many countries with which we are acquainted, and that have chapters of the IASP, that pain can be relieved.

To avoid the appearance of complacency, we emphasize that much more remains to be done for the relief of pain than has so far been accomplished from all sources, but that the association has, by its very existence, recognized and supported the dignity of the patient with pain. It is evident that that is not enough. No one expects to complete this task, but the principle of the association is that everyone should continue to contribute to it.

We thank the Council of the IASP for the wonderful opportunity to organize and display something of the state of knowledge on pain as it has existed and changed over the last 30 years. In so far as the association has been influential, so do we in turn feel privileged at the opportunity to edit the present volume.

We thank all the authors who provided chapters under strict conditions, agreeing to sacrifice some of their most attractive material in order to allow everyone else to have a fair opportunity to present their topics. We are grateful to Pfizer Limited for their generosity in funding this volume with an unrestricted grant, which meant that we were free to deal with any topic that we thought appropriate without reference to any of the interests of the donor.

We thank as well the other members of the editorial committee who joined us in the planning of this work and the staff of IASP Press, in particular the production editor, Elizabeth Endres, for outstanding assistance.

HAROLD MERSKEY
JOHN D. LOESER
RONALD DUBNER

The Paths of Pain 1975–2005, edited by
Harold Merskey, John D. Loeser, and Ronald
Dubner, IASP Press, Seattle, © 2005.

1

The History of Pain Concepts and Treatment before IASP[1]

Manfred Zimmermann

Neuroscience and Pain Research Institute, Heidelberg, Germany

A BACKGROUND TO THE MODERN HISTORY OF PAIN

The purpose of this chapter is to provide an overall historical and technical perspective on pain prior to the formation of the IASP in 1973 and the 1st World Congress on Pain in 1975. This perspective includes the social and cultural background and describes how pain was perceived. Its focus is on the main lines of medical thought about pain and the evolution of pain therapy in the five centuries preceding the foundation of IASP. This chapter does not deal with medieval or earlier times. Rey (1993) provides an excellent history of pain prior to and overlapping with the dates considered in this chapter.

SENSATIONS: FROM HEART TO BRAIN IN THE 15TH CENTURY

While the idea that the brain was the seat of perceptions had been promoted by a few philosophers and physicians, such as Pythagoras, Anaxagoras, and Galen in antiquity, or Avicenna (980–1037) and Albertus Magnus (1193–1280) in the middle ages, it did not replace Aristotle's postulate of the heart being the center for sensations and emotions until the Renaissance. This transition allowed pain to become a subject of interest for scientists investigating the brain.

Illustrations by Leonardo da Vinci (1452–1519) and Andreas Vesalius (1514–1564), based on systematic studies of autopsies, represented these novel ideas on brain function in great detail. According to da Vinci, the

---

[1]This article is adapted from a translation of Zimmermann (2001), with permission.

mind had its seat in the third ventricle of the brain, which was reached by sensations from the body and from the special sensory organs via the nerves and the spinal cord, represented in the form of tubes. In a drawing of a man with two bodies and two heads, Leonardo presented an allegory of pain and pleasure as a unitary concept of polar opposites, according to classical ideas described by Plato (Procacci and Maresca 1998). In view of these detailed anatomical presentations, it is surprising that brain functions continued to be associated with the brain *ventricles* (Clarke and Dewhurst 1972; Finger 1994). It took another 150 years until the gray and white matter of the brain was recognized as the functional substrate.

The shift in the concept of sensory functions from the heart to the brain is illustrated by the drawing in Fig. 1. Here, all the sensory organs are connected to the brain, including pain sensation indicated by the burning fire and by the snake biting the right arm of the person shown. Interestingly, the sensory pathways to the brain are connected to the heart as well, which may have been a tribute to the old views. This illustration is particularly important, because to my knowledge it is the first example that includes pain as part of the sensory systems, as symbolized by the fire and the snakebite. The drawing reminds us of the well-known drawing published 150 years later by Descartes, which will be discussed further below.

PAIN CONCEPTS IN THE 16TH CENTURY

Methods of relieving pain in the 16th century provided for the management of wounds with salves and other remedies. The *Feldbuch der Wundartzney* was an outstanding publication at the beginning of the modern period by Hans von Gerstdorff, a physician from Strassburg, who was working in the field as an army surgeon. In his book (von Gerstdorff 1976, originally published in 1517), he referred to ancient authorities such as Galen and Abu al-Qasim (Albucasis). The book contains 25 full-page woodcuts that display the therapeutic methods and tools available at the time. Von Gerstdorff advised that in caring for the wounded it is essential to pay attention to pain, stating that the caregiver should check to see if there is major pain or swelling and alleviate any pain and soreness.

For external pain treatment, von Gerstdorff recommended balsam (balm), bandages, and "Gliedwasser" (a term unknown in modern German, literally meaning "limb water"). The drug preparations contained substances such as galbanum and olibanum (resins similar to frankincense), sal ammoniac (ammonia), gum tragacanth, hypericum (St. John's wort), and rose oil. Some recipes even contained worms collected from the cemetery. In one of the

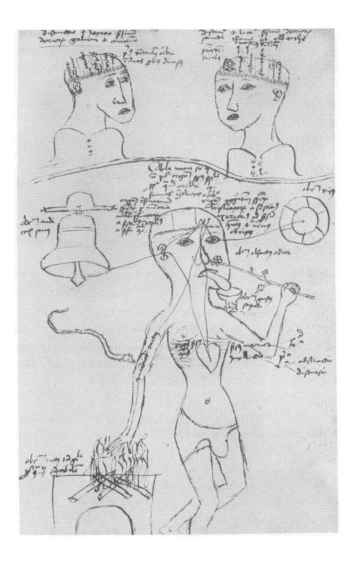

Fig. 1. Drawing showing the sensory systems of a human connected by lines (i.e. the sensory nerves) to both the heart and the brain. Hearing, vision, smell, taste, and pain are symbolized by pictograms, with pain being indicated by the fire affecting the hand and the snake biting the arm. The sensory connections to the brain express the concept prevailing since the Renaissance that the brain is the organ of sensation, while the bypass connections to the heart correspond to the antique view (promoted by Aristotle) that the heart is the seat of sensations, emotions, and mental functions. The two heads in the upper part express the functional subdivision of the brain, according to the cellular doctrine, in *Sensus communis, Phantasia, Imaginativa, Cogitativa, Aestimativa,* and *Memorativa.* The functional cells were associated with the brain ventricles. The drawing is contained on a fly-leaf in the book by Gerard de Harderwyck, *Epitomata seu reparationes totius philosophiae Aristotelis,* Part "De Sensu" (Cologne: H. Quentell, 1496). Reproduced from Clarke and Dewhurst (1972).

analgesic formulae, von Gerstdorff mentioned hemp (*Cannabis sativa*). Additives such as mastic gum and turpentine provided the preparations with a firm consistency. Such mixtures became fluid when warmed up, and could then be used to rinse the wound. Interestingly, an open skull wound was emphasized as a contraindication to this treatment, due to the risk of brain damage. For the treatment of recent or inflamed scars, von Gerstdorff recommended a bandage containing cantharidin (a vesicant derived from blister beetles).

Ambroise Paré (1510–1590), the great surgeon of the Renaissance period, was titled "Physician to the Kings of France." He provided detailed descriptions of the pain associated with wounds and surgery, and suggested methods for its relief. He specifically mentioned the different types of wounds induced by firearms and compared them with lacerations from more traditional weapons, pointing out that the bullet wounds were associated with much greater pain. He rejected the contemporary belief that the increased pain was due to poisoning from gunpowder.

The prevailing recommended treatment for bullet wounds was to apply boiling oil to cauterize them. In contrast, Paré discovered that ligation of vessels to stop bleeding and careful cleaning of the wounds resulted in much faster healing and much lower levels of pain. In 1564 he published his *Dix livres de la chirurgie* ("Ten books of surgery"), where he described these and many other new techniques for treating trauma. These books also contain many novel nonsurgical treatments and adjuvant techniques, such as advice on the reduction of dislocations, a description of a chair for steam baths to alleviate pain associated with urethral stones, and details of how to construct dentures, prosthetic noses, and mobile prostheses for missing hands and legs.

Paré was the first to describe pain from amputated limbs, named "phantom pain" by Silas Weir Mitchell 300 years later. Paré was particularly interested in devising better and more efficient methods of pain treatment. He emphasized the potential of drug preparations featuring opium as the main active ingredient. Paré used the name "anodyne" for pain-killing drugs, implying a justification for "symptomatic" pain treatment. By introducing symptomatic treatment, he resisted the common idea that pain was inflicted by God as a divine challenge.

Christianity associated salvation with the suffering of pain, holding that those who suffered pain during life on earth would be rewarded by access to Paradise. It was because of this positive interpretation of pain that doctors usually were not expected to make efforts to alleviate their patients' pain. In response to this prevailing attitude, Paré provided a somewhat sophisticated justification for his novel emphasis on pain treatment: "Even if a disease was sent to us by God, He gave us as well the remedies for the treatment, and if we use these remedies, we are glorifying God" (Rey 1993).

Paré was also greatly concerned with the treatment of pain induced by surgery, and he defined pain treatment as one of the important tasks of the surgeon. For example, he applied a tourniquet to block circulation in a limb before amputation to decrease sensation. One of his most important observations was that analgesia during and after surgery reduced various postoperative risks such as inflammation, fever, and gangrene. Another observation by Paré was that a positive and cooperative attitude on the part of the patient before surgery helped to improve the outcome of the operation, by which he anticipated today's beneficial concepts of pain coping. To improve the outcome of surgery, Paré considered it important that the patient be strengthened before surgery by relaxation and nourishment, and he even recommended delaying surgery in order to improve the patient's condition. In 1568 Paré published an article on how to treat the plague ("Traité de la peste"). In this publication, he listed the major symptoms of the plague, listing headache and kidney pain first.

PAIN IN THE THEORY AND PRACTICE OF MEDICINE IN THE 17TH CENTURY

In the 17th century, the theory of nervous system function was much promoted by René Descartes and Thomas Willis, dramatically changing the prevailing views on pain. Descartes (1596–1650) provided new concepts of the functional anatomy of the sensory organs and brain in his book *De Homine* (published posthumously in 1662). He may be considered the first analytical scientist in sensory physiology. In his famous allegorical picture he visualized the transmission of pain signals via the nerves and spinal cord as a bell-pull terminating in the brain ventricles and the pineal organ; this picture has been much used since it was reprinted in the original publication of the gate control theory of pain (Melzack and Wall 1965). For Descartes, the pineal organ was the tentative locus of the conscious perception of a pain stimulus. It was here that the signals of the outer world (*res extensa*) and the level of thinking and imagination (*res cogitans*) became connected to each other.

On the basis of this symbolic presentation, Descartes was considered to have introduced an extremely mechanistic view of nervous system and brain functions. I do not share this obvious criticism because in any modern textbook of neurophysiology, the same basic types of illustrations and interpretations are used to explain brain functions. Among Descartes' great innovations, he recognized for the first time the spatial mapping of the outer world in the brain and the basic principles of the brain's input-output functions.

Descartes never claimed to provide an explanation of mental functions (Procacci and Maresca 1998).

Thomas Willis (1622–1675) provided overwhelming evidence that the brain substance, including the cortex, is the substrate of sensory functions, and not the brain ventricles, as previously believed. For example, he localized the affective dimension of pain in the corpus striatum and corpus callosum. The motor and visceral reflexes associated with pain are initiated here and conducted via the cerebellum and brainstem, whereas the commands for the expression of pain are conducted to the facial muscles via the pons. Thus, it took 2000 years for Pythagoras's first association of pain sensation with the brain to become a generally established concept.

Thomas Sydenham (1624–1689) is known as a great reformer of medicine in England ("the English Hippocrates") and as the discoverer of the mechanism of the spread of disease in epidemic plague. He promoted the consistent and systematic treatment of pain. The analgesic drug laudanum, a composite of opium, saffron, cinnamon, and cloves in wine, was named by him. Based on his own experience as a pain patient, Sydenham strongly promoted laudanum as an indispensable basic tool of every physician. He complained that medicine performed without laudanum is rudimentary. According to him, laudanum was God's gift to console the suffering.

Sydenham gave the first comprehensive description of gout, a disease that he had himself. Apart from promoting the use of laudanum to treat the exacerbation of pain in gout, he also emphasized the role of lifestyle and diet in the pathogenesis and course of the disease. Thus, Sydenham was a pioneer of preventive measures in pain medicine.

The use of opium, consistently promoted by Sydenham, had strong opponents among his contemporaries. One of them was Georg Wolfgang Wedel (1645–1721), professor of medicine at the University of Jena in Germany. In 1684 Wedel published warnings that, among all the medications used by doctors, opium would require the doctor's most serious concern because of its dangerous and potentially lethal effects.

PHYSICS AND PSEUDOPHYSICS IN PAIN TREATMENT OF THE 18TH CENTURY

Applications of electricity and magnetism in medical therapy were prominent innovations in 18th-century medicine. Electricity generators using rotating glass disks had already been developed before 1700. Among the pioneers, the German physicist Otto von Guericke (1602–1686) published his experiments in 1672, and the British chemist and physicist Robert Boyle

(1627–1691), a founder of the Royal Society (1662), published his research on electricity in 1675. Within a short time, research on the nature of electricity and its propagation and remote actions had become an important topic in physics throughout Europe. This research received considerable support from the academies of science, which provided prizes for progress and discoveries in physics.

A breakthrough in medical use of electricity was initiated by the discovery of the Leyden jar (1745), which could be used for the storage and transportation of static electricity at high voltage. This was a glass bottle coated on the inside and outside with a metallic layer—a forerunner of the electric condenser, today a major element of electronic technology. The Leyden jar was charged by transiently connecting the metal layers with the poles of the generator. Several Leyden jars were charged for a treatment session, at which they were discharged through the patient's body, mostly at the site of the disease or of the pain. Discharges usually were associated with sparks; they evoked muscle and cardiovascular reflexes and sharp and strong sensations, often painful and frightening. This technology echoed the therapeutic use of electric fish known from ancient medicine.

A detailed description of treatment with electrical discharges was published in the 1766 book by Johann Gottlieb Schäffer (1720–1795), whose title translates to "Electrical medicine or the force and effect of electricity on the human body and diseases." Schäffer was a natural scientist as well as a medical practitioner. He used an electrostatic generator and Leyden jars to treat diseases associated with paralysis and pain (Fig. 2). According to Schäffer's description, the greatest therapeutic effect was obtained with "shaking electricity," when sparks were used to transmit the electricity to the patient, inducing strong muscular twitches, cardiovascular reflexes, and sensations that were usually painful. Schäffer also reported on the medical use of lightning during thunderstorms, which was conducted from the roof into the house with metal wires. Some of these applications had a fatal outcome for the patient or doctor, or both.

Schäffer's book contains impressive case descriptions of electrotherapy in paralysis, arthritis, rheumatism, gout, headache, cramps, and stroke. Some patients were free of symptoms after a single treatment, while others received repeated sessions. Schäffer explained the curative effects of electrical therapy mainly by the increases in blood flow. In addition, he claimed that nervous system functions become reactivated by external electricity, which would facilitate the return of normal function; this is still one of the principles of restorative neurology.

Electrotherapy continued to be used and developed for 250 years. In the late 19th century, Jean-Martin Charcot in Paris used a steam engine to

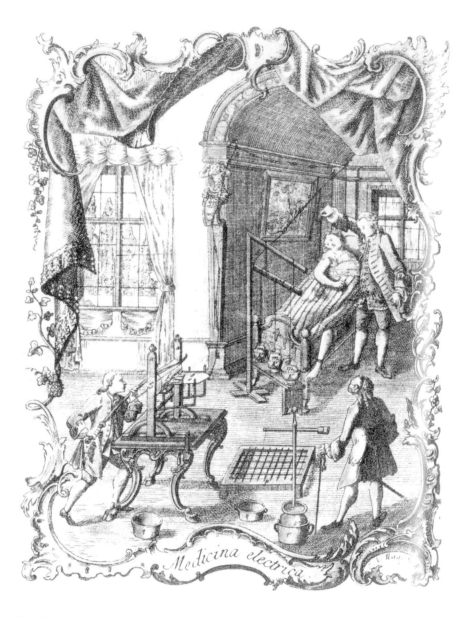

Fig. 2. Print showing the use of electricity to treat a patient, seen with his doctor in the rear cabinet. Electricity was produced by an electrostatic generator, consisting of rotating disk of glass or other insulating material. The electrical charge was conducted to and stored in Leyden jars (foreground right), which were carried to the patient. Electricity was then discharged to the patient's body via leads guided to the site of the disease (pain or paralysis) by the doctor. Figure reproduced from a facsimile reprint (1977) of Schäffer (1766).

operate an electrostatic generator to administer electrotherapy to psychiatric patients. Today, transcutaneous electrical nerve stimulation (TENS) has become a convenient small-scale version of electrotherapy for pain.

Another highlight of medicine originally associated with physics in the 18th century was presented by Franz Anton Mesmer (1734–1815), who claimed to utilize the physical forces of magnetism for medical treatment (Florey 1987). Today we know that Mesmer blatantly misinterpreted his observations. Mesmer is now partly credited with the discovery of hypnosis and related psychological forces in medicine, which are of great interest in modern pain medicine.

Mesmer was a student of metaphysics, theology, and medicine. His medical dissertation was on the influence of the planets on the human body. As a medical practitioner in Vienna, he founded the doctrine of "animal magnetism" and developed this idea into a new therapeutic method. Originally, Mesmer used iron magnets to treat various diseases, meeting with amazing success. He claimed that the therapeutic effect of the magnets were transmitted to the patient by the "fluidum," which was hypothesized in earlier physics to be the carrier of electrical and magnetic long-range effects. Mesmer soon observed that he could induce curative effects in patients just by directing his hands toward the patients, without using magnetized iron. He concluded that these effects originated from the magnetic forces originating from his own body.

In an attempt to amplify his magnetic forces, he used Leyden jars at room size, termed the "magnetic desk" or "baquet." He hosted ritual séances with groups of patients where he would play the glass harmonica, an instrument producing wonderful spheric sounds. The "fluidum" of physics was now reinterpreted as a carrier of cosmic vital forces. The rituals became more and more magical; female patients were particularly susceptible to these ritual acts, and were put into a trancelike state of "magnetic sleep." Physicians and charlatans increasingly used Mesmer's methods worldwide with variations of the magical rituals.

Mesmer was a kind of magician, but he was convinced that he was using scientific principles based on the physics of magnetism. However, Mesmer's methods were increasingly criticized as a pseudoscience, and in 1784 the Societé Royale in Paris rejected Mesmer's method as quackery. He was vindicated in 1812 by a medical committee guided by Wilhelm Christoph Hufeland, a highly respected medical professor in Berlin, and in 1831 the Paris Medical Academy also consented to Mesmer's posthumous vindication. In 1841 James Braid, an English physician, introduced the term "hypnosis" for the new therapeutic method unwittingly introduced by Mesmer.

DISCOVERIES IN THE 19TH CENTURY RELATING TO PAIN

PSYCHOPHYSICS OF EXPERIMENTAL PAIN

In the 19th century, pain became a subject in physiology. Magnus Blix (1849–1904) in Uppsala and Max von Frey (1852–1932) in Würzburg discovered that the spatial fine structure of cutaneous sensitivity consisted of discrete points at which sensations could be elicited by mechanical, thermal, or noxious stimuli (Handwerker and Brune 1987). They used calibrated hairs and bristles to exert defined mechanical stimuli to the skin of human subjects. The mosaic of pain points was different from that of the touch points. The conclusion from these psychophysical experiments was that specific sensory nerve endings exist in the skin for the sensation of painful stimuli. These "pain points" were associated anatomically with the intraepithelial free nerve endings.

Adolf Goldscheider (1858–1935) used the same instruments as von Frey to analyze cutaneous sensations, including pain. However, the conclusions formulated in his "intensity theory" or "summation theory" were at variance with those of von Frey; with increasing intensity of mechanical skin stimulation, the sensations reported by the subjects changed continuously from touch to pain (Goldscheider 1920). In Goldscheider's view, the neurophysiological information for touch and pain originate from the same set of nerve receptors.

While Goldscheider used the same equipment as von Frey to stimulate the skin, his stimulation paradigm included repetitive trains of stimulation and assessment of transitional phenomena during repetitive stimulation. Also, he included patients with abnormal skin sensations in his studies and accounted for their pathophysiological sensory phenomena when conceiving his summation theory. Goldscheider's observations and interpretations have been of great influence on subsequent pain theories, including the gate control theory (Melzack and Wall 1965).

THE DISCOVERY OF ETHER ANESTHESIA

In 1846 the first surgical operation using ether was conducted by John Collins Warren (1778–1856). The ether anesthesia was performed by William T.G. Morton (1819–1868), a dentist who had used this new type of anesthesia to completely suppress pain sensation during dental extraction. The report of Warren's cancer surgery without pain elicited a rush to use ether to prevent pain in various medical conditions (Fig. 3).

In Edinburgh, Sir James Young Simpson (1811–1870) used ether in childbirth as early as in 1847. In the same year he discovered chloroform as an alternative to ether. Childbirth under anesthesia was heavily criticized by Calvinistic ministers, who declaimed that the pain of childbirth was imposed by God on mankind, as stated in the Bible, when Adam and Eve were chased out of Paradise: "In pain shall you bear children." (The Hebrew word "etsev" can mean pain, toil, trouble, or grief.)

Ether anesthesia resulted in a wave of opposition. The early comprehensive review on the new method by Dieffenbach in 1847 (reprinted 1985) contains a detailed record of its unwanted effects, such as hallucinations, nightmares, cramps, and even death. However, artificially pain-free childbirth was finally accepted when Queen Victoria asked for anesthesia with chloroform in her eighth childbirth in 1853.

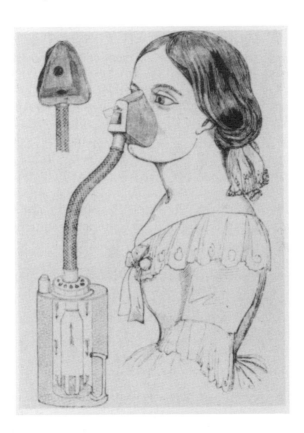

Fig. 3. Chloroform inhaler as developed and used by John Snow, Queen Victoria's anesthetist at her eighth childbirth (1853). The mouth and nose adapter was equipped with an expiration valve. The sectional drawing of the evaporator shows air being forced through the chloroform compartment. Figure from the book by John Snow, *On Chloroform and Other Anesthetics* (Bethesda, MD: National Library of Medicine, 1858), reproduced from Lyons and Petrucelli (1978).

The French physiologist François Magendie (1783–1855) opposed the use of ether in the Academy of Science in Paris. He strongly rejected the death-like state that enabled doctors to cut and scrape unrestricted by the patient's pain. Magendie's argument was that pain is one of the strongest driving forces of life that simply should not be removed. In addition, Magendie warned of the dangerous exacerbation of sensuality, comparable to the effects of animal magnetism, that would place women in particular at a risk similar to that of inebriation.

INCREASING SENSITIVITY TO PAIN IN HISTORY?

The anesthetic effect of nitrous oxide ("laughing gas") was reported as early as 1800 by the English chemist Sir Humphrey Davy (1778–1829), and that of ether was described in 1818 by the English physicist Michael Faraday (1791–1829). Both of these reports mentioned the possibility that anesthesia could be utilized for surgery (DeMoulin 1974).

To explain why these early reports did not immediately spark experiments with anesthesia for surgery, it has been argued that the pain sensitivity of humans may have been much lower at the time of these earlier reports. Mesmer's magnetic treatment was considered to have contributed to the increase in pain sensitivity of humans because it had introduced a powerful means by which to alleviate pain. The medical historian DeMoulin (1974) provided a critical post hoc analysis of indicators of pain sensitivity from the medical literature in the late 18th and early 19th centuries. He stated that there was no evidence for a change in pain sensitivity during this period, since he found examples of excruciating suffering as well as cases of remarkable tolerance of pain, such as in invasive medical procedures.

In contrast, Silas Weir Mitchell (1830–1914) provided evidence in favor of increasing pain sensitivity in his essay "Civilization and Pain" (Mitchell 1892). He concluded that progress in civilization implied an increase in pain sensitivity. The French surgeon René Leriche (1879–1955) adhered to the hypothesis that an increase in pain sensitivity occurred after the wide use of general anesthesia in medicine and childbirth. A similar hypothesis was promoted by Frederik Buytendijk (1948), who coined the term "algophobia" to denote increasing pain sensitivity, which he thought was due to the increasing medical options available by which to control pain.

Modern versions of the old issue of changing pain sensitivity have become important topics of today's medicine. To what extent has the sociocultural understanding of pain as a disease contributed to the rapid increase in the prevalence of chronic pain conditions such as low back pain, which has become a major reason for temporary or permanent disability or behaving as an invalid?

THE DISCOVERY OF LOCAL ANESTHESIA

Another sensational event, following the discovery of ether anesthesia, was the discovery of local anesthesia by Carl Koller (1857–1944) in Vienna. Koller used cocaine, a plant alkaloid extracted from South American coca plants. Cocaine, well known as a psychotropic substance, was traditionally used as an energizer by the Incas living at high altitudes in the Andes. An alcoholic extract from coca leaves became fashionable as a stimulating drink under the label "Vin Mariani" in France.

Sigmund Freud (1856–1939) in Vienna investigated the performance-enhancing and psychotropic effects of cocaine; he alerted the young ophthalmologist Carl Koller to the numbness that could be induced by cocaine in the oral cavity. Koller was aware of the need of a local anesthetic substance to perform invasive treatments on the eye that would prevent pain and disturbing reflexes. Although a publication by the physiologist von Anrep had appeared in 1879 in *Pflügers Archiv der gesamten Physiologie,* describing cocaine's local anesthetic effects in animal experiments, the enormous practical significance of this finding had remained unnoticed for several years.

Koller started experiments on animals and on himself and his colleagues, and within a short time he had evidence for rapid and complete local anesthesia in the eye. The first clinical application was a cataract operation under irrigation of the eye with a 2% cocaine solution, an operation that was completely pain free. A few days later, in September 1884, he asked a colleague traveling to the German Ophthalmology Congress in Heidelberg to present and demonstrate his findings, as he lacked the funds to travel to Heidelberg himself. In the same year, Koller (1884) published his discovery in *The Lancet.* Koller's biography was published 80 years later by his daughter, with reference to many important documents relating to the discovery and the broad foundation of local anesthesia in medicine (Koller-Becker 1963).

ISOLATION AND SYNTHESIS OF ANALGESIC SUBSTANCES

Some basic analgesic drugs for systemic use were also discovered in the 19th century: morphine, aspirin, antipyrine, and phenacetin.

Sertürner and morphine. In 1806 the young pharmacist Friedrich Wilhelm Sertürner (1783–1841) reported on his discovery and extraction of the sleep-inducing substance (*principium somniferum*) contained in opium, the extract of poppy juice used in medicine for centuries. He tested his extracts in heroic experiments on himself and his friends.

In those times pharmacy was not an academic profession but was learned in a four-year apprenticeship. Sertürner completed this apprenticeship and passed a final examination to obtain the qualifications necessary to conduct a pharmacy. He started his experiments on opium soon after completion of his training at the age of 20 years. The publication of his discovery (Sertürner 1806) remained unnoticed. He changed the subjects of his scientific interest, working on alkali and electricity. After nearly 10 years he resumed his investigation of opium extracts and used the new label "morphium" (derived from Morpheus, the Greek god of sleep) for the sleep-inducing substance (Sertürner 1817). This publication was widely acknowledged, and Sertürner became famous throughout Europe. The University of Jena awarded him the degree of Dr. Phil. in his absence, acknowledging the 1817 publication as his doctoral thesis. Subsequently, several other investigators, in particular from France, claimed priority in the discovery of morphine. These controversies were terminated in 1831 when the Institut de France awarded Sertürner a prize of 2,000 francs for his discovery of morphine.

The production of morphine was taken over by another pharmacist, Heinrich E. Merck in Darmstadt, starting in 1820. The laboratory of Merck's pharmacy was the origin of the E. Merck Company in Germany as well as Merck, Sharp and Dohme in the United States.

Development of aspirin, metamizol, and paracetamol (acetaminophen). Later, several other plant substances, which were traditionally used to alleviate pain, became the targets of drug development. The rationale was to identify and isolate the active molecule in a plant extract.

The Italian chemist Raffaele Piria (1815–1865) isolated salicylate, a glycoside, from willow bark, which had long been used as an analgesic. Salicylic acid was derived as a synthetic product from salicylate, the sodium salt which was produced industrially and became widely used from 1896 in Germany for the treatment of fever, polyarthritis, and sciatica (Handwerker and Brune 1987; Havertz et al. 1996). The final stage in the refinement of this drug was its acetylation, invented in 1897 by Felix Hoffmann, a chemist in the laboratory of the Bayer Company. The resulting acetylsalicylic acid, a powerful analgesic, was marketed by Bayer from 1899 under the label Aspirin. Aspirin was the first drug to be protected by a patent, and it remained the front-runner of analgesic drugs for more than 100 years.

Other synthetic analgesics were discovered in the search for drugs against fever. The first compound of the chemical group of pyrazolinones was antipyrine, jointly developed in 1884 by the chemist Ludwig Knorr and the pharmacologist Wilhelm Filehne at the University of Erlangen, followed by aminopyrine (Pyramidon) in 1896. A pyrazolone drug still used today is the sodium sulfonate of aminopyrine (known as metamizol sodium in Europe and as dipyrone in the United States and Britain).

The aniline derivatives, with acetanilide a prototype, also were originally developed as antipyretic drugs in 1887. However, their excellent analgesic effect soon became evident, changing the primary indication of these drugs to the treatment of pain. Phenacetin, most widely used as an over-the-counter analgesic, turned out to be nephrotoxic with prolonged use, and therefore was withdrawn from the market. Paracetamol (known as acetaminophen in the United States) was identified as an analgesic metabolite of phenacetin by Julius Axelrod in New York (1948) and became available as an analgesic drug in 1956.

Facsimile-reprints of key publications in German relating to the development of some of these drugs were published, together with an English translation, on the occasion of the 5th World Congress on Pain in Hamburg in 1987 (Handwerker and Brune 1987). They provide a direct glimpse into the pioneering era of analgesic drug development.

RECOGNIZING NEUROPATHIC PAIN IN A WAR

Great progress in the understanding of neuropathic pain was achieved by Weir Mitchell (1872) during the American Civil War. Again, war imposed major challenges on practitioners called on to treat painful wounds, similar to the work by Hans von Gerstdorff and Ambroise Paré described above. From 1863, Mitchell, a neurologist, provided detailed descriptions of post-traumatic neuralgias, phantom pain, and causalgias from cases he treated at the Philadelphia Hospital. For example, he observed patients with extreme hyperalgesia (or allodynia, according to modern taxonomy) following gunshot lesions of major nerves to the arms and legs. In some of these patients, severe amplification of burning pain occurred during excitement associated with sympathetic cardiovascular activation. Mitchell was the first to use the term *causalgia* for this syndrome, and he introduced innovative treatments including ice packs and baths, as well as bandages to protect against touch stimuli.

In the case of continuous excruciating pain, Mitchell routinely administered morphine injections several times a day. He administered a total of 40,000 morphine dosages within one year, and some patients received up to 500 injections per year. Mitchell reported on the excellent analgesic effect of the morphine. Interestingly, he administered morphine locally to the site of the lesion in cases of causalgia and therefore may be credited for the first observation of a peripheral opioid action.

Apart from his enthusiastic descriptions of the analgesia elicited by morphine treatment, he also reported on "very unfavorable physical and moral conditions" related to the use of morphine, i.e., the induction of dependence and addiction. Today he could have prevented such unfortunate outcomes by administering morphine at regular time intervals, following the guidelines introduced by the World Health Organization in 1986.

CHALLENGES AND CHANGING PAIN CONCEPTS DURING THE 20TH CENTURY

The first half of the 20th century left millions of patients in pain from injuries sustained in two world wars. Enormous new challenges arose with the need for treatment and care of those with old and new pain syndromes, and with increasing needs for medical education. After World War II, anesthesiologists and neurosurgeons were the first to respond to these challenges, resulting in rapidly increasing therapeutic skills and newly developed scientific concepts related to pain. First I will review the theoretical background that developed during the early 20th century.

CLINICAL RESEARCH ON PAIN

Sir Henry Head (1861–1940), a neurologist in London, criticized the specificity theory of skin sensation as formulated by Max von Frey (described above), because it was inadequate to explain clinical pain cases. Head used a different approach based on his clinical observations and his experience of sensory alterations following self-inflicted transections of some of his cutaneous small nerve branches. Accordingly, he formulated a new theory of the somatosensory system, outlining the *epicritic* and *protopathic* sensitivities of somatosensation (Head et al. 1905). Epicritic sensitivity referred particularly to well-localized touch sensations, while protopathic sensitivity referred to poorly localized, dull, disagreeable, and pathological sensations, which were, for the most part, related to the realm of pain sensations with a strong affective quality. According to Head, protopathic sensitivity was the first to reappear in the case of a regenerating nerve.

On the basis of electrophysiological studies by Erlanger and Gasser (1937), epicritic sensitivity was associated with the fast-conducting, large-diameter, myelinated A fibers in peripheral nerves. Protopathic sensitivity, on the other hand, was associated with the slowly conducting, nonmyelinated C fibers. An important basic observation by Head was that protopathic sensitivity was inhibited or masked by simultaneous activation of epicritic sensation. Later researchers found inconsistencies in Head's conception of a dual mechanism for cutaneous sensation, and it was nearly abandoned. More recently, in the context of neuropsychological investigations with brain imaging, interest is re-emerging in Head's conceptualization of these dual aspects of sensation.

Earlier work by Head (1893) was related to pain referral from the viscera to the body surface. The skin areas to which visceral sensations are referred were soon termed *Head's zones*, now explained physiologically by the convergence of visceral and cutaneous afferent fibers onto spinal cord neurons. Head's zones and other signs of pain referral remain basic principles in the diagnosis and assessment of internal diseases.

Otfried Foerster (1873–1941), a neurosurgeon and psychiatrist in Breslau, Germany, exploited therapeutic neurosurgery to study the human nervous system. He was one of the first surgeons to systematically use cordotomy (transection of the spinal anterolateral tract) for the treatment of pain. He carefully mapped the human dermatomes of therapeutic cases using spinal root transection or electrical stimulation. His clinical experience, enriched by ingenious conceptualization, was published in a valuable monograph on central pathways of pain (Foerster 1927), which is still essential reading material for the pain scientist and clinician. For example, he concluded from some clinical observations that spinal sensory transmission is under descending control from the brain.

The concepts of pain based on clinical studies by Head, Foerster, and others were further elaborated by William Noordenbos (1959) into a pain theory of central interactions, and his book *Pain* was a major support for the gate control theory (Melzack and Wall 1965), which was originally conceived without knowledge of his work.

René Leriche (1879–1955), a French surgeon, became a provocative and emphatic advocate of pain therapy in his lectures at the Collège de France, published in his book *Chirurgie de la douleur* (Leriche 1936). He coined the concept of pain as a disease (*douleur maladie*) to which multiple factors contribute. He emphasized excruciating chronic pain related to dysfunction of the sympathetic nervous system, and therefore he recommended interventions on the sympathetic nervous system. He criticized the overemphasis on pain as a tool in medical diagnosis, which often resulted in insufficient pain treatment and unnecessary suffering. He also criticized the fact that patients complaining of excruciating pain were often considered neurotic by doctors.

EXPERIMENTAL AND CLINICAL NEUROPHYSIOLOGY OF PAIN

Yngve Zotterman (1898–1982), a Swedish neurophysiologist, had recorded the first single nerve fiber action potentials in Lord Adrian's laboratory in Cambridge in 1926. Ten years later, Zotterman (1936) published the first action potentials recorded from a single nociceptive nerve fiber, probably a nonmyelinated C fiber, in the cat's tongue in response to noxious heating. He was the first to use, in pain research, the cathode ray oscilloscope, which had just been introduced in neurophysiology (Erlanger and Gasser 1937). From the 1950s, the functional characteristics of nociceptors were systematically explored in Edinburgh by the neurophysiologist Ainsley Iggo (born in 1922).

In the 1930s and 1940s, several contributions were published that became important for the development of pain concepts relevant to clinical phenomena. Thomas Lewis (1881–1945), a doctor of internal medicine in London, published his studies on pain, mostly conducted on human subjects and patients, in a stimulating monograph (Lewis 1942). His themes were visceral pain, referred pain, and primary and secondary hyperalgesia. He postulated the existence of a humoral nocifensive system based upon chemical mediators that slowly increased pain sensitivity in the environment of a primary lesion. Among the mediators he identified were histamine, bradykinin, and substance P. From his discoveries the concept of neurogenic inflammation emerged, which is now considered to contribute to pain-enhancing interactions between the nervous and immune systems in rheumatic and neuropathic diseases.

Innovative studies on the phenomenon of hyperalgesia were performed at Yale University by J.D. Hardy (a physiologist) and H.G. Wolff (a neurologist) on human subjects and patients (Hardy et al. 1950). These investigators identified central mechanisms in secondary hyperalgesia as mediators of progressively painful diseases. They built their ideas on a "neuronal pool" of variable excitability in the spinal cord, which had been conceptualized in 1943 by the surgeon William K. Livingston (1892–1966). Livingston treated and studied complex clinical pain phenomena during World War II, such as referred pain and causalgia, and emphasized their continual exacerbation if they were not treated consistently. In 1947 he initiated a pain project at the University of Oregon to study the physiology and psychology of pain in a clinical setting.

The concepts developed in about 1950 by Hardy, Wolff, Livingston, and others, relating to spinal mechanisms of hyperalgesia, were rediscovered and extended from about 1985 onwards, and now form part of our understanding of the central components of hyperalgesia and the progressive chronicity of pain.

NEW VISTAS ON PAIN SINCE 1950

After World War II enormous challenges arose relating to the medical care of the millions wounded during the war. The foremost pioneer of their care was John Bonica (1917–1994) in the United States, who established the first interdisciplinary pain clinic in 1947 to treat pain problems of wounded veterans (Bonica 1950). This clinic became part of the University of Washington in Seattle in 1960 and received worldwide recognition for its interdisciplinary treatment of pain problems. Bonica's *Management of Pain* (now in its third edition) became a bible for generations of doctors interested in pain treatment (Bonica 1953). It was Bonica's initiative and efforts that resulted in the foundation of the International Association for the Study of Pain (IASP) during the unforgettable International Symposium on Pain in Issaquah, Washington, May 21–26, 1973 (Bonica 1974).

At the same time there was renewed interest in the basic science of pain. The publication of the gate control theory by Ronald Melzack and Patrick Wall (1965) was aimed at an integration of the views of neurophysiology, psychology, and the huge variety of clinical phenomenon related to pain in patients, in an attempt to set up a coherent system of ideas. Although some of its neurophysiological details were later disproved (Zimmermann 1968), the gate control theory provided a new perspective on pain for medical scientists and is now considered the foundation of modern conceptions of pain.

The primary mission of the newly founded IASP was to further advance pain research and treatment at an international level. Since then, there has been great progress in all aspects of pain research, as described in this volume. The most important milestones, described fully in other chapters, were the discovery of endogenous opioids and central nervous system pain control systems, research on the neuromodulation of pain, oral and spinal administration of opioids for chronic pain, and work on psychological elements in chronic pain and pain therapy. More recently, other important topics have emerged, including the plasticity of the nervous system and progressive pain chronicity, risk factor models for pain, genetic determinants of pain and pain treatment, and interdisciplinary networks in the health system for the therapy and prevention of pain.

While postwar basic experimental pain research had resumed by approximately 1960, a phase of steadily growing clinical pain research began with the foundation of IASP. The early 1980s saw an upsurge of interdisciplinary basic, clinical, and psychological research, which resulted in the recognition of pain as a fundamental issue of medicine and health care.

REFERENCES

Bonica JJ. Organization and function of a pain clinic. *Northwest Med* 1950; 49:593–596.

Bonica JJ. *The Management of Pain.* Philadelphia: Lea & Febiger, 1953.

Bonica JJ (Ed). *International Symposium on Pain,* Advances in Neurology, Vol. 4. New York: Raven Press, 1974.

Buytendijk FJJ. *Über den Schmerz* (German trans). Bern: H. Huber, 1948.

Clarke E, Dewhurst K. *An Illustrated History of Brain Function.* Berkeley: University of California, 1972.

DeMoulin D. A historical-phenomenological study of bodily pain in Western man. *Bull Hist Med* 1974; 48:540–570.

Descartes R. *De Homine.* Leyden: Moyardus and Leffen, 1662.

Dieffenbach JF. *Der Aether gegen den Schmerz.* Berlin: A. Hirschwald, 1847; reprint 1985.

Erlanger J, Gasser HS. *Electrical Signs of Nervous Activity.* Philadelphia: University of Pennsylvania Press, 1937, 2nd ed. 1968.

Finger S. *Origins of Neuroscience: A History of Explorations into Brain Function.* New York: Oxford University Press, 1994.

Florey E. Franz Anton Mesmers magische Wissenschaft. *Konstanzer Blätter für Hochschulfragen* 1987; 94:5–32.

Foerster O. *Die Leitungsbahnen des Schmerzgefühls und die chirurgische Behandlung der Schmerzzustände.* Berlin: Urban & Schwarzenberg, 1927.

Goldscheider A. *Das Schmerzproblem.* Berlin: Springer, 1920.

Handwerker HO, Brune K (Eds). *Classical German Contributions to Pain Research.* Heidelberg: Gesellschaft zum Studium des Schmerzes für Deutschland, Österreich und die Schweiz, 1987.

Hardy JD, Wolff HG, Goodell H. Experimental evidence on the nature of cutaneous hyperalgesia. *J Clin Invest* 1950; 29:115–140.

Havertz B, Müller-Jahncke WD, Alstaedter R, Gotthold J. *Schmerz zwischen Steinzeit und Moderne: Ein Führer durch die Geschichte der Schmerztherapie.* Leverkusen: Bayer AG, 1996.

Head H. On disturbances of sensation with special reference to the pain of visceral disease. *Brain* 1893; 16:1–133.

Head H, Rivers WHR, Sherren J. The afferent nervous system from a new aspect. *Brain* 1905; 28:109–115.

Koller C. On the use of cocaine for producing anaesthesia on the eye. *Lancet* 1884; II:990–992.

Koller-Becker H. Carl Koller and cocaine. *Psychoanal Q* 1963; 32:309–373.

Leriche R. *La Chirurgie de la Douleur.* Paris: Masson, 1936.

Lewis T. *Pain.* New York: MacMillan Press, 1942.

Livingston WK. *Pain Mechanisms.* New York: MacMillan Press, 1943.

Lyons AS, Petrucelli RJ (Eds). *Medicine—An Illustrated History.* New York: Harry N. Abrams, 1978.

Melzack R, Wall PD. Pain mechanisms: a new theory. *Science* 1965; 150:971–979.

Mitchell SW. *Injuries to Nerves and Their Consequences.* Philadelphia: Lippincott, 1872.

Mitchell SW. Civilization and pain. *JAMA* 1892; 18:108.

Noordenbos W. *Pain.* Amsterdam: Elsevier, 1959.

Procacci P, Maresca M. Historical development of the concept of pain. *Pain Clin* 1998; 10:211–228.

Rey R. *History of Pain.* Paris: Editions La Decouverte, 1993.

Schäffer JG. *Die Electrische Medicin oder die Kraft und Wirkung der Electricität in den Menschlichen Körpern und dessen Krankheiten,* 2nd ed. Regensburg: Johann Leopold Montag, 1766. Facsimile ed. Lindau: Antiqua-Verlag, 1977.

Sertürner FW. Darstellung der reinen Mohnsäure (Opiumsäure) nebst einer chemischen Untersuchung des Opiums mit vorzüglicher Hinsicht auf einen darin neu entdeckten Stoff und die dahin gehörigen Bemerkungen. *Trommsdorffs J Pharmacie* 1806;14.

Sertürner FW. Über das Morphium, eine neue salzfähige Grundlage und die Mekonsäure, als Hauptbestandteile des Opiums. *Gilberts Annalen der Physik* 1817; 55:61.

Von Gerstdorff H. *Feldbuch der Wundartzney.* Strasburg: 1517. Facsimile ed. Lindau: Antiqua-Verlag, 1976.

World Health Organization. *Cancer Pain Relief.* Geneva: World Health Organization, 1986.

Zimmermann M. Dorsal root potentials after C-fibre stimulation. *Science* 1968; 160:896–898.

Zimmermann M. Zur Geschichte des Schmerzes. In: Zenz M, Jurna I (Eds). *Lehrbuch der Schmerztherapie.* Stuttgart: Wissenschaftliche Verlagsgesellschaft, 2001, pp 3–24.

Zotterman Y. Specific action potentials in the lingual nerve of the cat. *Scand Arch Physiol* 1936; 75:105–119.

Correspondence to: Professor Manfred Zimmermann, Dr.-Ing., Dr.med.h.c., Neuroscience and Pain Research Institute, Bonhoeffer Str. 17, 69123 Heidelberg, Germany. Email: manzimm@aol.com.

2

The History of the IASP: Progress in Pain since 1975

Michael R. Bond,[a] Ronald Dubner,[b] Louisa E. Jones,[c] and Marcia L. Meldrum[d]

[a]Emeritus Professor of Psychological Medicine, University of Glasgow, Glasgow, United Kingdom; [b]Department of Biomedical Sciences, University of Maryland Dental School, Baltimore, Maryland, USA; [c]International Association for the Study of Pain, Seattle, Washington, USA; [d]John C. Liebeskind History of Pain Collection, Louise M. Darling Biomedical Library, and Department of History, University of California, Los Angeles, California, USA

THE ORIGINS OF THE IASP

The International Association for the Study of Pain began in May 1973 with an exciting interdisciplinary meeting that brought together scientists and clinicians from 13 countries. Anesthesiologist and pain advocate John J. Bonica organized the meeting, held at a former convent in Issaquah, Washington, and invited 350 participants. Every session was a plenary, and more than one-third of the participants were speakers; the isolated setting ensured that conversation and debate continued after the formal presentations had ended. At the final session, the participants agreed unanimously to launch a multidisciplinary, professional organization dedicated to pain research and management and a journal, edited by Patrick D. Wall, to be called, simply, *PAIN*.

The new international group planned to come together at a World Congress on Pain every three years. Before the first such meeting convened in Florence in September 1975, Bonica, Wall, and Bonica's assistant, Louisa E. Jones, faced a massive organizational challenge. Bonica wrote the bylaws and oversaw the incorporation of the IASP, which was finalized on May 9, 1974. Wall negotiated the publication of *PAIN*, to begin as a quarterly journal with 400 pages a year, produced by Elsevier. Volume 1, Number 1 appeared in January 1975. Jones, working out of Bonica's office at the

University of Washington, solicited recommendations for members from those who had attended the Issaquah Symposium and sent out letters and membership applications. The initial dues were $25.

The enthusiasm and interest generated at Issaquah carried through that first congress. The association had grown to 1300 members from 35 countries by the opening day, and more than 800 registrants attended to hear 265 presentations. Wall gave the keynote address, "Modulation of Pain by Non-Painful Events." Several one-day special symposia were organized, including one on cancer pain that would lead to a redefinition of that problem and the development of the World Health Organization (WHO) analgesic ladder. Denise Albe-Fessard, the French physiologist, was chair of the Program Committee and was elected the IASP's first president, while John Bonica became president-elect. Jones was given both the elective office of treasurer and the staff position of executive secretary. Several committees were formed; among the most important were the Subcommittee on Taxonomy, chaired by Harold Merskey, then of the United Kingdom, and the Ad Hoc Committee on Ethical Issues, chaired by Manfred Zimmermann of Germany.

The IASP solidified its goals and aspirations over the next nine years. Bonica presented nine key objectives for the organization at the 2nd World Congress in Montreal in 1978, where 380 papers were presented. Merskey's group published its first list of pain definitions in *PAIN,* by then a bimonthly journal, in 1979. The first 11 national and regional chapters were organized. The initial spurt of membership growth gave way to a slower expansion; by 1981, there were just under 2000 members, and 1600 registrants from 41 countries attended the 3rd World Congress in Edinburgh. Responses to a member questionnaire indicated that IASP was meeting its obligations in an "impressive" manner.

The Edinburgh congress was highlighted by Hans Kosterlitz's talk on opioid peptides, one of the many new research directions in the pain field. Neurophysiologist Ainsley Iggo, who welcomed the IASP to his home city, became IASP president for the next three years. *PAIN,* under Wall's leadership, continued to grow in reputation and substance, becoming a monthly publication with 1200 pages a year in 1982. Zimmermann's committee addressed a key problem of public concern when it published ethical guidelines for research in conscious animals in 1983.

With the 4th World Congress in 1984, IASP returned to its origins in Seattle. Ronald Melzack became the fourth president and set as his goals the "revamping" of the committee structure and a meeting with all the national and regional chapter presidents. There were many other signs that the organization was coming to maturity. The first John J. Bonica Distinguished Lectureship honored Edward R. Perl of the University of North Carolina and his congress presentation, "Unraveling the Story of Pain." A major achievement of IASP's first decade was the publication of the first edition of the Committee on Taxonomy's "Classification of Chronic Pain" in *PAIN* in 1986. Several other long-term projects came to fruition during Melzack's tenure and were realized just before or during the 5th World Congress in Hamburg in 1987, including recognition by WHO as a nongovernmental organization and presentation of the first refresher course. In July of 1987, a cherished dream of John Bonica became a reality when several members of the IASP Council and the International Pain Foundation Board were granted a familial audience with Pope John Paul II, who later issued a Papal Letter recognizing the importance of the work of these organizations to end human suffering.

Under presidents Michael Cousins and Ulf Lindblom, IASP began an era of major growth. Cousins, like Melzack, envisioned the organization as becoming more proactive and oversaw the creation of a number of new task forces, including one on acute pain management, chaired by Brian Ready, and another to develop a curriculum for each of the many health professions engaged in pain management, chaired by Issy Pilowsky. The first curriculum outline, for medical schools, appeared in 1988. Other task forces reviewed standards for pain treatment facilities and for fellowship training in pain. Further new developments of this era were the addition of a Technical Corner, adding some scientific content to the *IASP Newsletter,* in 1988 and the organization of the first Special Interest Group (SIG), on Pain in Childhood, in 1989.

Cousins and Lindblom actively promoted IASP membership to clinicians and researchers from developing and poorly-resourced countries. The IASP Council recognized the need to provide assistance by reducing membership fees for these individuals and offered members in the richer nations opportunities to contribute to Adopt-a-Member or to Adopt-a-University-Library programs. As a result, IASP grew in size and diversity, boasting 25 national chapters at the 6th World Congress in Adelaide in 1990 and 30 by the 7th in Paris in 1993; membership had grown to just under 6000.

The mid-1990s, under presidents John D. Loeser and Jean-Marie Besson, saw the IASP logo appearing more and more often in print. A new quarterly bulletin, *Pain: Clinical Updates,* focusing on current medical topics and edited by Daniel B. Carr, first appeared in 1993. In 1990, Ronald Dubner joined Wall as chief co-editor of *PAIN,* and the journal bought another 800 pages that year, adding three double issues. The work of IASP Press, approved by the Council in 1993 and launched the following year under editor Howard L. Fields, opened the way for timely publication of books on important topics to the pain field, congress proceedings, committee and task force reports, and research symposia. In the first two years, the second editions of the *Classification of Chronic Pain* (1994) and the *Core Curriculum for Professional Education in Pain* (1995) were published, as well as *Back Pain in the Workplace* (1995). The Committee on Ethics guidelines for pain research in human subjects were published in *PAIN* in 1995. Recognizing the importance of preserving the field's history, John Liebeskind established a Pain Archival Collection at the University of California, Los Angeles, in 1995. The Internet offered a new venue for information sharing, and an IASP Web site, including *Pain: Clinical Updates,* ethical guidelines, and pain definitions, went online in 1996.

The 8th World Congress, held in Vancouver in August 1996, welcomed more than 4,000 members from 90 countries. By then, 54 chapters had been formed. The participants attended 25 plenaries and were able to choose from 80 workshops and 1,500 poster presentations. The recent deaths of John and Emma Bonica lent a touch of melancholy to the meeting, however, and Loeser in his presidential address pointed out how much was still unknown about pain mechanisms and treatment efficacy.

The 9th Congress in Vienna in 1999 and the 10th in San Diego in 2002 were also successes in terms of program content and attendance, with over 5,000 delegates. By 2004, the organization had a membership of 6,500 and 63 chapters. There were two regional federations of chapters, one in Europe and the other in Latin America. There were 13 active SIGs, the newest groups working on acute pain and on pain related to torture, organized violence, and war. The journal *PAIN* has increased in prestige and productivity, with 15 scheduled issues each year and double issues often added each year. Total published pages in 2003 reached 1800. Dubner became the sole chief editor in 1999 with Wall's retirement, and in 2003 he passed the stewardship of the journal on to Allan Basbaum. In the same year, Catherine Bushnell assumed the editorship of IASP Press. In 10 years IASP Press has published 45 books, many of which are essential reference volumes on pain theory and management. Presidents Barry Sessle and Michael Bond have pointed to the need for advocacy for the multidisciplinary approach and for better pain education in developing countries. As the organization in 2005 marks the 30th anniversary of the Florence meeting and the first publication of *PAIN,* we still face the challenges of incomplete knowledge about pain and inadequate pain management for patients around the world.

PROGRESS IN BASIC RESEARCH ON PAIN

The early 1970s saw the convergence of new knowledge on how the brain processed information about pain and the emergence of neuroscience as a new discipline. It is more than a coincidence that advances in anatomical, biochemical, physiological, pharmacological, behavioral, and molecular approaches to the study of the nervous system were paralleled by intense interest in the study of pain. The field attracted a number of sensory neurophysiologists, pharmacologists, neuroanatomists, and experimental psychologists who were interested in the study of pain. Some of the sensory neurophysiologists hypothesized that pain sensation involved the activation of specialized pathways in the peripheral and central nervous systems and that systematic study of primary afferent and spinal cord neurons encoding information from the skin and other target tissues would reveal the unique characteristics of these "specific" or specialized neurons and help explain the mechanisms of acute and persistent pain. The leading proponents of this approach were Iggo and Perl, whose findings of specialized receptors encoding the intensive, temporal, and spatial qualities of tissue-damaging stimuli were prominently reported and discussed at the early IASP congresses.

Other neuroscientists, such as Wall, Zimmermann, Dubner, William Willis, and Donald Price were primarily interested in the anatomical and functional properties of neurons in the spinal and medullary dorsal horns and how they coded information about tissue damage. Their studies revealed that different classes of specialized neurons in the dorsal horn (wide-dynamic-range and nociceptive-specific neurons) coded the quality, intensity, and temporal aspects of noxious stimulation. They also showed that these responses were subject to sensory modulation by non-noxious inputs from the environment and from other brain sites. The findings led to lively discussions about the organization of nociceptive systems in the brain at the IASP congresses. The gate control theory proposed by Wall and Melzack in 1965 emphasized the concept of sensory modulation at the level of the spinal cord and, in addition, introduced the idea of descending modulation from higher centers in the brain. In the 1970s, considerable research was generated to test the theory, which contrasted with the concept of specificity in nociceptive systems. Further excitement was generated by the findings of Liebeskind and Besson that the brainstem contained sites whose activation suppressed nocifensive behaviors in animals and diminished the responses of dorsal horn neurons. Their studies suggested that these effects could be blocked by "opiate" antagonist drugs, giving rise to the hypothesis that the brain may have its own opiate-dependent pain-suppressing systems. The discovery of opioid peptides in these pain-suppressing pathways by John Hughes, Hans Kosterlitz, and others in the 1970s provided support for this hypothesis.

Thus, the origins of the IASP in the 1970s coincided with major areas of discovery related to pain—the presence of specialized receptors, or nociceptors, in peripheral tissues that respond to tissue damage; the presence of specialized neurons in the spinal dorsal horn and its homologue in the trigeminal system that respond to tissue-damaging stimuli; the importance of segmental sensory modulation in spinal cord nociceptive pathways; and the discovery of endogenous opioid peptides in descending nociceptive pathways. Much of the rapid growth of the IASP in subsequent years is clearly related to the great interest in these findings and the need to move them from the "bench to the bedside" to help patients in pain. These important discoveries were also the foundation of subsequent exciting findings in the 1980s and 1990s that were clearly enhanced by the multidisciplinary nature of the pain field. This work includes (1) the molecular cloning of specialized receptors in peripheral tissues that respond to intense thermal and mechanical stimuli, to inflammatory mediators, and to acidic substances; (2) the enhancement of the responses of these receptors after tissue injury; (3) the discovery of unique sodium, calcium, and potassium channels in finely myelinated and unmyelinated nerve fibers that carry signals from nociceptors to the central nervous system; (4) the molecular cloning of mu, delta, and kappa opioid receptors in the nervous system that are components of descending pain-suppressing systems; (5) the activity-dependent plasticity or central sensitization in nociceptive pathways that amplifies persistent pain after tissue and nerve injury; (6) the molecular and cellular basis of such activity-dependent plasticity involving excitatory and inhibitory amino acids, neuropeptides, neurotrophins, second-messenger systems in cells, and calcium-dependent and -independent protein kinases that mediate receptor and protein phosphorylation and enhance targeted gene transcription; (7) the discovery of bimodal descending facilitatory as well as inhibitory pain-suppressing pathways whose activation is enhanced after tissue and nerve injury; and (8) the ability to utilize modern methodologies such as positron emission tomography and functional magnetic resonance imaging to image forebrain and other central structures activated after injury and correlate these findings with the sensory, affective, attentional, and cognitive functions of the brain. The remaining chapters in this book will elaborate on such findings and how they have been and will be translated into new approaches to the treatment of acute and chronic or persistent pain.

PROGRESS IN CLINICAL RESEARCH ON PAIN

The clinical management of pain at the time of the 1st World Congress of IASP in 1975 involved almost all the conditions that face clinicians today. As a result of discoveries in neuroscience, improvements in methods of investigation, and the development of treatment techniques, significant benefits have accrued to patients during the past 30 years; this is particularly true of the management of chronic pain, to which developments in psychological concepts and techniques have been applied. The development of new drugs for pain relief has, in contrast, been rather disappointing, but their methods of use have improved considerably, with definite benefits to those in pain.

In 1974 pain management was primarily a matter for physicians and nurses, and at that time anesthesiologists began to take a leading role in the development of new techniques and services. As described above, Bonica had developed a pain clinic with a multiprofessional team in Seattle. Elsewhere in the world, clinicians in other paramedical professions (except nursing) had not become involved in pain management to any extent. In addition to anesthesiologists, neurosurgeons had developed methods of pain relief over many years. The growth of pain management techniques owes much to anesthesiologists like Sampson Lipton and Mark Swerdlow from the United Kingdom and Mario Tiengo from Italy and to neurologist Peter Nathan from the United Kingdom and neurologist and anatomist Sydney Sunderland from Australia. Neurosurgeons included William H. Sweet and John D. Loeser from the United States, Ronald R. Tasker from Canada, William Noordenbos from the Netherlands, and Jan Gybels from Belgium. Therefore, the clinical developments within IASP began on a worldwide basis from its inception.

Independently from the work initiated by Bonica in the 1960s, the Hospice Movement was founded in 1967 by Cicely Saunders, a former nurse, social worker, and oncologist. The establishment of St. Christopher's Hospice in London began a worldwide movement that pioneered the rational use of opiates. This new standard of palliative care was marked by the development of the WHO treatment ladder for cancer pain relief, which had its origins at the IASP 1st World Congress on Pain and was initially published in 1986. It was based on collaboration between Jan Stjernswärd of WHO and Kathleen M. Foley and Vittorio Ventafridda of IASP. The benefits of their work and that of Saunders have been immense.

In the 1960s and early 1970s, anesthesiologists and neurosurgeons practiced a range of nerve block and nerve destruction techniques for pain relief, such as injection of the trigeminal ganglion with alcohol or its open surgical ablation. In addition, some surgeons practiced open cordotomy, although the percutaneous technique developed by Shealy and others in the mid 1960s for pain relief in terminal cancer rapidly replaced it. The latter method remained popular throughout the 1970s and 1980s, although it was partly replaced at that time by the technique of dorsal root entry zone (DREZ) lesions developed in the United States by Blaine Nashold. More recent cord stimulation techniques are based upon knowledge of the way in which nociceptive systems function in the spinal cord. Surgical techniques involving the brain have not played a significant part in physical approaches to pain relief to date, with the exception of pituitary adenolysis by alcohol injection, introduced by Italian anesthesiologist Guido Moricca in 1974 for the relief of severe pain in advanced cancer, a procedure that has now been replaced by alternative treatments.

Systematic analgesics have been used with increasing effectiveness since 1974. The development of new nonsteroidal anti-inflammatory drugs (NSAIDs), the oldest example of which is aspirin, added significantly to the list of drugs available for the treatment of acute and chronic pain. With their use, it has become clear that their effectiveness must be weighed against their adverse effects—for example, oral COX-1 inhibitors may cause gastric bleeding, impaired renal function, and effects on platelets, and more recently the COX-2 inhibitors, though less damaging to the stomach, have been found to have adverse effects upon the cerebrovascular circulation and the myocardium. The better use of analgesics has been due in part to improved techniques for evaluating potency. This advance, which has significantly reduced the somewhat "hit or miss" efforts of earlier prescribing habits, started with a series of clinical trials conducted in the 1960s and 1970s by John Dunbar in Northern Ireland. Much more recently, Henry J. McQuay and R. Andrew Moore in Oxford, United Kingdom, have established a reliable method for comparing the potency and the harmful effects of analgesic drugs. The measures they used are the NNT (number needed to treat for one patient to gain at least 50% pain relief) and the NNH (the number needed to harm). There has also been a movement toward adopting other drugs, which, although developed for different purposes, have been found to have pain-relieving properties. They include the anticonvulsants and antidepressants, particularly those with both serotoninergic and noradrenergic effects.

In addition to new compounds and better means of establishing drug potency, developments in techniques of drug administration have made pain control simpler, especially for patients. For example, the postoperative use of patient-controlled analgesia has resulted in less pain and less patient anxiety, given that patients using this technique are aware that they have some control over the pain experienced. Skin patches from which analgesics are absorbed steadily over time (for example, fentanyl and buprenorphine) and the formulation of long-acting analgesics are other developments that not only have reduced the need to take analgesics frequently on a daily basis but also have provided a method by which patients may control their own pain without frequent contact with doctors or other pain professionals. The use by anesthesiologists of spinal analgesia (e.g., intrathecal and epidural analgesia) and spinal cord stimulation during surgery and childbirth has contributed to greatly improved pain relief, as has the use of such methods to control pain in advanced cancer.

This brief review of the development of physical techniques would not be complete without mention of transcutaneous electrical nerve stimulation (TENS) and acupuncture. TENS was introduced in the 1970s and continues to be used widely. Respect for acupuncture, adopted from traditional Chinese medicine, grew in the late 1970s with evidence that acupuncture analgesia is linked to the activities of endogenous opioid peptides. Both techniques have a physiological basis because they alter the transmission of nociception at the level of the dorsal horn of the spinal cord, but the extent to which they will relieve pain is not entirely predictable.

The work of Melzack and Kenneth L. Casey led to the identification of three dimensions of pain, namely the sensory, the emotional, and the cognitive. That development, combined with the definition of pain as "an unpleasant sensory and emotional experience associated with actual or potential tissue damage, or described in terms of such damage" in IASP's definitions of chronic pain published under the direction of Merskey and others, led to a radical re-appraisal of the nature of pain and more particularly of ways in which pain should be managed. Improved clinical understanding and management were further facilitated by the *Classification of Chronic Pain,* the first edition produced by the Subcommittee on Taxonomy chaired by Merskey in 1986, with a second edition edited by Merskey and Bogduk in 1994. A new approach to the understanding of the pain experience has resulted in the establishment of the biopsychosocial model of pain and of multimodal treatment that takes into account the physical, psychological, behavioral, and social aspects of pain.

Interest in the relationship of personality and pain appeared in the work of Richard A. Sternbach of the United States and in that of Bond, Merskey, and Pilowsky in the United Kingdom. Pilowsky began to change this focus with his work on abnormal illness behavior. As early as 1968, psychologist Wilbert Fordyce and colleagues started to develop a formal behavior theory and practice for the management of pain. The use of behavior therapy opened up a new approach that has been expanded since that time.

It was soon accepted, however, that behavior could not be altered without consideration of cognitive functions. The introduction of cognitive theory by Dennis C. Turk and others in the early 1980s led to the well-established and valuable technique of cognitive-behavioral therapy, used chiefly in the management of chronic pain disorders, especially those in which psychological factors may be the main cause of disability. In more recent times, two further important aspects of chronic pain and contributors to its persistence, namely fear and anger, have been investigated, with acknowledgment that consideration of these emotions should be an integral part of pain assessment and management.

Other aspects of the individual and the family have also been explored with a view to improving pain management. They include the issues of ethnic origins, sex and gender, and social development. Increasing interest is being taken in specific groups within society, particularly the elderly and children.

The increased availability of methods for managing pain should be seen against a background of improved organization of pain treatment facilities. Some time ago, IASP defined the various types of pain management systems that might be used, which range from multimodal, university-based "super clinics," where research is conducted, to unimodal clinics, devoted to techniques practiced only by one type of specialists, such as anesthesiologists. In parallel, acute pain teams have been established in many general or university hospitals. The management of pain in the community by family physicians and others continues to be an area in need of development. The greatest improvements in methods of pain relief have occurred in developed countries, but nevertheless there are great variations between one country and another. The problems faced by developing countries are, in contrast, significantly greater, both in terms of education and in the need to establish adequate pain services. Recognizing this fact, IASP has in recent years significantly increased its aid for developing countries, with a particular emphasis on education and on the persuasion of governments and health deliverers with regard to the need for specific facilities for pain management. It has conducted that work through its members and chapters in these regions. Work in support of developing countries led to the establishment of an IASP Global Day Against Pain, and a major launch of this initiative involving collaboration by IASP, WHO, and the European Federation of IASP Chapters took place in Geneva in October 2004 with the slogan "Pain Treatment Should Be a Human Right." IASP is the leading professional forum for science, practice, and education in the field of pain. Its achievements in these areas during the past 30 years have been immense and have met or even exceeded the expectations of Bonica and others who founded it. The association flourishes and will continue to promote the study and treatment of pain in the years to come.

Correspondence to: Ronald Dubner, DDS, PhD, Department of Biomedical Sciences, University of Maryland Dental School, 666 West Baltimore Street, Room 5E-10, Baltimore, MD 21201, USA. Email: rnd001@dental.umaryland.edu.

The Paths of Pain 1975–2005, edited by
Harold Merskey, John D. Loeser, and Ronald
Dubner, IASP Press, Seattle, © 2005.

3

The Gate Theory, Then and Now

Fernando Cervero

Anaesthesia Research Unit, McGill University, Montreal, Quebec, Canada

THE GATE CONTROL THEORY

The gate control theory of pain mechanisms (Melzack and Wall 1965) has had a profound influence in the field of pain research and in the development of many pain therapies. In this chapter, presented on the 40th anniversary of the publication of that paper, I would like to give a historical perspective of the gate theory, discuss its basis and its modifications, and offer insight into its current state and its future. The account includes a few personal notes that give details of my involvement in some of the issues and debates. The starting point is the recognition that afferent inputs interact in the spinal dorsal horn and that this interaction can play a key role in the processing of pain-related information.

My first contact with the gate theory happened in 1968, three years after its publication, when I was finishing preclinical medical studies at Madrid University. This was a momentous time for my generation, and I have many memories from that year about events unrelated to pain research, including an enforced visit to the lugubrious headquarters of Franco's political police. I first read the gate theory when I was asked, as part of physiology coursework, to write an essay on the organization of presynaptic inhibition in the spinal cord. My interest in neuroscience was already high, but I became fascinated by the mechanism of presynaptic inhibition, which remains a neurobiological process that I find truly astonishing.

When I first read the Melzack and Wall paper I concentrated almost exclusively on the model that they proposed for the control of incoming sensory input into the spinal cord, and therefore I did not pay much attention to the discussion about specificity versus pattern interpretations of pain mechanisms. The specificity theory was presented in a very extreme way, and the existence of specific nociceptors was given a swift dismissal. The most innovative aspect of the theory was the idea of the "gating" of sensory inputs at the first synaptic relay, which by itself does not necessarily support or deny a specificity interpretation of the peripheral input. In fact, the division of the afferent input to the cord into "large" and "small" afferents, with the former being mainly tactile and the latter nociceptive, implies a considerable amount of peripheral specificity. What remained in my mind was the proposal of a presynaptic inhibitory mechanism responsible for pain-related interactions between sensory afferents in the substantia gelatinosa of the superficial dorsal horn. However, the original description of the gate theory also focused on the conflict between specificity and pattern interpretations of pain mechanisms, and this topic needs to be addressed here.

DESCARTES' BOY

One of the most enduring legacies of the gate theory has been an "anti-Descartes" movement, blaming Descartes, not very accurately, for being the founding father of the specificity theory. The original Melzack and Wall paper used Descartes' now-famous picture of a boy with his foot close to a fire to criticize the labeled-line mechanism of pain transmission. Yet, Descartes' writings (1664) and the picture in question address scientific questions far beyond those related to pain mechanisms. Descartes was a dualist, probably more by fear of the Catholic Church than by conviction, and so his book is about how the human body, as opposed to the soul, works. He proposed that the human body was a machine, and he used the technology of his time—mostly clockwork, optics, and mechanics—to illustrate some bodily functions, including how the brain deals with external stimuli. He suggested that such stimuli activate nerves in the periphery of the body, which transmit their signals to the brain, where, after being "reflected" by the pineal gland, they activate motor nerves that in turn move the appropriate muscles away from the stimulus. What Descartes was describing is the "reflex arc," so named as an acknowledgment of his idea of sensory signals being "reflected" in a mirror-like brain that directs them to motor nerves. This was quite revolutionary thinking at a time when all brain activity was though to be centrifugal and mediated by "animal spirits," and his idea of a "reflex arc" is a lasting interpretation of the way the brain reacts to external stimuli.

Descartes' picture also holds a lot of truth as an example of strict pain specificity. It implies the existence of sensors in the periphery capable of detecting noxious stimuli. His diagram suggests the presence of distributed sensory and motor pathways in the spinal cord and brain and implies a modular organization of sensory-motor transformations. Descartes' ideas can be regarded as partial or incomplete—it could not be otherwise from a book written in the 17th century—but should not be presented as utterly wrong. So, the next time you want to show a slide of Descartes' boy in your lecture, spare a thought for the man who discovered the "reflex arc" and was the first to hint that there could be nociceptors in the periphery and nociceptive pathways in the brain.

ONE PAIN OR MANY PAINS?

The central argument of the gate theory was to reject the specificity of pain pathways in favor of a pattern interpretation of pain perception. The presynaptic inhibition model was used to put forward ideas about convergent and nonspecific spinal cord neurons and about possible interactions between afferent drives. Yet, the presynaptic inhibition model is also what gave the Melzack and Wall paper its novelty and timeliness. Without it, the gate theory would have been only a restatement of previously proposed interpretations of pain mechanisms based on patterns of impulses in afferent fibers (Sinclair 1955; Noordenbos 1959; Weddell and Miller 1962).

The considerable amount of new information about pain mechanisms gathered in the intervening 40 years has relegated the specificity-pattern argument to a secondary role. It is no longer suggested that the sensory innervation of peripheral organs is mediated by nonspecific sensory receptors acting as intensity encoders. Studies of the sensory innervation of the viscera, which remained the last stand of the pattern interpretation (Jänig and Morrison 1986), have also demonstrated discrete classes of sensory receptors with distinct thresholds in the viscera, similar to those found in the skin, muscles, and joints (Cervero 1994). Equally, there can be no denial of the existence of neurons in the spinal cord driven mainly or exclusively by nociceptive stimuli and of centers in the brain directly activated by noxious stimuli. However, there is also substantial evidence for plasticity in the nociceptive sensory channel and for the existence of dynamic processes that can profoundly alter the functional properties of peripheral nociceptors and of nociceptive central neurons (Treede et al. 1992; Hunt and Mantyh 2001; Julius and Basbaum 2001). We have reached a point where neither a strict specificity model nor a pattern interpretation can account for all that it is known about pain mechanisms.

A more reasonable approach to the specificity-pattern controversy has been the realization that there are many forms of pain and that not all of them are mediated by the same mechanism. This question was not addressed by the original gate theory, which grouped together the sensory consequences of acute trauma with the altered sensations of neuropathic pain states. Today we recognize that different forms of pain are mediated by several mechanisms (Cervero and Laird 1991), which participate in various ways in the generation of nociceptive, inflammatory, or neuropathic pains. The specificity theory can explain fairly well the simpler forms of pain, such as a pinprick or the acute pain of a minor burn, as a direct activation of peripheral nociceptors and of specific nociceptive cells. However, complex pain experiences, including the pain of chronic inflammation or neuropathic pains, require the involvement of peripheral and central plasticity such that low-intensity stimuli evoke pain (i.e., secondary hyperalgesia or touch-evoked allodynia) (Cervero and Laird 1996). Even when considering the sensory innervation of the viscera, which can be very different to the innervation of somatic tissues (Cervero 1994, 1996), we also appreciate that diverse pain states can be expressed at different times through different mechanisms (Cervero and Jänig 1992).

THE RIGHTS AND WRONGS OF THE GATING MECHANISM

The word "gate" in the original description of the theory was not used to mean a "barrier closing the opening of a wall, road or passage" (Oxford English Dictionary), but was part of the jargon used in the mid-1960s by electrical engineers to describe the transistor circuit that, when activated, interrupts the passage of digital impulses through another circuit. This is precisely what the proposed diagram of the gate theory implies with the presynaptic inhibition model, a "gating" of nociceptive impulses by the activation of low-threshold mechanoreceptors and the deactivation of such gating by an intense nociceptive discharge (Fig. 1A). Whereas the concept of interaction between afferent inputs at spinal level has survived the test of time, the details of the mechanism proposed have not.

Testing by other laboratories of the presynaptic inhibitory mechanism proposed by the gate theory showed some fundamental flaws in the basic proposal. The "primary afferent hyperpolarization" induced by C-fiber activation, a central requirement of the gate theory, could not be confirmed by other authors, who demonstrated instead that both A and C fibers evoked primary afferent depolarization (PAD) (Franz and Iggo 1968; Zimmermann 1968; Whitehorn and Burgess 1973). The entire process of presynaptic inhibition induced by A or C afferents was found to be much more complex than the model proposed and appeared to depend on whether the afferent fiber originated from the skin, muscle, or viscera (Schmidt 1971). The hasty

Reciprocal Sensory Interaction in the Spinal Cord

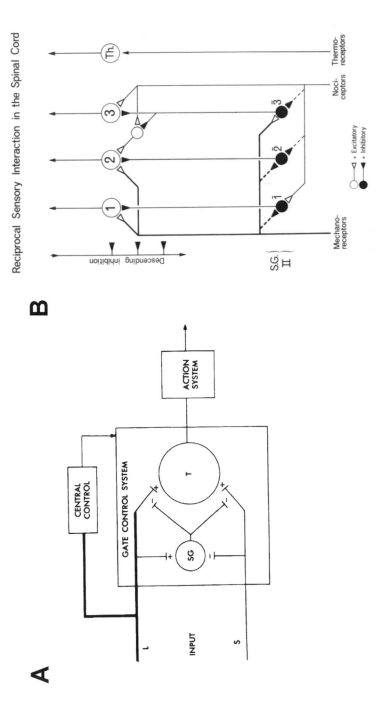

Fig. 1. (A) This figure, from the Melzack and Wall (1965) paper, was labeled: "Schematic diagram of the gate control theory of pain mechanisms." The now-famous diagram shows the presynaptic interaction model between large (L) and small (S) afferent fibers and the key role of substantia gelatinosa (SG) neurons controlling the activity of transmission (T) cells. (Reprinted with permission; © 1965 AAAS.) (B) The model proposed by Cervero and Iggo (1978) based on their data from SG neurons. The model is based on the hypothesis that SG neurons inhibit the activity of larger dorsal horn cells in a "reciprocal interaction" manner.

dismissal of the specificity of the afferent input to the central nervous system (CNS) and of the existence of separate categories of high-threshold sensory receptors proved to be mistaken as more and more laboratories showed that the afferent input to the CNS was not a continuum of thresholds, as Wall (1960) had suggested, but was mediated by discrete categories of specific sensory receptor (Belmonte and Cervero 1996). Finally, the discovery of nociceptor-specific neurons in the superficial dorsal horn (Christensen and Perl 1970) demonstrated a role for nociceptive channels in the transmission of pain-related information (Craig et al. 1994; Craig 2003).

Nevertheless, the gate theory had many positive effects. It stimulated a large amount of experimental work from several leading laboratories, which contributed a substantial body of data on the peripheral and spinal mechanisms of nociception. It emphasized the dynamic and plastic components of pain sensation and drew attention to pain modulation as opposed to an interpretation of pain exclusively as an alarm system. It also focused the attention of many researchers on the clinical aspects of pain, and away from physiological pain, which contributed a surge of studies on the effects of neuropathic lesions and on the development of animal models of inflammatory and neuropathic pain.

In 1976, 11 years after the publication of the gate theory, Peter Nathan published a comprehensive and scholarly review which concluded that, although the theory had been productive of further work, the mechanism proposed was incomplete or even flawed. He was also critical of the dismissal by the Melzack and Wall paper of the existing data, prior to 1965, on the functional properties of specific nociceptors. Nathan's review was sympathetic to the idea of pain modulation in the spinal cord and praised the gate theory for drawing attention to pathophysiological aspects of pain perception. But in the end it was a critical account, and this triggered an ardent reply by Pat Wall two years later (Wall 1978) in the form of a "restatement" of the theory, reforming those aspects of the original proposal that had been shown to be incompatible with subsequent data.

PAIN AND THE SUBSTANTIA GELATINOSA

My first steps in the field of pain research began in early 1975 when I joined Ainsley Iggo's laboratory as a postdoctoral fellow. The topic of my doctoral thesis was the transmission of sensory impulses by dorsal root ganglion cells, and it was only natural that I decided to continue my training in the laboratory of one of the leading authorities on the physiology of sensory afferents. By coincidence, I arrived in Iggo's laboratory only a few months after the founding of the International Association for the Study of Pain (IASP), and therefore my research work in his laboratory was presented at the first and second IASP world congresses in Florence (1975) and Montreal (1978). My two main projects in Iggo's laboratory were also directly relevant to fundamental aspects of the gate theory, and they both addressed the role of superficial dorsal horn neurons in the modulation of afferent inputs to the spinal cord.

The gate theory had given the small neurons of the substantia gelatinosa a key role in the control of the afferent input to the spinal cord. However, very little was known at the time about their functional responses or even about their contributions to the generation of presynaptic inhibition. On the other hand, Christensen and Perl (1970) had shown that the most superficial neurons of the dorsal horn, located in lamina I, were exclusively driven by peripheral nociceptors. Iggo's laboratory was engaged in a study of the actions of peripheral nociceptors on dorsal horn neurons, and therefore my first task was to study further the properties of lamina I cells. During this time I became interested in the organization of the superficial dorsal horn, and I persuaded Ainsley to start a major project aimed at recording the electrical activity of substantia gelatinosa neurons. Between 1975 and 1979, with the essential help of Hisashi Ogawa, Vince Molony, and Don Ensor, I was involved in two projects that would directly test the mechanisms proposed by the gate theory.

We first confirmed Christensen and Perl's discovery of nociceptor-specific cells in lamina I and extended their observations with descriptions of neuronal subcategories and of modulation of their nociceptive inputs by low-threshold stimulation. Preliminary results were presented at the first IASP Congress in Florence and published in the proceedings (Iggo et al. 1976), and a full paper appeared in the recently founded journal *PAIN* (Cervero et al. 1976). In the discussion section of our paper we debated the role in pain mechanisms of these neurons, which we called class 3 cells, and concluded: "If as we suggest, the class 3 cells are directly involved in pain mechanisms, our conclusions do not provide any support for the gate theory." There was not a great deal of love lost between Wall and Iggo, but with this statement I unwittingly joined those at the receiving end of Pat Wall's wrath.

Since those days, nociceptor-specific or class 3 neurons have been studied by many laboratories and have become an essential component of all interpretations of sensory processing in the spinal cord and, by extension, of pain mechanisms in general. The discovery of nociceptor-specific neurons has provided evidence for the existence of labeled lines in the CNS and is therefore fundamentally contradictory to pattern interpretations of pain mechanisms (Craig 2003). The presence of these cells along sensory pathways does not deny plasticity or modulation of nociceptive pathways, or the existence of other nonspecific lines, but shows that the brain uses a variety of means, including specific information, to assess the nature of a peripheral stimulus (Cervero 1986).

We then turned our attention to the small neurons of the substantia gelatinosa and made intra- and extracellular recordings of their activity. This was a laborious process and, as we found out along the way, one that also engaged the resources of several major laboratories around the world, including those of Ed Perl, Ron Dubner, and Pat Wall. In 1980 we published a fairly extensive review about the substantia gelatinosa and its role in pain mechanisms, summarizing the different results obtained by all the laboratories working on this topic (Cervero and Iggo 1980). There were nomenclature discrepancies between the various groups as well as fundamental differences and biases in the interpretation of results, which prevented a uniform view of data. We described "inverse" responses of substantia gelatinosa neurons to those found in the larger cells of the dorsal horn and produced an afferent interaction model based on the Sherringtonian idea of reciprocal innervation (Cervero and Iggo 1978; Cervero et al. 1979c). In a sense, our own data supported the idea of "gating" in the dorsal horn and gave a major role to substantia gelatinosa neurons, although the basic mechanism proposed was different (Fig. 1B). This information was presented at the second IASP congress in Montreal in 1978 and was the subject of several other publications (Cervero et al. 1977, 1978, 1979a,b,d; Molony et al. 1981).

It is puzzling that, from an electrophysiological point of view, the arguments about the responses of substantia gelatinosa neurons have never been resolved. The emphasis on electrophysiology of the late 1970s and early 1980s soon changed to a more neurochemical approach with the description of myriad potential transmitters and modulators in the superficial dorsal horn and more recently to purely molecular approaches. Even contemporary electrophysiological studies focus more on modulation and plasticity of inputs than on the descriptive aspects of neuronal input and output. And so, to this day, we still do not have a uniform view about the response properties of substantia gelatinosa neurons or a consensus about their role in pain processing.

The emphasis has currently moved to nonsynaptic communication between neurons and to a possible role of non-neuronal elements, such as glia or microglia, in nociceptive processing in the spinal cord (Watkins et al. 2001; Tsuda et al. 2003). However, we still focus on the first synaptic relay in the spinal cord as a key step in pain processing and continue to make assumptions about complex pain perceptions based only on dorsal horn data.

This legacy of the gate theory and of the prominence given to the substantia gelatinosa represents an obsession, perhaps mistaken, with the dorsal horn as a key player in pain processing and modulation.

PRESYNAPTIC INHIBITION REVISITED

The gate theory and much of the subsequent work on the role of the dorsal horn in pain mechanisms had firmly established in the minds of pain researchers that changes in pain perception, including the development of hyperalgesic states, were the consequence of, or at least were initiated by, neurobiological processes in the spinal cord. Key words by the late 1990s were plasticity, sensitization, and hyperalgesia, and the most popular animal models were of neuropathic or persistent inflammatory pain. Studies of dorsal horn processing in hyperalgesic states threw new light on one of the basic elements of the gate theory: the role of presynaptic inhibition in pain modulation.

A number of reports from Willis and Westlund's laboratory described an enhancement of dorsal root reflexes (DRRs) induced by an experimental inflammation of the joints (Rees et al. 1994, 1995; Sluka et al. 1995). DRRs were originally described in the 1940s and were known to be an overexpression of PAD, whereby an intense depolarization of the primary afferent leads to spiking activity that is conducted antidromically. The 1990s publications showed that experimental inflammation of a joint evoked an enhanced depolarization of fine afferent fibers, including those that innervated the inflamed joint. An obvious corollary was that if the spikes generated in the nociceptive afferent were also conducted orthodromically, the DRR mechanism could provide access to the nociceptive channel to low-threshold afferents capable of generating PAD in fine afferent fibers.

Based on these ideas, Jenny Laird and I published a review paper in *PAIN* proposing that tactile allodynia from areas of secondary hyperalgesia could be mediated by a presynaptic link between low- and high-threshold afferents (Cervero and Laird 1996). We had known for a long time that impulses in low-threshold mechanoreceptors with Aβ fibers evoke PAD of nociceptive afferents via a GABAergic presynaptic link between the two kinds of afferent fiber (Schmidt 1971; Rudomin 1990). We knew that this link contained at least one interneuron. Thus, in normal conditions, activation of low-threshold mechanoreceptors with Aβ afferents evokes presynaptic inhibition of nociceptive afferents (Calvillo 1978) and therefore reduces pain sensation (Fig. 2A). This is the basic starting point originally proposed by the gate theory.

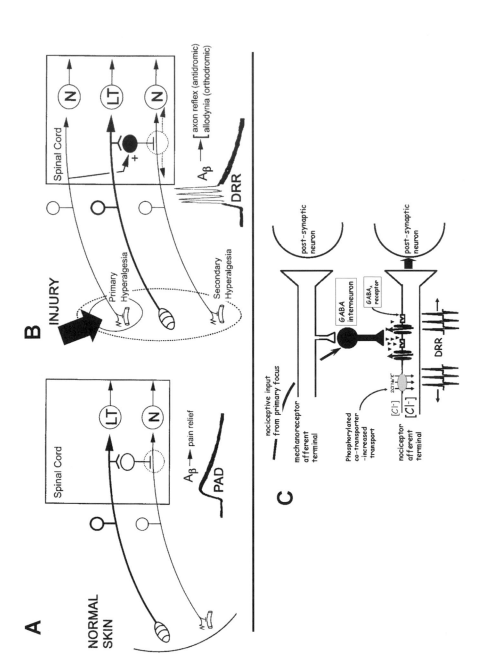

We also knew that following an injury, the nociceptors in the area close to the lesion are activated and sensitized (Treede et al. 1992). This mechanism includes the initial nociceptive discharge induced by the injury as well as persistent activity in the sensitized nociceptors and thus a continuous afferent barrage in these fibers. We suggested that this afferent barrage converges onto, among other places, the spinal substrate that mediates the presynaptic link between low-threshold mechanoreceptors and nociceptors. As a consequence of the increased and persistent barrage driving this system, excitability is increased such that, when the system is activated by low-threshold mechanoreceptors from areas surrounding the injury site, it produces a much more intense PAD in the nociceptive afferent terminals, reaching a depolarization level capable of generating spike activity. This activation would be conducted antidromically in the form of DRRs, but would also be conducted forward, activating the second-order neurons normally driven by nociceptors. The sensory consequence of this mechanism is pain evoked by the activation of low-threshold mechanoreceptors from an area of secondary hyperalgesia, that is, allodynia (Fig. 2B).

← **Fig. 2.** (A, B) The diagrams proposed by Cervero and Laird (1996) to illustrate their proposed model for the mechanisms of touch-evoked pain in (A) normal skin and (B) skin after an injury. Two types of afferent fiber are illustrated: large-caliber fibers, connected to low-threshold (LT) mechanoreceptors, and fine fibers connected to nociceptive (N) cells. The figure shows an axon reflex arrangement. PAD = primary afferent depolarization; DRR = dorsal root reflex. In normal skin, stimulation of Aβ afferents evokes PAD in C fibers and inhibits pain; in hyperalgesic skin the interneurons are sensitized (black neuron) by the nociceptive barrage, and Aβ-fiber stimulation evokes antidromic DRRs (and flare) and orthodromic activation of the C-fiber terminals (and allodynia). (C) Illustration of possible mechanisms that may account for the switch between PAD and DRRs in conditions that evoke allodynia. PAD in nociceptive primary afferent terminals is generated under normal circumstances when activity in mechanoreceptors activates GABAergic interneurons (black neuron) that release GABA onto the nociceptive terminal. The afferent terminal expresses GABA$_A$ receptors and has a high internal chloride concentration, maintained by the Na-K-Cl cotransporter. When GABA opens the chloride channel associated with the GABA$_A$ receptor, chloride ions flow out, partially depolarizing the membrane (PAD). Stimuli that evoke allodynia generate a sustained afferent barrage of nociceptive input from the peripheral focus, shown here as an arrow toward the area in which the GABAergic interneuron is found. This barrage may produce a release of neurotransmitters, for example, glutamate, acting on the nociceptive terminal to activate calcium-calmodulin-dependent protein kinase II (CaMKII), which is known to phosphorylate the cotransporter, thus increasing its activity. Enhanced activity in the cotransporter would also increase the intracellular chloride concentration, thus enhancing the depolarization produced by GABA$_A$-receptor activation. This enhanced depolarization could reach firing threshold, producing action potentials (DRRs) in the nociceptive afferent terminal. The DRRs would travel in both directions, as shown in the figure, toward the periphery and centrally toward the central synapses of nociceptive afferents on second-order neurons in the nociceptive pathway, thus evoking allodynia. Diagram based on a figure from Cervero et al. (2003).

We acknowledged in our paper that the presynaptic mechanism was part the original gate theory. We were bringing back ideas of presynaptically mediated interactions between afferent fibers to a field that had long abandoned this interpretation in favor of postsynaptic enhancements of excitability as an explanation for hyperalgesic states. We also acknowledged that the two interpretations were not mutually exclusive. In fact, some form of postsynaptic enhancement of excitability of the PAD-mediating interneuron was needed for the mechanism to work. We found the model attractive in that it seemed to bring together several pieces of evidence, old and new, that had previously been difficult to reconcile.

We are currently studying the mechanism by which peripheral injury changes the PAD-generating machinery such that sufficient depolarization occurs in the fine afferent terminal to reach the firing threshold and produce action potentials (Cervero et al. 2003). The mechanism that generates PAD in large myelinated afferent fibers in mammals is well established. Afferent input, or descending input from the brain, excites GABAergic spinal interneurons, which form axo-axonic synapses onto the central terminals of the primary afferent terminals. The primary afferent terminals express $GABA_A$ receptors, so that when GABA is released by the interneurons into the synaptic cleft, the chloride channel associated with the receptor opens.

Primary afferent neurons maintain a high internal chloride concentration because they express the Na-K-2Cl cotransporter, which transports chloride into the cell using the energy of the sodium gradient created by the Na-K-ATPase pump. Thus, when the chloride channel associated with the $GABA_A$ receptor opens, chloride flows out and the membrane depolarizes. A small depolarization of the membrane, or PAD, produces presynaptic inhibition because when an action potential arrives from the periphery along the axon of the primary afferent, the terminal is already depolarized, and the shift in membrane potential is reduced, which leads to less transmitter release at the synapse between the primary afferent terminal and the second-order neurons (Alvarez-Leefmans et al. 1998) (Fig. 2C).

A possible mechanism to explain the shift from PAD to DRRs would be modulation of the chloride concentration inside the primary afferent terminal. Preliminary results using knockout mice lacking the Na-K-2Cl transporter have shown that these animals have reduced or abolished tactile allodynia in areas of secondary hyperalgesia (Laird et al. 2004), which would support a role for the presynaptic inhibitory mechanism in the generation of hyperalgesic states. It remains to be seen whether this is only a mechanism for a short-term induction of tactile allodynia or if a similar process could also operate for the longer-lasting phases of allodynia characteristic of neuropathic and chronic inflammatory pain states.

FROM HERE TO ETERNITY

The gate theory has been with us for 40 years, and it appears that it will continue to provide grounds for debate for many years to come. The main point of the theory was a restatement of pattern interpretations of pain mechanisms, which has been found, in the intervening years, to be a great simplification for the CNS or even plainly wrong for the organization of the peripheral input to the spinal cord. Other details of the theory regarding the dorsal horn organization of presynaptic links between A and C fibers have also been proven incorrect. However, the gate theory has had an overall positive effect in the field of pain research and has helped to draw attention to previously forgotten aspects of pain modulation.

We still do not know how pain-related information is processed by the brain, although we recognize that both specific and convergent pathways participate in the process. We have learned that not all forms of pain are mediated by the same mechanism and that there is a considerable amount of plasticity along the nociceptive pathway. The role of central modulation, both excitatory and inhibitory, is also crucial in pain perception, as was brought to light by the gate theory. However, the debate between a strict specificity or pattern interpretation of pain mechanisms has been superseded, which makes the essence of the gate theory appear dated and obsolete.

On the other hand, by drawing attention to previously unexplored aspects of pain perception, most notably those of pathological states, the theory has contributed to a considerable surge in pain research, including the development of many models of pathological pain. It has also focused, perhaps excessively, on the dorsal horn as a site for pain modulation, and this spinal cord obsession is still very much with us. The failure to develop new analgesic drugs clearly based on spinal cord mechanisms, in spite of the huge amount of work on spinal neurochemistry, may indicate that the spinal cord focus of the gate theory was perhaps overoptimistic.

For years the gate theory has been a source of inspiration and a strong intellectual driving force for scientists and clinicians. Even those of us who have been critical of the underlying "pattern" theme of the theory recognize its influence in the pain field and its contribution to ideas about pain modulation and afferent interactions. Much has been written, both in praise and scorn, about the gate theory, but perhaps the best tribute that it ever received was given by Peter Nathan in his 1976 critical review: "Ideas need to be fruitful; they do not have to be right. And curiously enough, the two do not necessarily go together."

ACKNOWLEDGMENTS

I will always be indebted to Ainsley Iggo for introducing me to pain research, to good laboratory work, and to malt whisky. Without Vince Molony none of the work on substantia gelatinosa neurons that we carried out in Edinburgh would have been possible. Robert Schmidt has been a source of inspiration when it comes to questions of presynaptic inhibition (and fast cars), and I have always admired his extremely high standards. And I have shared so much with Jenny Laird that to acknowledge only her crucial role in this work seems silly. To all of them and to the many people who have helped me along the way: thanks!

REFERENCES

Alvarez-Leefmans FJ, Nani A, Márquez S. Chloride transport, osmotic balance, and presynaptic inhibition. In: Rudomin P, Romo R, Mendell LM (Eds). *Presynaptic Inhibition and Neural Control.* New York: Oxford University Press, 1998, pp 50–79.

Belmonte C, Cervero F (Eds). *Neurobiology of Nociceptors.* Oxford: Oxford University Press, 1996.

Calvillo O. Primary afferent depolarization of C-fibers in the spinal cord of the cat. *Can J Physiol Pharmacol* 1978; 56:154–157.

Cervero F. Dorsal horn neurones and their sensory inputs. In: Yaksh TL (Ed). *Spinal Afferent Processing.* New York: Plenum Press, 1986, pp 197–216.

Cervero F. Sensory innervation of the viscera: peripheral basis of visceral pain. *Physiol Rev* 1994; 74:95–138.

Cervero F. Visceral nociceptors. In: Belmonte C, Cervero F (Eds). *Neurobiology of Nociceptors.* Oxford: Oxford University Press, 1996, pp 220–240.

Cervero F, Iggo A. Reciprocal sensory interactions in the spinal cord. *J Physiol* 1978; 284:84–85P.

Cervero F, Iggo A. The substantia gelatinosa of the spinal cord: a critical review. *Brain* 1980; 103:717–772.

Cervero F, Jänig W. Visceral nociceptors: a new world order? *Trends Neurosci* 1992; 15:374–378.

Cervero F, Laird JMA. One pain or many pains? a new look at pain mechanisms. *News Physiol Sci* 1991; 6:268–273.

Cervero F, Laird JMA. Mechanisms of touch-evoked pain (allodynia): a new model. *Pain* 1996; 68:13–23.

Cervero F, Iggo A, Ogawa H. Nociceptor-driven dorsal horn neurones in the lumbar spinal cord of the cat. *Pain* 1976; 2:5–24.

Cervero F, Molony V, Iggo A. Extracellular and intracellular recordings from neurones in the substantia gelatinosa Rolandi. *Brain Res* 1977; 136:565–569.

Cervero F, Iggo A, Molony V. The tract of Lissauer and the dorsal root potential. *J Physiol* 1978; 282:295–305.

Cervero F, Iggo A, Molony V. An electrophysiological study of neurones in the Substantia Gelatinosa Rolandi of the cat's spinal cord. *Q J Exp Physiol* 1979a; 64:297–314.

Cervero F, Iggo A, Molony V. Segmental and intersegmental organisation of neurones in the Substania Gelatinosa Rolandi of the cat's spinal cord. *Q J Exp Physiol* 1979b; 64:315–326.

Cervero F, Molony V, Iggo A. Functional characteristics of neurones in the substantia gelatinosa Rolandi of the cat. In: Bonica JJ, Liebeskind JC, Albe-Fessard DG (Eds). *Proceedings of the Second World Congress on Pain,* Advances in Pain Research and Therapy, Vol. 3. New York: Raven Press, 1979c, pp 877–882

Cervero F, Molony V, Iggo A. Supraspinal linkages of substantia gelatinosa neurones: effects of descending impulses. *Brain Res* 1979d; 175:351–355.

Cervero F, Laird JMA, García-Nicas E. Secondary hyperalgesia and presynaptic inhibition: an update. *Eur J Pain* 2003; 7:345–351.

Christensen BN, Perl ER. Spinal neurons specifically excited by noxious or thermal stimuli: marginal zone of the dorsal horn. *J Neurophysiol* 1970; 33:293–307.

Craig AD. Pain mechanisms: labeled lines versus convergence in central processing. *Annu Rev Neurosci* 2003; 26:1–30.

Craig AD, Bushnell MC, Zhang E-T, Blomqvist A. A thalamic nucleus specific for pain and temperature sensation. *Nature* 1994; 372:770–773.

Descartes R. *L'homme.* Paris: Chez Jacques Le Gras, 1664.

Franz DN, Iggo A. Dorsal root potentials and ventral root reflexes evoked by nonmyelinated fibers. *Science* 1968; 162:1140–1142.

Hunt SP, Mantyh PW. The molecular dynamics of pain control. *Nat Rev Neurosci* 2001; 2:83–91.

Iggo A, Ogawa H, Cervero F. Inhibition of nociceptor driven dorsal horn neurones in the cat. In: Bonica JJ, Albe-Fessard DG (Eds). *Proceedings of the First World Congress on Pain,* Advances in Pain Research and Therapy, Vol. 1. New York: Raven Press, 1976, pp 99–104.

Jänig W, Morrison JFB. Functional properties of spinal visceral afferents supplying abdominal and pelvic organs with special emphasis on visceral nociception. In: Cervero F, Morrison JFB (Eds). *Visceral Sensation,* Progress in Brain Research, Vol. 67. Amsterdam: Elsevier, 1986, pp 87–114.

Julius D, Basbaum AI. Molecular mechanisms of nociception. *Nature* 2001; 413:203–210.

Laird JMA, García-Nicas E, Delpire EJ, Cervero F. Presynaptic inhibition and spinal pain processing: a possible role of the NKCC1 cation-chloride co-transporter in hyperalgesia. *Neurosci Lett* 2004; in press.

Melzack R, Wall PD. Pain mechanisms: a new theory. *Science* 1965; 150:971–979.

Molony V, Steedman WM, Cervero F, Iggo A. Intracellular marking of identified neurones in the superficial dorsal horn of the cat spinal cord. *Q J Exp Physiol* 1981; 66:211–233.

Nathan PW. The gate-control theory of pain. A critical review. *Brain* 1976; 99:123–158.

Noordenbos W. *Pain.* Amsterdam: Elsevier, 1959.

Rees H, Sluka KA, Westlund KN, Willis WD. Do dorsal root reflexes augment peripheral inflammation? *Neuroreport* 1994; 5:821–824.

Rees H, Sluka KA, Westlund KN, Willis WD. The role of glutamate and GABA receptors in the generation of dorsal root reflexes by acute arthritis in the anaesthetised rat. *J Physiol* 1995; 484:437–445.

Rudomin P. Pre-synaptic inhibition of muscle spindle and tendon organ afferents in the mammalian spinal cord. *Trends Neurosci* 1990; 13:499–505.

Schmidt RF. Pre-synaptic inhibition in the vertebrate nervous system. *Rev Physiol Biochem Pharm* 1971; 63:21–101.

Sinclair DC. Cutaneous sensation and the doctrine of specific energy. *Brain* 1955; 78:584–614.

Sluka KA, Willis WD, Westlund KN. The role of dorsal root reflexes in neurogenic inflammation. *Pain Forum* 1995; 4:141–149.

Treede R-D, Meyer RA, Raja SN, Campbell JN. Peripheral and central mechanisms of cutaneous hyperalgesia. *Prog Neurobiol* 1992; 38:397–421.

Tsuda M, Shigemoto-Mogami Y, Koizumi S, et al. P2X4 receptors induced in spinal microglia gate tactile allodynia after nerve injury. *Nature* 2003; 424:778–783.

Wall PD. Cord cells responding to touch, damage, and temperature of skin. *J Neurophysiol* 1960; 23:197–210.

Wall PD. The gate control theory of pain mechanisms. A re-examination and re-statement. *Brain* 1978; 101:1–18.

Watkins LR, Milligan ED, Maier SF. Glial activation: a driving force for pathological pain. *Trends Neurosci* 2001; 24:450–455.

Weddell G, Miller S. Cutaneous sensibility. *Ann Rev Physiol* 1962; 24:199–222.

Whitehorn D, Burgess PR. Changes in polarization of central branches of myelinated mechanoreceptor and nociceptor fibers during noxious and innocuous stimulation of the skin. *J Neurophysiol* 1973; 36:226–237.

Zimmermann M. Dorsal root potentials after C-fiber stimulation. *Science* 1968; 160:896–898.

Correspondence to: Professor Fernando Cervero, MD, PhD, DSc, Anaesthesia Research Unit, McGill University, McIntyre Medical Building, Room 1207, 3655 Promenade Sir William Osler, Montreal, Quebec H3G 1Y6, Canada. Tel: 514-398-5764; Fax: 514-398-8241; email: fernando.cervero@mcgill.ca.

The Paths of Pain 1975–2005, edited by
Harold Merskey, John D. Loeser, and Ronald
Dubner, IASP Press, Seattle, © 2005.

4

Molecular Basis of Receptors

Michael S. Gold

*Department of Biomedical Sciences, Dental School; Program in Neuroscience;
and Department of Anatomy and Neurobiology, Medical School, University
of Maryland, Baltimore, Maryland, USA*

Thirty years ago, John Bonica wrote in his introduction to the proceedings of the 1st World Congress on Pain that the major problem before the pain community was inadequately treated chronic pain (Bonica 1976). Bonica went on to point out that one of the reasons for this problem was a lack of knowledge—with a limited mechanistic understanding of chronic pain, appropriate treatment was impossible. Researchers took up Bonica's challenge, and their success has been nothing short of astonishing. This chapter represents an attempt to highlight three decades of phenomenal achievement. To accomplish this task in a relatively limited amount of space, I will focus on one specific area, the molecular biology of receptors in primary afferent neurons.

In 1975 our mechanistic understanding of chronic pain was extremely limited. It was 17 years since Crick and Watson had published the structure of DNA, and 10 years after the galvanizing paper by Melzack and Wall (1965) had inspired many young scientists to devote their careers to pain research. The existence of a subpopulation of primary afferent neurons that was selectively activated by noxious stimuli had been firmly established a few years earlier by the work of Burgess and Perl (1967) and Iggo (1969). Pharmacological studies had established the concepts of "neurotransmitter" and "receptor," and it was becoming clear that the nervous system utilized more than just six major neurotransmitters. It was also clear that there must be specialized structures that enabled the peripheral nervous system to transduce environmental stimuli (thermal, mechanical, and chemical) into an electrical signal, but at a mechanistic level, we knew nothing about these structures.

TECHNOLOGICAL ADVANCES PAVED THE WAY
FOR PROGRESS IN NEUROBIOLOGY

Progress in our mechanistic understanding of nociception was dependent on major technological advances that occurred in three main areas: electrophysiology, biochemistry, and molecular biology. The work of Hodgkin and Huxley in the early 1950s had established the ionic basis of fundamental electrophysiological properties of neural tissue such as the resting membrane potential, the action potential and action potential conduction. Throughout the first half of the century, investigators perfected the use of glass microelectrodes to enable intracellular recording from excitable tissues. When used in combination with the operational amplifier, first developed in the 1950s, these electrodes made it possible to record the relatively small ionic currents in mammalian neurons. Application of these recording techniques to primary afferent neurons in vivo enabled characterization of the electrophysiological and histological properties of damage-sensing primary afferents, and this work began in earnest at the end of the 1970s. The seminal work of Sakmann and Nehrer in the early 1980s (Hamill et al. 1981) led to a major advance in the realm of electrophysiology with the discovery of the patch-clamp recording configuration. With this approach, it was possible to study the behavior of a single molecule in real time, and therefore to characterize many of the critical properties of ion channels that serve as receptors in primary afferent neurons. Of course, it would have been impossible to deal with the vast amounts of data generated with these approaches had there not been simultaneous advances in computing.

Prior to developments that occurred in the 1980s, advances in the areas of biochemistry and molecular biology were largely the result of "brute force" approaches to isolating, purifying, and sequencing cellular proteins. During the late 1970s and early 1980s, techniques were developed that enabled the isolation of cellular mRNA, which could then be used as a template with which to synthesize complementary DNA (cDNA) in a test tube. Transcripts originally encoded by the mRNA could be inserted into the DNA of a plasmid used to transform bacteria, resulting in a cDNA "library" with each bacterial colony containing a "clone" of an mRNA transcript. Techniques were also developed that enabled transfection of cDNA into different cell types. These transfection approaches enabled researchers to take advantage of the host cells' transcriptional and translational "machinery" so that these cells would generate the proteins encoded by the foreign cDNA. This method of inducing cells to express foreign proteins is called heterologous expression, and it enabled researchers to study the function of the proteins expressed in this way in relative isolation. If, for example, researchers were interested in identifying the receptor encoding a specific inflammatory mediator, they could screen transfected cells for a response to the inflammatory mediator of interest. This screening process, called expression cloning, would enable identification of genes encoding many of the receptors present in sensory neurons.

Once a gene was identified, it was possible to deduce the amino acid sequence of the encoded protein. Knowledge of protein sequence enabled the generation of antibodies that were used in conjunction with physiological approaches to further establish structure-function relationships for specific proteins and more importantly, the localization of proteins at a cellular and subcellular level. A major advance occurred in 1985 with the discovery of a process that enabled the rapid amplification of small fragments of DNA: polymerase chain reaction (PCR; Mullis et al. 1986). This technique fueled an explosion in the rate at which the genes encoding specific proteins were identified. It also enabled researchers to manipulate, or mutate, the genes encoding specific proteins, which, when used with heterologous expression, enabled researchers to identify the function of specific sequences and even single amino acids of the protein of interest.

CHEMORECEPTORS: TWENTY YEARS OF PROGRESS

Prior to 1975, traditional pharmacological approaches employed well into the second half of the 20th century not only had established the concept of a receptor as a specialized structure that enabled specific chemicals to produce biological effects, but had enabled the classification of receptor subtypes. The ability of specific classes of molecules (i.e., agonists) to produce the same or similar effects (such as muscle contraction or an increase in heart rate) and more importantly, the ability of other classes of molecules (i.e., antagonists) to block the actions of agonists made it clear that there were several distinct classes of receptors subserving specific biological functions. Furthermore, biochemical and electrophysiological approaches had established the distinction between ionotropic receptors (those coupled to ion channels) and metabotropic receptors (those coupled to second-messenger pathways). The importance of second-messenger pathways to nociception had been recently underscored by the discovery in the early 1970s that aspirin-like compounds worked by blocking an enzyme, cyclooxygenase. Thus, one important mechanism whereby inflammatory mediators like bradykinin produce hyperalgesia is via activation of a receptor that initiates the activation of a second-messenger cascade, resulting in the liberation of arachidonic acid, the substrate for cyclooxygenase. Within this framework, and with the knowledge that many of the chemicals released at sites of tissue injury could reproduce the pain and hyperalgesia of tissue injury when injected into naive tissue, researchers were well aware that there must be specific receptors in damage-sensing neurons that mediated both neural activation and sensitization. And while it was appreciated that the molecular identification of the chemoreceptors responsible for the activation of damage-sensing neurons may facilitate the identification of antagonists and therefore foster novel ways to treat pain, progress in our understanding of chemoreceptors had been relatively slow prior to 1983.

However, the year 1983, with the cloning of the first G-protein-coupled receptor (GPCR), marked a significant turning point in the rate of progress in this area (Nathans and Hogness 1983). Because the topology of GPCRs is relatively conserved, the first GPCR cloned served as a prototype for the cloning of all subsequent receptors, thereby enabling the rapid identification of both structure and function of genes cloned from a number of tissues, including the primary afferent neuron. The first guanine nucleotide-binding protein (G-protein) was cloned two years after the first GPCR (Gilman 1987). Identification of the genes encoding G-proteins and a GPCR were critical discoveries, not only because they led to the elucidation of the cellular pathways underlying the transduction of light and subsequently odorants, but because it would turn out that many of the chemicals, in particular inflammatory mediators such as bradykinin, prostaglandin, histamine, and serotonin, that activate as well as sensitize primary afferent neurons do so via GPCRs. It also turned out that several receptors responsible for the actions of analgesics such as opioids are also coupled to G-proteins. Thus, by 1990, there was compelling evidence that inflammatory hyperalgesia reflects, at least in part, inflammatory-mediator-induced activation of GPCRs on damage-sensing primary afferent neurons. GPCR activation results in the activation of adenylate cyclase, an increase in the second messenger cyclic adenosine monophosphate (cAMP), and the subsequent activation of the cAMP-dependent protein kinase, PKA. Antinociceptive compounds such as morphine were then shown to attenuate inflammatory hyperalgesia via activation of another GPCR on damage-sensing primary afferent neurons, resulting in the inhibition of adenylate cyclase, a decrease in cAMP, and the subsequent inhibition of PKA (Levine and Reichling 1999).

Further clarification of the mechanism of opioid antinociception would come in 1992 with the cloning of the first of three opioid receptors, the δ-opioid receptor, which was isolated with an expression-cloning approach (Evans et al. 1992; Kieffer et al. 1992). The μ- and κ-opioid receptors were cloned soon thereafter by investigators who located sequences in rat brain cDNA libraries that were homologous to that of the δ-opioid receptor. The subsequent demonstration (Stein 2003) that all three opioid receptors are present in subpopulations of damage-sensing primary afferent neurons continues to justify efforts into the development of peripherally acting opioids that could provide pain relief while avoiding some of the more troubling side effects of centrally acting opioids.

By 1995, the molecular biological tools were in place to enable investigators to pursue the notion that the function of primary afferent neurons, in particular damage-sensing primary afferent neurons, implied that these cells would express proteins found in no other tissue of the body (Akopian and Wood 1995). The generation of a subtractive cDNA library in which mRNA from a number of nonsensory tissues is used to remove nonspecific species from a DRG-derived cDNA library is a powerful tool to address this idea. This approach led to the identification of two ion channels, an ionotropic or ligand-gated ion channel and a voltage-gated ion channel, that have proven to be critical for the function of damage-sensing primary afferents. Adenosine triphosphate (ATP) was the ligand for the ionotropic receptor. This receptor, called $P2X_3$, was ideally situated to enable primary afferents to respond rapidly to tissue damage, given that ATP is released from all injured cells. SNS, the sensory-neuron-specific voltage-gated sodium channel (now called $Na_V1.8$) was the ion channel isolated with the subtractive library approach. Subsequent research has confirmed that both channels are only expressed in primary afferent neurons and preferentially in damage-sensing afferents (Burnstock 2000; Gold 2000). Because of this unique pattern of distribution and the evidence suggesting that both ion channels contribute to the pain associated with peripheral tissue injury, both channels remain potential targets for novel therapeutic interventions.

It had long been appreciated that the active ingredient in chili peppers, called capsaicin, is effective in both causing pain (the "burn" associated with hot peppers) as well as relieving it. Modern electrophysiological and biochemical techniques indicated that capsaicin has a direct action on primary afferent neurons. The receptor responsible for the actions of capsaicin was ultimately identified in 1997, using calcium imaging as a way to screen capsaicin-responsive cells in a heterologous expression system (Caterina et al. 1997). This receptor was originally called VR1 for vanilloid receptor 1, but was subsequently renamed TRPV1 ("V" for vanilloid) because it is a member of a larger family of receptors that was originally identified as homologous to the channel responsible for a transient receptor potential observed following a brief activation of the *Drosophila* retina (Jordt et al. 2003).

The cloning of TRPV1 was a critical milestone not only because of the therapeutic potential suggested by the actions of capsaicin, but because it turned out to be the first molecule identified that is gated (i.e., opened and closed) by changes in temperature. Under resting conditions the channel is activated by temperatures in the noxious range (i.e., >43°C). However, the thermosensitivity of the channel is modulated by a number of different compounds including protons and inflammatory mediators such as bradykinin and nerve growth factor (NGF), each of which appears to utilize a distinct cellular pathway in order to influence the properties of TRPV1. Importantly, an inflammatory-mediator-induced shift in the thermal sensitivity of TRPV1 may enable this channel to contribute to the ongoing burning pain associated with tissue injury. Consistent with this suggestion is the observation that TRPV1 is critical for the expression of inflammatory thermal hyperalgesia. Thus, blocking TRPV1 may be an effective way to attenuate inflammatory pain. However, the real therapeutic potential of TRPV1 lies in the fact that prolonged receptor activation results in desensitization of afferent terminals. Importantly, this desensitization affects mechanical and chemical stimuli, in addition to thermal stimuli. While its mechanism remains to be fully elucidated, this desensitization appears to occur subsequent to a TRPV1-induced increase in intracellular calcium and is likely to reflect the "dying back" of afferent terminals. Thus, TRPV1 activation has the potential to attenuate the more troubling mechanical hypersensitivity associated with chronic inflammation. Furthermore, because TRPV1 expression develops in mechanically sensitive afferents spared by a partial nerve injury, activation of this receptor may be used to treat the mechanical hypersensitivity associated with neuropathic pain (Jordt et al. 2003).

CHEMORECEPTORS: THE STATE OF THE ART
AND FUTURE DIRECTIONS

To say that primary afferent neurons express a rich array of both ionotropic and metabotropic chemoreceptors would be an understatement. Metabotropic receptors have more recently been subdivided on the basis of the second-messenger cascade initiated by receptor activation. The most extensively studied of these include the heterotrimeric GPCRs (i.e., seven-transmembrane or serpentine receptors), but other subgroups include receptors bearing intrinsic protein tyrosine kinase domains (i.e., Trk receptors), receptors that associate with cytosolic tyrosine kinases (i.e., non-tyrosine kinase receptors such as cytokine receptors, integrins), and protein serine/threonine kinases (i.e., transforming growth factor [TGF]-β receptors). Not only do primary afferents express each of these major subtypes of chemoreceptor, but they also express multiple isoforms of these receptors. For example, sensory neurons contain all seven ionotropic ATP receptors (Kage et al. 2002; Wood 2004), three of the four acid-sensitive ion channels (Wood 2004), multiple ionotropic glutamate receptor subunits including AMPA (GluR1–3) Kainate (GluR5) and NMDA (NR1, NR2B–C) (Sato et al. 1993; Kerchner et al. 2002; Marvizon et al. 2002), multiple nicotinic receptor subtypes (resulting in four pharmacologically distinct current types) (Genzen et al. 2001), and the only ionotropic serotonin receptor (5-HT3) (Wu et al. 2001). Similarly, evidence suggests that sensory neurons also contain at least 21 isoforms of metabotropic receptors for the classic neurotransmitters: five cholinergic receptors (Tata et al. 2000), four adrenergic receptors (Nicholas et al. 1993; Xie et al. 2001), eight serotonergic receptors (Wu et al. 2001), and four dopaminergic receptors (Xie et al. 1998). Sensory neurons also contain four metabotropic amino acid receptors comprising two glutamate (Crawford et al. 2000; Berent-Spillson et al. 2004) and two GABA receptors (Towers et al. 2000), two metabotropic purinergic receptors (Ruan and Burnstock 2003), multiple metabotropic receptors for inflammatory mediators including prostanoids (three EP receptors and one IP receptor) (Hingtgen and Vasko 1994; Mizumura et al. 1996), bradykinin receptors (Seabrook et al. 1997), histamine receptors (Kashiba et al. 1999), two adenosine receptors (Hu and Li 1997), endothelin receptors (Pomonis et al. 2001), two proteinase-activated receptors (de Garavilla et al. 2001; Dai et al. 2004), and an almost countless number of peptide receptors (Hökfelt et al. 1997). Finally, it is clear that primary afferents also express a number of the more recently identified tyrosine kinase receptors, including all three of the classic high-affinity Trk receptors (TrkA–C), the low-affinity Trk receptor p75, at least three subtypes of the glial-cell-line-derived neurotrophic factor (GDNF) family receptor (Sah et al. 2003), and a number of non-tyrosine kinase receptors for inflammatory cytokines (Wood 2004). And while each of these receptors is differentially distributed among subpopulations of sensory neurons, it is clear that any given sensory neuron expresses multiple receptor subtypes. More importantly, tissue injury has been shown to result in changes in the receptors expressed, in patterns of expression, and in the cellular distribution of the receptors expressed.

Chemoreceptor research is presently focused on addressing three major gaps in our understanding of chemoreceptor processes: (1) second-messenger pathways activated by chemoreceptor occupancy, (2) receptor trafficking, and (3) receptor influences on transcription and translation. The level of analysis in each of these areas varies according to the present state of the art.

In the case of second-messenger pathways, the questions facing researchers today are relatively subtle. It has long been appreciated that receptor activation can initiate a cascade of cellular processes involving the liberation or release of other molecules such as Ca^{2+}, cAMP, or arachidonic acid, called second messengers, that determine the immediate consequences of receptor activation and enable the brief application of an agonist to produce effects that far outlast the agonist half-life in tissue. In the hope of identifying additional intracellular targets such as cyclooxygenase that can be used to more specifically block the actions of inflammatory mediators, researchers have discovered a tremendous amount about the specific sequence of events that occurs following chemoreceptor activation. For example, NGF is a molecule originally shown to be critical for the survival and directed growth of neurons in the peripheral nervous system. Work from a number of laboratories in the early 1990s led to the discovery that NGF is increased at the site of an injury and plays a critical role in the development of inflammatory hyperalgesia. Yet the second-messenger signaling that underlies the actions of NGF is extraordinarily complex. Binding to its high-affinity receptor TrkA, NGF may initiate a number of distinct cellular processes via distinct second-messenger pathways, ultimately influencing gene expression (e.g., see Fukuoka et al. 2001), protein translation (e.g., see Ji et al. 2002), or the modulation of plasma membrane proteins (e.g., see Zhang et al. 2002). And herein lie the more subtle questions to be addressed about second-messenger signaling regarding exactly how these signaling pathways interact and whether each pathway is essentially independent or whether blocking one pathway results in compensatory changes in the others. Similarly, it is unknown whether there is any subcellular segregation of distinct pathways. Furthermore, the relationship between receptor activation and specific second-messenger pathway activation remains to be determined. This relationship is particularly relevant for receptors like the TrkA receptor in light of observations indicating that there is constitutive NGF release and TrkA-receptor activation in the adult that is necessary for the maintenance of afferent phenotype (Sah et al. 2003), while at the same time endogenous mediators like estrogen can influence TrkA expression (Sohrabji et al. 1994), and environmental influences like inflammation can influence NGF expression (Woolf et al. 1994).

The gaps in our knowledge about receptor trafficking are considerably larger than those for second-messenger pathways. Receptor trafficking is a term used to describe the targeting of receptors at specific places in the plasma membrane. While this line of research is relatively new, the concept that receptors must be targeted to specific places in the membrane was implicit in the observation that chemical sensitivity was greatest at afferent terminals rather than along axons or at the cell body. Significant progress has been made in this field for specific classes of receptors, particularly for nicotinic acetylcholine receptors at the neuromuscular junction and for ionotropic glutamate receptors in postsynaptic membranes in the central nervous system (Li and Sheng 2003; Lu and Je 2003). Whole families of molecules have been identified that are involved in the anchoring of receptors to particular sites in the plasma membrane as well as in establishing proximal relationships between receptors and other modulatory proteins. However, it remains to be determined whether any of the intricate machinery involved in receptor trafficking in hippocampal dendrites is involved in receptor trafficking in sensory neurons. That is, while a number of ionotropic glutamate receptor subunits are both present and specifically distributed within primary sensory neurons, these neurons do not express proteins normally found in dendrites. More fundamentally, we know virtually nothing about the cellular machinery that underlies the functional relationship between chemoreceptors (and any other receptor for that matter) and other ion channels. Given the evidence that injury can produce profound changes in these functional relationships (i.e., Gold et al. 2003), identification of underlying mechanisms may yield novel targets for useful therapeutic interventions.

Prior to the 1990s, evidence for connections between tissue damage, receptor activation, and changes in gene expression (transcription) and protein synthesis (translation) were rather indirect. The birth of modern endocrinology in the mid-1800s provided the foundation for the link between chemical actions and protein synthesis. During this same period, it became clear that tissue injury, particularly nerve injury, was associated with changes in nervous tissue, most notably neural sprouting. The molecular basis for protein synthesis was established in the 1950s, as was the link between the genetic code and the synthesis of specific proteins. By the mid 1960s the first neurotrophic factors were isolated, providing the first chemicals that appeared to specifically influence transcription and translation in the peripheral nervous system. By the early 1990s, NGF was shown to be involved in nociceptive processing, although as noted above, it was not until the mid-1990s that it was shown to underlie transcriptional and translational events associated with tissue injury. Since that time, a number of additional molecules have been identified that influence transcription and translation in a similar manner. Thus, while there has been great progress in our understanding of receptor-mediated influences on transcription and translation, there remain significant gaps in our knowledge. That is, while we now recognize many molecules underlying signal transduction at both transcriptional and translational levels and we know a great deal about the transcriptional regulation of a number of specific genes, we do not know which factors influence the selective transcription of specific genes or the selective translation of specific mRNAs. And we are only just beginning to understand how selectivity is achieved when only a limited number of transcription factors have been identified.

An issue related to both trafficking and translation is a process referred to as receptor internalization. Many receptors, particularly serpentine GPCRs, undergo endocytosis following receptor activation and the subsequent initiation of specific second-messenger pathways. Internalized receptors are then either recycled to the cell membrane or shipped back to the cell body in phagocytic vesicles. There are several theories concerning the function of receptor internalization, including proposals that (1) it is a mechanism of desensitization, (2) it enables the "recharging" of used receptors, and (3) it enables signaling to the cell body about activity at peripheral terminals. While there is evidence in support of each of these theories, researchers have begun to harness the therapeutic potential implicit in the third by using this signaling pathway as a way to deliver toxic molecules to neuronal cell bodies, thereby producing a highly specific lesion (Khasabov et al. 2002). This approach has been used to eliminate specific subpopulations of sensory neurons as well as central neurons, and may prove to be an effective treatment for intractable pain.

THERMORECEPTORS: SEVEN YEARS OF PROGRESS

Psychophysical studies conducted in the mid-1960s suggested that there may be discrete populations of afferents enabling the detection or temperature changes across the spectrum of noxious cold to noxious heat. This suggestion was confirmed with single-unit electrophysiological studies conducted in the late 1960s and early 1970s that indicated that there were four and possibly five discrete classes of afferents activated by temperatures over very specific temperature ranges encompassing noxious cold, innocuous cool, innocuous warm, painful heat, and extremely painful heat. These early observations suggested there should be at least two, but perhaps as many as five, distinct receptors underlying this afferent activity. But the revolution in our understanding of thermosensation would have to wait until 1997 and the molecular identification of the first thermoreceptor, TRPV1 (Caterina et al. 1997).

Within a year and a half of reporting the discovery of TRPV1, the same group identified a TRPV1 homologue that was originally called VRL-1, for vanilloid receptor-like molecule 1, and has subsequently been renamed TRPV2 (Caterina and Julius 2001). This receptor is not sensitive to changes in pH or capsaicin but is activated at very high temperatures (approximately 52°C). TRPV2 is expressed in a different population of sensory neurons than TRPV1 and therefore was hypothesized to underlie the thermal sensitivity observed in high-threshold Aδ fibers and to subserve the sensation of extremely painful heat. Consistent with this suggestion was the observation that like the sensitization of high-threshold Aδ-fibers, repeated thermal activation of TRPV2 sensitized the receptor such that it became activated at temperatures as low as 40°C.

A third TRP family member was identified in 2000 (Strotmann et al. 2000). This channel was originally shown to be gated by changes in osmolality and was called OTRPC4. More recently, it was demonstrated that this channel is also responsive to innocuous warming; because of this property and its homology to TRPV1, the channel was renamed TRPV4. The presence of TRPV4 in keratinocytes led to the suggestion that innocuous warming was transduced in keratinocytes that then signaled to primary afferent neurons via an undetermined mechanism. However, recent data indicate that functional TRPV4 channels are present in sensory neurons. Concomitant with the recognition that TRPV4 has thermal sensitivity, a third heat-sensitive TRPV homologue, called TRPV3, was also found in keratinocytes and was shown to be activated by innocuous warming (Jordt et al. 2003). It has yet to be determined which, if either, of these TRP channels is ultimately responsible for the sensation of warming.

Several different approaches were employed in the isolation and characterization of receptors responsive to cooling. Calcium imaging and electrophysiological recordings from isolated sensory neurons constituted the first attempt to identify, at a mechanistic level, these proteins (Reid and Flonta 2001a,b). These in vitro studies suggested that at least two distinct ionic mechanisms underlie the response to cooling. One mechanism involved a cooling-induced activation of a nonselective cation channel, resulting in the direct depolarization of the neuronal membrane. Heterologous expression of an amiloride-sensitive epithelial sodium channel (ENaC) (Askwith et al. 2001) indicated that these cation channels could function as cold transducers. However, another cation channel was subsequently identified that appeared to have properties more similar to what was expected of a cooling receptor. The molecule was called TRPM8 (because of its homology to the TRPM subfamily of TRP channels) and CMR1 (for cold and menthol receptor-1) and is now called TRPM8 by convention. TRPM8 is selectively expressed in a subset of sensory neurons, is activated by relatively small decreases in temperature, and is sensitized by menthol.

The second mechanism for cold transduction suggested by in vitro studies involved the closing of a potassium channel normally active at the resting membrane potential (i.e., a "leak" channel). Such a change would result in membrane depolarization secondary to a decrease in a hyperpolarizing current. Heterologous expression of a member of the two-pore potassium channel family, TREK-1, suggests that this channel could underlie such a response because the channel opens with an increase in temperature and closes in response to a decrease in temperature (Maingret et al. 2000). Nevertheless, at present, the weight of pharmacological, electrophysiological, and molecular biological data supports a role for TRPM8 in the transduction of cooling.

The most recently identified sensory neuron ion channel may be a transducer for noxious cold stimuli. This molecule was also identified with a database screen for TRP channel homologues, a process now referred to as "cloning in silica." The channel was originally called ANKTM1 because of the presence of 14 N-terminal ankyrin domains followed by six transmembrane domains. The channel was subsequently renamed TRPA1. Heterologous expression of the channel indicated that it was activated at lower temperatures than TRPM8 and therefore might subserve the function as noxious cold transducer (but see Thut et al. 2003). Subsequent analysis of TRPA1 suggests that this channel is more widely expressed than was first thought. More interesting, however, is that the channel appears to function better as a complement to TRPV1 to the extent that it is activated by isothiocyanate and cinnamaldehyde, constituents of pungent foods like cinnamon oil, mustard oil, and horseradish. Importantly, because TRPA1 is activated by inflammatory mediators like bradykinin and is expressed in a subset of TRPV1-expressing sensory neurons, it is likely that activation of this channel also contributes to inflammatory pain (Bandell et al. 2004; Jordt et al. 2004).

Two important themes have emerged over the last seven years during which six molecules were identified that together encompass the entire range of thermal sensitivity. First, there are specific classes of chemicals that increase the thermal sensitivity of thermosensitive channels. These observations have prompted searches for endogenous ligands that may also influence channel gating. And second, these channels subserve multiple functions in sensory neurons and other cells.

MECHANORECEPTORS: IN SEARCH OF THE ELUSIVE TRANSDUCER

Several early lines of evidence suggest that mechanoreception in sensory neurons would reflect activation of one or more discrete molecules present in afferent endings (Lewin and Stucky 2000). First, there were early observations indicating that several classes of low-threshold mechanoreceptor remained mechanically sensitive following removal of specialized endings. Second, data from nerve injury models indicated that mechanosensitivity developed in the cut ends of primary afferents, suggesting that a transducer made in the primary afferent was inserted into the "new" afferent terminals. Third, early patch-clamp studies revealed the existence of stretch-activated channels, which, while present in all cell types, provided a direct mechanism for ion flux in response to mechanical deformation of cell membranes (Hamill and McBride 1996). Fourth, research into the mechanosensitivity of other mechanically sensitive tissues indicated the existence of specialized ion channels that are opened and closed in response to changes in extracellular forces. And fifth, mutagenesis studies in the flat worm *C. elegans* revealed a family of molecules, called the degenerins (of which ENaC is a family member), that were necessary for mechanosensitivity. Several of these molecules encode ion channels that have vertebrate homologues expressed in sensory neurons (Lewin and Stucky 2000).

The relative contribution of putative mechanotransducers to mechanosensation has been most extensively studied in mutant mice. The first of these to be assessed was a channel called BNaC1 (also termed BNC1, MDEG, and ASIC-2) for brain sodium channel 1, a mammalian homologue of a degenerin-related ion channel. In BNaC1 null mutant mice, there was a marked and specific deficit in the mechanical sensitivity of low-threshold rapidly adapting afferents, suggesting that this channel contributes to the mechanosensitivity of a specific class of afferents. However, other channels must also contribute to mechanical transduction, given that the majority of mechanically sensitive afferents were unaffected by the loss of BNaC1 (Price et al. 2000).

Because ASIC-3 (acid-sensing ion channel 3, also known as DRASIC) is another degenerin family member, the contribution of this channel to mechanotransduction was also assessed in null mutant mice (Price et al. 2002). As with BNaC1 null mutants, ASIC-3 null mutants also demonstrated deficits in mechanosensitivity of distinct afferent populations. However, the phenotype was markedly different. In ASIC-3 null mutants, there was an increase in the sensitivity of low-threshold mechanosensitive afferents and a decrease in the response of damage-sensing afferents to noxious pinch. This channel was shown to be present in the endings of several low-threshold afferents, including those terminating in Meissner corpuscles and in the lanceolate nerve endings surrounding hair follicles. ASIC-3 was also present in some, but not all, free nerve endings. A subsequent analysis of ASIC-3 and ASIC-1 null mutant mice indicated that neither channel contributes to mechanically evoked currents in isolated sensory neurons. One possible explanation for the less than clear results obtained with any of the ASIC null mutant mice is that these channels may be formed by subunits encoded by different genes (i.e., ASIC-3 and BNaC1 may be assembled together to form a functional channel), a process referred to as heteromultimerization, resulting in a channel referred to as a heteromultimer. As a result, mechanosensitivity my reflect activation of different heteromultimers of ASIC channel subunits, which not only include ASIC-1–3, but a splice variant of ASIC-1 (i.e., ASIC1-β) and the β and γ subunits of an ENaC channel (which have also been localized in afferent endings in hairy skin) (Krishtal 2003). Furthermore, given the likelihood of compensatory changes in channel expression in null mutants, the loss of a single subunit in a complex may be compensated for by an increase in the expression of another subunit.

Several other ion channels have also shown to have mechanical sensitivity. The first of these to be identified was a potassium channel called TREK-1, for TWIK-related potassium channel, where TWIK stands for tandem of P domains in a weak inward rectifier potassium channel (Patel et al. 2001). TREK-1 was cloned in 1996 based on homology to TWIK. While TREK-1 was originally shown to be activated by arachidonic acid and inhibited by cAMP, it was subsequently shown to be activated by membrane stretch, by osmotic swelling, and by molecules that cause membrane crenation. Two more mechanosensitive two-pore potassium channels, TREK-2 and TRAAK, were subsequently described. These channels are also activated by membrane stretch and by crenators. Both TREK-1 and TRAAK-1 expression have been demonstrated in sensory neurons. Nevertheless, it remains to be determined whether either of these channels underlies the mechanosensitivity of primary afferent neurons (Patel et al. 2001).

TRPV4 is another channel that may serve as a mechanotransducer. Compelling evidence from both knockout and knockdown studies in vivo and in vitro suggests that the channel underlies the response to hypertonicity in primary afferent neurons (Nilius et al. 2004). However, the observation that TRPV4 null mutant mice respond poorly to intense mechanical stimuli suggests that the channel may also be involved in mechanotransduction (Nilius et al. 2004).

The ionotropic ATP receptor $P2X_3$ is one of the most promising candidates for a receptor primarily responsible for mechanotransduction in specific populations of primary afferent neurons. $P2X_3$ is particular intriguing because it is enriched in damage-sensing neurons, although $P2X_1$ and $P2X_2$ receptors may also contribute to mechanotransduction (North 2003). This receptor is present in the terminals of afferents and appears to underlie the rapid response to mechanical damage to surrounding tissue. This channel is most likely to contribute to mechanotransduction in visceral structures such as the bladder and colon. There is evidence for a calcium-dependent vesicular release of ATP from bladder urothelial cells that is evoked by both distension and cell swelling (Birder et al. 2003), and similar observations have been made in the colon (Wynn et al. 2003). In $P2X_3$ null mutant mice, the bladder becomes hyporeflexive and distension-evoked afferent activity is markedly attenuated, while ATP release is normal (Vlaskovska et al. 2001), and in the colon, distension-evoked afferent activity is attenuated by P2X-receptor antagonists (Wynn et al. 2003). Other mechanotransduction mechanisms are likely to underlie afferent activation in somatic tissue, because attenuation of $P2X_3$ with antagonists, antisense knockdown, and gene knockout have no influence on mechanical thresholds in naive tissue. However, given evidence of an increase in $P2X_3$ expression in the presence of both nerve injury and inflammation, this mechanism may become more important under these pathophysiological conditions (North 2003).

SUMMARY AND CONCLUSIONS

Over the last 30 years, our understanding of nociceptive processing in general and of the transduction of noxious stimuli in particular has moved from a rudimentary concept of a receptor to a detailed knowledge not just of the genes encoding whole families of receptors and consequently the amino acid sequence underlying the receptor structure, but of specific amino acids responsible for receptor function. We now know the molecular identity of receptors responsible for the transduction of a wide array of both endogenous and exogenous compounds as well as thermal stimuli that run the temperature range between noxious cold to noxious heat. While our understanding of mechanical transduction is still limited, a number of molecules and pathways have been identified that are likely to contribute to this process. It is dismaying to note that our ability to treat chronic pain not only has failed to keep pace with this virtual explosion of knowledge, but has in fact progressed little in the last 30 years. Worse still is the fact that Bonica had the same lament in his introduction to the proceedings of the 1st World Congress on Pain. Nevertheless, I remain optimistic that all of this progress will pay off very soon. Targets have been identified, high-throughput screening systems have been developed, novel delivery systems are being implemented, clinical protocols have been refined, patient populations have been defined, the basis for and impact of individual differences can be more appropriately addressed, and the public is better informed and more appropriately prepared to implement novel therapeutic interventions. Thus, my optimism stems from the fact that the tools are in place at almost every level to ensure the translation of our basic understanding into novel and effective therapeutic interventions for the chronic pain patient.

ACKNOWLEDGMENTS

I would like to thank Dr. Michael Caterina and Natasha Flake for helpful discussions during the preparation of this manuscript. Some of the work described in this manuscript was supported by NIH grants P50 AR049555 and P01 NS41384.

REFERENCES

Akopian AN, Wood JN. Peripheral nervous system-specific genes identified by subtractive cDNA cloning. *J Biol Chem* 1995; 270:21264–21270,

Askwith CC, Benson CJ, Welsh MJ, Snyder PM. DEG/ENaC ion channels involved in sensory transduction are modulated by cold temperature. *Proc Natl Acad Sci USA* 2001; 98:6459–6463.

Bandell M, Story GM, Hwang SW, et al. Noxious cold ion channel TRPA1 is activated by pungent compounds and bradykinin. *Neuron* 2004; 41:849–857.

Berent-Spillson A, Robinson AM, Golovoy D, et al. Protection against glucose-induced neuronal death by NAAG and GCP II inhibition is regulated by mGluR3. *J Neurochem* 2004; 89:90–99.

Birder LA, Barrick SR, Roppolo JR, et al. Feline interstitial cystitis results in mechanical hypersensitivity and altered ATP release from bladder urothelium. *Am J Physiol Renal Physiol* 2003; 285:F423–F429.

Bonica JJ. Introduction to the First World Congress on Pain: goals of IASP and the World Congress. In: Bonica JJ, Albe-Fessard D (Eds). *Proceedings of the First World Congress on Pain,* Advances in Pain Research and Therapy, Vol. 1. New York: Raven, 1976, pp xxvii–xxxix.

Burgess PR, Perl ER. Myelinated afferent fibers responding specifically to noxious stimulation of the skin. *J Physiol (Lond)* 1967; 190:541–562.

Burnstock G. P2X receptors in sensory neurones. *Br J Anaesth* 2000; 84(4):476–488.

Caterina MJ, Julius D. The vanilloid receptor: a molecular gateway to the pain pathway. *Annu Rev Neurosci* 2001; 24:487–517.

Caterina MJ, Schumacher MA, Tominaga M, et al. The capsaicin receptor: a heat-activated ion channel in the pain pathway. *Nature* 1997; 389:816–824.

Crawford JH, Wainwright A, Heavens R, et al. Mobilisation of intracellular Ca^{2+} by mGluR5 metabotropic glutamate receptor activation in neonatal rat cultured dorsal root ganglia neurones. *Neuropharmacology* 2000; 39:621–630.

Dai Y, Moriyama T, Higashi T, et al. Proteinase-activated receptor 2-mediated potentiation of transient receptor potential vanilloid subfamily 1 activity reveals a mechanism for proteinase-induced inflammatory pain. *J Neurosci* 2004; 24:4293–4299.

de Garavilla L, Vergnolle N, Young SH, et al. Agonists of proteinase-activated receptor 1 induce plasma extravasation by a neurogenic mechanism. *Br J Pharmacol* 2001; 133:975–987.

Evans CJ, Keith DE Jr., Morrison H, Magendzo K, Edwards RH. Cloning of a delta opioid receptor by functional expression. *Science* 1992; 258(5090):1952–1955.

Fukuoka T, Kondo E, Dai Y, Hashimoto N, Noguchi K. Brain-derived neurotrophic factor increases in the uninjured dorsal root ganglion neurons in selective spinal nerve ligation model. *J Neurosci* 2001; 21:4891–4900.

Genzen JR, Van Cleve W, McGehee DS. Dorsal root ganglion neurons express multiple nicotinic acetylcholine receptor subtypes. *J Neurophysiol* 2001; 86:1773–1782.

Gilman AG. G proteins: transducers of receptor-generated signals. *Annu Rev Biochem* 1987; 56:615–649.

Gold MS. Sodium channels and pain therapy. *Curr Opin Anaesthesiol* 2000; 13(5):565–572.

Gold MS, Weinreich D, Kim CS, et al. Redistribution of Na(V)1.8 in uninjured axons enables neuropathic pain. *J Neurosci* 2003; 23:158–166.

Hamill OP, McBride DW Jr. The pharmacology of mechanogated membrane ion channels. *Pharmacol Rev* 1996; 48:231–252.

Hamill OP, Marty A, Neher E, Sakmann B, Sigworth FJ. Improved patch-clamp techniques for high-resolution current recording from cells and cell-free membrane patches. *Pflugers Arch* 1981; 391:85–100.

Hingtgen CM, Vasko MR. Prostacyclin enhances the evoked-release of substance P and calcitonin gene-related peptide from rat sensory neurons. *Brain Res* 1994; 655:51–60.

Hökfelt T, Zhang X, Xu ZQ, et al. Phenotype regulation in dorsal root ganglion neurons after nerve injury: focus on peptides and their receptors. In: Borsook D (Ed). *Molecular Neurobiology of Pain,* Progress in Pain Research and Management, Vol. 9. Seattle: IASP Press, 1997, pp 115–143.

Hu HZ, Li ZW. Modulation by adenosine of GABA-activated current in rat dorsal root ganglion neurons. *J Physiol* 1997; 501 (Pt 1):67–75.

Iggo A. Cutaneous thermoreceptors in primates and sub-primates. *J Physiol* 1969; 200:403–430.

Ji RR, Samad TA, Jin SX, Schmoll R, Woolf CJ. p38 MAPK activation by NGF in primary sensory neurons after inflammation increases TRPV1 levels and maintains heat hyperalgesia. *Neuron* 2002; 36:57–68.

Jordt SE, McKemy DD, Julius D. Lessons from peppers and peppermint: the molecular logic of thermosensation. *Curr Opin Neurobiol* 2003; 13:487–492.

Jordt SE, Bautista DM, Chuang HH, et al. Mustard oils and cannabinoids excite sensory nerve fibres through the TRP channel ANKTM1. *Nature* 2004; 427:260–265.

Kage K, Niforatos W, Zhu CZ, et al. Alteration of dorsal root ganglion P2X3 receptor expression and function following spinal nerve ligation in the rat. *Exp Brain Res* 2002; 147:511–519.

Kashiba H, Fukui H, Morikawa Y, Senba E. Gene expression of histamine H1 receptor in guinea pig primary sensory neurons: a relationship between H1 receptor mRNA-expressing neurons and peptidergic neurons. *Brain Res Mol Brain Res* 1999; 66:24–34.

Kerchner GA, Wilding TJ, Huettner JE, Zhuo M. Kainate receptor subunits underlying presynaptic regulation of transmitter release in the dorsal horn. *J Neurosci* 2002; 22:8010–8017.

Khasabov SG, Rogers SD, Ghilardi JR, et al. Spinal neurons that possess the substance P receptor are required for the development of central sensitization. *J Neurosci* 2002; 22:9086–9098.

Kieffer BL, Befort K, Gaveriaux-Ruff C, Hirth CG. The delta-opioid receptor: isolation of a cDNA by expression cloning and pharmacological characterization. *Proc Natl Acad Sci USA* 1992; 89(24):12048–12052.

Krishtal O. The ASICs: signaling molecules? Modulators? *Trends Neurosci* 2003; 26:477–483.

Levine JD, Reichling DB. Peripheral mechanisms of inflammatory pain. In: Wall PD, Melzack R (Eds). *Textbook of Pain,* 4th ed. New York: Harcourt, 1999, pp 59–84.

Lewin GR, Stucky CL. Sensory neuron mechanotransduction: regulation and underlying molecular mechanisms. In: Wood JN (Ed). *Molecular Basis of Pain Induction.* New York: Wiley-Liss, 2000, pp 129–144.

Li Z, Sheng M. Some assembly required: the development of neuronal synapses. *Nat Rev Mol Cell Biol* 2003; 4:833–841.

Lu B, Je HS. Neurotrophic regulation of the development and function of the neuromuscular synapses. *J Neurocytol* 2003; 32:931–941.

Maingret F, Lauritzen I, Patel AJ, et al. TREK-1 is a heat-activated background K(+) channel. *Embo J* 2000; 19:2483–2491.

Marvizon JC, McRoberts JA, Ennes HS, et al. Two N-methyl-D-aspartate receptors in rat dorsal root ganglia with different subunit composition and localization. *J Comp Neurol* 2002; 446:325–341.

Melzack R, Wall PD. Pain Mechanisms: a new theory. *Science* 1965; 150:971–979.

Mizumura K, Koda H, Kumazawa T. Opposite effects of increases in intracellular cyclic AMP on the heat and bradykinin responses of canine visceral polymodal receptors in vitro. *Neurosci Res* 1996; 25:335–341.

Mullis K, Faloona F, Scharf S, et al. Specific enzymatic amplification of DNA in vitro: the polymerase chain reaction. *Cold Spring Harb Symp Quant Biol* 1986; 51(Pt 1):263–273.

Nathans J, Hogness DS. Isolation, sequence analysis, and intron-exon arrangement of the gene encoding bovine rhodopsin. *Cell* 1983; 34(3):807–814.

Nicholas AP, Poeribone V, Hökfelt T. Distributions of mRNAs for alpha-2 adrenergic receptor subtypes in rat brain: an in situ hybridization study. *J Comparative Neurol* 1993; 328:575–594.

Nilius B, Vriens J, Prenen J, Droogmans G, Voets T. TRPV4 calcium entry channel: a paradigm for gating diversity. *Am J Physiol Cell Physiol* 2004; 286:C195–C205.

North RA. The P2X3 subunit: a molecular target in pain therapeutics. *Curr Opin Investig Drugs* 2003; 4:833–840.

Patel AJ, Lazdunski M, Honore E. Lipid and mechano-gated 2P domain K(+) channels. *Curr Opin Cell Biol* 2001; 13:422–428.

Pomonis JD, Rogers SD, Peters CM, Ghilardi JR, Mantyh PW. Expression and localization of endothelin receptors: implications for the involvement of peripheral glia in nociception. *J Neurosci* 2001; 21:999–1006.

Price MP, Lewin GR, McIlwrath SL, et al. The mammalian sodium channel BNC1 is required for normal touch sensation. *Nature* 2000; 407:1007–1011.

Price M, McIlwrath S, Xie J, et al. The DRASIC cation channel contributes to the detection of cutaneous touch and acid stimuli in mice. *Neuron* 2002; 35:407.

Reid G, Flonta M. Cold transduction by inhibition of a background potassium conductance in rat primary sensory neurones. *Neurosci Lett* 2001a; 297(3):171–174.

Reid G, Flonta ML. Physiology. Cold current in thermoreceptive neurons. *Nature* 2001b; 413(6855):480.

Ruan HZ, Burnstock G. Localisation of P2Y1 and P2Y4 receptors in dorsal root, nodose and trigeminal ganglia of the rat. *Histochem Cell Biol* 2003; 120:415–426.

Sah DW, Ossipo MH, Porreca F. Neurotrophic factors as novel therapeutics for neuropathic pain. *Nat Rev Drug Discov* 2003; 2:460–472.

Sato K, Kiyama H, Park HT, Tohyama M. AMPA, KA and NMDA receptors are expressed in the rat DRG neurones. *Neuroreport* 1993; 4:1263–1265.

Seabrook GR, Bowery BJ, Heavens R, et al. Expression of B1 and B2 bradykinin receptor mRNA and their functional roles in sympathetic ganglia and sensory dorsal root ganglia neurones from wild-type and B2 receptor knockout mice. *Neuropharmacology* 1997; 36:1009–1017.

Sohrabji F, Miranda RC, Toran-Allerand CD. Estrogen differentially regulates estrogen and nerve growth factor receptor mRNAs in adult sensory neurons. *J Neurosci* 1994; 14:459–471.

Stein C. Opioid receptors on peripheral sensory neurons. *Adv Exp Med Biol* 2003; 521:69–76.

Strotmann R, Harteneck C, Nunnenmacher K, Schultz G, Plant TD. OTRPC4, a nonselective cation channel that confers sensitivity to extracellular osmolarity. *Nat Cell Biol* 2000; 2(10):695–702.

Tata AM, Vilaro MT, Mengod G. Muscarinic receptor subtypes expression in rat and chick dorsal root ganglia. *Brain Res Mol Brain Res* 2000; 82:1–10.

Thut PD, Wrigley D, Gold MS. Cold transduction in rat trigeminal ganglia neurons in vitro. *Neuroscience* 2003; 119:1071–1083.

Towers S, Princivalle A, Billinton A, et al. GABAB receptor protein and mRNA distribution in rat spinal cord and dorsal root ganglia. *Eur J Neurosci* 2000; 12:3201–3210.

Vlaskovska M, Kasakov L, Rong W, et al. P2X3 knock-out mice reveal a major sensory role for urothelially released ATP. *J Neurosci* 2001; 21:5670–5607.

Wood JN. Recent advances in understanding molecular mechanisms of primary afferent activation. *Gut* 2004; (53 Suppl 2):9–12.

Woolf CJ, Safieh GB, Ma QP, Crilly P, Winter J. Nerve growth factor contributes to the generation of inflammatory sensory hypersensitivity. *Neuroscience* 1994; 62:327–331.

Wu S, Zhu M, Wang W, et al. Changes of the expression of 5-HT receptor subtype mRNAs in rat dorsal root ganglion by complete Freund's adjuvant-induced inflammation. *Neurosci Lett* 2001; 307:183–186.

Wynn G, Rong W, Xiang Z, Burnstock G. Purinergic mechanisms contribute to mechanosensory transduction in the rat colorectum. *Gastroenterology* 2003; 125:1398–1409.

Xie GX, Jones K, Peroutka SJ, Palmer PP. Detection of mRNAs and alternatively spliced transcripts of dopamine receptors in rat peripheral sensory and sympathetic ganglia. *Brain Res* 1998; 785:129–135.

Xie J, Ho Lee Y, Wang C, Mo Chung J, Chung K. Differential expression of alpha 1-adrenoceptor subtype mRNAs in the dorsal root ganglion after spinal nerve ligation. *Brain Res Mol Brain Res* 2001; 93:164–172.

Zhang YH, Vasko MR, Nicol GD. Ceramide, a putative second messenger for nerve growth factor, modulates the TTX-resistant Na(+) current and delayed rectifier K(+) current in rat sensory neurons. *J Physiol* 2002; 544:385–402.

Correspondence to: Michael S. Gold, PhD, University of Maryland Dental School, 666 W. Baltimore Street, Room 5-A-12, Baltimore, MD 21201, USA. Tel: 410-706-0909; Fax: 410-706-0865; email: msg001@dental.umaryland.edu.

The Paths of Pain 1975–2005, edited by
Harold Merskey, John D. Loeser, and Ronald
Dubner, IASP Press, Seattle, © 2005.

5

The Study of the Genetics of Pain in Humans and Animals

Jeffrey S. Mogil

*Department of Psychology and Centre for Research on Pain,
McGill University, Montreal, Canada*

PAIN GENETICS: TWO QUESTIONS

As of the founding of IASP in 1975, only a handful of studies documenting rodent strain differences in pain and analgesic sensitivity had been published, and this year saw the first systematic attempts to study opioid genetics (Baran et al. 1975; Shuster 1975). From modest beginnings, however, research into "pain genetics" has exploded, especially in the last decade. Although research did not produce the panacea some had expected, it is true that the techniques of molecular and classical genetics allow the study of biological phenomena in a fundamentally new manner. Whereas the 20th century saw the study of biology largely at the level of the protein—visualizing, measuring, or altering protein levels or functions—the 21st century will see the study of biology at its most proximal levels, that of DNA and RNA molecules. This is in some sense a step backwards, since it is proteins and not genes that directly perform the "work" of biology. Nonetheless, the tools of genetics have allowed biological investigations that are simply not possible at the protein level due to lack of appropriately selective pharmacological ligands or antibodies. Two genetic approaches engendering considerable excitement among basic scientists studying pain are transgenic knockout mice and microarray-based gene expression profiling (see Mogil and McCarson 2000 for a review of their utilities). In the former, genetic engineering of embryonic stem cell DNA is used to produce a mouse that lacks all expression of a targeted gene. One then tests the null mutant mouse on one or more nociceptive assays. Differences compared to "wild-type" counterparts are taken as evidence for the involvement of the targeted gene in the processing of pain in that assay. In the latter technique, mRNAs from pain-relevant tissues taken from subjects experiencing and not experiencing pain are hybridized in a competitive fashion to a "chip" containing probes for thousands of known and unknown genes. Using this technique one can identify virtually every gene whose expression differs significantly between the experimental conditions. Transgenic knockout experiments have discovered or confirmed the direct involvement of well over 100 genes in the processing of nociception in mice, and microarray studies will greatly (and quickly) expand this number. A review of the application of transgenic and microarray technology to pain research is beyond the scope of this chapter (see Mogil and Grisel 1998; Costigan et al. 2004; Malmberg and Zeitz 2004 for reviews). It is clear, though, that these and other methods of studying and altering DNA sequences and mRNA levels will eventually afford a full answer to one key question of pain genetics: which genes are relevant to pain?

There is however a second question, one answerable only by the genetics of Gregor Mendel. This question asks: of the pain-relevant genes, which ones are responsible for individual differences in the perception of pain? This question is multifaceted, because the genes in question might affect variability in the susceptibility to developing pain syndromes, variability in the perceptual severity (sensory and affective) of pain, and/or variability in the behavioral responses to pain. Genes contributing to the genetic portion of such variability cannot easily be identified using transgenic knockout or microarray techniques. Knockout strategies consider genes largely in isolation, and produce gross ablations—complete removal of gene expression, in every tissue and at all developmental stages—that represent poor models of the more subtle changes that likely characterize most pain traits. Microarray studies, in turn, are limited by the inability to distinguish cause from effect. Genes found to be upregulated in rats exhibiting behavioral signs of chronic pain might indeed contribute to producing the pain, but they might also be upregulated *by* the pain itself or as a reaction to changes in the expression of yet other genes. In fact, there are only two techniques that can identify genes that are the root causes of (the genetic component of) pain variability: genetic linkage mapping and genetic association. The application of these techniques to pain in humans and laboratory animals will be the focus of this chapter.

THE NATURE (AND NURTURE) OF PAIN VARIABILITY IN HUMANS AND ANIMALS

There is no doubt that both clinical and experimental pain are highly variable phenomena. Broadly similar traumatic or infectious insults (e.g., car accidents, stroke, and herpes zoster) only produce neuropathic pain in a small minority of people (e.g., Richards 1967; Andersen et al. 1995; Cluff and Rowbotham 1998), suggesting that those people might be susceptible or "prone" to developing chronic pain. This suggestion is difficult to prove, however, because no two injuries or infections are precisely the same. But even for experimental pain, where the application of the noxious stimulus is standardized, researchers have observed surprisingly large ranges of pressure pain thresholds (e.g., Isselee et al. 1997), of pain tolerances in the cold-pressor test (e.g., Chen et al. 1989), and of visual analogue scale (VAS) ratings of thermal stimuli (e.g., Coghill et al. 2003).

To what extent do such individual differences in pain behaviors truly reflect differential pain perception in these subjects rather than simply differences in sociocultural variables (e.g., machismo) or scale usage? That is, are subjects giving higher pain ratings actually in more pain? One recent study addressing this issue was performed by Coghill and colleagues (2003), who stimulated 17 subjects lying in a functional magnetic resonance imaging (fMRI) scanner with a thermode applied to the lower leg. VAS intensity ratings in these subjects ranged from 1.0 to 8.9 on a 10-point scale. The blood oxygenation level-dependent (BOLD) activity in various cortical regions known to be activated by noxious stimuli (i.e., anterior cingulate gyrus, somatosensory area 1, and prefrontal cortex) was compared in subjects with the highest and lowest ratings, and indeed, the pain-sensitive subjects showed higher activations in these areas. Thus, at least to the extent that fMRI truly reflects cortical activations from noxious stimulation, these interindividual differences were "real" and not an artefact of scale usage.

Finally, it should be noted that individual differences in experimental pain might be directly related to individual differences in clinical pain, given that patients with a wide range of pain disorders (e.g., fibromyalgia, musculoskeletal pain, headache, temporomandibular disorder, irritable bowel syndrome, and vulvodynia) show enhanced experimental pain sensitivities compared to controls. This correlation even holds within patient groups, such that those with worse clinical pain have lower experimental pain thresholds and tolerances (see Edwards et al. 2003). The mediating factor might be diffuse noxious inhibitory controls (DNIC), with those normal subjects showing greater DNIC responses scoring lower on the bodily pain subscale of the Short Form-36 (SF-36) health survey questionnaire, and higher on the general health subscale (Edwards et al. 2003).

The existence of variability does not necessarily imply that genetic factors are associated with that variability. Variability in pain, like that in any other biological phenomenon, is mediated by some combination of nature, nurture, and their interaction. The literature abounds with environmental explanations of pain variability, and of the tendency of pain behavior and

certain pain pathologies to "run in families." These include personality variables (e.g., Pud et al. 2004), coping styles (e.g., Jamner and Schwartz 1986),
anxiety levels (e.g., Sternbach 1975), expectancies (Benedetti and Amanzio
1997), blood pressure (in normotensives) (e.g., Bruehl et al. 1992), social
learning (e.g., Edwards et al. 1985), and other factors in the family environment (Payne and Norfleet 1986). All of these factors are themselves affected
by genes, of course, but it is also possible—and given the existing animal
data (see below), likely—that some genetic variants are directly responsible
for at least some of the observed variability.

The gold-standard technique for partitioning trait variability into its genetic and environmental components is the twin study, which directly com-
pares monozygotic (100% genetically identical) with dizygotic (50% genetically identical) twin pairs. Twin studies have been conducted in a number of
diseases defined by painful symptoms—migraine, headache, dysmenorrhea,
abdominal pain, back pain, irritable bowel, arthritis, and fibromyalgia—and
in most cases the heritability (i.e., the percentage variance due to inherited
factors) is substantial (see Mogil 1999; MacGregor 2004). However, two
studies reported that genetic factors did not account for twin similarity in
widespread musculoskeletal pain in Finnish children (Mikkelsson et al. 2001)
or temporomandibular joint pain (Michalowicz et al. 2000). In all these
studies, what was being evaluated was the presence or absence of a painful
disorder, *not* pain severity or duration. Thus, only one study is directly
relevant to the question at hand, by MacGregor and colleagues (1997), who
studied pressure pain thresholds in adult female twin pairs. Although thresholds in twin pairs were highly correlated, the excess correlation in monozygotic twins over dizygotic twins was quite small, suggesting that shared
environmental factors accounted for the bulk of the variability in this pain
trait. The authors point out that this finding may have been strongly influenced by the fact that the twins were tested for pressure pain sensitivity
together, on the same day (MacGregor 2004).

The issue of heritability of pain in humans is still unresolved. This
situation is unlikely to change substantially in the near future, especially for
neuropathic pain syndromes, because it is difficult to identify cohorts of
twins in which *both* members of the twin pair have suffered a particular
injury. However, one can look for indirect evidence of heritability. A recent
study reported on the prevalence of neuropathic pain in patients who underwent coronary artery bypass graft surgery (Bruce et al. 2003). This surgery
requires two separate incisions, a sternotomy and a saphenectomy, and both
are associated with a certain frequency of iatrogenic neuropathic pain. The
authors reported a frequency of chronic pain secondary to the sternotomy of
12%, and secondary to the saphenectomy of 9%. But 18% of patients had

chronic pain at *both* locations. As Devor (2004) recently pointed out, the chances of developing iatrogenic chronic pain at both locations, if the two events were independent, are only $0.12 \times 0.09 = 0.01$ (1%). The large excess of patients with both chest and leg pain suggests (but certainly does not prove) that these patients were predisposed to developing chronic pain after nerve injury.

The situation is much clearer in animal models of pain. Both rats and mice display clear and robust individual differences in apparent nociceptive sensitivity, as inferred by their behavior on any number of algesiometric assays (see Mogil 1999). Moreover, this variability is moderately-to-highly heritable in almost every assay (median heritability estimate across 22 assays: 46%), as assessed by selective breeding experiments or by the comparison of inbred (genetically identical) strains derived using multigenerational brother-sister matings (Lariviere et al. 2002). Remarkable qualitative differences between strains have been observed as well, including strain-dependent brainstem neuroanatomy (Clark and Proudfit 1992) and strain-dependent neurochemistry of opiate pain inhibition (Rady et al. 1998).

Again, it is appropriate to ask to what extent these differences truly represent genetically based differences in nociceptive processing versus morphological or behavioral artefacts. It is impossible, of course, to rule out all possible competing explanations of such strain differences, but we can point to some pertinent negative data. There is no significant correlation (Spearman's $r = -0.15$) between latencies to respond to the application of a noxious tail clip and tail diameter of 12 inbred mouse strains (Lariviere et al. 2002). The robust strain differences in licking behavior in the late/tonic phase (10–60 minute) after formalin injection observed between C57BL/6J (sensitive) and A/J (resistant) mice are not accompanied by significant differences in formalin-induced edema, whether assessed via hindpaw weight, hindpaw thickness, or histologically (Mogil et al. 1998). Furthermore, none of our nociception phenotypes show significant genetic correlation (based on strain means) with any of the following measures in at least five common inbred strains (see Mouse Phenome Database at http://aretha.jax.org/pub-cgi/phenome): body weight at 7 weeks, locomotor activity, exploratory behavior, balance beam coordination, "wildness," or systolic blood pressure. There are some rather high genetic correlations between certain nociception phenotypes and anxiety levels measured with the elevated zero maze test; the importance of these correlations is difficult to evaluate at present because the data sets have only five strains in common. Also, with seven common strains, capsaicin-induced licking behavior correlates highly (Spearman's $r = 0.93$) with basal heart rate (beats per minute); the possible significance of this finding is unclear.

The best evidence that behavioral strain differences on nociceptive assays really do reflect differential nociceptive processing comes from recent anatomical and electrophysiological studies. One study investigated the genetic correlation between formalin-induced licking behavior and c-*fos* immediate-early gene expression in the spinal cord dorsal horn (Bon et al. 2002). It is well known that the c-*fos* gene is expressed in neurons transsynaptically stimulated by tonic noxious stimuli; in the spinal cord after formalin stimulation one sees punctate staining of Fos-protein immunoreactivity throughout the dorsal horn, but especially in laminae I/II and V/VI (see Harris 1998). We found an extremely high correlation (r = 0.94; Spearman's r = 1) between tonic-phase licking and Fos-protein immunoreactivity in the deep (but not superficial) dorsal horn among eight mouse strains (Bon et al. 2002). This high correlation suggests that the behavioral differences are accompanied by strain-dependent processing of the noxious stimulus in appropriate pain-relevant neural pathways. In a just-completed study, we studied heat-evoked activity of primary afferent nociceptors (mechano-heat-sensitive C fibers) of AKR/J and C57BL/6J mice in the isolated skin-saphenous nerve preparation. These strains were chosen because their withdrawal latencies to thermal heat in the paw-withdrawal test differ by at least twofold (Mogil et al. 1999). C fibers from the behaviorally sensitive C57BL/6J strain displayed significantly lower firing thresholds to heat, and significantly higher firing rates compared to those from AKR/J mice (J.S. Mogil et al., unpublished manuscript). In this particular case, the strain difference in behavioral response (withdrawal latency) is explainable at the level of primary afferent functioning. There is no need to invoke more complex behavioral or motoric strain differences, although they might also play a role.

PAIN GENETICS IN HUMANS

Twin studies are studies of genetic epidemiology, designed to address the question of whether inherited genetic factors play an important role in trait variability. They are not useful, however, in identifying the trait-relevant genes themselves, or the variants of those genes responsible for the variability. To these ends one needs to employ either genetic linkage mapping or genetic association approaches (e.g., Lander and Schork 1994). The techniques, which rely on similar assumptions, are both based on the phenomenon of homologous recombination during meiosis. They differ in important practical ways, however. Linkage mapping seek to demonstrate co-inheritance, through successive generations, of genomic marker alleles with trait variability. That is, an attempt is made to identify which of a set of markers spanning the genome is inherited along with the trait being studied. The responsible gene near the "linked" markers can then be tracked down by a process known as positional cloning. Association studies seek to demonstrate increased frequencies of genomic marker alleles in "cases" compared to "controls" (or, for quantitative traits, in high versus low responders). The genomic markers used in either case are di- or trinucleotide repeats, or single-nucleotide polymorphisms (SNPs). In their most common forms, linkage mapping requires the "phenotyping" and "genotyping" of multigenerational pedigrees whereas association studies are performed on unrelated individuals, but new linkage and association study designs involving sibling pairs and parents (e.g., affected sib pair linkage or transmission disequilibrium test association) are becoming increasingly common (see Risch 2000). The major practical difference is that linkage mapping can be performed without any prior assumptions whatsoever, whereas association studies are designed to evaluate the candidacy of particular genes identified beforehand.

Researchers applying either approach face serious challenges, with linkage mapping in humans found to be effective only for single-gene disorders with no genetic heterogeneity, and association studies plagued by failures to replicate. An ongoing debate concerns the extent to which the failure to replicate existing association studies can be attributed to ethnic stratification confounds, statistical underpowering, or publication bias (see Lohmueller et al. 2003). A long-term solution has already been identified, but it remains cost-prohibitive for the moment. So-called linkage disequilibrium mapping (Risch and Merikangas 1996) combines the best features of both techniques; it is essentially a full-genome search for association. Because of the "haplotype block" structure of the genome (Gabriel et al. 2002), it is not necessary to search for association with every single SNP (which occur on average every 1,000 base pairs), but rather to 300,000–1,000,000 representative SNPs defining each haplotype block. Nonetheless, SNP genotyping costs will need to decrease further—from the current cost of about US$0.20 per genotype—before studies genotyping many hundreds of pain patients at hundreds of thousands of markers are routinely conducted.

Despite these obstacles, a small number of human genes have been implicated in pain-related traits. Linkage mapping and positional cloning efforts have identified the responsible gene and variants causing hereditary sensory and autonomic neuropathies (HSANs), all featuring loss of sensitivity to pain, and causing two rare, familial forms of migraine. These conditions and the responsible genes are listed in Table I. What is striking is the variety of biological functions represented by these genes, including trophic factors, receptors, ion channels, biosynthetic enzymes, and signal transduction molecules. This ought to remind us that the pain pathway contains many, many molecular components, and that dysfunction of any one of them could have catastrophic implications for the processing and perception of pain.

The pain pathologies described in Table I afflict an extremely small number of people, and there is evidence that the genes causing these pathologies may not affect pain perception in the "normal" range of variation. For example, although 8 years have passed since *NTRK1* (previously, *TRKA*) was reported as the gene responsible for HSAN IV (congenital insensitivity to pain with anhidrosis), no subsequent study has implicated this gene in causing variability in any other pain-related trait. This outcome is likely because although over 37 different mutations of *NTRK1* are known, they are virtually all rare "private" mutations (except in certain population isolates), none with a high enough allelic frequency to explain much variability in the population at large (Indo 2001). For this particular gene, however, two mutations were found to be fairly common in Japanese and Israeli-Bedouins, respectively (see Indo 2001). The gene responsible for familial hemiplegic migraine type 1 was found to be *CACNA1A*, which codes for the α_{1A} subunit of the P/Q-type calcium channel (Ophoff et al. 1996). Many attempts have been made subsequently to implicate this or related genes in idiopathic migraine, but without obvious success (Estevez and Gardner 2004), suggestive of a greater complexity and heterogeneity of the more common pathology.

Thus, in pain research we cannot rely on linkage mapping or positional cloning of rare, inherited disorders to shed light on which genes may be profitably tested for their relationship to more common pain syndromes via association study. There are only two other alternatives. One is to prioritize candidate pain variability genes, conduct association studies on as many high-priority genes as time and funding allow, and hope for the best. Indeed, a reasonable strategy for prioritizing genes for pain-related association studies has been recently proposed (Belfer et al. 2004). This strategy considers the strength of the conventional evidence supporting the involvement of the gene's protein product in pain processing, the frequency of known minor variants in the gene, and the likelihood that those variants themselves have functional consequences. In fact, several association studies of pain traits with complex genetics have been performed; positive (if not necessarily replicated) findings are shown in Table II. Of these, only one has definite relevance to pain processing per se, the association between *COMT* gene variants and experimental pain produced by hypertonic saline (Zubieta et al. 2003). In this study, four subjects with the minor Met/Met genotype at amino acid 158 of catechol-*O*-methyltransferase were found to display higher McGill Pain Questionnaire ratings to 5% hypertonic saline infused into the masseter muscle than did subjects with Met/Val or Val/Val genotypes. The differences in pain sensitivity among genotypes were accompanied by differences in μ-opioid activation in multiple brain areas, as evidenced using [^{11}C]-carfentanil positron emission tomography.

Although this finding is important, it represents the one positive finding in a series of (unpublished) negative association studies. There is another strategy with perhaps a higher likelihood of success: performing human association studies on genes implicated in pain variability by linkage mapping studies in animals. The first of these animal-to-human "translations" was recently published (Mogil et al. 2003). In this study, linkage mapping of inhibition by U50,488 (a selective κ-opioid agonist) of thermal nociception

Table I
Single genes causing hereditary pain-related pathologies in humans

Pathology*	MIM†	Gene‡	Location	Protein Function	Reference
FHM1	141500	CACNA1A	19p13	Calcium channel subunit	Ophoff et al. 1996
FHM2	602481	ATP1A2	1q21–q23	Ion pump subunit	DeFusco et al. 2003
HSAN I	162400	SPTLC1	9q22.1–q22.3	Sphingolipid biosynthesis	Bejaoui et al. 2001
HSAN II	201300	HSN2	12p13	Unknown	Lafreniere et al. 2004
HSAN III/FD	223900	IKBKAP	9q31	Transcriptional regulation	Anderson et al. 2001
HSAN IV/CIPA	256800	NTRK1	1q21–q22	Neurotrophin receptor	Indo et al. 1996
HSAN V	none§	NGFB	1p13.1	Neurotrophin	Einarsdottir et al. 2004

* Many pathologies feature pain as a symptom; listed here are pathologies in which pain is the defining symptom, and not secondary to some other known defect (e.g., inflammation or musculoskeletal disease). Abbreviations: FHM1, familial hemiplegic migraine, type 1; FHM2, familial hemiplegic migraine, type 2; HSAN I, hereditary sensory and autonomic neuropathy, type I; HSAN II, hereditary sensory and autonomic neuropathy, type II (neurogenic acroosteolysis); HSAN III/FD, hereditary sensory and autonomic neuropathy, type III (familial dysautonomia); HSAN IV/CIPA, hereditary sensory and autonomic neuropathy, type IV (congenital insensitivity to pain with anhidrosis); HSAN V, hereditary sensory and autonomic neuropathy, type V.
† Mendelian Inheritance in Man (MIM) entry number.
‡ Abbreviations: ATP1A2, sodium/potassium transporting ATPase (Na$^+$/K$^+$ pump), α$_2$ subunit; CACNA1A, P/Q-type voltage-dependent calcium channel, α$_{1A}$ subunit; IKBKAP, inhibitor of κ light polypeptide gene enhancer in B cells, kinase complex-associated protein; HSN2, protein associated with HSAN2 (unknown function); NGFB, nerve growth factor, β subunit; NTRK1, neurotrophic tyrosine receptor kinase, type 1 (tyrosine receptor kinase A); SPTLC1, serine palmitoyltransferase, long-chain base subunit 1.
§ HSAN V is too rare and poorly characterized to be listed.

Table II
Genes whose polymorphic alleles are associated with variable pain
or analgesia phenotypes in humans

Phenotype*	Gene†	Variant‡	Protein Function§	Reference
CRPS/RSD	HLA-DQB1	n.r.	MHC	Kemler et al. 1999
	HLA-DRB1	15(2)		Mailis and Wade 1994
	HLA-DRB1	13		van Hilten et al. 2000
β-Endorphin affinity	OPRM	A118G	G-protein-coupled receptor	Bond et al. 1998
Fibromyalgia	COMT	V158M	Biogenic amine metabolism	Gursoy et al. 2003
	HTR2A	T102C	G-protein-coupled receptor	Bondy et al. 1998
	SLC6A4	44-bp ins/del	Biogenic amine transporter	Offenbaecher et al. 1999
Hypertonic saline pain	COMT	V158M	Biogenic amine metabolism	Zubieta et al. 2003
Low back pain	IL1+IL1RN	C889T + G1812A	Cytokine + cytokine modulator	Solovieva et al. 2004
Migraine	>12 genes			Estevez and Gardner 2004
Pentazocine analgesia	MC1R	R151C/ D294H/ R160W	G-protein-coupled receptor	Mogil et al. 2003
Pelvic pain syndrome	IL-10	G1082A	Cytokine	Shoskes et al. 2002

(continues on facing page)

in a cross between two inbred mouse strains revealed the existence of a gene on distal mouse chromosome 8 conferring variable analgesic sensitivity on female but not male mice. Convergent lines of evidence suggested that the gene in question was *Mc1r*, encoding the melanocortin-1 receptor. A small association study then confirmed that variants of the human *MC1R* gene affected analgesic sensitivity to the κ-opioid-acting drug, pentazocine, again in women but not men (Mogil et al. 2003). A number of other promising "translational" studies are ongoing. Thus, a brief consideration of the genetics of pain in animals is warranted here.

PAIN GENETICS IN ANIMALS

A full account of our work in the mouse and that of others in the rat is beyond the scope of this chapter, and this topic has been reviewed on a

Table II
(continued)

Phenotype*	Gene†	Variant‡	Protein Function§	Reference
Postherpetic neuralgia	*HLA-A+* *HLA-B+* *HLA-DRB1*	*3303 + *4403 + *1302	MHC	Sato et al. 2002
Vulvar vestibulitis	*IL1RN*	86-bp VNTR	Cytokine modulator	Jeremias et al. 2000

* The choice of listed phenotypes is somewhat arbitrary, including pathologies in which pain is the defining symptom, but excluding pathologies like arthritis, where genes associated with disease susceptibility or severity, but not pain levels per se, have been identified. Abbreviation: CRPS/RSD = complex regional pain syndrome/reflex sympathetic dystrophy.

† Abbreviations: *COMT*, catechol-*O*-methyl-transferase; *HLA*, human lymphocyte antigen; *HTR2A*, serotonin receptor, type 2A; *IL1*, interleukin-1 complex; *IL1RN*, interleukin-1 receptor antagonist; *MC1R*, melanocortin-1 receptor; *OPRM*, μ-opioid receptor; *SLC6A4*, solute carrier, family 6, member 4 (serotonin transporter).

‡ Variants are listed either as gene single nucleotide polymorphisms (SNPs), protein isozymes, HLA alleles, or HLA serological specificities, following the format of the reference in question. For SNPs and protein isozymes the "consensus" nucleotide (allele) or amino acid is listed first, followed by the position from the start codon or amino acid number, followed by the "minor" nucleotide (allele) or amino acid. In some cases, the variants might be directly involved in producing trait variability; in others they are simply in linkage disequilibrium with the true functional variant. Abbreviations: n.r., not reported; 44-bp ins/del, 44-base-pair insertion or deletion; 86-bp VNTR, variable number of an 86-base-pair tandem repeat in second intron.

§ MHC = major histocompatibility complex.

number of prior occasions (see, e.g., Mogil 1999, 2004). As mentioned above, our laboratory has studied a wide variety of nociceptive and antinociceptive traits in a common set of 11–12 inbred mouse strains, and every trait thus far examined displays at least moderate heritability. Because the same strains were used each time, we can investigate genetic correlations among them. Pain traits showing similar strain distribution patterns (i.e., with the same strains sensitive and the same strains resistant) are genetically correlated, implying that the same gene or genes are responsible for trait variability in each case. In turn, this genetic correlation implies similar physiological mediation underlying each trait. Using this strategy, we have provided evidence for the existence of at least five fundamental pain "types": (1) acute thermal (including cold) nociception, (2) tonic chemical nociception, (3) thermal hypersensitivity following spontaneous nociception, (4) thermal hypersensitivity in the absence of spontaneous nociception, and (5) mechanical hypersensitivity (Lariviere et al. 2002). The status of acute mechanical nociception remains unclear. Recent data suggest that cold allodynia is genetically independent from both thermal and mechanical hypersensitivity (S.E. Crager, S.B. Smith, and J.S. Mogil, unpublished data). Other (nongenetic) data have also been collected supporting the independence of physiological mechanisms underlying hypersensitivity to different evoking stimulus modalities (e.g., Meller 1994).

I believe that this fact presents a serious challenge for pain research. Much ongoing research in the field measures neuropathic "pain behaviors," which in fact are mechanical, thermal, and cold hypersensitivity states. Almost no current work attempts to measure spontaneous chronic nociception in rodent models, largely because there is no agreement over what behaviors should be trusted as indicating its presence. If the genetic and physiological mediation of mechanical, thermal, and cold hypersensitivity can all be qualitatively dissociated, it seems reasonable to assume that spontaneous nociception in neuropathic animals will eventually be as well. To the extent that these different symptoms of neuropathic pain feature independent underlying mechanisms, the basic science knowledge we are rapidly collecting about genes, molecules, and mechanisms underlying, say, thermal hypersensitivity may apply *specifically* to thermal hypersensitivity, and not to spontaneous pain itself. This disconnect might explain some of the well-known failures to translate basic science knowledge into the clinic (e.g., Hill 2000). That is, it is possible that certain drugs really *are* efficacious in humans, but only against hypersensitivity states, not against the chronic spontaneous pain that one might expect to largely drive patients' global pain scores in clinical trials.

Despite this caveat, much progress is being made in identifying, by linkage mapping, genes responsible for variability on murine nociceptive assays. We reported in 1997 that a region on mouse chromosome 4—a so-called quantitative trait locus (QTL)—was linked to variable hot-plate sensitivity between DBA/2 and C57BL/6 strains (Mogil et al. 1997). This linkage was far stronger in male than in female mice, and pharmacological evidence suggested that the gene in question might be *Oprd1*, coding for the δ-opioid receptor. A recent study has also provided evidence for *OPRD1*'s involvement in thermal pain in humans, again with stronger effects in males (Kim et al. 2004). In recent work (J.S. Mogil et al., unpublished manuscript), we found that variability among 13 mouse strains in Hargreaves and colleagues' test of paw withdrawal can be explained in terms of calcitonin gene-related peptide levels, and strain-dependent expression of the *Calca* gene. Attempts to "translate" this finding to humans are ongoing. As regards chemical/inflammatory nociception, we reported the existence of two QTLs on mouse chromosomes 9 and 10 (Wilson et al. 2002); using a set of overlapping congenic strains (Fortin et al. 2001), we have now localized one of the genes to a <3-cM region containing only 15 known genes. Finally, Seltzer and colleagues (2001) mapped a QTL for autotomy behavior following nerve transection to a small region of mouse chromosome 15.

THE FUTURE OF PAIN GENETICS

We are on the verge of an explosion of pain genetics data. More and more laboratories are entering the field, especially in human genetics. Although there are some pitfalls to avoid (Max 2004), I encourage people to join the search, especially since real progress will require independent replication of association study findings. The potential rewards include the chance to truly individualize existing pain therapy, the opportunity to identify truly novel molecular targets for development of new pain therapies, and the ability to truly "cure" pain pathologies via gene therapy.

REFERENCES

Andersen G, Vestergaard K, Ingeman-Nielsen M, Jensen TS. Incidence of central post stroke pain. *Pain* 1995; 61:187–193.

Anderson SL, Coli R, Daly IW, et al. Familial dysautonomia is caused by mutations of the *IKAP* gene. *Am J Hum Genet* 2001; 68:753–758.

Baran A, Shuster L, Eleftheriou BE, Bailey DW. Opiate receptors in mice: genetic differences. *Life Sci* 1975; 17:633–640.

Bejaoui K, Wu C, Scheffler MD, et al. *SPTLC1* is mutated in hereditary sensory neuropathy, type 1. *Nat Genet* 2001; 27:261–262.

Belfer I, Wu T, Kingman A, et al. Candidate gene studies of human pain mechanisms: a method for optimizing choice of polymorphisms and sample size. *Anesthesiology* 2004; 100(6):1562–1572.

Benedetti F, Amanzio M. The neurobiology of placebo analgesia: from endogenous opioids to cholecystokinin. *Prog Neurobiol* 1997; 52:109–125.

Bon K, Wilson SG, Mogil JS, Roberts WJ. Genetic evidence for the correlation of deep dorsal horn Fos protein immunoreactivity with tonic formalin pain behavior. *J Pain* 2002; 3:181–189.

Bond C, LaForge KS, Tian M, et al. Single-nucleotide polymorphism in the human mu opioid receptor gene alters beta-endorphin binding and activity: possible implications for opiate addiction. *Proc Natl Acad Sci USA* 1998; 95:9608–9613.

Bondy B, Spaeth M, Offenbaecher M, et al. The *T102C* polymorphism of the 5-HT$_{2A}$-receptor gene in fibromyalgia. *Neurobiol Dis* 1999; 6:433–439.

Bruce J, Drury N, Poobalan AS, et al. The prevalence of chronic chest and leg pain following cardiac surgery: a historical cohort study. *Pain* 2003; 104:265–273.

Bruehl S, Carlson CR, McCubbin JA. The relationship between pain sensitivity and blood pressure in normotensives. *Pain* 1992; 48:463–467.

Chen ACN, Dworkin SF, Haug J. Human pain responsivity in a tonic pain model: psychological determinants. *Pain* 1989; 37:143–160.

Clark FM, Proudfit HK. Anatomical evidence for genetic differences in the innervation of the rat spinal cord by noradrenergic locus coeruleus neurons. *Brain Res* 1992; 591:44–53.

Cluff RS, Rowbotham MC. Pain caused by herpes zoster infection. *Neurol Clin* 1998; 16:813–832.

Coghill RC, McHaffie JG, Yen Y-F. Neural correlates of interindividual differences in the subjective experience of pain. *Proc Natl Acad Sci USA* 2003; 100:8538–8542.

Costigan M, Griffin RS, Woolf CJ. Microarray analysis of the pain pathway. In: Mogil JS (Ed). *The Genetics of Pain,* Progress in Pain Research and Management, Vol. 28. Seattle: IASP Press, 2004, pp 65–84.

Dawkins JL, Hulme DJ, Brahmbhatt SB, et al. Mutations in SPTLC1, encoding serine palmitoyltransferase, long chain base subunit-1, cause hereditary sensory neuropathy type I. *Nat Genet* 2001; 27:309–312.

Einarsdottir E, Carlsson A, Minde J, et al. A mutation in the nerve growth factor beta gene (*NGFB*) causes loss of pain perception. *Hum Mol Genet* 2004; 13:799–805.

Estevez M, Gardner KL. Update on the genetics of migraine. *Hum Genet* 2004; 114:225–235.

DeFusco M, Marconi R, Silvestri L, et al. Haploinsufficiency of *ATP1A2* encoding the Na^+/K^+ pump alpha$_2$ subunit associated with familial hemiplegic migraine type 2. *Nat Genet* 2003; 33:192–196.

Devor M. Evidence for heritability of pain in patients with traumatic neuropathy. *Pain* 2004; 108:200–201.

Edwards PW, Zeichner A, Kuczmierczyk AR, Boczkowski J. Familial pain models: the relationship between family history of pain and current pain experience. *Pain* 1985; 21:379–384.

Edwards RR, Ness TJ, Weigent DA, Fillingim RB. Individual differences in diffuse noxious inhibitory controls (DNIC): association with clinical variables. *Pain* 2003; 106:427–437.

Estevez M, Gardner KL. Update on the genetics of migraine. *Hum Genet* 2004; 114:225–235.

Fortin A, Diez E, Rochefort D, et al. Recombinant congenic strains derived from A/J and C57BL/6J: a tool for genetic dissection of complex traits. *Genomics* 2001; 74:21–35.

Gabriel SB, Schaffner SF, Nguyen H, et al. The structure of haplotype blocks in the human genome. *Science* 2002; 296:2225–2229.

Gursoy S, Erdal E, Herken H, et al. Significance of catechol-O-methyltransferase gene polymorphism in fibromyalgia syndrome. *Rheumatol Int* 2003; 23:104–107.

Harris JA. Using c-fos as a neural marker of pain. *Brain Res Bull* 1998; 45:1–8.

Hill R. NK1 (substance P) receptor antagonists—why are they not analgesic in humans? *Trends Pharmacol Sci* 2000; 21:244–246.

Indo Y. Molecular basis of congenital insensitivity to pain with anhidrosis (CIPA): mutations and polymorphisms in TRKA (*NTRK1*) gene encoding the receptor tyrosine kinase for nerve growth factor. *Hum Mutat* 2001; 18:462–471.

Indo Y, Tsuruta M, Hayashida Y, et al. Mutations in the TRKA/NGF receptor gene in patients with congenital insensitivity to pain with anhidrosis. *Nat Genet* 1996; 13:485–488.

Isselee H, De Laat A, Lesaffre E, Lysens R. Short-term reproducibility of pressure pain thresholds in masseter and temporalis muscles of symptom-free subjects. *Eur J Oral Sci* 1997; 105:583–587.

Jamner LD, Schwartz GE. Self-deception predicts self-report and endurance of pain. *Psychosom Med* 1986; 48:211–223.

Jeremias J, Ledger WJ, Witkin SS. Interleukin 1 receptor antagonist gene polymorphism in women with vulvar vestibulitis. *Am J Obstet Gynecol* 2000; 182:283–285.

Kemler MA, van de Vusse AC, van den Berg-Loonen EM, et al. *HLA-DQ1* associated with reflex sympathetic dystrophy. *Neurology* 1999; 53:1350–1351.

Kim H, Neubert JK, San Miguel A, et al. Genetic influence on variability in human acute experimental pain sensitivity associated with gender, ethnicity and psychological temperament. *Pain* 2004; 109(3):488–496.

Lafreniere RG, MacDonald ML, Dube MP, et al. Identification of a novel gene (*HSN2*) causing hereditary sensory and autonomic neuropathy type II through the study of Canadian genetic isolates. *Am J Hum Genet* 2004; 74:1064–1073.

Lander ES, Schork NJ. Genetic dissection of complex traits. *Science* 1994; 265:2037–2048.

Lariviere WR, Wilson SG, Laughlin TM, et al. Heritability of nociception. III. Genetic relationships among commonly used assays of nociception and hypersensitivity. *Pain* 2002; 97:75–86.

Lohmueller KE, Pearce CL, Pike M, et al. Meta-analysis of genetic association studies supports a contribution of common variants to susceptibility to common disease. *Nat Genet* 2003; 33:177–182.

MacGregor AJ. The heritability of pain in humans. In: Mogil JS (Ed.). *The Genetics of Pain, Progress in Pain Research and Management*, Vol. 28. Seattle: IASP Press, 2004, pp 151–170.

MacGregor AJ, Griffiths GO, Baker J, Spector TD. Determinants of pressure pain threshold in adult twins: evidence that shared environmental influences predominate. *Pain* 1997; 73:253–257.

Mailis A, Wade J. Profile of Caucasian women with possible genetic predisposition to reflex sympathetic dystrophy: a pilot study. *Clin J Pain* 1994; 10:210–217.

Malmberg AB, Zeitz KP. Studies of pain mechanisms in genetically manipulated mice. In: Mogil JS (Ed). *The Genetics of Pain, Progress in Pain Research and Management*, Vol. 28. Seattle: IASP Press, 2004, pp 21–48.

Max MB. Assessing pain candidate gene studies. *Pain* 2004; 109(1–2):1–3.

Meller ST. Thermal and mechanical hyperalgesia: a distinct role for different excitatory amino acid receptors and signal transduction pathways? *APS J* 1994; 3:215–231.

Michalowicz BS, Pihlstrom BL, Hodges JS, Bouchard TJ Jr. No heritability of temporomandibular joint signs and symptoms. *J Dent Res* 2000; 79:1573–1578.

Mikkelsson M, Kaprio J, Salminen JJ, et al. Widespread pain among 11-year-old Finnish twin pairs. *Arthritis Rheum* 2001; 44:481–485.

Mogil JS. The genetic mediation of individual differences in sensitivity to pain and its inhibition. *Proc Natl Acad Sci USA* 1999; 96:7744–7751.

Mogil JS. Complex trait genetics of pain in the laboratory mouse. In: Mogil JS (Ed). *The Genetics of Pain, Progress in Pain Research and Management*, Vol. 28. Seattle: IASP Press, 2004, pp 123–149.

Mogil JS, Grisel JE. Transgenic studies of pain. *Pain* 1998; 77:107–128.

Mogil JS, McCarson KE. Finding pain genes: bottom-up and top-down approaches. *J Pain* 2000; 1(Suppl 1):66–80.

Mogil JS, Richards SP, O'Toole LA, et al. Genetic sensitivity to hot-plate nociception in DBA/2J and C57BL/6J inbred mouse strains: possible sex-specific mediation by $\delta2$ opioid receptors. *Pain* 1997; 70:267–277.

Mogil JS, Lichtensteiger CA, Wilson SG. The effect of genotype on sensitivity to inflammatory nociception: characterization of resistant (A/J) and sensitive (C57BL/6) inbred mouse strains. *Pain* 1998; 76:115–125.

Mogil JS, Wilson SG, Bon K, et al. Heritability of nociception. I. Responses of eleven inbred mouse strains on twelve measures of nociception. *Pain* 1999; 80:67–82.

Mogil JS, Wilson SG, Chesler EJ, et al. The melanocortin-1 receptor gene mediates female-specific mechanisms of analgesia in mice and humans. *Proc Natl Acad Sci USA* 2003; 100:4867–4872.

Offenbaecher M, Bondy B, de Jonge S, et al. Possible association of fibromyalgia with a polymorphism in the serotonin transporter gene regulatory region. *Arthritis Rheum* 1999; 42:2482–2488.

Ophoff RA, Terwindt GM, Vergouwe MN, et al. Familial hemiplegic migraine and episodic ataxia type-2 are caused by mutations in the Ca^{2+} channel gene *CACNL1A4*. *Cell* 1996; 87:543–552.

Payne B, Norfleet MA. Chronic pain and the family: a review. *Pain* 1986; 26:1–22.

Pud D, Eisenberg E, Sprecher E, et al. The tridimensional personality theory and pain: harm avoidance and reward dependence traits correlate with pain perception in healthy volunteers. *Eur J Pain* 2004; 8:31–38.

Rady JJ, Elmer GI, Fujimoto JM. Opioid receptor selectivity of heroin given intracerebro-ventricularly differs in six strains of inbred mice. *J Pharmacol Exp Ther* 1998; 288:438–445.

Richards RL. Causalgia. A centennial review. *Arch Neurol* 1967; 16:339–350.

Risch NJ. Searching for genetic determinants in the new millennium. *Nature* 2000; 405:847–856.

Risch N, Merikangas K. The future of genetic studies of complex human diseases. *Science* 1996; 273:1516–1517.

Sato M, Ohashi J, Tsuchiya N, et al. Association of HLA-A*3303-B*4403-DRB1*1302 haplo-type, but not of TNFA promoter and NKp30 polymorphism, with postherpetic neuralgia (PHN) in the Japanese population. *Genes Immun* 2002; 3:477–481.

Seltzer Z, Wu T, Max MB, Diehl SR. Mapping a gene for neuropathic pain-related behavior following peripheral neurectomy in the mouse. *Pain* 2001; 93:101–106.

Shoskes DA, Albakri Q, Thomas K, Cook D. Cytokine polymorphisms in men with chronic prostatitis/chronic pelvic pain syndrome: association with diagnosis and treatment re-sponse. *J Urol* 2002; 168:331–335.

Shuster L. Genetic analysis of morphine effects: activity, analgesia, tolerance and sensitization. In: Eleftheriou BE (Ed). *Psychopharmacogenetics*. New York: Plenum Press: New York, 1975, pp 73–97.

Slaugenhaupt SA, Blumenfeld A, Gill SP, et al. Tissue-specific expression of a splicing mutation in the *IKBKAP* gene causes familial dysautonomia. *Am J Hum Genet* 2001; 68:598–605.

Solovieva S, Leino-Arjas P, Saarela J, et al. Possible association of interleukin 1 gene locus polymorphisms with low back pain. *Pain* 2004; 109:8–19.

Sternbach RA. Psychophysiology of pain. *Int J Psychiatry Med* 1975; 6:63–73.

van Hilten JJ, van de Beek WJ, Roep BO. Multifocal or generalized tonic dystonia of complex regional pain syndrome: a distinct clinical entity associated with HLA-DR13. *Ann Neurol* 2000; 48:113–116.

Wilson SG, Chesler EJ, Hain HS, et al. Identification of quantitative trait loci for chemical/inflammatory nociception in mice. *Pain* 2002; 96:385–391.

Zubieta J-K, Heitzeg MM, Smith YR, et al. COMT *val158met* genotype affects μ-opioid neurotransmitter responses to a pain stressor. *Science* 2003; 299:1240–1243.

Correspondence to: Jeffrey S. Mogil, PhD, Department of Psychology, McGill University, 1205 Dr. Penfield Avenue, Montreal, Quebec H3A 1B1, Canada. Tel: 514-398-6085; Fax: 514-398-4896; email: jeffrey.mogil@mcgill.ca.

The Paths of Pain 1975–2005, edited by
Harold Merskey, John D. Loeser, and Ronald
Dubner, IASP Press, Seattle, © 2005.

6

Physiology and Anatomy of the Spinal Cord Pain System

William D. Willis, Jr.

*Department of Neuroscience and Cell Biology, University of Texas
Medical Branch, Galveston, Texas, USA*

The state of knowledge of the anatomy and physiology of the spinal cord pain system near the time when the International Association for the Study of Pain was founded is reflected in the proceedings of the 1st World Congress on Pain held in 1975 (Bonica and Albe-Fessard 1976). This chapter summarizes what was known at that time and discusses advances in this field between 1975 and 2005.

PRIMARY AFFERENT NOCICEPTORS

In 1975. Numerous finely myelinated (Aδ) and unmyelinated (C) primary afferent nociceptive axons are found in peripheral nerves of experimental animals (Handwerker 1976; Perl 1976). The microneurography technique permits recordings from nociceptors in human subjects (Torebjörk and Hallin 1976; Van Hees 1976). The sensitization of C nociceptors following strong stimulation or administration of inflammatory substances is well recognized (Handwerker 1976; Perl 1976). Sensitization results in the development of spontaneous activity, reduced thresholds, and increases in responses to suprathreshold stimulation in nociceptors.

Since 1975. In humans, activation of C-fiber nociceptors by intraneural microstimulation elicits dull or burning pain sensation (or sometimes itch) that is referred accurately to the receptive fields of the stimulated nociceptors (Ochoa and Torebjörk 1989). Mechanically insensitive nociceptors in peripheral nerves were described first in joint nerves (Schaible and Schmidt 1985) and later in cutaneous (Handwerker et al. 1991) and visceral (Häbler et al. 1990) nerves. These "sleeping nociceptors" "awakened" when the afferents were sensitized during inflammation (Schaible and Schmidt 1985; Davis et al. 1993). Sensitization of nociceptors was proposed to account for primary hyperalgesia (Meyer and Campbell 1981).

Peripheral sensitization of nociceptors (reviewed by Willis and Coggeshall 2004) follows triggering of signal transduction cascades in the nociceptors by increases in intracellular calcium concentration and other second messengers, leading to activation of protein kinases (PKC, PKA, and p38 MAPK). The protein kinases phosphorylate membrane proteins involved in nociceptive transduction.

TRPV1 (vanilloid) receptors are responsive to capsaicin, as well as to heat and protons, and are among the proteins activated in nociceptors sensitized to heat stimuli (Caterina and Julius 2001). In transgenic mice lacking TRPV1 receptors, some responses to noxious heat or chemical stimuli are eliminated or reduced, whereas others are unaffected. The responses retained may be due to the presence of other transient receptor potential (TRP) receptors, such as TRPV2 receptors, which are activated at higher temperatures than TRPV1 (Davis et al. 2000).

Responses of nociceptors can also be sensitized to mechanical stimuli. The molecular basis for transduction of noxious mechanical stimuli is still being explored. Recently, mechanically sensitive cation channels in mammalian sensory neurons have been identified. They belong to a family of proteins called degenerin/epithelial (DEG/ENaC) sodium channels, which have been found in cutaneous mechanoreceptors and in axon endings that may belong to nociceptors (García-Añoveros et al. 2001).

ANATOMY OF LISSAUER'S TRACT AND THE DORSAL HORN

In 1975. The afferent projections to and the organization of the spinal cord dorsal horn (with morphological and physiological similarities to the medullary dorsal horn; see Sessle, this volume) were reviewed by Kerr (1976). Aδ and C afferent fibers enter Lissauer's tract and then send collaterals into the superficial dorsal horn to synapse. The substantia gelatinosa was believed to a closed system, connecting only with itself. Both laminae II and III were believed to belong to the substantia gelatinosa. Features of the neuropil of the substantia gelatinosa are the paucity of myelinated axons and the presence of complex synaptic arrangements formed by terminals of primary afferent fibers (glomeruli). Fine afferent fibers end chiefly on neurons in laminae I and II, whereas large myelinated afferents project to deeper layers of the dorsal horn.

Since 1975. Many details about the organization of the dorsal horn have been documented since 1975, and several opinions have been corrected (reviewed by Willis and Coggeshall 2004). For example, lamina II can be equated with the substantia gelatinosa, is subdivided into outer (II_o) and inner (II_i) parts, and is not a closed system. Synaptic endings that contain large dense-core vesicles are common in laminae I and II_o. Finely myelinated afferents project mainly to laminae I and V, unmyelinated afferents to laminae I and II, and large myelinated afferents to laminae III–VI. Unmyelinated primary afferents can end on the dorsally projecting dendrites of neurons in the deep dorsal horn.

The dense-core vesicles found in many synaptic terminals in the superficial dorsal horn store and release neuropeptides, such as substance P and calcitonin gene--related peptide (CGRP). These peptides contribute to nociceptive processing (see review by Willis and Coggeshall 2004). However, the same nerve terminals also contain clear, round vesicles for storage and release of glutamate. Immunocytochemical staining of identified spinothalamic tract (STT) cells labeled intracellularly with horseradish peroxidase has shown that synaptic endings on these STT cells can contain glutamate, substance P (Fig. 1A), CGRP (Fig. 1B), γ-aminobutyric acid (GABA), catecholamines, or serotonin (reviewed by Willis and Coggeshall 2004). Some of these endings are located on dorsally projecting dendrites of neurons whose cell bodies are in the deep dorsal horn. For example, the substance P- and CGRP-containing synaptic endings in Fig. 1A and B were found in lamina III in contact with the dendrites of a labeled STT cell whose soma was at the border between laminae IV and V (Fig. 1C).

The iontophoretic release of neurotransmitters near a primate STT neuron can result in excitatory or inhibitory responses. For example, excitatory amino acids acting at *N*-methyl-D-aspartate (NMDA) or non-NMDA (AMPA) receptors produce a dose-related excitation of spinothalamic tract cells (reviewed by Willis and Coggeshall 2004). Combined iontophoretic application of substance P with an excitatory amino acid can greatly enhance and prolong the excitatory effect of amino acids. The inhibitory amino acids GABA and glycine produce a powerful inhibition of STT cells, as do serotonin and norepinephrine. Opioids generally also produce an inhibition.

Interestingly, the intrinsic neurons of the substantia gelatinosa lack neurokinin-1 (NK1) receptors and do not respond to substance P (Bleazard et al. 1994). Instead, peptidergic synaptic transmission in the substantia gelatinosa involves NK1 receptors on the dendrites of neurons whose cell bodies are in lamina I or in deeper laminae, including laminae III and IV (Naim et al. 1997), and which extend into lamina II (see Fig. 1).

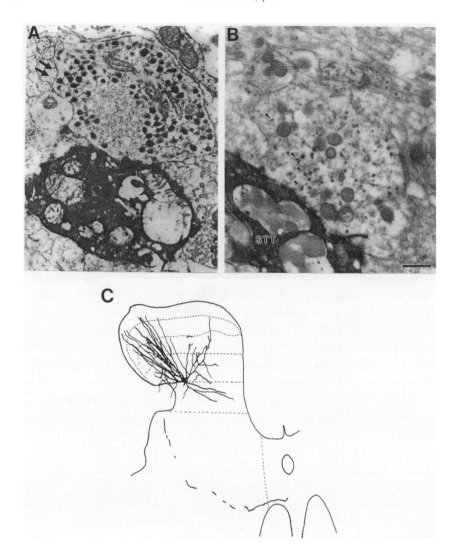

Fig. 1. Synaptic endings containing substance P (SP) or calcitonin gene-related peptide (CGRP) contacting dendrites of a labeled spinothalamic tract (STT) cell in the primate spinal cord. The STT cell was injected intracellularly with horseradish peroxidase after the neuron was identified by antidromic activation from the contralateral ventral posterior lateral thalamic nucleus. (A) A labeled dendrite in the electron micrograph is postsynaptic to a terminal that contains SP, shown by immunolabeling of numerous dense-core vesicles. (B) Another synaptic ending contacting the same STT cell contains CGRP, which was immunostained with 15-nm gold particles, some of which are indicated by arrowheads. Many gold particles are associated with dense-core vesicles. Calibration bar = 0.5 μm. (From Carlton et al. 1990.) (C) A drawing of the same STT cell. The cell body is in lamina IV, near the border with lamina V, and numerous dendrites extend as far dorsally as lamina I. The axon is shown crossing in the ventral commissure. The synapses in A and B were located on dendrites within lamina III.

GATE CONTROL THEORY

In 1975. Key features of the gate theory of pain are: (1) injury activates Aδ and C fibers; (2) these nerve impulses excite central transmission cells; (3) central transmission cells also receive excitatory and inhibitory inputs from other types of afferents; (4) the activity of central transmission cells is influenced by connections from descending pathways that originate in the brainstem and cerebral cortex; and (5) pain perception occurs in response to apparent injury when the "initial gate and subsequent stages of the transmission pathway are favorably set for the exhibition of this state" (Wall 1976).

In support of the gate theory is the effectiveness of stimulation of large afferent fibers, either in peripheral nerves or in the dorsal column, in relieving pain (Long 1976). Experimental studies demonstrate that nociceptive dorsal horn neurons are inhibited by afferent volleys in large afferent fibers or by stimulation of the dorsal column (Foreman et al. 1976; Iggo et al. 1976). Some of the criticisms of the gate theory were directed at evidence that conflicted with the predicted role of presynaptic inhibition in the gate mechanism. However, postsynaptic inhibition could play an equivalent role.

Since 1975. The use of transcutaneous electrical nerve stimulation (TENS) and spinal cord stimulation for pain relief has been reviewed (Hansson and Lundeberg 1999; Simpson 1999). Hansson and Lundeberg (1999) felt that there was still insufficient proof of the clinical effectiveness of TENS. Furthermore, it is unclear to what extent favorable results can be related to the mechanism suggested by the gate theory. For example, in monkeys, repetitive stimulation of the large myelinated axons in a peripheral nerve produced only a slight inhibition of the responses of STT cells to volleys in C fibers, whereas raising the strength of stimulation so that small, as well as large, myelinated axons were activated had a strong inhibitory action, and higher stimulus strengths that also excited C fibers were even more effective (Fig. 2; Chung et al. 1984).

Another inhibitory system triggered by noxious, rather than innocuous, stimulation has been termed "diffuse noxious inhibitory controls" or DNICs (Le Bars et al. 1979a,b). DNICs are activated by stimulation of Aδ and C nociceptors and involve a supraspinal loop through the dorsal reticular nucleus in the medulla (Villanueva et al. 1988). DNICs may have contributed to the inhibition of the C-fiber responses of primate STT cells in the experiments mentioned above (Chung et al. 1984).

Wall's statement about the important role of descending modulatory pathways in regulating nociceptive transmission in the dorsal horn is reflected in numerous studies of the "endogenous analgesia system" (see Besson

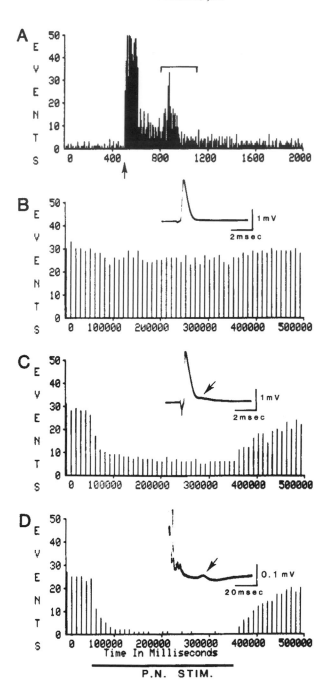

Time In Milliseconds

P.N. STIM.

and Chaouch 1987; Willis and Coggeshall 2004). There are also descending pathways that facilitate nociceptive transmission in the spinal cord (Willis and Coggeshall 2004).

RESPONSES OF NOCICEPTIVE DORSAL HORN NEURONS, INCLUDING STT CELLS

In 1975. Lamina I neurons in the cat spinal cord that respond only to noxious stimuli ("high-threshold" or HT neurons) can be inhibited following activation of large afferent fibers (Iggo et al. 1976). Rat dorsal horn neurons that respond only to innocuous stimuli ("low-threshold or LT neurons") are located in the nucleus proprius. Cells excited by innocuous and noxious stimuli ("wide-dynamic-range" or WDR neurons) and HT cells were in both lamina I and the nucleus proprius. Cells that respond to joint movement were in the deep dorsal horn and ventral horn (Giesler et al. 1976). Similar results were obtained for primate STT neurons (Willis 1976).

Since 1975. The majority of primate STT neurons in lamina I and in the nucleus proprius of the dorsal horn are of the WDR type, although many HT STT cells are also found in lamina I and in the deeper laminae of the dorsal horn (Owens et al. 1992). Some lamina I STT cells respond to innocuous thermal stimuli (Craig et al. 2001).

Recordings from primate STT cells can model the sensory responses of human subjects to intradermal injection of capsaicin, providing evidence about the possible roles of WDR and HT STT cells in pain, primary heat hyperalgesia and secondary mechanical allodynia and hyperalgesia (see Willis and Coggeshall 2004). Following a capsaicin injection, humans report severe pain that lasts 10–30 minutes (LaMotte et al. 1991). As the pain recedes, primary heat hyperalgesia develops in the skin near the capsaicin injection site where capsaicin sensitizes nociceptive endings to heat. Large regions of skin surrounding the area of primary hyperalgesia develop secondary

---

←— **Fig. 2.** Inhibition of the responses of a primate STT cell to volleys in C fibers of the sural nerve by repetitive stimulation of different fiber groups in the tibial nerve. (A) Summed responses of the cell to repeated stimulation of the sural nerve at the time indicated by the arrow. The stimuli were at a strength that activated C fibers, and they were repeated 10 times. The horizontal bracket shows the C-fiber component of the response, which was integrated in the histograms in B–D, where the responses to C-fiber volleys are shown as vertical lines. The responses in B–D were evoked every 10 seconds. During the 5-minute time period indicated by the horizontal bar below D, the tibial nerve was stimulated at a frequency of 2 Hz at several different stimulus strengths. The neurograms above the histograms show that the afferent volleys included just Aβ fibers in panel B, Aβ and Aδ fibers (see arrow) in panel C, and A plus C fibers (see arrow) in panel D. (From Chung et al. 1984.)

mechanical allodynia and hyperalgesia over a period of about 15 minutes. These sensory changes last for hours.

Primate STT cells show a greatly enhanced firing rate during the time when humans experience severe pain, increased responses and a lowered threshold to heat stimuli applied near the injection site, and enhanced responses to innocuous and mildly noxious mechanical stimuli applied in the secondary area (Simone et al. 1991; Dougherty and Willis 1992). The enhanced responses to stimulation of the skin in the secondary area following a capsaicin injection must result from plastic changes within the central nervous system, since the nociceptive afferent fibers that supply the secondary area do not become sensitized; the responsible central process has been termed "central sensitization" (see Willis and Coggeshall 2004). During central sensitization, there is an enhancement of the discharges of the cells evoked by volleys in cut dorsal rootlets (Simone et al. 1991) or by iontophoretic release of excitatory amino acids (Dougherty and Willis 1992), stimuli that are independent of any sensitization of nociceptive afferents.

The activity of both WDR and HT primate STT cells increases following a capsaicin injection, but the increased discharges in WDR neurons continue for more than 5 minutes after the injection, paralleling the duration of acute pain in human subjects, whereas the discharge rate of most HT STT cells returns to the baseline level within about 2–3 minutes (Simone et al. 1991). HT STT cells often show a reduction in firing rate after the initial increase (Dougherty and Willis 1992). Both WDR and HT cells can contribute to the immediate and intense pain that follows an injection of capsaicin, but the discharges of only WDR cells help explain the sustained pain that lasts 10–30 minutes after the injection (Simone et al. 1991). Laird and Cervero (1989) found that HT dorsal horn neurons in rats are much less likely to show central sensitization of their responses to mechanical stimuli than are WDR neurons.

Capsaicin-induced central sensitization is triggered by the release of glutamate and peptides from nociceptive primary afferent fibers (see Willis and Coggeshall 2004). These molecules trigger a number of signal transduction cascades in nociceptive dorsal horn neurons, such as STT cells, leading to activation of several protein kinases (CaMKII, PKA, PKC, and PKG). These protein kinases phosphorylate proteins that participate in the sensitization process, including NR1 subunits of NMDA receptors (Zou et al. 2000) and GluR1 subunits of AMPA receptors (Fang et al. 2003). Similarly, NR2B subunits in the spinal cord are phosphorylated after inflammation is produced by an injection of complete Freund's adjuvant into the skin (Guo et al. 2002). Central sensitization appears to be a spinal cord form of long-term potentiation (Willis 2002; see Ji et al. 2003).

NEURONS OF ORIGIN OF THE SPINOTHALAMIC
AND OTHER ASCENDING NOCICEPTIVE TRACTS

In 1975. At autopsy following cordotomies to relieve pain, chromatolytic neurons were observed in laminae I and IV–IX, but not in laminae II–III, and rarely in the ventral horn. Most of the chromatolytic cell bodies were contralateral to the cut axons. It was concluded that the STT arises from cells dispersed over many laminae (Smith 1976).

Since 1975. Retrograde labeling studies in monkeys show that primate STT neurons projecting to the ventral posterior lateral nucleus are chiefly in laminae I and IV–VI, although some are in laminae II–III and VII–X (reviewed by Willis and Coggeshall 2004); most project contralaterally. STT neurons that project to the central lateral nucleus of the intralaminar complex are located in laminae VI and VII (see Willis and Coggeshall 2004).

Although it has been proposed that all or almost all lamina I STT cells project to a medial thalamic nucleus recently renamed VMpo (Craig et al. 1994), this hypothesis has been refuted (Willis et al. 2002). Graziano and Jones (2004) have recently reported that there is no VMpo nucleus, showing that the area indicated by Craig et al. (1994) is actually part of the ventral posterior medial nucleus and that there are lamina I projections to several thalamic nuclei, including the ventrobasal complex.

PROJECTION OF THE SPINOTHALAMIC TRACT

In 1975. Axons of primate STT cells at an upper lumbar level are scattered in the anterolateral white matter of the spinal cord. The axons have a somatotopic organization: axons located dorsolaterally have more caudal receptive fields, and axons located ventromedially have more rostral receptive fields (Willis 1976). The axons of presumed human STT cells at various levels of the human neuraxis, including the spinal cord, midbrain, and thalamus, have been demonstrated by stimuli that evoke sensory reports of warmth, cold, or pain, referred to the contralateral side (Tasker et al. 1976). Mayer et al. (1975) found that pain sensations can be produced reliably when axons in the anterolateral quadrant of the human spinal cord are stimulated at a frequency greater than 5 Hz at a sufficient intensity. The relatively refractory periods of the axons in the lateral funiculus that produce pain are between 1.0 and 1.5 ms, suggesting that the stimulated axons are large myelinated fibers and therefore that pain can be evoked when WDR neurons are activated.

Since 1975. Apkarian, Hodge, and colleagues proposed that the primate STT can be subdivided into dorsolateral and ventral components (reviewed by Willis and Coggeshall 2004). The dorsolateral component is suggested to arise from neurons of lamina I. However, when Craig (2000) labeled the axons of lamina I neurons anterogradely following injections of a marker into the superficial dorsal horn of cats and monkeys, the labeled axons were concentrated in the middle of the lateral funiculus. This is the location of axons that are at least partially responsible for thermal sensation in cats, according to Norrsell (1983), and so it seems reasonable to presume that the lamina I component of the STT contributes to thermal sensations, as well as to pain.

In a study of the locations of the axons of primate STT neurons using antidromic microstimulation, Zhang et al. (2000) found that, at T7–9, most of the axons of neurons with cell bodies in lamina I were at the level of the dentate ligament, whereas those of STT cells whose somas were in the deep dorsal horn were in the ventral part of the lateral funiculus. In the C6–8 segments, the axons of STT cells of the superficial dorsal horn shifted more ventrally.

Pain relief by anterolateral cordotomy requires that the lesion interrupts most of the anterolateral quadrant, extending dorsal to the dentate ligament (Nathan et al. 2001; see also Gybels and Sweet 1989), implying a role in pain of STT neurons in both the superficial and deep dorsal horn.

ASCENDING NOCICEPTIVE PATHWAYS OTHER THAN THE STT

In 1975. Nociceptive pathways other than the STT recognized in 1975 include the spinoreticular tract and the postsynaptic dorsal column pathway

---

Fig. 3. Effect of lesions of the dorsal column on the responses of neurons in the rat ventral posterior lateral (VPL) thalamic nucleus to noxious visceral stimuli. In panel I, parts A–C show the recording site for a VPL neuron, the cutaneous receptive field of the neuron, and spinal cord lesions made during the experiment. The upper row of peristimulus time histograms in panel I, parts D and E, are responses of the VPL neuron to graded intensities of mechanical stimuli applied to the cutaneous receptive field and to graded colorectal distensions. The middle row of histograms show the effect of a lesion of the dorsal column, and the lowermost one the effect of an additional lesion of the lateral column. Panel I, part F shows the action potential of the cell throughout the experiment. (From Al-Chaer et al. 1996a.) In Panel II, A, the upper row of histograms shows the responses of a neuron in the VPL nucleus of a rat to graded distensions of the duodenum. There was little change in the responses after a midline lesion of the dorsal column. However, the responses were nearly eliminated by two lesions placed bilaterally in the dorsal column at the level of the dorsal intermediate septum. Part B shows the action potential of the cell at different times during the experiment. The lesions, receptive field, and recording site are shown in Panel II, parts C–E. (From Feng et al. 1998.) ⟶

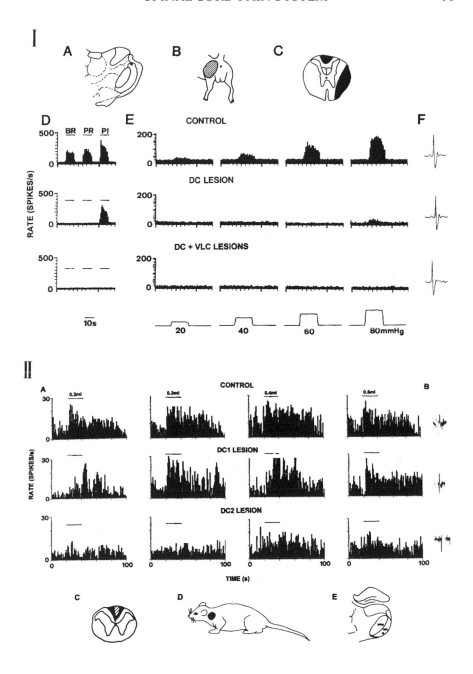

(Angaut-Petit 1976; Fields and Anderson 1976). Although the spino-cervicothalamic pathway has been shown to have a nociceptive component in cats and monkeys, the role of this pathway in humans was questioned (Kerr 1976).

Since 1975. Willis and Coggeshall (2004) have reviewed these and other nociceptive pathways. Responses to noxious stimulation of the skin have been recorded from thalamic projection neurons in the nucleus gracilis of cats and monkeys, suggesting a potential role of the dorsal column-medial lemniscus pathway in pain.

Because of clinical evidence that a midline lesion of the dorsal column in humans can alleviate pelvic cancer pain, experimental studies were undertaken to determine if there is a visceral pain pathway in this part of the cord. These studies demonstrated that the dorsal column is more important for visceral nociception than is the STT (Fig. 3; Al-Chaer et al. 1996a,b; Feng et al. 1998; Palecek et al. 2002). Postsynaptic dorsal column (PSDC) neurons, rather than collaterals of primary afferent fibers that ascend directly to the medulla through the dorsal column, are responsible for the electrophysiological responses to noxious visceral stimuli that can be recorded from the ventral posterior lateral thalamic nucleus or from the nucleus gracilis (Al-Chaer et al. 1996b). Anterograde tracing has shown that the axons of PSDC neurons in the sacral cord project near the midline of the dorsal column, whereas axons of PSDC neurons at a midthoracic level ascend near the dorsal intermediate septum (Wang et al. 1999). For this reason, lesions at the midline in the cervical or thoracic spinal cord are effective in preventing nociceptive responses to stimulation of pelvic visceral organs (Fig. 3, panel I), whereas dorsal column lesions need to be placed more laterally in the cervical or upper thoracic cord to prevent responses to noxious stimulation of abdominal viscera (Fig. 3, panel II).

ACKNOWLEDGMENTS

Experimental work done in the author's laboratory has been supported by research grants from the National Institutes of Health (NS 09743 and NS 11255). The author thanks Griselda Gonzales for her assistance with the illustrations and Kelli Gondesen for help with the experiments.

REFERENCES

Al-Chaer ED, Lawand NB, Westlund KN, Willis WD. Visceral nociceptive input into the ventral posterolateral nucleus of the thalamus: a new function for the dorsal column pathway. *J Neurophysiol* 1996a; 76:2661–2674.

Al-Chaer ED, Lawand NB, Westlund KN, Willis WD. Pelvic visceral input into the nucleus gracilis is largely mediated by the postsynaptic dorsal column pathway. *J Neurophysiol* 1996b; 76:2675–2690.

Angout-Petit D. An electrophysiological investigation of the dorsal column system: its possible role in nociception. In: Bonica JJ, Albe-Fessard DG (Eds). *Proceedings of the First World Congress on Pain,* Advances in Pain Research and Therapy, Vol. 1. New York: Raven Press, 1976, pp 239–243.

Besson JM, Chaouch A. Peripheral and spinal mechanisms of nociception. *Physiol Rev* 1987; 67:67–186.

Bleazard L, Hill RG, Morris R. The correlation between the distribution of the NK1 receptor and the actions of tachykinin agonists in the dorsal horn of the rat indicates that substance P does not have a functional role on substantia gelatinosa (lamina II) neurons. *J Neurosci* 1994; 14:7655–7664.

Bonica JJ, Albe-Fessard DG (Eds). *Proceedings of the First World Congress on Pain,* Advances in Pain Research and Therapy, Vol. 1. New York: Raven Press, 1976.

Carlton SM, Westlund KN, Zhang D, Sorkin LS, Willis WD. Calcitonin gene-related peptide containing primary afferent fibers synapse on primate spinothalamic tract cells. *Neurosci Lett* 1990; 109:76–81.

Caterina MJ, Julius D. The vanilloid receptor: a molecular gateway to the pain pathway. *Annu Rev Neurosci* 2001; 24:487–517.

Chung JM, Lee KH, Hori Y, Endo K, Willis WD. Factors influencing peripheral nerve stimulation produced inhibition of primate spinothalamic tract cells. *Pain* 1984; 19:277–293.

Craig AD. Spinal location of ascending lamina I axons in the macaque monkey. *J Pain* 2000; 1:33–45.

Craig AD, Bushnell MC, Zhang ET, Blomqvist A. A thalamic nucleus specific for pain and temperature sensation. *Nature* 1994; 372:770–773.

Craig AD, Krout K, Andrew D. Quantitative response characteristics of thermoreceptive and nociceptive lamina I spinothalamic neurons in the cat. *J Neurophysiol* 2001; 86:1459–1480.

Davis JB, Gray J, Gunthorpe MJ, et al. Vanilloid receptor-1 is essential for inflammatory thermal hyperalgesia. *Nature* 2000; 405:183–187.

Davis KD, Meyer RA, Campbell JN. Chemosensitivity and sensitization of nociceptive afferents that innervate the hairy skin of monkey. *J Neurophysiol* 1993; 69:1071–1081.

Dougherty PM, Willis WD. Enhanced responses of spinothalamic tract neurons to excitatory amino acids accompany capsaicin-induced sensitization in the monkey. *J Neurosci* 1992; 12:883–894.

Fang L, Wu J, Zhang X, Lin Q, Willis WD. Increased phosphorylation of the GluR1 subunit of spinal cord α-amino-3-hydroxy-5-methyl-4-isoxazole propionate receptor in rats following intradermal injection of capsaicin. *Neuroscience* 2003; 122:237–245.

Feng Y, Cui M, Al-Chaer ED, Willis WD. Epigastric antinociception by cervical dorsal column lesions in rats. *Anesthesiology* 1998; 89:411–420.

Fields HL, Anderson SD. Comparison of spinoreticular and spinothalamic projections in the cat. In: Bonica JJ, Albe-Fessard DG (Eds). *Proceedings of the First World Congress on Pain,* Advances in Pain Research and Therapy, Vol. 1. New York: Raven Press, 1976, pp 179–283.

Foreman RD, Beall JE, Applebaum AE, Coulter JD, Willis WD. Inhibition of primate spinotha-
lamic tract neurons by electrical stimulation of dorsal column or peripheral nerve. In: Bonica JJ,
Albe-Fessard DG (Eds). *Proceedings of the First World Congress on Pain,* Advances in
Pain Research and Therapy, Vol. 1. New York: Raven Press, 1976, pp 405–410.

García-Añoveros J, Samad TA, Zuvela-Jelaska L, Woolf CJ, Corey DP. Transport and localization of the DEG/ENaC ion channel BNaC1α to peripheral mechanosensory terminals of
dorsal root ganglia neurons. *J Neurosci* 2001; 21:2678–2686.

Giesler GJ Jr, Menetrey D, Besson JM. Response properties of dorsal horn neurons to noxious
and nonnoxious stimuli in the spinal rat. In: Bonica JJ, Albe-Fessard DG (Eds). *Proceedings of the First World Congress on Pain,* Advances in Pain Research and Therapy, Vol. 1.
New York: Raven Press, 1976, pp 105–110.

Graziano A, Jones EG. Widespread thalamic terminations of fibers arising in the superficial
medullary dorsal horn of monkeys and their relation to calbindin immunoreactivity. *J
Neurosci* 2004; 24:248–256.

Guo W, Zou S, Guan Y, et al. Tyrosine phosphorylation of the NR2B subunit of the NMDA
receptor in the spinal cord during the development and maintenance of inflammatory
hyperalgesia. *J Neurosci* 2002; 22:6208–6217.

Gybels JM, Sweet WH. *Neurosurgical Treatment of Persistent Pain.* Basel: Karger, 1989.

Häbler HJ, Jänig W, Koltzenburg M. Activation of unmyelinated afferent fibres by mechanical
stimuli and inflammation of the urinary bladder in the cat. *J Physiol* 1990; 425:545–562.

Handwerker HO. Influences of algogenic substances and prostaglandins on the discharges of
unmyelinated cutaneous nerve fibers identified as nociceptors. In: Bonica JJ, Albe-Fessard
DG (Eds). *Proceedings of the First World Congress on Pain,* Advances in Pain Research
and Therapy, Vol. 1. New York: Raven Press, 1976, pp 41–45.

Handwerker HO, Kilo S, Reeh PW. Unresponsive afferent nerve fibres in the sural nerve of the
rat. *J Physiol* 1991; 435:229–242.

Hansson P, Lundeberg T. Transcutaneous electrical nerve stimulation, vibration, and acupuncture as pain-relieving measures. In: Wall PD, Melzack R (Eds). *Textbook of Pain,* 4th ed.
New York: Churchill Livingstone, 1999; pp 1341–1351.

Iggo A, Ogawa H, Cervero F. Inhibition of nociceptor-driven dorsal horn neurons in the cat. In:
Bonica JJ, Albe-Fessard DG (Eds). *Proceedings of the First World Congress on Pain,*
Advances in Pain Research and Therapy, Vol. 1. New York: Raven Press, 1976, pp 99–104.

Ji RR, Kohno T, Moore KA, Woolf CJ. Central sensitization and LTP: do pain and memory
share similar mechanisms? *Trends Neurosci* 2003; 26:696–705.

Kerr FWL. Segmental circuitry and spinal cord nociceptive systems. In: Bonica JJ, Albe-
Fessard DG (Eds). *Proceedings of the First World Congress on Pain,* Advances in Pain
Research and Therapy, Vol. 1. New York: Raven Press, 1976, pp 75–89.

Laird JMA, Cervero F. A comparative study of the changes in receptive-field properties of
multireceptive and nocireceptive rat dorsal horn neurons following noxious mechanical
stimulation. *J Neurophysiol* 1989; 62:854–863.

LaMotte RH, Shain CN, Simone DA, Tsai EFP. Neurogenic hyperalgesia: psychophysical
studies of underlying mechanisms. *J Neurophysiol* 1991; 66:190–211.

Le Bars D, Dickenson AH, Besson JM. Diffuse noxious inhibitory controls (DNIC). I. Effects
on dorsal horn convergent neurones in the rat. *Pain* 1979a; 6:283–304.

Le Bars D, Dickenson AH, Besson JM. Diffuse noxious inhibitory controls (DNIC). II: Lack of
effect on non-convergent neurones, supraspinal involvement and theoretical implications.
Pain 1979b; 6:305–327.

Long DM. Use of peripheral and spinal cord stimulation in the relief of chronic pain. In: Bonica
JJ, Albe-Fessard DG (Eds). *Proceedings of the First World Congress on Pain,* Advances in
Pain Research and Therapy, Vol. 1. New York: Raven Press, 1976, pp 395–403.

Mayer DJ, Price DD, Becker DP. Neurophysiological characterization of the anterolateral
spinal cord neurons contributing to pain perception in man. *Pain* 1975; 1:51–58.

Meyer RA, Campbell JN. Myelinated nociceptive afferents account for the hyperalgesia that follows a burn to the hand. *Science* 1981; 213:1527–1529.

Naim M, Spike RC, Watt C, Shehab SAS, Todd AJ. Cells in laminae III and IV of the rat spinal cord that possess the neurokinin-1 receptor and have dorsally directed dendrites receive a major synaptic input from tachykinin-containing primary afferents. *J Neurosci* 1997; 17:5536–5548.

Nathan PW, Smith M, Deacon P. The crossing of the spinothalamic tract. *Brain* 2001; 124:793–803.

Norrsell U. Unilateral behavioral thermosensitivity after transection of one lateral funiculus in the cervical spinal cord of the cat. *Exp Brain Res* 1983; 53:71–80.

Ochoa J, Torebjörk HE. Sensations evoked by intraneural microstimulation of C nociceptor fibres in human skin nerves. *J Physiol* 1989; 415:583–599.

Owens CM, Zhang D, Willis WD. Changes in the response states of primate spinothalamic tract cells caused by mechanical damage of the skin or activation of descending controls. *J Neurophysiol* 1992; 67:1509–1527.

Palecek J, Palecková V, Willis WD. The roles of pathways in the spinal cord lateral and dorsal funiculi in signaling nociceptive somatic and visceral stimuli in rats. *Pain* 2002; 96:297–307.

Perl ER. Sensitization of nociceptors and its relation to sensation. In: Bonica JJ, Albe-Fessard DG (Eds). *Proceedings of the First World Congress on Pain,* Advances in Pain Research and Therapy, Vol. 1. New York: Raven Press, 1976, pp 17–28.

Schaible HG, Schmidt RF. Effects of an experimental arthritis on the sensory properties of fine articular afferent units. *J Neurophysiol* 1985; 54:1109–1122.

Simone DA, Sorkin LS, Oh U, et al. Neurogenic hyperalgesia: central neural correlates in responses of spinothalamic tract neurons. *J Neurophysiol* 1991; 66:228–246.

Simpson BA. Spinal cord and brain stimulation. In: Wall PD, Melzack R. *Textbook of Pain,* 4th ed. New York: Churchill Livingstone, 1999, pp 1353–1381.

Smith MC. Retrograde cell changes in human spinal cord after anterolateral cordotomies: location and identification after different periods of survival. In: Bonica JJ, Albe-Fessard DG (Eds). *Proceedings of the First World Congress on Pain,* Advances in Pain Research and Therapy, Vol. 1. New York: Raven Press, 1976, pp 91–98.

Tasker RR, Organ LW, Rowe IH, Hawrylyshyn P. Human spinothalamic tract: stimulation mapping in the spinal cord and brainstem. In: Bonica JJ, Albe-Fessard DG (Eds). *Proceedings of the First World Congress on Pain,* Advances in Pain Research and Therapy, Vol. 1. New York: Raven Press, 1976, pp 251–257

Torebjörk HE, Hallin RG. A new method for classification of C-unit activity in intact human skin nerves. In: Bonica JJ, Albe-Fessard DG (Eds). *Proceedings of the First World Congress on Pain,* Advances in Pain Research and Therapy, Vol. 1. New York: Raven Press, 1976, pp 29–34.

Villanueva L, Bouhassira D, Bing Z, Le Bars D. Convergence of heterotopic and nociceptive information onto subnucleus reticularis dorsalis neurons in the rat medulla. *J Neurophysiol* 1988; 60:980–1009.

Wall PD. Modulation of pain by nonpainful events. In: Bonica JJ, Albe-Fessard DG (Eds). *Proceedings of the First World Congress on Pain,* Advances in Pain Research and Therapy, Vol. 1. New York: Raven Press, 1976, pp 1–16.

Wang CC, Willis WD, Westlund KN. Ascending projections from the area around the spinal cord central canal: a *Phaseolus vulgaris* leucoagglutinin study in rats. *J Comp Neurol* 1999; 415:341–367.

Willis WD. Spinothalamic system: physiological aspects. In: Bonica JJ, Albe-Fessard DG (Eds). *Proceedings of the First World Congress on Pain,* Advances in Pain Research and Therapy, Vol. 1. New York: Raven Press, 1976, pp 215–223.

Willis WD. Long-term potentiation in spinothalamic neurons. *Brain Res Rev* 2002; 40:202–214.

Willis WD, Coggeshall RE. *Sensory Mechanisms of the Spinal Cord.* New York: Kluwer, 2004.

Willis WD, Zhang X, Honda CN, Giesler GJ. A critical review of the role of the proposed VMpo nucleus in pain. *J Pain* 2002; 3:79–94.

Zhang X, Wenk HN, Honda CN, Giesler GJ. Locations of spinothalamic tract axons in cervical and thoracic spinal cord white matter in monkeys. *J Neurophysiol* 2000; 83:2869–2880.

Zou X, Lin Q, Willis WD. Enhanced phosphorylation of NMDA receptor 1 subunits in spinal cord dorsal horn and spinothalamic tract neurons after intradermal injection of capsaicin in rats. *J Neurosci* 2000; 20:6989–6997.

Correspondence to: William D. Willis, Jr., MD, PhD, Department of Neuroscience and Cell Biology, University of Texas Medical Branch, 301 University Boulevard, Galveston, TX 77555-1069, USA. Tel: 409-772-2103; Fax: 409-772-4687; email: wdwillis@utmb.edu.

The Paths of Pain 1975–2005, edited by
Harold Merskey, John D. Loeser, and Ronald
Dubner, IASP Press, Seattle, © 2005.

7

Plasticity in Central Nociceptive Pathways

Ronald Dubner

*Department of Biomedical Sciences, University of Maryland Dental School,
Baltimore, Maryland, USA*

The emergence of the study of chronic persistent pain had its origins before the establishment of the International Association for the Study of Pain in 1973 and the first World Congress on Pain in 1975. The greatest impetus for this research was the devoted efforts of two giants in medicine, Patrick Wall and John J. Bonica. Their goal was the same: to help the patient in persistent pain with little hope for relief, let alone cure. However, the strategies they used to achieve their goal were quite different. Wall, although he was a physician who saw patients with chronic pain, was primarily a basic neuroscientist who was concerned about the then-prevalent thinking in neurophysiology that the nervous system was a system of immutable specialized pathways, each carrying out unique functions related to sensation or motor behavior. He rejected the idea that the underlying mechanisms of persistent pain after injury could be explained by such a rigid neural organization.

Bonica was an anesthesiologist who treated thousands of pain patients and saw chronic persistent pain as "a malefic force that often imposes severe emotional, physical, economic, and sociologic stresses on the patient as well as his family as well as on society" (Bonica 1976). He not only tackled the problem clinically, but also used his own emotional, spiritual, and physical strength to convince government agencies, scientists, and clinicians to band together to eliminate or reduce these terrible conditions that afflicted millions of people worldwide, lessening the quality of human life and costing billions of dollars annually in health services. He concluded that adequate knowledge of chronic pain conditions would only come from the combined efforts of research scientists and clinicians who exchanged their facts and ideas and tested hypotheses that would lead to new knowledge and ulti-mately to improved treatments for persistent pain. At a meeting in Issaquah, Washington, in 1973, Bonica realized his multidisciplinary vision by bring-ing together 350 physicians, scientists, and other health professionals from 13 countries, representing almost every basic science and clinical discipline interested in the study of pain. Besides the sharing of a multitude of research knowledge and ideas that propelled the field forward at a rapid pace, the meeting led to the formation of the IASP under Bonica's forceful direction, and to the beginnings of the journal, *Pain,* the first multidisciplinary journal devoted to the study of pain, under Wall's innovative and dynamic editorship.

THE STATE OF PAIN RESEARCH IN THE EARLY 1970S

Insight into the state of the pain research field in the early 1970s can be gained from a perusal of the proceedings of the Issaquah conference (Bonica 1974) and those of the 1st World Congress on Pain (Bonica and Albe-Fessard 1976). These meetings were preceded in the late 1960s and early 1970s by the discovery and thorough analysis of specialized receptors in target tissues (mainly the skin at that time) that responded almost exclu-sively and in a stimulus-intensity-dependent fashion to tissue-damaging stimu-lation (Bessou and Perl 1969; Iggo and Ogawa 1971; Burgess and Perl 1973). The gate control theory of pain published in 1965 by Melzack and Wall was a prominent discussion point at these meetings since it had led to an avalanche of studies testing its hypotheses. Among new discoveries were specialized peripheral receptors that signaled tissue damage and a class of spinal cord dorsal horn neurons that responded exclusively to intense forms of mechanical and thermal stimulation (Christensen and Perl 1970; Handwerker et al. 1975). These findings supported the view that pain infor-mation was coded by a unique neural apparatus that transmitted the physical and chemical attributes of tissue damage in an immutable fashion to at least the level of the dorsal horn. Similar findings were reported for the trigeminal system innervating the face and mouth, both at the level of primary afferent neurons and in the trigeminal homologue of the spinal dorsal horn in the brainstem (see Sessle, this volume).

However, it was puzzling to many that the responses of these special-ized neurons in the spinal dorsal horn were subject to sensory modulation by input from nerve fibers that were not part of this unique system. For ex-ample, activation of Aβ mechanoreceptive afferent fibers inhibited or sup-pressed the activity of these neurons (Iggo et al. 1976). Furthermore,

Liebeskind and colleagues (1974) published their exciting findings that the brain appeared to have endogenous opioid-dependent pain-suppressing systems originating in the brainstem and other levels of the central nervous system (CNS) that could be activated to suppress behavioral responses to painful input. Liebeskind also presented evidence at the Issaquah meeting, based on studies he had conducted with Jean-Marie Besson in Paris, that the responses of spinal dorsal horn neurons activated by noxious stimulation could be suppressed by stimulation of this descending system (Liebeskind et al. 1974). It was also becoming clear that inputs from the cerebral cortex could modify the output of dorsal horn neurons, including those that responded to noxious stimulation (Coulter et al. 1976). Other findings supported the idea that deafferentation led to a loss of central inhibition leading to hyperactivity in the spinal cord and its homologue in the trigeminal system, the trigeminal nucleus caudalis or medullary dorsal horn. These findings let to the decision that the major theme of the 1st World Congress would be "modulation."

For many reasons, I have outlined the multidisciplinary nature and the state of the field in the early 1970s as an introduction to the major topic of this paper, activity-dependent plasticity in the nervous system. First, a number of findings presented at that time were predictive of our present state of knowledge. Second, I want to contrast modulation with plasticity. Third, it is clear that the strong interest by Bonica and Wall in chronic pain conditions and their influence on these meetings was a strong impetus for basic science research at the time. It ultimately led to the development of new animal models of persistent pain and the study of peripheral and central nervous system changes after tissue or nerve injury (the simplest definition of plasticity). Fourth, it is also clear that plasticity was on the agenda even at that time. The findings of peripheral sensitization produced by tissue injury in spinal and trigeminal afferent fibers (Bessou and Perl 1969; Beitel and Dubner 1976) are clearly a form of activity-dependent plasticity. The discovery of ectopic discharges from neuromas formed after nerve transection is another form of plasticity (Wall and Gutnick 1974), and these findings influenced the development of animal models of nerve injury, discussed below. Finally, the discoveries of various forms of modulation in nociceptive pathways suggested the possibility that CNS synaptic connectivity and receptor sensitivity may change after injury and may form the underlying basis of what we now refer to as activity-dependent plasticity in the nervous system and central sensitization in pain transmission pathways (Woolf 1983; Woolf and Wall 1986; Dubner 1991).

SENSORY MODULATION

Sensory modulation of pain transmission in the CNS refers to excitatory and inhibitory signals from other sites that modify the encoding of sensory information in ascending nociceptive pathways. In contrast, activity-dependent plasticity refers to changes in anatomical and functional connectivity produced by activity that outlasts the stimulus and includes molecular changes in gene and protein expression as well as in post-translational processing. The concept of sensory modulation was embodied in the gate control theory, which recognized the importance of sensory convergence, inhibition, and descending control in contributing to the transmission of signals related to tissue damage in the nervous system (Melzack and Wall 1965). Although the gate theory proposed some specific mechanisms that have not withstood the test of time, it predicted that certain types of neuronal responses were necessary in order to account for many of the sensory features of persistent and pathological pain. Some quotes from Wall's chapter in the proceedings of the Issaquah meeting (Wall 1974) are illustrative:

> "If the cells which send messages to the head and tend to put the sensorium into a pain posture are fired by both noxious and innocuous stimuli, then we have possible explanations for some of the curious concomitants of pain such as tenderness. These cells can be examined under conditions of pathology to see if the time course of their discharge imitates that of pain triggered by gentle stimuli ..."

Thus, a prediction of the neural events that could account for mechanical allodynia associated with inflammatory and neuropathic pain, and a concept that encouraged the discovery of animal models of persistent pain. Again:

> "... the presence of inhibition which is triggered by particular afferent stimuli. It is this fact which opened the possibility of explaining some pains by the absence of this inhibition and of generating new therapies by stimulating the inhibition either by electrical ... or by chemical stimulation."

Thus, a prediction of approaches to attenuate persistent pain by amplification of inhibitory afferent and descending systems, and a concept that has encouraged drug discovery of agents that enhance central inhibition. Again: "Some afferents trigger excitation followed by further excitation ..." Thus, the prediction that activity could lead to enhanced activity, a prediction of activity-dependent plasticity, which plays a dominant role in hyperexcitability or central sensitization.

Finally: "we must ask in a particular patient if the descending controls from the brain are in their normally functioning state or are they amplifying the central effects of the afferent barrage." Further: "The discovery of the nature, location and pharmacology of the descending controls probably offers the most powerful chance for the development of future understanding and therapy." Thus, the prediction of descending facilitation, which had not yet been reported, and its importance in deep-tissue persistent pain conditions such as fibromyalgia, temporomandibular disorders, and irritable bowel syndrome. The final quote above points to a prediction still to be judged in the future.

ACTIVITY-DEPENDENT PLASTICITY IN NOCICEPTIVE SYSTEMS

The last three decades since the origins of the IASP have produced three major areas of discovery that contribute significantly to our understanding of persistent pain and its management. I like to refer to these as *sensory coding,* or how the nervous system extracts stimulus feature information such as quality, intensity, and duration from the environment; *descending modulation,* or how that information is modified by control systems in the brain; and *activity-dependent neuronal plasticity,* or how persistent neuronal activity leads to changes in neural function and resulting amplification of pain. In the remainder of this chapter I would like to focus on the discoveries related to plasticity that have enhanced our knowledge of central mechanisms of sensory coding and descending modulation and our understanding of persistent pain. Evidence for central neuronal plasticity during the formative years of the IASP was completely lacking. A discussion of peripheral nervous system plasticity is provided by Gold (this volume).

The gate control theory and other models lacked adequate explanations for hyperalgesia and allodynia following injury. Important discoveries were made in the 1980s and early 1990s on neuronal plasticity in response to the persistent neuronal barrage associated with tissue and nerve injury (Woolf 1983; Woolf and Wall 1986; Dubner 1991; Torebjork et al. 1992). We now know that pain that persists for days, or even just hours, leads to long-term changes in the CNS that amplify and prolong the pain.

Much of this new knowledge came about following the development of animal models of tissue and nerve injury that produced hyperalgesia and allodynia. My colleagues and I at the National Institutes of Health (NIH) at that time used the injection of complete Freund's adjuvant (CFA) or carrageenan to produce inflammation of the rat hindpaw. We used paw-withdrawal latency as a measure of inflammatory hyperalgesia and allodynia (Hargreaves et al. 1987; Iadarola et al. 1988). Other models of inflammation have been developed to help discover the underlying mechanisms of persistent inflammatory pain (Dubner and Ren 1999). Models of hyperalgesia and allodynia produced by nerve injury also were developed (Bennett and Xie 1988; Seltzer et al. 1990; Kim and Chung 1991) and have significantly enhanced our understanding of neuropathic pain. The "Bennett" model was discovered in our laboratory at the NIH, and I had the pleasure of collaborating in the discovery of the "Seltzer "model in Jerusalem.

What are the CNS mechanisms responsible for hyperalgesia associated with tissue and nerve injury? One can study spinal dorsal horn neuronal activity to examine changes in excitability after tissue or nerve injury. One measure of an increase in excitability is an enlargement of the receptive fields (RFs) of neurons. We and others have shown that an increased peripheral barrage produced by electrical stimulation, inflammation, or nerve injury leads to an enlargement of RFs and increased excitability in response to mechanical and thermal stimulation (Menetrey and Besson 1982; Cook et al. 1987; Hylden et al. 1989). The enlargement in RF size, which parallels the time course of development of the inflammatory hyperalgesia, can be seen as early as 4 hours after the injection of the inflammatory agent. RF enlargement leads to more neurons activated by a stimulus than the number activated in the absence of RF expansion. The increase in neuronal activity may ultimately be perceived as more intense pain or hyperalgesia. Similar findings of increased excitability have been found at the level of the trigeminal system (see Sessle, this volume). Woolf, Wall, and colleagues referred to the increase in excitability in the spinal dorsal horn as "central sensitization," and that term has received wide acceptance in the pain literature. Unfortunately, the term has often been confused with phenomena such as "wind-up" (Mendell 1966), which is an example of sensory modulation. The same term also has been used to describe psychophysical measures of increases in response to noxious stimuli where the underlying mechanism is unknown. It is clear, however, based in studies in the last decade, that central sensitization is a form of activity-dependent plasticity at the spinal cord and trigeminal levels that mechanistically resembles plasticity seen in the hippocampus and cerebral cortex related to learning and memory (Woolf and Salter 2000; Ji et al. 2003).

Central sensitization in the spinal cord appears to involve excitation at receptor sites activated by excitatory amino acids and neuropeptides such as substance P and brain-derived neurotrophic factor (BDNF) (Ren et al. 1992; Woolf and Salter 2000). Transient pain, the normal response to acute noxious stimuli, is largely mediated by glutamate acting at its AMPA (α-amino-

3-hydroxy-5-methyl-4-isoxazole propionic acid) receptor on dorsal horn neurons, providing a rapid, protective pain-warning system in the brain. The channel of this ionotropic receptor is selective mainly for sodium. If the injury persists, glutamate continues to be released from the central endings of nociceptive afferent neurons along with substance P. The metabotropic glutamate receptor and the neurokinin-1 receptor, activated by glutamate and substance P, respectively, are G-protein-coupled receptors that lead to the activation of second-messenger systems, resulting in the release of calcium from intracellular stores. With the initiation of synaptic depolarization via the above receptors, the voltage-dependent magnesium block of the *N*-methyl-D-aspartate (NMDA) ion channel is removed, and glutamate release results in the influx of calcium into the cell and the activation of calcium-dependent kinases including protein kinase C and Src. Calcium is a critical player in the process because many protein kinases in the cell are dependent upon calcium influx or calcium release from intracellular stores for their activation. These protein kinases participate in the phosphorylation of membrane-bound receptors and ion channels. Finally, BDNF, a neurotrophin acting at tyrosine receptor kinase B (trk B), is released and plays a role in phosphorylating proteins in subunits of the NMDA receptor. The NMDA receptor is the best-characterized glutamate receptor, and its phosphorylation is a major factor in central sensitization and the resulting hyperalgesia. Phosphorylation of the NMDA receptor sensitizes the receptor so that its subsequent responsiveness to synaptically released glutamate is enhanced, increasing synaptic strength and allowing subthreshold inputs to reach threshold levels. This amplification of the response alters receptive field properties and increases sensitivity to subsequent stimulation, resulting in allodynia and hyperalgesia.

The prevailing hypothesis has been that the activity of calcium-dependent kinases was dependent on the influx of calcium into cells through calcium-permeable channels of the NMDA and AMPA receptors, as well as through voltage-gated calcium channels in the cell membrane (Woolf and Salter 2000). Our recent data indicate that the initiation of behavioral hyperalgesia and allodynia and central sensitization in the spinal dorsal horn requires activation of Group I metabotropic glutamate receptors and possibly other G-protein-coupled receptors on dorsal horn neurons and their coupling to the NMDA receptor (Guo et al. 2002). These findings suggest the importance of mGluR-NMDA coupling in the priming of the NMDA receptor for the initiation of central sensitization.

It has been known since the early 1990s that NMDA-receptor antagonists significantly attenuate the hyperalgesia induced by tissue inflammation and by partial nerve injury (Ren et al. 1992; Tal and Bennett 1994). If an

NMDA-receptor antagonist such as MK-801 is injected intrathecally, thus having its effect at the spinal level, there is a dose-dependent attenuation of the hyperalgesia. Similarly, the expanded receptive fields of pain transmission neurons following inflammation can be blocked or reduced by the administration of NMDA-receptor antagonists (Ren et al. 1992).

Inflammation of the rat hindpaw also produces increases in the expression of genes that code for neuropeptides such as the opioid peptides, dynorphin and enkephalin, with a time course that parallels the behavioral hyperalgesia (Iadarola et al. 1988; Ruda et al. 1988; Dubner and Ruda 1992). The neurons showing increased gene expression are localized to the superficial laminae and to the neck of the dorsal horn, the two regions of the dorsal horn that contain neurons involved in pain transmission. In animal models of nerve injury, there also is a large increase in dynorphin gene expression that parallels the behavioral hyperalgesia (Draisci et al. 1991).

The increased sensitivity of excitatory amino acids during the development of inflammation also appears to be related to transcriptional, translational, and post-translational changes. NMDA receptors are heteromers mainly of NR1 and NR2 subunits. There are three regions of alternative splicing, named N1, C1, and C2 cassettes, on the NR1 protein. In other systems, serine residues (896/897) on the C1 cassette are phosphorylated upon activation of protein kinases (Tingley et al. 1997). The AMPA receptor consists of four subunits, namely GluR1–4. The GluR1 subunit has two serine phosphorylation sites (831 and 845) that have been carefully studied in other systems (Mammen et al. 1997). Our recent studies have shown an increase in total NR1 and GluR1 proteins and an upregulation of GluR1 mRNAs after CFA-induced inflammation (Zhou et al. 2001; Guo et al. 2005). The increase in total protein levels suggests an increased turnover related to enhanced synaptic transmission in the spinal dorsal horn due to the inflammation. Our studies have also shown an increase in the phosphorylation of NR1 serine 896, GluR1 serine 831, and GluR1 serine 845 after CFA inflammation (Guo et al. 2005). In addition, CFA inflammation leads to tyrosine phosphorylation of the NR2B subunit of the NMDA receptor, without any changes in transcription or translation of this subunit (Guo et al. 2002). The post-translational changes of the NR1, NR2, and GluR1 subunits occur typically within 10 minutes of the onset of inflammation, correlate highly with the onset of behavioral hyperalgesia, and are dependent on the persistence of primary afferent drive (Guo et al. 2002, 2005). The studies cited indicate that these changes are important in the *initiation* of inflammatory hyperalgesia and central sensitization; however, their roles in the *maintenance* of the hyperalgesia and central sensitization are less clear.

We proposed a model a number of years ago in which increased nociceptor activity at the site of tissue or nerve injury leads to spinal cord dorsal horn hyperexcitability and behavioral hyperalgesia (Dubner 1991). Although the mechanisms of increased activity arising from the sites of tissue and nerve injury are different, both types of injury increase the neuronal barrage reaching the CNS. Increased neural activity from the periphery will enhance depolarization or excitation at receptor sites. The result is an expansion of receptive fields and hyperexcitability that leads to an increase in pain. This hyperexcitability, or central sensitization, if excessive, can lead to a pathological state by promoting excitotoxicity, cell dysfunction, and a loss of inhibitory mechanisms (Moore et al. 2002). The combined effects of excessive excitation and loss of inhibition would further contribute to the expansion of receptive fields, hyperexcitability, and amplification and prolongation of pain.

These findings of central sensitization have important clinical implications. We can now develop strategies to reduce the peripheral barrage originating at the site of injury or to reduce its effects on nociceptive neurons in the CNS. It appears that persistent pain is not only initiated, but sometimes maintained, by residual peripheral nerve activity associated with the injury (Gracely et al. 1992; Guo et al. 2002, 2005). A number of studies have also shown that central sensitization is of greater magnitude and more prolonged after deep tissue injury of muscle or viscera. This finding has important implications for chronic pain conditions associated with deep tissues such as temporomandibular disorders, low back pain, and fibromyalgia, where pain spreads to distant and multiple sites.

DESCENDING MODULATION AFTER TISSUE INJURY

The studies I have described above have focused almost entirely on the role of primary afferent neurons and intrinsic spinal cord neurons in dorsal horn neuronal plasticity. The role of the third major component system in the dorsal horn, the axon terminals of descending pathways, has recently received attention in the study of persistent pain produced by injury. Descending mechanisms are important because they provide neural networks by which cognitive, attentional, and emotional aspects of the pain experience modulate pain transmission at the spinal and trigeminal levels.

Considerable evidence now shows that descending circuitry is enhanced after tissue inflammation and nerve injury and involves inhibitory and facilitatory mechanisms (Porreca et al. 2002; Ren and Dubner 2002). The origins of our knowledge of endogenous descending modulatory circuitry and recent findings on its role in hyperalgesia and descending facilitation are discussed in detail by Ossipov and Porreca (this volume). We and others have demonstrated, however, that following inflammation, brainstem descending inhibitory pathways become progressively more involved in suppressing incoming sensory signals originating from primary hyperalgesic zones (Schaible et al. 1991; Ren and Dubner 1996; Danziger et al. 1999; Hurley and Hammond 2000; Terayama et al. 2000).

We have studied the molecular, cellular, and neurochemical mechanisms that underlie descending modulation after inflammation. We asked the following question: Are these changes merely a reflection of enhanced activity ascending from spinal cord levels to the brainstem, or is there also an increase in excitability at the level of the rostral ventromedial medulla (RVM) (i.e., activity-dependent plasticity)? The dynamic changes in descending inhibition after inflammation can be examined over time by monitoring nocifensive responses in lightly anesthetized rats during stimulation of the RVM (Terayama et al. 2000; Guan et al. 2002). In these studies, we have demonstrated that dynamic temporal changes in synaptic activation occur in the brainstem after inflammation. Early in the development of inflammation there is increased descending facilitation, which reduces the net effect of the inhibition. Over time, the level of descending inhibition increases, or descending facilitation decreases, leading to a net enhancement of antinocifensive behavior.

What are the cellular mechanisms that underlie these changes? Excitatory amino acids (EAAs) mediate descending modulation in response to transient noxious stimulation and early inflammation (Heinricher et al. 1999; Urban and Gebhart 1999), and they appear to be involved in the development of RVM excitability associated with inflammation and persistent pain (Terayama et al. 2000; Miki et al. 2002; Guan et al. 2002). At 3 hours post-inflammation, low doses of NMDA facilitate the response of the inflamed hindpaw to noxious heat, supporting previous findings that descending facilitatory effects are NMDA dependent and occur early after inflammation (Urban and Gebhart 1999). Higher doses of NMDA 3 hours after inflammation only produce inhibition. At 24 hours post-inflammation, NMDA produces only inhibition in a dose-dependent fashion. These effects are blocked by administration of NMDA-receptor antagonists. AMPA produces dose-dependent and time-dependent levels of inhibition at all doses at 3 and 24 hours post-inflammation. These effects are blocked by an AMPA-receptor antagonist. These findings indicate a leftward shift of the dose-response curves of NMDA- and AMPA-produced inhibition at 24 hours post-inflammation as compared to 3 hours. The leftward shift of the dose-response curves of these EAA-receptor agonists parallels the time-dependent enhancement of net descending inhibition produced by RVM electrical stimulation, which is also attenuated by NMDA-receptor antagonists (Terayama et al. 2000). The results suggest that the time-dependent functional changes in descending modulation are mediated, in part, by enhanced EAA neurotransmission.

Rats with inflammatory hyperalgesia exhibit an increased sensitivity to opioid analgesics (Neil et al. 1986; Hylden et al. 1991). Typically, there is a leftward shift of the dose-response curve for opioids from the inflamed hyperalgesic paw when compared to the non-inflamed paw (Hylden et al. 1991). Hurley and Hammond (2000) have demonstrated enhancement of the descending inhibitory effects of μ and δ_2 opioid receptor agonists microinjected into the RVM during the development and maintenance of persistent inflammatory hyperalgesia. It is likely that opioid peptide activation and γ-aminobutyric acid (GABA) disinhibition (Fields and Basbaum 1999) are also important in the initiation and maintenance of RVM plasticity.

In recent studies we have examined whether transcriptional, translational, and post-translational changes occur in the RVM after inflammation and whether they may underlie the changes in sensitivity we have observed. Increases in gene expression of subunits of the NMDA and AMPA receptors could lead to more receptors trafficking to the cell membrane and could enhance their participation in the sensitization. Changes in the affinity of the receptors for glutamate and other receptor agonists could also occur due to the phosphorylation of receptor subunits. Examination of the mRNA and protein expression of the NR1, NR2A, and NR2B subunits of the NMDA receptor in the RVM revealed an upregulation that parallels the time course of the RVM excitability changes (Miki et al. 2002). Western blot analysis also reveals a time-dependent increase in the AMPA receptor GluR1 subunit levels in the RVM as compared to naive animals (Guan et al. 2003). Using an antibody that recognizes the phospho-GluR1 subunit at the serine 831 residue, Western blots also demonstrated that GluR1 phosphoprotein levels were increased as early as 30 minutes after inflammation, suggesting that post-translational receptor phosphorylation may also contribute to the enhanced AMPA transmission (Guan et al. 2004). More recently, we used immunoprecipitation and Western blot methodology to demonstrate that there is also an increase in phosphorylation of the NR2A subunit of the NMDA receptor (Turnbach et al. 2003). These findings support our hypothesis that activity-dependent plasticity takes place at the RVM level and involves changes in EAA-receptor gene and protein expression and increased phosphorylation of these receptors.

This activity-induced plasticity in pain-modulating circuitry after inflammation complements the activity-dependent neuronal plasticity in ascending pain transmission pathways discussed earlier. Inflammation leads to peripheral sensitization of nociceptors and central sensitization or activity-dependent plasticity of spinal nociceptive neurons. The increased neuronal barrage at the spinal level activates spinomedullary projection neurons, which in turn activates glutamatergic, opioidergic, and presumably GABAergic neurons at the brainstem level and causes a similar but not identical form of activity-dependent plasticity. It is likely that transmission sites at multiple levels in nociceptive pathways exhibit enhanced sensitivity in the face of a persistent neuronal barrage associated with tissue or nerve injury.

CONCLUSION

We have come a long way since the findings of the early 1970s and the beginnings of the IASP. The visions of Wall and Bonica have led to significant new knowledge of the underlying mechanisms of persistent pain, and it is clear that the multidisciplinary nature of the pain field has been a major factor in these advances. I quote Patrick Wall again from his chapter in the proceedings of the Issaquah conference as he guides us into the future (Wall 1974):

"In the challenge of pain, the clinician and the basic scientist ... play ... an interdependent role. It is the job of the clinician to collect and describe the phenomena of the real world. ... He must organize his facts in terms of questions and see to it that the basic scientist understands the facts. He must be ready to collect more facts and to check theories against facts. The basic scientist must grapple with the entirety of the real facts and not just select the easy and convenient phenomena and ignore or deny the uneasy ones. This then I see to be the shape of the future, not a collaboration in which everyone does everybody else's job but a mutual feeling and encouragement for the benefit of the patients."

REFERENCES

Beitel RE, Dubner R. Responses of unmyelinated (C) polymodal nociceptors to thermal stimuli applied to monkey's face. *J Neurophysiol* 1976; 39:11660–11675.

Bennett GJ, Xie Y. A peripheral mono-neuropathy in rat that produces disorders of pain sensation like those seen in man. *Pain* 1988; 33:87–107.

Bessou P, Perl ER. Response of cutaneous sensory units with unmyelinated fibers to noxious stimuli. *J Neurophysiol* 1969; 32:1025–1043.

Bonica JJ (Ed). *International Symposium on Pain,* Advances in Neurology, Vol. 4. New York: Raven Press, 1974.

Bonica JJ. Introduction to the First World Congress on Pain. In: Bonica JJ, Albe-Fessard DG (Eds). *Proceedings of the First World Congress on Pain,* Advances in Pain Research and Therapy, Vol. 1. New York: Raven Press, 1976, pp xxvii–xxxix.

Bonica JJ, Albe-Fessard DG (Eds). *Proceedings of the First World Congress on Pain,* Advances in Pain Research and Therapy, Vol. 1. New York: Raven Press, 1976.

Burgess PR, Perl ER. Cutaneous mechanoreceptors and nociceptors. In: Iggo A (Ed). *Somatosensory System,* Handbook of Sensory Physiology, Vol. 2. Heidelberg: Springer, 1973, pp 29–78.

Christensen BN, Perl ER. Spinal neurons specifically excited by noxious or thermal stimuli: marginal zone of the dorsal horn. *J Neurophysiol* 1970; 33:293–307.

Cook AJ, Woolf CJ, Wall PD, McMahon SB. Dynamic receptive field plasticity in rat spinal cord dorsal horn following C-primary afferent input. *Nature* 1987; 325:151–153.

Coulter JD, Foreman RD, Beall, JE, Willis WD. Cerebral cortical modulation of primate spinothalamic neurons. In: Bonica JJ, Albe-Fessard DG (Eds). *Proceedings of the First World Congress on Pain,* Advances in Pain Research and Therapy, Vol. 1. New York: Raven Press, 1976, pp 271–277.

Danziger N, Weil-Fugazza J, Le Bars D, Bouhassira D. Alteration of descending modulation of nociception during the course of monoarthritis in the rat. *J Neurosci* 1999; 19:2394–2400.

Draisci G, Kajander KC, Dubner R, Bennett GJ, Iadarola MJ. Up-regulation of opioid gene expression in spinal cord evoked by experimental nerve injuries and inflammation. *Brain Res* 1991; 50:186–192.

Dubner R. Neuronal plasticity and pain following peripheral tissue inflammation or nerve injury. In: Bond MR, Charlton JE, Woolf CJ (Eds). *Proceedings of the 6th World Congress on Pain.* Amsterdam: Elsevier, 1991, pp 263–276.

Dubner R, Ren K. Assessing transient and persistent pain in animals. In: Wall PD, Melzack R (Eds). *Textbook of Pain,* 4th ed. London: Churchill Livingstone, 1999, pp 359–369.

Dubner R, Ruda MA. Activity-dependent neuronal plasticity following tissue injury and inflammation. *Trends Neurosci* 1992; 15:96–103.

Fields HL, Basbaum AI. Central nervous system mechanisms of pain modulation. In: Wall PD, Melzack R (Eds). *Textbook of Pain,* 4th ed. London: Churchill Livingstone, 1999, pp 309–329.

Gracely RH, Lynch SA, Bennett GJ. Painful neuropathy: altered central processing maintained dynamically by peripheral input. *Pain* 1992; 51:175–194.

Guan Y, Terayama R, Dubner R, Ren K. Plasticity in excitatory amino acid receptor-mediated descending pain modulation after inflammation. *J Pharmacol Exp Ther* 2002; 300:513–520.

Guan Y, Guo W, Zou S-P, Dubner R, Ren K. Inflammation-induced upregulation of AMPA receptor subunit expression in brain stem pain modulatory circuitry. *Pain* 2003; 104:401–413.

Guan Y, Guo W, Robbins MT, Dubner R, Ren K. Changes in AMPA receptor phosphorylation in the rostral ventromedial medulla after inflammation. *Neurosci Lett* 2004; 366(2):201–205.

Guo W, Zou S-P, Guan Y, et al. Tyrosine phosphorylation of the NR2B subunit of the NMDA receptor in the spinal cord during the development and maintenance of inflammatory hyperalgesia. *J Neurosci* 2002; 22:6208–6217.

Guo W, Zou S-P, Ikeda T, Dubner R. Rapid and lasting increase in serine phosphorylation of rat spinal cord NMDAR1 and GluR1 subunits after peripheral inflammation. *Thalamus Relat Syst* 2005; in press.

Handwerker HO, Iggo A, Zimmermann M. Segmental and supraspinal actions on dorsal horn neurons responding to noxious and non-noxious skin stimuli. *Pain* 1975; 1:147–165.

Hargreaves K, Dubner R, Brown F, Flores C, Joris JA. New and sensitive method for measuring thermal nociception in cutaneous hyperalgesia. *Pain* 1987; 32:77–88.

Heinricher MM, McGaraughty S, Farr DA. The role of excitatory amino acid transmission within the rostral ventromedial medulla in the antinociceptive actions of systemically administered morphine. *Pain* 1999; 81:57–65.

Hurley RW, Hammond DL. The analgesic effects of supraspinal mu and delta opioid receptor agonists are potentiated during persistent inflammation. *J Neurosci* 2000; 20:1249–1259.

Hylden JLK, Nahin RL, Traub RJ, Dubner R. Expansion of receptive fields of spinal lamina I projection neurons in rats with unilateral adjuvant-induced inflammation: the contribution of dorsal horn mechanisms. *Pain* 1989; 37:229–243.

Hylden JLK, Thomas DA, Iadarola MJ, Dubner R. Spinal opioid analgesic effects are enhanced in a model of unilateral inflammation/hyperalgesia: possible involvement of noradrenergic mechanisms. *Eur J Pharmacol* 1991; 194:135–143.

Iadarola MJ, Brady LS, Draisci G, Dubner R. Enhancement of dynorphin gene expression in spinal cord following experimental inflammation: stimulus specificity, behavioral parameters and opioid receptor binding. *Pain* 1988; 35:313–326.

Iggo A, Ogawa H. Primate cutaneous thermal nociceptors. *J Physiol* 1971; 216:77P.

Iggo A, Ogawa H, Cervero F. Inhibition of nociceptor-driven dorsal horn neurons in the cat. In: Bonica JJ, Albe-Fessard DG (Eds). *Proceedings of the First World Congress on Pain,* Advances in Pain Research and Therapy, Vol. 1. New York: Raven Press, 1976, pp 99–104.

Ji R-R, Kohno T, Moore KA, Woolf CJ. Central sensitization and LTP: do pain and memory share similar mechanisms? *Trends Neurosci* 2003; 26:696–706.

Kim SH, Chung JM. Sympathectomy alleviates mechanical allodynia in an experimental animal model for neuropathy in the rat. *Neurosci Lett* 1991; 134:131–134.

Liebeskind JC, Mayer DJ, Akil H. Central mechanisms of pain inhibition: studies of analgesia from focal brain stimulation. In: JJ Bonica (Ed). *International Symposium on Pain,* Advances in Neurology, Vol. 4. New York: Raven Press, 1974, pp 261–268.

Mammen AL, Kameyama K, Roche KW, Huganir RL. Phosphorylation of the alpha-amino-3-hydroxy-5-methylisoxazole-4-propionic acid receptor GluR1 subunit by calcium/calmodulin-dependent kinase II. *J Biol Chem* 1997; 272:32528–32533.

Melzack R, Wall PD. Pain mechanisms: a new theory. *Science* 1965; 150:971–979.

Mendell LM. Physiological properties of unmyelinated fiber projection to the spinal cord. *Exp Neurol* 1966; 16:316–332.

Menetrey D, Besson JM. Electrophysiological characteristics of dorsal horn cells in rats with cutaneous inflammation resulting from chronic arthritis. *Pain* 1982; 13:343–364.

Miki K, Zhou QQ, Guo W, et al. Changes in gene expression and neuronal phenotype in brain stem pain modulatory circuitry after inflammation. *J Neurophysiol* 2002; 87:750–760.

Moore KA, Kohno T, Karchewski LA, et al. Partial nerve injury promotes a selective loss of GABAergic inhibition in the superficial dorsal horn of the spinal cord. *J Neurosci* 2002; 22:6724–6731.

Neil A, Kayser V, Gacel G, Besson J-M, Guilbaud G. Opioid receptor types and antinociceptive activity in chronic inflammation: both kappa and mu opiate agonistic effects are enhanced in arthritic rats. *Eur J Pharmacol* 1986; 130:203–208.

Porreca F, Ossipov MH, Gebhart GF. Chronic pain and medullary descending facilitation. *Trends Neurosci* 2002; 25:319–325.

Ren K, Dubner R. Enhanced descending modulation of nociception in rats with persistent hindpaw inflammation. *J Neurophysiol* 1996; 76:3025–3037.

Ren K, Dubner R. Descending modulation in persistent pain: an update. *Pain* 2002; 100:1–6.

Ren K, Hylden JLK, Williams GM, Ruda MA, Dubner R. The effects of a non-competitive NMDA receptor antagonist, MK-801, on behavioral hyperalgesia and dorsal horn neuronal activity in rats with unilateral inflammation. *Pain* 1992; 50:331–344.

Ruda MA, Iadarola MJ, Cohen LV, Young WS III. In situ hybridization histochemistry and immunocytochemistry reveal an increase in spinal dynorphin biosynthesis in a rat model of peripheral inflammation and hyperalgesia. *Proc Natl Acad Sci USA* 1988; 85:622–626.

Schaible HG, Neugebauer V, Cervero F, Schmidt RF. Changes in tonic descending inhibition of spinal neurons with articular input during the development of acute arthritis in the cat. *J Neurophysiol* 1991; 66:1021–1032.

Seltzer Z, Dubner R, Shir Y. A novel behavioral model of neuropathic pain disorders produced in rats by partial sciatic nerve injury. *Pain* 1990; 43:205–218.

Tal M, Bennett GJ. Neuropathic pain sensations are differentially sensitive to dextrorphan. *Neuroreport* 1994; 5:1438–1440.

Terayama R, Guan Y, Dubner R, Ren K. Activity-induced plasticity in brain stem pain modulatory circuitry after inflammation. *Neuroreport* 2000; 11:1915–1919.

Tingley WG, Ehlers MD, Kameyama K, et al. Characterization of protein kinase A and protein kinase C phosphorylation of the N-methyl-D-aspartate receptor NR1 subunit using phosphorylation site-specific antibodies. *J Biol Chem* 1997; 272:5157–5166.

Torebjork HE, Lundberg LER, LaMotte RH. Central changes in processing of mechanoreceptive input in capsaicin-induced secondary hyperalgesia in humans. *J Physiol (Lond)* 1992; 448:765–780.

Turnbach ME, Guo W, Dubner R, Ren K. Inflammation induces tyrosine phosphorylation of the NR2A subunit and serine phosphorylation of the NR1 subunits in the rat rostral ventromedial medulla. *Soc Neurosci Abstr* 2003; 29.

Urban MO, Gebhart GF. Supraspinal contributions to hyperalgesia. *Proc Natl Acad Sci USA* 1999; 96:7687–7692.

Wall PD. The future of attacks on pain. In: JJ Bonica (Ed.) *International Symposium on Pain, Advances in Neurology*, Vol. 4. New York: Raven Press, 1974, pp 301–308.

Wall PD, Gutnick M. Properties of afferent nerve impulses originating from a neuroma. *Nature (Lond)* 1974; 248:740–743.

Woolf CJ. Evidence for a central component of post-injury pain hypersensitivity. *Nature* 1983; 306:686–688.

Woolf CJ, Salter MW. Neuronal plasticity: increasing the gain in pain. *Science* 2000; 288:1765–1768.

Woolf CJ, Wall PD. Relative effectiveness of C primary afferent fibers of different origins in evoking a prolonged facilitation of the flexor reflex in the rat. *J Neurosci* 1986; 6:1433–1442.

Zhou QQ, Imbe H, Zou S, et al. Selective upregulation of the flip-flop splice variants of AMPA receptor subunits in the rat spinal cord after hindpaw inflammation. *Mol Brain Res* 2001; 88:186–193.

Correspondence to: Ronald Dubner, DDS, PhD, Department of Biomedical Sciences, University of Maryland Dental School, 666 West Baltimore Street, Room 5E-10, Baltimore, MD 21201, USA. Email: rnd001@dental.umaryland.edu.

The Paths of Pain 1975–2005, edited by
Harold Merskey, John D. Loeser, and Ronald
Dubner, IASP Press, Seattle, © 2005.

8

Descending Modulation of Pain

Michael H. Ossipov and Frank Porreca

*Department of Pharmacology, University of Arizona Health Sciences Center,
Tucson, Arizona, USA*

At the time of the founding of the International Association for the Study of Pain (IASP) in 1973, the concept that endogenous mechanisms may modulate pain was only beginning to take root. The gate control theory of Melzack and Wall (1965) had been published a scant 8 years earlier. The publication of this theory is considered to be the first attempt to provide for an endogenous physiological mechanism through which pain may be modulated. At about the same time that the gate control theory was presented, it was discovered that the microinjection of morphine into the midbrain periaqueductal gray (PAG), or electrical stimulation of this region, produced powerful antinociception (Tsou and Jang 1964; Reynolds 1969). These discoveries were rapidly followed by the characterization of stereospecific receptors for opioids and by the identification of endogenous peptides that activated these receptors (Pert and Snyder 1973; Simon 1973; Terenius 1973; Hughes et al. 1975). The rapid succession of these important discoveries represented a quantum leap in our understanding of mechanisms that mediate and control pain and ushered in the current era of intense pain research. With the birth of the IASP, the concept that pain may be a sensory modality independent of the five senses began to receive acceptance, and the field of pain research as a discipline in its own right was born. This chapter provides an overview of advances made in understanding descending pain modulation systems from the time of the first IASP congress to our current state of knowledge, with an eye toward future avenues of exploration.

DESCENDING MODULATION OF PAIN

THE PERIAQUEDUCTAL GRAY

Electrophysiological techniques and single-unit recordings from the spinal dorsal horn and from the medullary trigeminal nucleus demonstrated that selective primary afferent neurons respond specifically to noxious or tissue-damaging stimuli. The primary afferent nociceptors synapse onto second-order neurons in trigeminal and spinal laminae I, II, and V and project to higher centers including the thalamus and cortical sites (Giesler et al. 1979; Sessle 1999, 2000). In turn, these supraspinal sites modulate the activity of nociceptive neurons of the spinal cord (Wall 1967). The firing frequency of dorsal horn units in response to cutaneous stimuli is enhanced by spinal transection or cold block of the spinal cord (Wall 1967). Electrical stimulation of the PAG produced antinociception powerful enough to allow a laparotomy in rats without any overt signs of behavioral distress and outlasting the period of stimulation (Reynolds 1969). Systematic electrical stimulation of brain loci revealed that the PAG, lateral hypothalamus, dorsomedial nucleus of the thalamus, septal nucleus, ventral tegmentum, and ventrobasal thalamic complex attenuate responses to noxious mechanical and thermal stimuli (Mayer and Liebeskind 1974). Stimulation applied in the PAG produced consistent antinociception analogous to 10 mg/kg of morphine (Mayer and Liebeskind 1974). Electrical stimulation of the PAG also inhibited increased activity of spinal wide-dynamic-range neurons in response to noxious stimuli (Hayes et al. 1979). Electrical stimulation of the PAG was also shown to block intractable pain in humans (Hosobuchi et al. 1977). The medullary trigeminal nucleus is analogous to the spinal dorsal horn with regard to nociceptive and sensory functions, and many observations regarding spinal nociceptive processing also apply to this nucleus (Dubner and Bennett 1983; see also Sessle, this volume). For example, PAG stimulation attenuates nociceptive-induced activity of trigeminal neurons (Hayashi et al. 1984).

Like electrical stimulation, the microinjection of morphine into the ventrolateral aspect of the PAG also produces robust behavioral signs of antinociception (Jacquet and Lajtha 1973). A detailed survey of 403 injection sites revealed that morphine applied into the ventrolateral PAG produces a very robust, naloxone-reversible inhibition of responses to noxious pinch (Yaksh et al. 1976). Furthermore, there is considerable overlap of PAG sites responsive to morphine with those that block dorsal horn unit responses or behavioral reflexes to peripheral noxious stimuli in response to focal electrical stimulation (Lewis and Gebhart 1977; Yeung et al. 1977; Bennett and Mayer 1979; Hayes et al. 1979). The PAG is known to receive inputs from the hypothalamus, cortical regions, and the limbic system and to communicate with spinally projecting structures (Fields 2004). Taken together, these studies laid the foundation establishing the PAG as a principal site of descending modulation of pain.

THE ROSTROVENTROMEDIAL MEDULLA

It was evident that the PAG interacts with other brainstem structures in order to modulate nociception because direct spinopetal projections from the PAG are sparse. Several sites have been identified as receiving communications from the PAG and contributing to its antinociceptive actions, including the A5 (locus ceruleus), A6, and A7 noradrenergic nuclei (Westlund et al. 1983). Overwhelming evidence shows that the rostroventromedial medulla (RVM), which includes the serotonergic nucleus raphe magnus (NRM) and the nucleus gigantocellularis pars alpha, is a principal relay in the integration of ascending nociceptive inputs with descending inputs from rostral sites to modulate nociception (for review, see Fields and Basbaum 1999; Fields 2004). The RVM is defined anatomically as the region of the medulla between the pyramids, from the ventral surface to the top of the facial nucleus and extending rostrocaudally from the caudal aspect of the superior olive to the rostral aspect of the inferior olive (Fields and Heinricher 1985). Direct, reciprocal communications between the RVM and the PAG have been identified, as well as projections to the RVM from the A5 and A7 noradrenergic nuclei (see Fields and Basbaum 1999 for review). Electrical stimulation and morphine microinjection into the RVM produced behavioral antinociception and inhibited dorsal horn unit responses to noxious peripheral stimuli (Basbaum and Fields 1978; Fields and Basbaum 1978). The RVM is also a major source of bulbospinal projections that terminate in laminae I, II, and V of the spinal dorsal horn. These projections are found principally in the dorsolateral funiculus (DLF) and also in the ventrolateral funiculus (VLF). Lesions of the DLF block the inhibition of dorsal horn unit responses to noxious stimuli caused by electrical stimulation of the RVM (Basbaum and Fields 1978; Fields and Basbaum 1978). Lidocaine injections made either medially or laterally in the RVM only partly blocked antinociception elicited by electrical stimulation of the PAG, whereas application of lidocaine at both medial and lateral sites produced a complete blockade (Gebhart et al. 1983; Sandkühler and Gebhart 1984). Likewise, lesions of the RVM or excitatory amino acid antagonists microinjected into the RVM also blocked antinociception elicited from the PAG (Behbehani and Fields 1979; Aimone and Gebhart 1986). Because the earliest indications were that the RVM is a final relay in the descending inhibition of nociception, this aspect of RVM function has received the most attention.

Later studies, described below, revealed the dual nature of this region, which is now considered to be important for both the inhibition and facilitation of nociception (see Dubner, this volume).

PAIN-MODULATORY CIRCUITRY IN THE RVM

Extensive studies by Fields and colleagues have characterized three classes of neurons within the RVM, based on their electrophysiological responses to noxious heat and correlated to the tail-flick reflex in the rat (Fields et al. 1983; Fields and Basbaum 1999). Extracellular recordings performed within the RVM revealed that on-cells accelerate their firing rate just prior to the nociceptive tail-flick reflex and that off-cells cease firing at the same time (Fields et al. 1983). The activity of on-cells is increased by nociceptive stimuli whereas that of off-cells is decreased (Fields et al. 1983; Fields and Heinricher 1985). A third class of cells, the neutral cells, do not demonstrate any consistent changes with noxious stimuli, and might be related to processes other than modulation of nociception. Antinociceptive doses of morphine given systemically or into the PAG or RVM result in increased off-cell activity and suppressed on-cell activity (Fields et al. 1983; Heinricher et al. 1994). Suppression of the off-cell pause is necessary for the antinociceptive effect of opioids from supraspinal sites, whereas inhibition of on-cell activity is not a critical component of antinociception (Heinricher et al. 1994; Fields and Basbaum 1999). It was established that the bulbospinal projections of the off-cells account for descending inhibition of nociception from the RVM, and that these neurons represent a key component of endogenous pain control systems (Fields and Basbaum 1999).

In addition to its inhibitory functions, the RVM also facilitates nociceptive inputs (see Gebhart 2004). Electrical stimulation applied at low current intensities facilitated, while high current intensities inhibited, dorsal horn unit responses and behavioral reflexes to noxious cutaneous thermal stimuli (Zhuo and Gebhart 1990, 1992). Facilitatory RVM stimulation also produced a leftward shift of the stimulus-response function of dorsal horn neurons in response to graded heating of the skin, indicating a facilitation of nociceptive inputs (Zhuo and Gebhart 1992). Furthermore, the microinjection of neurotensin or glutamate into the RVM produced a biphasic facilitation and inhibition of behavioral and electrophysiological responses to cutaneous or visceral noxious stimuli (Urban and Gebhart 1999; Gebhart 2004).

Just as the off-cells mediate descending inhibition, evidence supports the concept that on-cells mediate descending facilitation. The electrophysiological characteristics of on-cells are consistent with a pronociceptive function (Fields and Basbaum 1999; Heinricher et al. 2003). Moreover, manipulations that facilitate responses to nociceptive stimuli also increase on-cell activity (Fields and Basbaum 1999; Heinricher et al. 2003). For example, prolonged delivery of a noxious thermal stimulus increased on-cell firing rates and facilitated nociceptive reflexes (Morgan and Fields 1994). The facilitated tail-flick reflex was abolished by lidocaine in the RVM (Morgan and Fields 1994). Naloxone-precipitated withdrawal is also associated with enhanced on-cell activity along with enhanced nociceptive tail-flick responses that are also abolished by lidocaine in the RVM (see Fields and Basbaum 1999).

RVM FACILITATION IN INFLAMMATORY PAIN

Hyperalgesia caused by inflammatory processes, which may serve as a protective mechanism to allow healing of an injury, is mediated in part through descending facilitation arising from the RVM. Secondary hyperalgesia of the tail was elicited in rats by formalin injection into the hindpaw or by electrical stimulation of the RVM (Calejesan et al. 1998). This hyperalgesia was abolished by pharmacological blockade of facilitatory serotonergic spinal projections from the RVM (Calejesan et al. 1998). Neurogenic inflammation caused a leftward shift in the stimulus-response function of dorsal horn units to noxious thermal and mechanical stimuli that was blocked by lidocaine or ibotenic acid injected into the RVM or by lesions of the DLF (Pertovaara 1998; Urban et al. 1999). Increases in RVM activity associated with facilitation caused by hindpaw inflammation are time-dependent, indicating a dynamic plasticity of this region in response to persistent pain, and may be due to an upregulation of N-methyl D-aspartate (NMDA) receptors in the RVM (Terayama et al. 2000). These studies provide evidence that prolonged noxious stimulation may cause an activation of descending facilitatory fibers arising from the RVM, which in turn leads to enhanced pain-related behaviors. Inflammation also produces neuronal hyperexcitability and pronociceptive neuroplastic changes in the trigeminal nucleus (Yu et al. 1993; Ren and Dubner 1999).

DESCENDING FACILITATION FROM THE
RVM MEDIATES NEUROPATHIC PAIN

Behavioral signs of neuropathic pain in rats with peripheral nerve injury have been abolished by spinal cord transection or hemisection, indicating that supraspinal sites mediate these states of enhanced pain (Kauppila 1997;

Bian et al. 1998; Sung et al. 1998). Lesions of the DLF or microinjection of lidocaine or of a CCK-2 antagonist into the RVM of nerve-injured rats abolished injury-induced tactile and thermal hyperesthesias (Pertovaara et al. 1996; Kovelowski et al. 2000; Ossipov et al. 2000a; Burgess et al. 2002). The RVM neurons that drive nerve-injury-induced hyperalgesias are activated by cholecystokinin (CCK), and these neurons correlate with functioning of the RVM on-cells (Heinricher et al. 1994, 2001). Microinjection of the cytotoxin saporin conjugated to dermorphin selectively destroyed RVM neurons expressing μ-opioid receptors; the internalization of the receptor was used as a portal through which saporin was imported into the neuron (Porreca et al. 2001; Burgess et al. 2002). This manipulation, performed either 7 days prior to spinal nerve ligation (SNL) or once tactile and thermal hyperesthesias were well established, prevented or reversed the behavioral signs of neuropathic pain, respectively (Porreca et al. 2001; Burgess et al. 2002). In situ hybridization studies also showed a reduction in RVM neurons expressing μ-opioid receptor mRNA (Porreca et al. 2001; Burgess et al. 2002).

DESCENDING FACILITATION UPREGULATES SPINAL DYNORPHIN

Abnormal pain resulting from peripheral nerve injury has been linked to an upregulation of spinal dynorphin content and to an enhanced release of excitatory neurotransmitters from primary afferent neurons, both of which appear to be secondary to neuroplastic changes that include enhanced descending facilitation from the RVM. We have hypothesized that an initiation phase of neuropathic pain is driven by activity from primary afferent fibers, whereas the maintenance phase is mediated by these central neuroplastic adaptations (Ossipov et al. 2001; Burgess et al. 2002; Porreca et al. 2002). It is well established that elevated levels of spinal dynorphin and its fragments play a prominent pronociceptive role in chronic pain states (Dubner and Ruda 1992; Wagner and DeLeo 1996; Burgess et al. 2002). Strains of mice that do not normally show upregulation of spinal dynorphin or mutants with deletions of the gene coding for prodynorphin also do not develop behavioral signs of neuropathic pain (Wang et al. 2001; Gardell et al. 2003). Behavioral signs of neuropathic pain were blocked by spinal injection of dynorphin antiserum 10 days, but not 2 days, after SNL; given that spinal dynorphin content peaks 10 days after SNL, spinal dynorphin may not be required for the initial onset of neuropathic pain, but is critical to its maintenance (Malan et al. 2000; Wang et al. 2001; Burgess et al. 2002; Gardell et al. 2004). Critically, manipulations that block bulbospinal pain-facilitatory pathways in animals with nerve injury abolish both neuropathic pain behaviors and spinal dynorphin upregulation (Burgess et al. 2002; Gardell et al. 2004). Lesions of the DLF or dermorphin-saporin microinjection into the RVM prevented both behavioral manifestations of neuropathic pain and upregulation of spinal dynorphin (Burgess et al. 2002; Gardell et al. 2004). Thus, descending facilitation is required for elevation of spinal dynorphin levels that serve to enhance nociceptive inputs and maintain, but not initiate, an enhanced pain state following peripheral nerve injury.

The stimulated release of neuropeptides from spinal cord and trigeminal preparations or from cultured DRG neurons has emerged as a useful tool to assess the function of peptidergic neurons and as an indicator of enhanced primary afferent activity in neuropathic pain states (Chen et al. 1996; Ulrich-Lai et al. 2001; Jenkins et al. 2003). It was recently found that peripheral nerve injury enhances the capsaicin-evoked release of calcitonin gene-related peptide (CGRP) from primary afferent terminals, which may provide a mechanism driving injury-induced enhanced pain (Gardell et al. 2004). Importantly, pharmacological addition of *des*-Tyr dynorphin to the perfusion medium enhanced the capsaicin-evoked release of CGRP, whereas dynorphin antiserum attenuated the same (Claude et al. 1999; Gardell et al. 2002, 2004). The disruption of descending facilitation from the RVM either through the microinjection of dermorphin-saporin conjugate into the RVM or through ablation of the DLF in rats with SNL also blocked capsaicin-evoked enhanced release of CGRP (Gardell et al. 2004). These manipulations also prevent the upregulation of spinal dynorphin and stop behavioral signs of neuropathic pain (Ossipov et al. 2000b, 2001; Porreca et al. 2001, 2002; Burgess et al. 2002; Gardell et al. 2004). Taken together, these observations provide firm evidence that neuropathic pain states are maintained, at least in part, by increased sensitivity of primary afferent neurons to noxious stimuli. In addition, it is hypothesized that persistent nociceptive inputs elicits supraspinal neuroplastic changes that result in a tonic descending facilitation of nociceptive inputs that is mediated by an upregulation of spinal dynorphin content. Thus, increased spinal dynorphin serves to promote excitatory transmitter release, which in turn maintains and perpetuates a chronic pain state (Gardell et al. 2004).

DESCENDING FACILITATION IS A NEUROPLASTIC CONSEQUENCE OF NERVE INJURY

The studies summarized above present abundant evidence that enhanced abnormal pain is driven by the activation of a tonic spinopetal pain-facilitatory system. In the normal state, acute nociceptive inputs are relayed rostrally from second-order neurons projecting to the thalamus from the spinal cord or trigeminal nucleus contralateral to the input (Basbaum et al. 1978; Hayashi et al. 1984). Recent studies have begun to address the contribution of ascending projections to the maintenance of the neuropathic pain state. Substance P conjugated to saporin (SP-SAP) given spinally markedly reduced the population of neurons that express the neurokinin-1 (NK1) receptor in the spinal dorsal horn, which represent a substantial portion of nociceptive-responsive spinothalamic tract neurons (Nichols et al. 1999; Suzuki et al. 2002). The selective, but partial, ablation of the NK1-expressing neurons with SP-SAP abolished behavioral signs of neuropathic pain without altering acute nociceptive responses (Nichols et al. 1999). Furthermore, ablation of NK1-expressing neurons of the spinal dorsal horn by SP-SAP abolished sensitization of the wide-dynamic-range (WDR) neurons induced by nerve injury or peripheral inflammation (Suzuki et al. 2002). Similar results were observed after spinal administration of the 5HT3-receptor antagonist ondansetron, which blocks the activity of the descending serotonergic pain facilitatory system from the RVM (Suzuki et al. 2002). Moreover, SP-SAP produced a reduction in Fos expression in the deeper, but not superficial, laminae of the spinal cord in response to formalin injection, implying the role of a descending facilitatory input to neurons of the deeper laminae (Suzuki et al. 2002). Ascending persistent nociceptive inputs through the nociceptive lamina I neurons that express the NK1 receptor may activate descending pain-facilitatory systems that are expressed electrophysiologically as enhanced activity of the WDR of the deeper laminae and behaviorally as tactile and thermal hyperesthesias (Suzuki et al. 2002).

There is also the possibility that other systems may be activated. Some of the NK1-expressing neurons of lamina I send collateral projections to the deeper laminae of the dorsal horn, where they may directly excite WDR cells (Cheunsuang and Morris 2000). The WDR neurons may correspond to the postsynaptic dorsal column (PSDC) neurons that project to the nucleus gracilis. These neurons normally mediate light touch and vibration but may become sensitized in persistent pain states (Giesler et al. 1984; Al-Chaer et al. 1997). A sensitized PSDC projection to the nucleus gracilis might make this region more responsive to tactile inputs from the large-diameter Aβ primary afferent fibers (Bennett et al. 1983). The nucleus gracilis demonstrates significant neuroplastic changes in response to peripheral nerve injury, including de novo expression of substance P, CGRP, and neuropeptide Y (NPY) (Noguchi et al. 1995; Miki et al. 1998). Upregulation of NPY in the nucleus gracilis was abolished by dorsal rhizotomy, and by ipsilateral, though not contralateral, lesions of the dorsal columns (Sun et al. 2001;

Ossipov et al. 2002). Similarly, tactile, but not thermal, hyperesthesia after SNL was abolished by lidocaine or NPY antagonists given into the ipsilateral, and not the contralateral, nucleus gracilis and by ipsilateral lesions of the dorsal columns (Sun et al. 2001; Ossipov et al. 2002). Peripheral nerve injury caused sensitization of WDR neurons of the ventroposterolateral nucleus of the thalamus (VPL), which was abolished by lesions of the dorsal columns or of the nucleus gracilis (Miki et al. 2000). Nociceptive inputs from the spinothalamic tract and somatosensory inputs from the dorsal column and from medial lemniscal pathways converge in the thalamus, which has projections to limbic and cortical sites (Ma et al. 1987); these findings suggest possible mechanisms by which descending pain-facilitatory systems may be engaged, although experimental evidence is lacking at this point.

As noted above, CCK in the RVM appears to promote pain, and enhanced CCK activity in response to persistent noxious stimulation may be partly responsible for engaging descending facilitatory pathways from the RVM. Intra-RVM microinjection of CCK enhanced behavioral responses to colorectal distension in normal rats, but not in rats with colonic inflammation, whereas administration of CCK antagonists enhanced morphine antinociception in rats with inflammation, but not in normal rats, indicating a maximal activation of endogenous CCK mechanisms in the RVM by inflammation (Friedrich and Gebhart 2003). Furthermore, intra-RVM microinjection of CCK antagonists abolished behavioral signs of enhanced pain due to SNL or inflammation but not those due to acute noxious stimuli (Kovelowski et al. 2000; Friedrich and Gebhart 2003). These studies suggest that endogenous CCK promotes descending facilitation of nociceptive inputs in the chronic pain state. CCK has been identified in the PAG and the RVM, and some of the CCK-expressing neurons projecting from the RVM to the spinal cord also express 5HT (Mantyh and Hunt 1984; Liu et al. 1994). Such a projection may contribute to the observed enhanced release of spinal CCK after nerve injury or inflammation (Gustafsson et al. 1998). Taken together, these studies provide growing evidence that tonic pain states are maintained by a spinobulbospinal excitatory system, where incoming pain causes supraspinal neuroplastic changes that in turn serve to facilitate further nociceptive inputs that maintain enhanced pain states (Porreca et al. 2002).

CONCLUSIONS

Tremendous progress in our understanding of mechanisms that modulate pain has been made in the years since the 1st World Congress on Pain was held in 1975. At that time, many exciting discoveries were made that established the existence of endogenous mechanisms that inhibit the expression of pain. Further studies have established that the PAG appears to be a central collection and processing site for nociceptive inputs and for integration of descending information from limbic and cortical sites, which may partly explain the observations that environmental, psychological, and emotional cues alter pain responses. More detailed explorations have revealed that the RVM is the major relay in descending inhibition of pain, but that it also relays a pain-facilitatory system. Increasing evidence suggests that pain facilitation from the RVM may serve a protective role in conditions of wound healing, but may also become maladaptive, permitting long-lasting, abnormal pain that persists after the initial insult has terminated. Neuropathic pain is an important example of this maladaptive pain state. With our increased understanding of the pathways that may underlie these enhanced pain states, we are now able to focus on the neuromodulators that mediate enhanced pain. Prime examples are CCK at supraspinal sites and dynorphin at spinal sites, which enhance release of neuropeptides from primary afferent nerve terminals. Armed with these advances in our understanding of pain regulatory systems, pain researchers cannot help but be optimistic that significant novel therapeutic advances will soon be available for the treatment of chronic pain.

REFERENCES

Aimone LD, Gebhart GF. Stimulation-produced spinal inhibition from the midbrain in the rat is mediated by an excitatory amino acid neurotransmitter in the medial medulla. *J Neurosci* 1986; 6:1803–1813.

Al-Chaer ED, Westlund KN, Willis WD. Sensitization of postsynaptic dorsal column neuronal responses by colon inflammation. *Neuroreport* 1997; 8:3267–3273.

Basbaum AI, Fields HL. Endogenous pain control mechanisms: review and hypothesis. *Ann Neurol* 1978; 4:451–462.

Basbaum AI, Clanton CH, Fields HL. Three bulbospinal pathways from the rostral medulla of the cat: an autoradiographic study of pain modulating systems. *J Comp Neurol* 1978; 178:209–224.

Behbehani MM, Fields HL. Evidence that an excitatory connection between the periaqueductal gray and nucleus raphe magnus mediates stimulation produced analgesia. *Brain Res* 1979; 170:85–93.

Bennett GJ, Mayer DJ. Inhibition of spinal cord interneurons by narcotic microinjection and focal electrical stimulation in the periaqueductal central gray matter. *Brain Res* 1979; 172:243–257.

Bennett GJ, Seltzer Z, Lu GW, et al. The cells of origin of the dorsal column postsynaptic projection in the lumbosacral enlargements of cats and monkeys. *Somatosens Res* 1983; 1:131–149.

Bian D, Ossipov MH, Zhong C, et al. Tactile allodynia, but not thermal hyperalgesia, of the hindlimbs is blocked by spinal transection in rats with nerve injury. *Neurosci Lett* 1998; 241:79–82.

Burgess SE, Gardell LR, Ossipov MH, et al. Time-dependent descending facilitation from the rostral ventromedial medulla maintains, but does not initiate, neuropathic pain. *J Neurosci* 2002; 22:5129–5136.

Calejesan AA, Ch'ang MH, Zhuo M. Spinal serotonergic receptors mediate facilitation of a nociceptive reflex by subcutaneous formalin injection into the hindpaw in rats. *Brain Res* 1998; 798:46–54.

Chen JJ, Barber LA, Dymshitz J, et al. Peptidase inhibitors improve recovery of substance P and calcitonin gene-related peptide release from rat spinal cord slices. *Peptides* 1996; 17:31–37.

Cheunsuang O, Morris R. Spinal lamina I neurons that express neurokinin 1 receptors: morphological analysis. *Neuroscience* 2000; 97:335–345.

Claude P, Gracia N, Wagner L, et al. Effect of dynorphin on ICGRP release from capsaicin-sensitive fibers. *Abstracts of the 9th World Congress on Pain*. Seattle: IASP Press, 1999, p 262.

Dubner R, Bennett GJ. Spinal and trigeminal mechanisms of nociception. *Annu Rev Neurosci* 1983; 6:381–418.

Dubner R, Ruda MA. Activity-dependent neuronal plasticity following tissue injury and inflammation. *Trends Neurosci* 1992; 15:96–103.

Fields HL. State-dependent opioid control of pain. *Nat Rev Neurosci* 2004; 5:565–575.

Fields HL, Basbaum AI. Brainstem control of spinal pain-transmission neurons. *Annu Rev Physiol* 1978; 40:217–248.

Fields HL, Basbaum AI. Central nervous system mechanisms of pain modulation. In: Wall PD, Melzack R (Eds). *Textbook of Pain*. Edinburgh: Churchill Livingstone, 1999, pp 309–329.

Fields HL, Heinricher MM. Anatomy and physiology of a nociceptive modulatory system. *Philos Trans R Soc Lond B Biol Sci* 1985; 308:361–374.

Fields HL, Bry J, Hentall I, et al. The activity of neurons in the rostral medulla of the rat during withdrawal from noxious heat. *J Neurosci* 1983; 3:2545–2552.

Friedrich AE, Gebhart GF. Modulation of visceral hyperalgesia by morphine and cholecystokinin from the rat rostroventral medial medulla. *Pain* 2003; 104:93–101.

Gardell LR, Wang R, Burgess SE, et al. Sustained morphine exposure induces a spinal dynorphin-dependent enhancement of excitatory transmitter release from primary afferent fibers. *J Neurosci* 2002; 22:6747–6755.

Gardell LR, Vanderah TW, Gardell SE, et al. Enhanced evoked excitatory transmitter release in experimental neuropathy requires descending facilitation. *J Neurosci* 2003; 23:8370–8379.

Gardell LR, Ibrahim M, Wang R, et al. Mouse strains that lack spinal dynorphin upregulation after peripheral nerve injury do not develop neuropathic pain. *Neuroscience* 2004;123:43–52.

Gebhart GF. Descending modulation of pain. *Neurosci Biobehav Rev* 2004; 27:729–737.

Gebhart GF, Sandkühler J, Thalhammer JG, et al. Inhibition of spinal nociceptive information by stimulation in midbrain of the cat is blocked by lidocaine microinjected in nucleus raphe magnus and medullary reticular formation. *J Neurophysiol* 1983; 50:1446–1459.

Giesler GJ Jr, Menetrey D, Basbaum AI. Differential origins of spinothalamic tract projections to medial and lateral thalamus in the rat *J Comp Neurol* 1979; 184:107–26.

Giesler GJ Jr, Nahin RL, Madsen AM. Postsynaptic dorsal column pathway of the rat. I. Anatomical studies. *J Neurophysiol* 1984; 51:260–275.

Gustafsson H, de Araujo Lucas G, Schott E, et al. Peripheral axotomy influences the in vivo release of cholecystokinin in the spinal cord dorsal horn-possible involvement of cholecystokinin-B receptors. *Brain Res* 1998; 790:141–150.

Hayashi H, Sumino R, Sessle BJ. Functional organization of trigeminal subnucleus interpolaris: nociceptive and innocuous afferent inputs projections to thalamus cerebellum and spinal cord and descending modulation from periaqueductal gray. *J Neurophysiol* 1984; 51:890–905.

Hayes RL, Price DD, Ruda M, et al. Suppression of nociceptive responses in the primate by electrical stimulation of the brain or morphine administration: behavioral and electrophysiological comparisons. *Brain Res* 1979; 167:417–421.

Heinricher MM, Morgan MM, Tortorici V, et al. Disinhibition of off-cells and antinociception produced by an opioid action within the rostral ventromedial medulla. *Neuroscience* 1994; 63:279–288.

Heinricher MM, McGaraughty, S, Tortorici, V. Circuitry underlying antiopioid actions of cholecystokinin within the rostral ventromedial medulla. *J Neurophysiol* 2001; 85:280–286.

Heinricher MM, Pertovaara A, Ossipov MH. Descending modulation after injury. In: Dostrovsky DO, Carr DB, Koltzenburg M (Eds). *Proceedings of the 10th World Congress on Pain, Progress in Pain Research and Management*, Vol. 24. Seattle: IASP Press, 2003, pp 251–260.

Hosobuchi Y, Adams JE, Linchitz R. Pain relief by electrical stimulation of the central gray matter in humans and its reversal by naloxone. *Science* 1977; 197:183–186.

Hughes J, Smith TW, Kosterlitz HW, et al. Identification of two related pentapeptides from the brain with potent opiate agonist activity. *Nature* 1975; 258:577–580.

Jacquet YF, Lajtha A. Morphine action at central nervous system sites in rat: analgesia or hyperalgesia depending on site and dose. *Science* 1973; 182:490–492.

Jenkins DW, Sellers LA, Feniuk W, et al. Characterization of bradykinin-induced prostaglandin e2 release from cultured rat trigeminal ganglion neurones *Eur J Pharmacol* 2003; 469:29–36.

Kauppila T. Spinalization increases the mechanical stimulation-induced withdrawal reflex threshold after a sciatic cut in the rat. *Brain Res* 1997; 770:310–312.

Kovelowski CJ, Ossipov MH, Sun H, et al. Supraspinal cholecystokinin may drive tonic descending facilitation mechanisms to maintain neuropathic pain in the rat. *Pain* 2000; 87:265–273.

Lewis VA, Gebhart GF. Evaluation of the periaqueductal central gray (PAG) as a morphine-specific locus of action and examination of morphine-induced and stimulation-produced analgesia at coincident PAG loci. *Brain Res* 1977; 124:283–303.

Liu H, Chandler S, Beitz AJ, et al. Characterization of the effect of cholecystokinin (CCK) on neurons in the periaqueductal gray of the rat: immunocytochemical and in vivo and in vitro electrophysiological studies. *Brain Res* 1994; 642:83–94.

Ma W, Peschanski M, Ralston HJ III. The differential synaptic organization of the spinal and lemniscal projections to the ventrobasal complex of the rat thalamus. Evidence for convergence of the two systems upon single thalamic neurons. *Neuroscience* 1987; 22:925–934.

Malan TP, Ossipov MH, Gardell LR, et al. Extraterritorial neuropathic pain correlates with multisegmental elevation of spinal dynorphin in nerve-injured rats. *Pain* 2000; 86:185–194.

Mantyh PW, Hunt SP. Evidence for cholecystokinin-like immunoreactive neurons in the rat medulla oblongata which project to the spinal cord. *Brain Res* 1984; 291:49–54.

Mayer DJ, Liebeskind JC. Pain reduction by focal electrical stimulation of the brain: an anatomical and behavioral analysis. *Brain Res* 1974; 68:73–93.

Melzack R, Wall PD. Pain mechanisms: a new theory. *Science* 1965; 150:971–979.

Miki K, Fukuoka T, Tokunaga A, et al. Calcitonin gene-related peptide increase in the rat spinal dorsal horn and dorsal column nucleus following peripheral nerve injury: up-regulation in a subpopulation of primary afferent sensory neurons. *Neuroscience* 1998; 82:1243–1252.

Miki K, Iwata K, Tsuboi Y, et al. Dorsal column-thalamic pathway is involved in thalamic hyperexcitability following peripheral nerve injury: a lesion study in rats with experimental mononeuropathy. *Pain* 2000; 85:263–271.

Morgan MM, Fields HL. Pronounced changes in the activity of nociceptive modulatory neurons in the rostral ventromedial medulla in response to prolonged thermal noxious stimuli. *J Neurophysiol* 1994; 72:1161–1170.

Nichols ML, Allen BJ, Rogers SD, et al. Transmission of chronic nociception by spinal neurons expressing the substance P receptor. *Science* 1999; 286:1558–1561.

Noguchi K, Kawai Y, Fukuoka T, et al. Substance P induced by peripheral nerve injury in primary afferent sensory neurons and its effect on dorsal column nucleus neurons. *J Neurosci* 1995; 15:7633–7643.

Ossipov MH, Lai J, Malan TP Jr, et al. Spinal and supraspinal mechanisms of neuropathic pain. *Ann N Y Acad Sci* 2000a; 909:12–24.

Ossipov MH, Sun H, Malan TP, et al. Mediation of spinal nerve injury induced tactile allodynia by descending facilitatory pathways in the dorsolateral funiculus in rats. *Neurosci Lett* 2000b; 290:129–132.

Ossipov MH, Lai J, Malan TP Jr, et al. Tonic descending facilitation as a mechanism of neuropathic pain. In: Hansson PT, Fields HL, Hill RG, et al. (Eds). *Neuropathic Pain: Pathophysiology and Treatment,* Progress in Pain Research and Management, Vol. 21. Seattle: IASP Press, 2001, pp 107–124.

Ossipov MH, Zhang ET, Carvajal C, et al. Selective mediation of nerve injury-induced tactile hypersensitivity by neuropeptide Y. *J Neurosci* 2002; 22:9858–9867.

Pert CB, Snyder SH. Opiate receptor: demonstration in nervous tissue. *Science* 1973; 179:1011–1014.

Pertovaara A. A neuronal correlate of secondary hyperalgesia in the rat spinal dorsal horn is submodality selective and facilitated by supraspinal influence. *Exp Neurol* 1998; 149:193–202.

Pertovaara A, Wei H, Hamalainen MM. Lidocaine in the rostroventromedial medulla and the periaqueductal gray attenuates allodynia in neuropathic rats. *Neurosci Lett* 1996; 218:127–130.

Porreca F, Burgess SE, Gardell LR, et al. Inhibition of neuropathic pain by selective ablation of brainstem medullary cells expressing the mu-opioid receptor. *J Neurosci* 2001; 21:5281–5288.

Porreca F, Ossipov MH, Gebhart GF. Chronic pain and medullary descending facilitation. *Trends Neurosci* 2002; 25:319–325.

Ren K, Dubner R. Central nervous system plasticity and persistent pain *J Orofac Pain* 1999; 13:155–163; discussion 164–171.

Reynolds DV. Surgery in the rat during electrical analgesia induced by focal brain stimulation. *Science* 1969; 164:444–445.

Sandkühler J, Gebhart GF. Relative contributions of the nucleus raphe magnus and adjacent medullary reticular formation to the inhibition by stimulation in the periaqueductal gray of a spinal nociceptive reflex in the pentobarbital-anesthetized rat. *Brain Res* 1984; 305:77–87.

Sessle BJ. Neural mechanisms and pathways in craniofacial pain *Can J Neurol Sci* 1999; 26(Suppl 3):S7–11.

Sessle BJ. Acute and chronic craniofacial pain: brainstem mechanisms of nociceptive transmission and neuroplasticity and their clinical correlates *Crit Rev Oral Biol Med* 2000; 11:57–91.

Simon EJ. In search of the opiate receptor. *Am J Med Sci* 1973; 266:160–168.

Sun H, Ren K, Zhong CM, et al. Nerve injury-induced tactile allodynia is mediated via ascending spinal dorsal column projections. *Pain* 2001; 90:105–111.

Sung B, Na HS, Kim YI, et al. Supraspinal involvement in the production of mechanical allodynia by spinal nerve injury in rats. *Neurosci Lett* 1998; 246:117–119.

Suzuki R, Morcuende S, Webber M, et al. Superficial NK1-expressing neurons control spinal excitability through activation of descending pathways. *Nat Neurosci* 2002; 5:1319–1326.

Terayama R, Guan Y, Dubner R, et al. Activity-induced plasticity in brain stem pain modulatory circuitry after inflammation. *Neuroreport* 2000; 11:1915–1919.

Terenius L. Characteristics of the "receptor" for narcotic analgesics in synaptic plasma membrane fraction from rat brain. *Acta Pharmacol Toxicol (Copenhagen)* 1973; 33:377–384.

Tsou K, Jang CS. Studies on the site of analgesic action of morphine by intracerebral microinjection. *Sci Sin* 1964; 13:1099–1109.

Ulrich-Lai YM, Flores CM, Harding-Rose CA, et al. Capsaicin-evoked release of immunoreactive calcitonin gene-related peptide from rat trigeminal ganglion: evidence for intraganglionic neurotransmission. *Pain* 2001; 91:219–226.

Urban MO, Gebhart GF. Supraspinal contributions to hyperalgesia. *Proc Natl Acad Sci USA* 1999; 96:7687–7692.

Urban MO, Zahn PK, Gebhart GF. Descending facilitatory influences from the rostral medial medulla mediate secondary, but not primary hyperalgesia in the rat. *Neuroscience* 1999; 90:349–352.

Wagner R, DeLeo JA. Pre-emptive dynorphin and N-methyl-D-aspartate glutamate receptor antagonism alters spinal immunocytochemistry but not allodynia following complete peripheral nerve injury. *Neuroscience* 1996; 72:527–534.

Wall PD. The laminar organization of dorsal horn and effects of descending impulses. *J Physiol* 1967; 188:403–423.

Wang Z, Gardell LR, Ossipov MH, et al. Pronociceptive actions of dynorphin maintain chronic neuropathic pain. *J Neurosci* 2001; 21:1779–1786.

Westlund KN, Bowker RM, Ziegler MG, et al. Noradrenergic projections to the spinal cord of the rat. *Brain Res* 1983; 263:15–31.

Yaksh TL, Yeung JC, Rudy TA. Systematic examination in the rat of brain sites sensitive to the direct application of morphine: observation of differential effects within the periaqueductal gray. *Brain Res* 1976; 114:83–103.

Yeung JC, Yaksh TL, Rudy TA. Concurrent mapping of brain sites for sensitivity to the direct application of morphine and focal electrical stimulation in the production of antinociception in the rat. *Pain* 1977; 4:23–40.

Yu XM, Sessle BJ, Hu JW. Differential effects of cutaneous and deep application of inflammatory irritant on mechanoreceptive field properties of trigeminal brain stem nociceptive neurons *J Neurophysiol* 1993; 70:1704–1707.

Zhuo M, Gebhart GF. Characterization of descending inhibition and facilitation from the nuclei reticularis gigantocellularis and gigantocellularis pars alpha in the rat. *Pain* 1990; 42:337–350.

Zhuo M, Gebhart GF. Characterization of descending facilitation and inhibition of spinal nociceptive transmission from the nuclei reticularis gigantocellularis and gigantocellularis pars alpha in the rat. *J Neurophysiol* 1992; 67:1599–1614.

Correspondence to: Frank Porreca, PhD, Departments of Pharmacology and Anesthesiology, University of Arizona Health Sciences Center, Tucson, AZ 85724, USA. Tel: 520-626-7421; Fax: 520-626-4182; email: frankp@ u.arizona.edu.

The Paths of Pain 1975–2005, edited by
Harold Merskey, John D. Loeser, and Ronald
Dubner, IASP Press, Seattle, © 2005.

9

Orofacial Pain

Barry J. Sessle

*Faculty of Dentistry and Centre for the Study of Pain,
University of Toronto, Toronto, Ontario, Canada*

The face and mouth have special biological, emotional, and psychological meaning and represent sites of some of the most common pains in the body (see Lipton et al. 1993; LeResche 2001). This chapter reviews briefly what has been learned about the processes, diagnosis, and management of these pains since the first IASP World Congress on Pain, and cites review articles that can be consulted for specific references.

PERIPHERAL TRIGEMINAL OROFACIAL NOCICEPTIVE PROCESSES

GENERAL FEATURES

Prior to the early 1970s, a few studies in animals had shown the existence of nociceptors associated with small myelinated (Aδ) and unmyelinated (C-fiber) primary afferents (see Willis, this volume), but little information was available of their properties in the orofacial region. By the time of the 1st World Congress on Pain, Dubner's group had described the properties of different types of Aδ- and C-fiber nociceptive afferents supplying the primate facial skin, and several studies had provided some anatomical and physiological definition of pulp afferents (see Dubner et al. 1978; Dubner 1985). Subsequent studies have provided details of nociceptive orofacial afferents also supplying the cornea, the mucosa, the cerebrovasculature, and musculoskeletal tissues (see below). Like nociceptors elsewhere in the body (see Willis, this volume), those in the orofacial region are associated with a diverse population of Aδ- and C-fiber afferents that detect and encode intense physical, thermal, and chemical events associated with actual or near tissue damage (Darian-Smith 1966; Dubner et al. 1978; Dubner 1985). However, there are some differences between orofacial and spinal sensory systems (see Table I).

Table I

Trigeminal sensory systems: differences from spinal sensory systems

A. *Peripheral Tissues and Innervation*
1. Tissues unique to the craniofacial region (e.g., tooth pulp, cornea)
2. Higher innervation density in many craniofacial tissues than in most spinally innervated tissues
3. Shorter conduction distances of peripheral nerve pathways
4. Slower conduction velocities of peripheral nerve fibers
5. Higher ratio of myelinated to unmyelinated fibers
6. Lower proportion of sympathetic efferents
7. Certain craniofacial receptors (e.g., some periodontal mechanoreceptors and jaw muscle spindles) have their primary afferent cell bodies *within* the CNS

B. *Central Nervous System*
1. Complete representation of the face and mouth at most rostrocaudal levels of VBSNC, and a dual representation of some tissues in the Vc
2. Distinctive brainstem termination patterns of some nociceptive afferents
3. Transitional regions between the Vc and Vi and between the Vc and CDH, with distinctive properties (e.g., bilateral afferent inputs to Vc/Vi)
4. Prominence of a "deep bundle" fiber system in the Vc (connects caudal and rostral levels of the VBSNC), but absence of Lissauer's tract
5. Significant ipsilateral as well as contralateral projections from the VBSNC to the thalamus

C. *Pain Conditions Specific to the Craniofacial Region*
1. Headaches (e.g., migraine, cluster headache)
2. Toothaches (e.g., pulpitis pain)
3. Trigeminal neuralgia
4. Miscellaneous (e.g., atypical facial pain, burning mouth syndrome, atypical odontalgia)

Abbreviations: CDH = upper cervical dorsal horn; VBSNC = trigeminal brainstem sensory nuclear complex; Vc = subnucleus caudalis; Vi = subnucleus interpolaris.

The cell bodies of most primary afferents innervating facial cutaneous, intraoral (e.g., mucosa, periodontium, tooth pulp), musculoskeletal, and cerebrovascular tissues occur in the trigeminal (V) ganglion. Hand-in-hand with analogous findings in the spinal somatosensory system, trigeminal studies using in vivo and in vitro recordings and molecular and immunocytochemical approaches have shown that these cell bodies synthesize the vast array of chemicals that help define the role of primary afferent nociceptive neurons in encoding pain (Cooper 2005; see Gold, this volume). These include calcitonin gene-related peptide (CGRP), substance P, somatostatin, neurokinin A, and nerve growth factor, and the afferents may express serotonergic, cholinergic, opiate, purinergic, bradykinin, histamine, anandamide, prostaglandin, or acid-sensitive receptors and ion channels, as well as adrenoreceptors and the capsaicin-sensitive TRPV1 or insensitive (e.g., TRPV2) receptors. In addition, receptors also exist for chemical mediators long thought to be involved in nociceptive transmission or modulation within the central nervous system (CNS), such as glutamate, opiate, and γ-aminobutyric acid (GABA) receptors. Sex differences occur in the peripheral actions of glutamate and morphine (Sessle 2000; Cairns 2005; Cooper 2005), suggesting that peripherally based physiological mechanisms may contribute to the sex differences in the prevalence of many chronic pain conditions.

Most of these receptors and chemical mediators have only been identified in the last decade and shown to be involved in the activation, sensitization, or modulation of orofacial nociceptors. The findings highlight the complexity of the peripheral mechanisms underlying pain, but also reveal a number of potential targets that hold out promise for the development of new and more effective therapeutic approaches to manage acute and chronic orofacial pain.

SPECIFIC OROFACIAL NOCICEPTIVE AFFERENTS

Facial cutaneous and oral mucosal tissues receive a dense innervation that includes high-threshold mechanoreceptive afferents (most of which conduct in the Aδ range), Aδ mechanothermal nociceptive afferents, and Aδ and C-fiber polymodal nociceptive afferents. Many of these nociceptive afferents can be activated or sensitized by algesic chemical, mechanical, or thermal stimuli and express several of the receptors and ion channels outlined above (Cooper 2005). The *temporomandibular joint (TMJ)* and *masticatory muscles* also are supplied by Aδ- and C-fiber afferents that may respond to a wide range of peripheral stimuli, including heavy pressure and algesic chemicals such as glutamate, hypertonic saline, capsaicin, and mustard oil (Cairns 2005). Small-diameter afferents also supply the *cerebrovasculature* and *dura*, and many can be activated by noxious stimuli. The modulation of these afferents by peripheral neurochemical processes (e.g., 5HT, CGRP) appear to be important factors in the initiation and control of certain types of headaches such as migraine (Messlinger 2005; Burstein, this volume).

The *cornea* is a unique tissue found only in the orofacial region. Aδ and C fibers penetrate into the corneal epithelium. They respond to a wide range of mechanical, thermal, and chemical stimuli, and despite their low activation thresholds, their input to the CNS can evoke pain (Belmonte 2005).

The *tooth pulp* is another unique orofacial tissue that warrants particular emphasis. It is also exquisitely sensitive to stimulation but unlike the cornea, it is highly vascular. It is encased by dentine, which is also very sensitive. Pain is the predominant sensation evoked by dentinal or pulpal stimuli.

The pulp is richly innervated by Aδ- and C-fiber afferents, but it also receives some Aβ afferents and sympathetic efferents (see Dubner et al. 1978; Sessle 1987; Matthews and Sessle 2001; Hu 2004; Narhi 2005). With the advent of improved anatomical techniques for defining nerve fibers, it was becoming clear by the time of the 1st World Congress on Pain that dentine is also innervated (see Dubner et al. 1978). However, the extent to which this dentinal innervation accounted for dentinal sensitivity remained unresolved, although several theories existed (see Dubner et al. 1978). Over the past 30 years, little evidence has emerged in support of two of the main theories proposing that a dentinal stimulus produces pain by a direct excitation of the fibers within dentinal tubules or through a transduction mechanism involving the cells (odontoblasts) that form a layer beneath the dentine and are responsible for its formation. The relatively limited investigation brought to bear on this issue suggests instead that most stimuli activate intradental nerve fibers indirectly through a hydrodynamic mechanism. This proposal, first championed by Bränström over 30 years ago, argues that dentinal stimulation produces strong capillary forces in the dentinal tubules that deform the tissue and mechanically activate the fibers (Bränström and Åström 1972; see also Dubner et al. 1978; Matthews and Sessle 2001).

It was not until after the early 1970s that the physiological properties of intradental afferents started to receive detailed attention, most notably in the laboratories of Anderson and Matthews, Edwall and Olgart, and more recently Narhi (see Dubner et al. 1978; Matthews and Sessle 2001; Narhi 2005). The afferents were shown to be sensitive to a wide range of dental stimuli that produce pain in humans. As with nociceptors elsewhere in the body, most of these afferents are polymodal, but they include some "silent" nociceptors (see Willis, this volume). Since the 1980s, electrophysiological recordings in animals and correlated studies in humans also have indicated that activation of intradental A and C fibers may induce different types of pain sensations, namely sharp and dull pain, respectively. Recent studies have suggested that many A fibers terminate in the tubules within dentine and are responsible for dentine's sensitivity, probably through a hydrodynamic mechanism, whereas C fibers predominate in the pulp and may be activated only if the dental stimulus reaches the pulp (Narhi 2005). Furthermore, intradental Aβ and Aδ fibers appear to respond in a similar way to dental stimulation and thus may belong to the same functional group. Elsewhere in the body, Aβ afferents are not normally nociceptive, and it is unclear whether these intradental afferents represent a notable exception or whether their sensitivity has been altered by the experimental procedures required for their recording.

Tissue injury and inflammation can lead to neurochemical changes and nerve sprouting and may induce peripheral sensitization of intradental afferents that can result in extremely intense toothache (Byers and Narhi 1999; Hu 2004; Narhi 2005). As in other tissues, the changes in afferent sensitivity are due to several different inflammatory mediators and intraneural chemicals, and many of the receptor mechanisms outlined above also characterize the pulp. Nonetheless, unlike other tissues, inflammation of the pulp occurs in a noncompliant environment (since it is encased by dentine) with a high extracellular tissue pressure; this may account for the exquisite sensitivity of pulp afferents.

CENTRAL TRIGEMINAL NOCICEPTIVE PROCESSES

BRAINSTEM NOCICEPTIVE TRANSMISSION

The trigeminal brainstem sensory nuclear complex (VBSNC) is the projection site of orofacial nociceptive primary afferents and most other V afferents. Its second-order neurons project directly or indirectly to the thalamus and to several brainstem areas (e.g., the parabrachial nucleus, cerebellum, cranial nerve motor nuclei, and the reticular formation) and also contribute to intrinsic projections terminating within the complex itself. The VBSNC consists of the main sensory nucleus and the spinal tract nucleus, and the latter is subdivided into three subnuclei: the oralis, interpolaris, and caudalis (Fig. 1). The subnucleus caudalis (Vc) is a laminated structure resembling the spinal dorsal horn. By the early 1970s, anatomical, clinical, and behavioral findings were suggesting that the Vc is the crucial brainstem substrate for orofacial nociceptive processing. Paradoxically, neuronal recordings from the Vc performed through the 1960s had detected only a few neurons activated by noxious stimulation, but by the time of the 1st World Congress on Pain, it was becoming evident that the Vc contains substantial populations of nociceptive neurons (Darian-Smith 1966; Dubner et al. 1978). It soon became clear that the Vc has several morphological as well as physiological similarities with the spinal dorsal horn, to the extent that the Vc was subsequently termed the medullary dorsal horn (see Dubner et al. 1978; Gobel et al. 1981; Dubner and Bennett 1983; Dubner 1985; Sessle 1987). In general, the similarities have also been borne out by the application of more recently developed immunocytochemical techniques. In view of the similarity of many features of the Vc with those of the spinal dorsal horn, which are detailed by Willis in this volume, the following will only briefly summarize these features and also note some important differences (Table I).

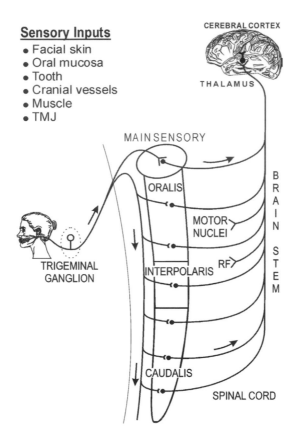

Sensory Inputs
- Facial skin
- Oral mucosa
- Tooth
- Cranial vessels
- Muscle
- TMJ

Fig. 1. Major somatosensory pathway from the face and mouth. Trigeminal primary afferents project via the trigeminal ganglion to second-order neurons in the trigeminal brainstem sensory nuclear complex. These neurons may project to neurons in higher levels of the brain (for example, in the thalamus) or in brainstem regions such as cranial nerve motor nuclei or the reticular formation (RF). Not shown are the projections of some cervical nerve and cranial nerve VII, IX, X, and XII afferents to the trigeminal complex and the projection of many VII, IX, and X afferents to the solitary tract nucleus. (Reprinted from Sessle 2000.)

Several lines of evidence since the early 1970s indicate that the Vc is critical in trigeminal brainstem nociceptive processing (see Sessle 2000; Woda 2003; Hu and Woda 2005). For example, two classes of nociceptive neurons, based on their cutaneous mechanoreceptive field and response properties, occur in the superficial and deep laminae of the Vc: high-threshold or nociceptive-specific (NS) neurons and wide-dynamic-range (WDR) neurons. NS neurons receive small-diameter nociceptive afferent inputs, while WDR neurons receive both large- and small-diameter inputs. The large mechanosensitive primary afferents terminate throughout the VBSNC, including laminae

III and IV of the Vc, whereas the small myelinated or unmyelinated primary afferents terminate almost exclusively in the Vc, most densely in laminae I and II and the paratrigeminal islands, and only sparsely in the deep laminae of the Vc and dorsomedial portions of rostral regions of the VBSNC (Dubner and Bennett 1983; Bereiter et al. 2000; Sessle 2000). Studies of the past 25 years have shown that some of these afferents stain positive for substance P, CGRP, and neurotrophins, whereas others stain negative for the neuropeptides but positive for the cell surface marker, isolectin B4; these IB4 afferents have a different distribution in the Vc compared with the spinal dorsal horn (see Bereiter et al. 2000). Several receptor types associated with nociceptive processing are localized in the afferent endings or neurons in the Vc, e.g., neurokinin, opiate, GABA, purinergic, TRPV1, estrogen, and N-methyl D-aspartate (NMDA) and non-NMDA receptors. The Vc also is characterized by a substantia gelatinosa (SG) similar to that of the spinal dorsal horn (see Willis, this volume). Briefly, the axons of most SG neurons terminate locally within the VBSNC and release neuromodulatory substances such as enkephalin or GABA. The SG represents one of the main sites by which peripheral afferents and brain centers modulate somatosensory transmission (Gobel et al. 1981; Dubner and Bennett 1983; Sessle 2000). There are also intrinsic projections that connect different components of the VBSNC; these include the "deep bundles" by which many Vc neurons project to and influence the activity of neurons in more rostral components of the VBSNC.

The Vc has also provided a unique opportunity for recording from nociceptive second-order neurons and relating their activity to pain behavior in the same awake animal. In the 1980s, Dubner's group spearheaded such studies, documenting that NS and WDR neurons with a cutaneous receptive field play an important role in our ability to localize, detect, and discriminate cutaneous noxious stimuli (Dubner and Bennett 1983; Dubner 1985). Subsequent studies revealed that most of the NS and WDR neurons of the Vc can nonetheless be excited by afferents from deep tissues (e.g., the tooth pulp, cerebrovasculature, TMJ, and jaw muscle) as well as by cutaneous (or mucosal) afferent inputs (see Sessle 1987, 2000; Dostrovsky et al. 1991). Such features are thought to contribute to central sensitization and referred pain, and they underscore the inadvisability of using "convergent" neurons as an alternative term for WDR neurons, since NS neurons typically also reveal extensive afferent convergence.

Despite the similarities between the Vc and spinal dorsal horn, the long-held concept that these two structures are homologous may need revision in view of emerging evidence that, unlike the spinal dorsal horn, some tissues (e.g., the cornea and the cerebrovasculature) are dually represented in the Vc, in its rostral and caudal regions; these two regions also may be differentially involved in autonomic and muscle reflex responses to noxious stimulation of some orofacial tissues (Bereiter et al. 2000; Sessle 2000; Dubner and Ren 2004). Furthermore, since the 1st World Congress on Pain, it has become increasingly apparent that the Vc is not the only component of the VBSNC with a nociceptive role (Dubner et al. 1978; Sessle 1987, 2000; Woda 2003). Some orofacial nociceptive behaviors may persist after Vc lesions, and lesions of VBSNC rostral components (e.g., the subnucleus oralis) may disrupt some pain behaviors. Moreover, the rostral components have substantial numbers of NS and WDR neurons with an intraoral or perioral nociceptive receptive field (including tooth pulp). More recent support comes from findings that the rostral components contribute to ascending and reflex nociceptive pathways and manifest neurochemical markers for nociceptive processes (see Sessle 2000; Woda 2003). Nonetheless, these rostral regions receive only sparse direct input from small-diameter primary afferents and lack the modulatory SG substrate characteristic of the Vc; indeed, their nociceptive functions may be dependent on the functional integrity of the Vc, given that studies in the last decade have documented that the Vc, especially via its SG, exerts a modulatory influence on the subnucleus oralis through NMDA and purinergic receptor mechanisms within the Vc itself (Sessle 2000; Chiang et al. 2003; Woda 2003).

Although these various findings indicate that the Vc is crucial both to nociceptive processing and, as noted below, to the induction of central sensitization in the rostral VBSNC, more research is needed on the specific functional roles of the different regions of the Vc itself as well as its transition with the cervical dorsal horn. Further research is also needed on the relative roles of the rostral and caudal VBSNC components in orofacial nociceptive mechanisms and on the extent to which homology exists between the components of the VBSNC and the spinal nociceptive system.

THALAMOCORTICAL NOCICEPTIVE TRANSMISSION

By the time of the 1st World Congress on Pain, only limited attention had been given to thalamic processing related to orofacial pain, and most of this interest had centered on tooth-pulp-induced thalamic activity (see Dubner et al. 1978). This focus was subsequently broadened, building upon the information obtained of nociceptive processing in the VBSNC and of thalamic processing of spinal nociceptive inputs. Studies in awake as well as anesthetized animals revealed that many nociceptive neurons occur in the thalamic nucleus ventroposterior medialis (VPM) and that these neurons generally have properties similar to those described for NS and WDR neurons in the subthalamic relays such as the Vc and the spinal dorsal horn, including convergence of cutaneous and deep afferent inputs (Craig and Dostrovsky 1997). Their receptive field and response properties and their connections with the overlying somatosensory cerebral cortex suggest that most are involved in the sensory-discriminative dimension of pain. Nociceptive neurons receiving orofacial inputs also occur in other thalamic areas (e.g., the medial nuclei and nucleus submedius), but they are usually considered to be involved more in the affective or motivational dimensions of pain. A limited number of studies have also documented NS and WDR neurons in the primary face somatosensory cerebral cortex that respond to noxious facial or tooth pulp stimuli in a manner suggesting a role in the sensory-discriminative dimension of pain. Nociceptive neurons also occur in other cortical regions such as the anterior cingulate cortex, which has been implicated in the affective or motivational dimension of pain (see Bushnell, this volume).

NOCICEPTIVE REFLEX AND BEHAVIORAL RESPONSES

As well as projecting to thalamocortical regions involved in pain perception, many neurons in the VBSNC relay to brainstem or higher brain centers involved in reflex or more complex behavioral responses to noxious orofacial stimuli. By the time of the 1st World Congress on Pain, it was well known that orofacial pain could be associated with reflex changes in blood pressure, heart rate, breathing, and salivation evoked by noxious orofacial stimulation, and indeed several behavioral paradigms had been developed in humans and animals on the basis of these autonomic responses in order to study the effects of noxious orofacial stimuli (see Dubner et al. 1978). Human behavioral paradigms have been expanded since the 1970s, and now include measures of facial expression, subjective reports (using tools such as the pressure pain threshold, quantitative sensory testing, and the McGill Pain Questionnaire), and motor responses (see Rainville 2001; Svensson and Sessle 2004). Studies of the past three decades have also provided insights into some of the underlying reflex circuits and sensorimotor mechanisms of orofacial nociceptive reflexes and behaviors (see Bereiter et al. 2000; Sessle 2000; Svensson and Sessle 2004), showing for example that some neurons, especially in the rostral components of the VBSNC, are involved in the reflex circuits underlying the jaw-opening reflex, whereas the Vc is crucial in cardiac, adrenal, and respiratory changes and in the prolonged nociceptive reflex responses of jaw-opening and jaw-closing muscles as well as more complex pain-avoidance behaviors that can be evoked by noxious orofacial stimulation. Behavioral models of orofacial pain have also recently been developed in animals to replicate inflammatory or neuropathic pain conditions.

For example, models applying inflammatory irritants such as Freund's adjuvant, formalin, or mustard oil to facial skin, tooth pulp, and musculoskeletal tissues, or chronic constriction injury of trigeminal nerve branches, have been applied to studies of the pathogenesis of these conditions and to studies of modulatory influences on nociceptive transmission and pain behavior (Ren and Dubner 1999; Sessle 2000; Iwata et al. 2004; Svensson and Sessle 2004).

TRIGEMINAL NOCICEPTIVE MODULATION AND MODIFICATION

In the 1950s and 1960s it became evident that somatosensory transmission in the trigeminal and spinal systems was subject to segmental (afferent) and descending modulatory influences, but the scarce information available until the 1970s of nociceptive neural elements in the CNS limited our understanding of how these influences could operate in terms of modification of sensation and specifically in pain control (Darian-Smith 1966). At the time of the 1st World Congress on Pain, pain scientists and clinicians were avidly discussing the modulatory mechanisms proposed in the gate control theory of pain and their clinical implications (see Cervero, this volume). Discussion was especially colored by the recent discovery of intrinsic brain pathways capable of exerting descending control over the transmission of nociceptive signals in the CNS and by reports of the analgesic effectiveness of acupuncture (see Meyerson and Linderoth, this volume).

Orofacial pain research was at the forefront of the ensuing surge of interest into pain modulation, guided by the discovery of NS and WDR neurons in the Vc and related reflex events, as described above. The studies during and since the 1970s focused on the VBSNC, with more limited attention given to thalamic and cortical modulatory processes related to orofacial pain. The modulatory mechanisms and their implications in modification of sensation and in pain control are generally analogous to those described for spinal nociceptive transmission (see Willis, this volume), and so will be only briefly described.

INHIBITORY INFLUENCES

The intricate organization of the VBSNC and its variety of inputs from peripheral tissues and from different parts of the brain provide a particularly important substrate for numerous interactions between the various inputs. The Besson, Dubner, and Sessle groups were the first to document that electrical or chemical stimulation of the periaqueductal gray matter or rostroventral medulla/nucleus raphe magnus (NRM) activates descending pathways that project to the VBSNC and can inhibit trigeminal brainstem neuronal and related reflex and behavioral responses to noxious orofacial stimulation in experimental animals (see Dubner et al. 1978). Other powerful modulatory effects on trigeminal nociceptive transmission were subsequently discovered, including pathways emanating from the locus ceruleus, pontine parabrachial area, anterior pretectal nucleus, thalamic nucleus submedius, and cerebral cortex (e.g., somatosensory and motor areas; Ren and Dubner 1999; Sessle 1999a; Maixner 2001). Clinical studies have also reported relief of pain in pain patients by stimulation of some of these structures (see Meyerson and Linderoth, this volume). These descending pathways exert their effects by the release from their endings within the Vc of certain neurochemicals (e.g., 5HT) or by causing other chemicals (e.g., enkephalins, GABA) to be released from the endings of interneurons intrinsic to the VBSNC (e.g., in the SG of the Vc). These pathways and chemical processes are involved in the analgesia associated with, for example, deep brain stimulation and placebo; they can be modulated by sleep/wake state and may be up- or downregulated in pain states (Ren and Dubner 1999; Sessle 1999; Maixner 2001; Meyerson and Linderoth, this volume).

As in the spinal system (see Willis, this volume), so-called segmental or afferent influences also modulate trigeminal nociceptive transmission, especially through the interneuronal circuitry and neurochemical substrate of the Vc (Sessle 1999a; Maixner 2001). These influences include inputs into the CNS from nociceptive as well as non-nociceptive afferents, and also from visceral afferents (e.g., baroreceptors). The modulation by nociceptive inputs underlies the powerful descending inhibitory noxious control effects exerted on trigeminal nociceptive neurons, and these effects may contribute to the analgesia reported for acupuncture and transcutaneous electrical nerve stimulation (TENS; see Meyerson and Linderoth, this volume).

FACILITATORY INFLUENCES

Nociceptive transmission in the trigeminal and spinal systems can be enhanced by alterations to the peripheral afferent inputs to the CNS that may result from inflammation or trauma of peripheral tissues and nerves. This feature further emphasizes the plasticity of the neural circuitry underlying nociceptive transmission, i.e., that it is not "hard-wired." Little attention had been given to this topic up to the 1st World Congress on Pain, and even though plasticity in brainstem and higher centers (e.g., the somatosensory cortex) of the trigeminal system was documented in the 1980s, these findings were largely limited to non-nociceptive neurons (Sessle 1987; Kaas 1991). It was not until the early 1990s that collaborative studies by the Sessle and Woda groups in particular first detailed plasticity in trigeminal nociceptive pathways. Utilizing electrophysiological recordings of brainstem neurons and peripheral application of algesic inflammatory agents, they documented the particular efficacy of inputs from deep musculoskeletal tissues (e.g., the TMJ, masticatory muscle) and tooth pulp in inducing spontaneous activity, lowering activation threshold, expanding the receptive field, and enhancing peripherally evoked responses of NS and WDR neurons of the Vc (Hu et al. 1992; see Sessle 1999b, 2000; Woda 2003). Subsequent studies utilizing immunocytochemical and pharmacological approaches as well as electro-physiological recordings documented the neurochemical processes underly-ing these neuroplastic changes and the associated nociceptive behavior, show-ing that they can occur with nerve injury as well as with peripheral inflammation or injury (Ren and Dubner 1999; Sessle 2000; Woda 2001; Dubner and Ren 2004; Iwata et al. 2004). These changes and underlying neurochemical processes in many respects replicate the central sensitization described in spinal nociceptive pathways which are thought to contribute to persistent pain and its common characteristics of spontaneous pain, allodynia and hyperalgesia, and pain spread and referral (see Dubner, this volume).

Studies in the trigeminal system have also been amongst the first to show that purinergic as well as NMDA and non-NMDA receptor mecha-nisms are involved in central sensitization and that central depressive influ-ences (e.g., opioid-related) can normally be "triggered" by noxious orofacial stimulation and may serve to limit the sensitization (see Ren and Dubner 1999; Sessle 2000; Chiang et al. 2003). It is also noteworthy that trigeminal central sensitization is not limited to the Vc. It also has been shown in nociceptive neurons in the subnucleus oralis and in higher brain regions such as the VPM thalamus, although the Vc is responsible for their expres-sion of central sensitization by way of its projections to both structures (Chiang et al. 2003).

The trigeminal studies also documented the close interplay between sensory and motor pathways in prolonged pain. The nociceptive behavior associated with trigeminal central sensitization includes prolonged increases in both jaw-opening and jaw-closing muscle activity that involves a reflex pathway via the Vc, and noxious stimulation of jaw muscles may also modify the normal alternating activity of the jaw-opening and jaw-closing muscles during mastication. These and other findings in the past 15 years have un-dermined the credibility of long-held concepts related to the etiology of musculoskeletal pain, e.g., the so-called vicious cycle whereby muscle hyperactivity leads to pain, which produces more muscle hyperactivity, and so on. Rather, a concept of pain adaptation has been proposed, in which pain limits mobility and thereby aids healing (see Lund et al. 2001; Svensson and Sessle 2004).

CLINICAL FINDINGS

By the time of the 1st World Congress on Pain, many of the diagnostic and therapeutic approaches used today to manage chronic and especially acute orofacial pain were already available. Nonetheless, the last 30 years have seen refinements in local anesthetic techniques, new or improved diagnostic paradigms, improved pharmacological and physiological approaches to pain management, and recognition and application of biopsychosocial approaches. Given the space limitations of this chapter and topics covered in related chapters, these clinical developments will only be briefly highlighted below, together with information gained over this period on the etiology and pathogenesis of selected pain conditions.

ETIOLOGY AND PATHOGENESIS

The characterization of peripheral sensitization and central sensitization noted above represents important advances over the past 30 years because many pain conditions may involve one or both phenomena. For example, the acute pain and sensitivity of injured orofacial tissue, such as that of a "hot tooth" that gives an exaggerated response to mechanical or thermal stimuli applied to the inflamed tooth, can be explained by peripheral and central sensitization. Likewise, the pain and limitations in jaw movements that are characteristic of temporomandibular disorders (TMD) may result from sensitization phenomena producing states of allodynia and hyperalgesia as well as changes in jaw-opening and jaw-closing muscle activity (see Sessle 1999b; Svensson and Sessle 2004). In addition, the presence of a superficial as well as a deep receptive field in most Vc nociceptive neurons, plus the efficacy of deep nociceptive afferent inputs in inducing Vc central sensitization (Sessle 1999b, 2000; Woda 2003), which includes an expansion of both the cutaneous and deep receptive field, represent neuronal features thought to contribute to the poor localization and referral of deep pain that is a feature of TMD. This supposition is consistent with similar concepts of pain referral in the spinal nociceptive system (Mense and Simons 2001).

Despite these new insights, the etiology and pathogenesis of most chronic pain conditions manifested in the orofacial region remain an enigma. Nerve damage or changes in neural function have been implicated in the etiology of conditions such as such as trigeminal neuralgia, atypical facial pain, atypical odontalgia, and burning mouth syndrome. Studies of the past two decades have revealed that damage to afferent fibers or deafferentation may trigger several different mechanisms. These include sprouting of the afferents into peripheral tissues and even neuroma formation, the initiation of abnormal impulses in the injured afferents, the development of functional contacts between sympathetic efferents and nociceptive afferents, phenotypic changes in the afferents, structural reorganization and central sprouting of the endings in the CNS of primary afferents, changes in central inhibition, and most recently, changes in CNS microglia; most of these processes induce central sensitization (Sessle 2000; Woda 2001; Tsuda et al. 2003). Although study of these changes in trigeminal nociceptive pathways has been much more limited than in spinal nociceptive pathways, recent approaches using nerve injury, as well as acute or chronic inflammation of orofacial tissues, have revealed some comparable physiological and neurochemical changes in trigeminal nociceptive processing in association with exaggerated orofacial pain behavior (Ren and Dubner 1999; Sessle 2000; Woda 2001; Dubner and Ren 2004; Iwata et al. 2004). A particular challenge is to clarify which of these changes are specifically applicable to each of the chronic orofacial pain conditions noted above.

CLASSIFICATION, ASSESSMENT, AND MANAGEMENT

Several revised classification schemes for orofacial pain have appeared in the last decade, the most notable being those of IASP (Merskey and Bogduk 1994), the American Academy of Orofacial Pain (Okeson 1996), and the International Headache Society (2004). Also notable is the disagreement between them on some features. A move towards a mechanisms-based classification of orofacial pain has also recently been advocated, but application of such a scheme is stymied by a lack of clear definition of the specific mechanisms applicable to the development and maintenance of most chronic pain conditions.

As noted above, many of the current measures to diagnose and manage orofacial pain were in place at the time of the 1st World Congress on Pain. Acupuncture, TENS, and other less traditional approaches have since become available, although their efficacy generally has not been the subject of rigorous scientific testing. The past 30 years have also seen the development or improvement of a number of diagnostic and assessment approaches that have been specifically developed for chronic as well as acute orofacial pain conditions or have found extensive application in the orofacial region, such as the pressure pain threshold, visual analogue scales, the McGill Pain

Questionnaire, quantitative sensory testing, and magnetic resonance imaging (see Rainville 2001; Jääskeläinen 2004; Svensson and Sessle 2004).

In the case of one of the most common pains in the body, toothache, several forms are still categorized as they were in the 1970s, and most acute pulpal conditions associated with pain are managed with standard dental approaches (Holland 2001; Svensson and Sessle 2004). Nonetheless, improved understanding of nociceptive mechanisms in the pulp and other peripheral tissues has guided the few advances in the past 30 years in local anesthetic approaches and in physical and pharmacological therapies that have been beneficial for managing most toothaches and other forms of acute orofacial pain (Holland 2001; Svensson and Sessle 2004).

Temporomandibular disorders (TMD) are very common chronic pains, with a prevalence of around 10% (Lipton et al. 1993; LeResche 2001). The last 15 years has seen some notable advances in this field, with a focus on specificity and sensitivity of diagnostic and management approaches and the development of the Research Diagnostic Criteria for TMD, which has assisted in the classification and diagnosis of these conditions (Dworkin and LeResche 1992; Widmer et al. 1994; Stohler and Zarb 1999; Svensson and Sessle 2004). These advances have stemmed from a change in conceptualization of these conditions that had started by the time of the 1st World Congress on Pain. It reflected a paradigm shift away from local factors (e.g., dental occlusion) to psychosocial factors as being of greatest importance in most cases. Extensive research has subsequently shown that occlusion generally has very little to do with the cause of the great majority of TMD, that occlusal balancing and most occlusal splints have very little scientific basis for their use in TMD, and that most TMD conditions can be adequately managed by relatively simple, irreversible techniques (see Stohler and Zarb 1999; Okeson 2003; Forssell and Kalso 2004; Svensson and Sessle 2004). While the etiology of TMD is still unknown, sensitization phenomena may be involved in its pathogenesis (Sessle 1999b, 2000), and female gender, depression, and multiple other pain conditions in particular have been identified in the past decade as significant risk factors.

Trigeminal neuralgia is much less common than TMD, and studies since the 1970s have confirmed an incidence of around 4 cases per 100,000 individuals (see LeResche 2001; Zakrzewska and Harrison 2002). Although there is no satisfactory laboratory model, animal studies in the past 30 years have resulted in proposals that the etiology and pathogenesis of trigeminal neuralgia are based largely on peripherally induced generation of ectopic action potentials in trigeminal nerve branches and on changes in central inhibition (see Fromm and Sessle 1991; Zakrzewska and Harrison 2002). No diagnostic tests have sufficient specificity and sensitivity for trigeminal neuralgia, so its diagnosis remains largely based on clinical history, signs, and symptoms. A continuing concern is its differential diagnosis, because clinicians often misdiagnose trigeminal neuralgia and may institute therapies that are ineffective or indeed exacerbate the condition. Since the 1st World Congress on Pain, additional surgical approaches aimed at the trigeminal ganglion or rootlets have been developed (e.g., thermocoagulation, glycerol gangliolysis, microvascular decompression), and while considerable success rates have been reported, there have been no randomized controlled trials of the surgical approaches, and neuralgia recurrence and unpleasant sensory deficits are not uncommon. Consequently, pharmacological management with anticonvulsants developed before the 1st World Congress on Pain (e.g., carbamazepine) remain the mainstay of treatment for trigeminal neuralgia, although not all patients benefit from their use (Fromm and Sessle 1991; Zakrzewska and Harrison 2002).

Postherpetic neuralgia is more common than trigeminal neuralgia, and typically develops in the ophthalmic nerve and midthoracic spinal segments following the rash characteristic of herpes zoster. Evidence suggests that central as well as peripheral factors are involved in its etiology and pathogenesis (Fine 2001; Watson 2005). Since the 1st World Congress on Pain, antiviral therapy has been introduced, with moderate success, to prevent its clinical features, including pain. There have also been randomized controlled trials documenting the efficacy of tricyclic antidepressants in relieving postherpetic neuralgia, and recent studies also suggest that other approaches such as gabapentin and topical therapies such as capsaicin and local anesthetics may be useful in some patients (Fine 2002; Watson 2004).

Atypical facial pain, atypical odontalgia, and burning mouth syndrome are chronic orofacial pain conditions that have less clear diagnostic signs than those noted above and are even more problematic in their management. Atypical facial pain is particularly ill-defined and is usually diagnosed by elimination. However, there have been recent attempts to define these conditions in a more positive and integrated manner (Woda and Pionchon 1999; Sharav 2005). They are not uncommon (e.g., prevalence of 1% or more for burning mouth syndrome), but their etiology and pathogenesis remain unclear. A general consensus has been developing since the 1st World Congress on Pain that some or all of these enigmatic conditions may be neuropathic because there is often a history of orofacial trauma, and so several of the mechanisms implicated in neuropathic pain have been invoked to account for or at least contribute to these conditions (Woda 2001; Sharav 2005). However, this opinion is not borne out in every case because psychophysical and other testing for changes typical of neuropathic pain conditions generally reveal limited objective changes. Additional risk factors include sex and age because most cases are women in the perimenstrual period. Earlier claims of the psychogenic origin of these conditions have been tempered by studies in the 1980s and 1990s (Ship et al. 1995; Woda 2001; Sharav 2005) that have documented that psychological disturbances may be the result and not the cause of symptoms in most patients; this finding is not dissimilar to most other chronic pain conditions associated with an unknown etiology and uncertainty of treatment success. These conditions also are often incorrectly diagnosed, or therapies are applied that are not beneficial or indeed exacerbate the condition. Management, however, is problematic even for correctly diagnosed cases, and these conditions still have no well-established and effective therapeutic approaches (Sharav 2005).

Improvements in diagnostic and management approaches for the persistent pain conditions in the face and mouth will rely heavily on advances in basic and clinical research that will clarify their underlying mechanisms in animal models and on randomized controlled trials of existing and newly developed approaches. Emerging technologies, particularly in imaging, sensory testing, biological markers, and molecular biology, hold out promise of improved therapeutic approaches for these conditions.

ACKNOWLEDGMENTS

Studies of the author are supported by grants DE04786 and DE15420 of the U.S. National Institute of Dental and Craniofacial Research and by grant MT4918 of the Canadian Institutes of Health Research. The author is also the recipient of a Canada Research Chair.

REFERENCES

Belmonte C. Ocular nociceptors. In: Schmidt RF, Willis WD (Eds). *Pain Encyclopedia.* Heidelberg: Springer-Verlag, 2005, in press.

Bereiter DA, Hiraba H, Hu JW. Trigeminal subnucleus caudalis beyond homologies with the spinal dorsal horn. *Pain* 2000; 88:221–224.

Bränström M, Åström A. The hydrodynamics of the dentine: its possible relationship to dentinal pain. *Int Dent J* 1972; 22:219–227.

Byers MR, Narhi MVO. Dental injury models: experimental tools for understanding neuroinflammatory interactions and polymodal nociceptor functions. *Crit Rev Oral Biol Med* 1999; 10:4–39.

Cairns B. Nociceptors in the orofacial region—TMJ and muscle. In: Schmidt RF, Willis WD (Eds). *Pain Encyclopedia.* Heidelberg: Springer-Verlag, 2005, in press.

Chiang CY, Hu B, Park SJ, et al. Purinergic and NMDA-receptor mechanisms underlying tooth pulp stimulation-induced central sensitization in trigeminal nociceptive neurons. In: Dostrovsky JO, Carr DB, Koltzenburg M (Eds). *Proceedings of the 10th World Congress on Pain*, Progress in Pain Research and Management, Vol. 24, Seattle: IASP Press, 2003, pp 345–354.

Cooper. Nociceptors in the orofacial region—skin/mucosa. In: Schmidt RF, Willis WD (Eds). *Pain Encyclopedia.* Heidelberg: Springer-Verlag, 2005, in press.

Craig AD, Dostrovsky JO. Processing of nociceptive information at supraspinal levels. In: Yaksh TL, Lynch C III, Zapol WM, et al. (Eds). *Anesthesia: Biological Foundations.* Philadelphia: Lippincott-Raven, 1997, pp 625–642.

Darian-Smith I. Neural mechanisms of facial sensation. *Int Rev Neurobiol* 1966; 9:301–395.

Dostrovsky JO, Davis KD, Kawakita K. Central mechanisms of vascular headaches. *Can J Physiol Pharmacol* 1991; 69:652–658.

Dubner R. Recent advances in our understanding of pain. In: Klineberg I, Sessle BJ (Eds). *Oro-Facial Pain and Neuromuscular Dysfunction: Mechanisms and Clinical Correlates.* Oxford: Pergamon Press, 1985, pp 3–19.

Dubner R, Bennett GJ. Spinal and trigeminal mechanisms of nociception. *Annu Rev Neurosci* 1983; 6:381–418.

Dubner R, Ren K. Brainstem mechanisms of persistent pain following injury. *J Orofac Pain* 2004; 18: 299–305.

Dubner R, Sessle BJ, Storey AT. *The Neural Basis of Oral and Facial Function.* New York: Plenum Press, 1978.

Dworkin SF, LeResche L. Research diagnostic criteria for temporomandibular disorders: review, criteria, examinations and specifications, critique. *J Craniomandib Disord* 1992; 6:301–355.

Fine P. Neve blocks. In: Watson CPN, Gershon AA (Eds). *Herpes Zoster and Postherpetic Neuralgia,* 2nd ed, Pain Research and Management, Vol. 11. Amsterdam: Elsevier, 2001.

Forssell H, Kalso E. Application of principles of evidence-based medicine to occlusal treatment for temporomandibular disorders: are there lessons to be learned? *J Orofac Pain* 2004; 18:9–22.

Fromm GH, Sessle BJ. *Trigeminal Neuralgia: Current Concepts Regarding Pathogenesis and Treatment.* Stoneham: Butterworth-Heinemann, 1991.

Gobel S, Hockfield S, Ruda MA. Anatomical similarities between medullary and spinal dorsal horns. In: Kawamura Y, Dubner R (Eds). *Oral-Facial Sensory and Motor Functions.* Tokyo: Quintessence, 1981, pp 211–223.

Holland GR. Management of dental pain. In: Lund JP, Lavigne GJ, Dubner R, Sessle BJ (Eds). *Orofacial Pain: From Basic Science to Clinical Management.* Chicago: Quintessence, 2001, pp 211–220.

Hu JW. Tooth pulp. In: Miles TS, Nauntofte B, Svensson P (Eds). *Clinical Oral Physiology.* Copenhagen: Quintessence, 2004, pp 141–163.

Hu JW, Woda A. Trigeminal brainstem nuclear complex, physiology. In: Schmidt RF, Willis WD (Eds). *Pain Encyclopedia.* Heidelberg: Springer-Verlag, 2005, in press.

Hu JW, Sessle BJ, Raboisson P, Dallel R, Woda A. Stimulation of craniofacial muscle afferents induces prolonged facilitatory effects in trigeminal nociceptive brainstem neurones. *Pain* 1992; 48:53–60.

International Headache Society. The International Classification of Headache Disorders, 2nd ed. *Cephalalgia* 2004; 24(Suppl).

Iwata K, Tsuboi Y, Shima A, et al. Central neuronal changes after nerve injury: neuroplastic influences of injury and aging. *J Orofac Pain* 2004; 18:293–298.

Jääskeläinen SK. Clinical neurophysiology and quantitative sensory testing in the investigation of orofacial pain and sensory function. *J Orofac Pain* 2004; 18:85–107.

Kaas JH. Plasticity of sensory and motor maps in adult mammals. *Annu Rev Neurosci* 1991; 14:137–167.

LeResche L. Epidemiology of orofacial pain. In: Lund JP, Lavigne GJ, Dubner R, Sessle BJ (Eds). *Orofacial Pain: From Basic Science to Clinical Management.* Chicago: Quintessence, 2001, pp 15–25.

Lipton JA, Ship JA, Larach-Robinson D. Estimated prevalence and distribution of reported orofacial pain in the United States. *J Am Dent Assoc* 1993; 124:115–121.

Lund JP. Pain and movement. In: Lund JP, Lavigne GJ, Dubner R, Sessle BJ (Eds). *Orofacial Pain: From Basic Science to Clinical Management*. Chicago: Quintessence, 2001, pp 151–163.

Matthews B, Sessle BJ. Peripheral mechanisms of orofacial pain. In: Lund JP, Lavigne GJ, Dubner R, Sessle BJ (Eds). *Orofacial Pain: From Basic Science to Clinical Management*. Chicago: Quintessence, 2001, pp 37–46.

Maixner W. Pain modulatory systems. In: Lund JP, Lavigne GJ, Dubner R, Sessle BJ (Eds). *Orofacial Pain: From Basic Science to Clinical Management*. Chicago: Quintessence, 2001, pp 79–91.

Mense S, Simons DG. *Muscle Pain: Understanding its Nature, Diagnosis and Treatment*. Philadelphia: Lippincott Williams and Wilkins, 2001.

Merskey H, Bogduk N (Eds). *Classification of Chronic Pain: Descriptions of Chronic Pain Syndromes and Definitions of Pain Terms,* 2nd ed. Seattle: IASP Press, 1994.

Messlinger K. Nociceptors in the orofacial region—vessels/dura. In: Schmidt RF, Willis WD (Eds). *Pain Encyclopedia*. Heidelberg: Springer-Verlag, 2005, in press.

Narhi MVO. Nociceptors in the dental pulp. In: Schmidt RF, Willis WD (Eds). *Pain Encyclopedia*. Heidelberg: Springer-Verlag, 2005, in press.

Okeson JP (Ed). *Orofacial Pain: Guidelines for Assessment, Diagnosis and Management*. Chicago: Quintessence, 1996, pp 45–52.

Okeson JP. *Management of Temporomandibular Disorders and Occlusion*, 5th ed. St. Louis: Mosby, 2003.

Rainville P. Measurement of pain. In: Lund JP, Lavigne GJ, Dubner R, Sessle BJ (Eds). *Orofacial Pain, From Basic Science to Clinical Management*. Chicago: Quintessence, 2001, pp 95–105.

Ren K, Dubner R. Central nervous system plasticity and persistent pain. *J Orofac Pain* 1999; 13:155–163.

Sessle BJ. The neurobiology of orofacial and dental pain. *J Dent Res* 1987; 66:962–981.

Sessle BJ. Somatosensory transmission in the trigeminal brainstem complex and its modulation by peripheral and central neural influences. In: Lydic R, Baghdoyan HA (Eds). *Handbook of Behavioral State Control: Cellular and Molecular Mechanisms*. Boca Raton, FL: CRC Press, 1999a, pp 445–461.

Sessle BJ. The neural basis of temporomandibular joint and masticatory muscle pain. *J Orofac Pain* 1999b; 13:238–245.

Sessle BJ. Acute and chronic craniofacial pain: brainstem mechanisms of nociceptive transmission and neuroplasticity, and their clinical correlates. *Crit Rev Oral Biol Med* 2000; 11:57–91.

Sharav Y. Atypical facial pain, etiology, pathogenesis and management. In: Schmidt RF, Willis WD (Eds). *Pain Encyclopedia*. Heidelberg: Springer-Verlag, 2005, in press.

Ship JA, Grushka M, Lipton JA, et al. An update on burning mouth syndrome. *J Am Dent Assoc* 1995; 126:842–853.

Stohler CS, Zarb GA. On the management of temporomandibular disorders: a plea for a low-tech, high-prudence approach. *J Orofac Pain* 1999; 13:255–261.

Svensson P, Sessle BJ. Orofacial pain. In: Miles TS, Nauntofte B, Svensson P (Eds). *Clinical Oral Physiology*. Copenhagen: Quintessence, 2004, pp 93–139.

Tsuda M, Shigemoto-Mogami Y, Koizumi S, et al. P2X4 receptors induced in spinal microglia gate tactile allodynia after nerve injury. *Nature* 2003; 424(6950):778–783.

Watson CPN. Postherpetic neuralgia: etiology, pathogenesis, and management. In: Schmidt RF, Willis WD (Eds). *Pain Encyclopedia*. Heidelberg: Springer-Verlag, 2005, in press.

Widmer CG, McCall WD, Lund JP. Adjunctive diagnostic tests. In: Zarb GA, Carlsson GE, Sessle BJ, Mohl ND (Eds). *Temporomandibular Joint and Masticatory Muscle Disorders*. Copenhagen: Munksgaard, 1994, pp 510–525.

Woda A. Mechanisms of neuropathic pain. In: Lund JP, Lavigne GJ, Dubner R, Sessle BJ (Eds). *Orofacial Pain: From Basic Science to Clinical Management*. Chicago: Quintessence, 2001, pp 67–78.

Woda A. Pain in the trigeminal system: from orofacial nociception to neural network modeling. *J Dent Res* 2003; 82(10):764–768.

Woda A, Pionchon P. A unified concept of idiopathic orofacial pain: clinical features. *J Orofac Pain* 1999; 13:172–184.

Zakrzewska JM, Harrison SD (Eds). *Assessment and Management of Orofacial Pain*. Amsterdam: Elsevier, 2002.

Correspondence to: Barry J. Sessle, MDS, PhD, DSc, Faculty of Dentistry, University of Toronto, 124 Edward Street, Toronto, ON, Canada M5G 1G6. Tel: 416-979-4921 Ext. 4336; Fax: 416-979-4936; email: barry.sessle@utoronto.ca.

The Paths of Pain 1975–2005, edited by
Harold Merskey, John D. Loeser, and Ronald
Dubner, IASP Press, Seattle, © 2005.

10

A Thirty-Year Perspective on the Pathophysiology of Migraine Pain

Rami Burstein, Dan Levy, and Moshe Jakubowski

Departments of Anesthesia and Critical Care, Beth Israel Deaconess Medical Center; Department of Neurobiology and the Program in Neuroscience, Harvard Medical School, Boston, Massachusetts, USA

Migraine is a heterogeneous neurological disorder characterized as a recurring, episodic, unilateral headache. Migraine pain usually throbs (Anthony 1993) and typically intensifies during physical activities that increase intracranial pressure (e.g., bending over or coughing) (Blau and Dexter 1981; Rasmussen et al. 1991). The pain is associated with a high incidence of nausea and a predominance of hypersensitivity to light (photophobia) and noise (phonophobia). Symptoms of lesser prevalence include aversion to odors (osmophobia), vomiting, fatigue, red eyes, tearing, nasal congestion, and frequent yawning. A migraine attack may be precipitated by endogenous factors (hormonal changes, psychosocial stress, sleep deficit or surplus, or hunger), or by exogenous factors (certain kinds of food or the stimulation of different sensory modalities). An attack can be preceded by abnormal visual, sensory, motor, and/or speech functions (migraine with aura) or may start with no warning signs (migraine without aura).

VASCULAR THEORIES

EXTRACRANIAL VASCULAR THEORY

For many years, migraine headache has been thought to be related to dilation of extracranial arteries. The theory was, as cited extensively in medical textbooks, that abnormal vasodilation during migraine causes mechanical activation of perivascular stretch receptors, resulting in throbbing headache (Wolff 1963). This view was based on observations that extracranial arteries are vasodilated, edematous, and partially damaged during

migraine (Wolff et al. 1953; Wolff 1963). However, the extracranial vascular theory has fallen out of favor because clinical studies have yielded no
convincing evidence for any significant extracranial vasodilation during migraine, nor have they shown that vasodilation can produce headache
(Zwetsloot et al. 1991; Moskowitz and Macfarlane 1993).

INTRACRANIAL VASCULAR THEORY

The prevailing view today is that migraine headache is a neurovascular
disorder of intracranial origin that involves meningeal blood vessels and the
pain fibers that innervate them. This theory has originated from reports that
electrical and mechanical stimulation of dural vasculature (but not of the
surface of the brain) produced referred head pain in awake patients undergoing craniotomy (Penfield and McNaughton 1940; Ray and Wolff 1940).
Three types of referred pain were reported: (1) periorbital pain (by stimulating the superior sagittal sinus or blood vessels of the floor of the anterior
fossa); (2) parietal/temporal pain (by stimulating the middle meningeal artery); and (3) occipital pain (by stimulating the dura at the floor of the
posterior fossa, and the sigmoid, transverse and occipital sinuses). It should
be emphasized that no sensation other than pain was evoked by stimulation
of these structures and that stimulation of nonvascular areas of the dura was
largely ineffective in inducing pain sensation. These findings fit well with
the pattern of dural innervation, whereby sensory nerves that originate in
trigeminal and upper cervical ganglia closely follow meningeal blood vessels but not nonvascular areas of the dura (Penfield and McNaughton 1940).
It was not until the 1980s that the nature of dural innervation was proved to
be nociceptive. We now know that the dura is richly innervated by axons
with unmyelinated (C) fibers and thinly myelinated (Aδ) fibers that originate
in the trigeminal ganglion and in C1–C3 dorsal root ganglia (Mayberg et al.
1981; Keller et al. 1985; Andres et al. 1987; Moskowitz and Macfarlane
1993). These pain fibers contain vasoactive neuropeptides such as substance
P and calcitonin gene-related peptide (CGRP) (Uddman et al. 1985; Keller
and Marfurt 1991). These lines of evidence promoted the theory that the
headache phase of migraine is mediated by activation of nociceptors that
innervate meningeal blood vessels (i.e., meningeal nociceptors), and provided the basis for developing animal models of neurovascular head pain
with intracranial origin.

EXPERIMENTAL ACTIVATION OF TRIGEMINOVASCULAR PATHWAYS

The first animal model of neurovascular head pain employed the paradigm of electrical or mechanical stimulation of the dural sinuses (Davis and Dostrovsky 1986; Strassman et al. 1986). Using anatomical, physiological, histological, and pharmaceutical techniques, such animal studies have demonstrated the presence of dura-sensitive neurons in brain and spinal cord structures, such as the medullary dorsal horn, thalamus, hypothalamus, and periaqueductal gray (PAG) (Strassman et al. 1986, 1994; Davis and Dostrovsky 1988; Zagami and Lambert 1990; Goadsby and Zagami 1991; Kaube et al. 1993; Malick et al. 2001; Levy and Strassman 2002; Benjamin et al. 2004). In the medullary dorsal horn (Burstein et al. 1998; Yamamura et al. 1999) and thalamus (Davis and Dostrovsky 1988; Zagami and Lambert 1990), the majority of these trigeminovascular neurons respond to noxious skin stimuli either preferentially (wide-dynamic-range neurons) or exclusively (high-threshold neurons). Administration of antimigraine drugs such as ergotamines, triptans, or CGRP antagonists inhibits responses to electrical stimulation of the dura in dura-sensitive neurons in the medullary dorsal horn (Zagami and Lambert 1990; Lambert et al. 1992; Goadsby and Hoskin 1996; Hoskin et al. 1996). The acute stimulation of dural sinuses as a model for neurovascular head pain with intracranial origin has identified the trigeminovascular system and established the potential involvement of each of its elements in vascular headache and its associated symptoms. However, acute electrical or mechanical stimulation of the dura does not induce migraine in humans, and can only evoke a short burst of activity in peripheral and central trigeminovascular neurons.

In recent years, it has become apparent that many types of prolonged or chronic pain are associated with long-lasting activation and sensitization of peripheral nociceptors and/or central nociceptive neurons in the dorsal horn. A new animal model for long-lasting headache of migraine was developed that incorporated these concepts into basic research on migraine pathophysiology. This model involves prolonged activation and subsequent sensitization of the trigeminovascular system in response to a brief exposure of the dura to a mixture of inflammatory agents consisting of serotonin, bradykinin, histamine, and prostaglandin (Strassman et al. 1996). These agents activate and sensitize somatic and visceral nociceptors in rats (Beck and Handwerker 1974; Mizumura et al. 1987; Neugebauer et al. 1989; Steen et al. 1992; Davis et al. 1993) and are potent algesics in humans (Armstrong et al. 1957; Hollander et al. 1957; Guzman et al. 1962; Sicuteri 1967), capable of inducing headache (Sicuteri 1967).

PERIPHERAL SENSITIZATION

Using an animal model, Strassman et al. (1996) found that a brief chemical irritation of the dura activates and sensitizes meningeal nociceptors (first-order trigeminovascular neurons) over a long period of time, rendering them responsive to mechanical stimuli to which they showed only minimal or no response prior to their sensitization. During migraine, such *peripheral* sensitization is likely to mediate the throbbing pain and its aggravation during routine physical activities such as coughing, sneezing, bending over, rapid shaking one's head, holding one's breath, climbing up the stairs, or walking. By the end of a migraine attack, when meningeal nociceptors are presumably no longer sensitized, their sensitivity to fluctuations in intracranial pressure returns to normal, and the patient no longer feels throbbing.

CENTRAL SENSITIZATION

Brief stimulation of the dura with inflammatory agents also activates and sensitizes second-order trigeminovascular neurons located in the medullary dorsal horn that receive convergent input from the dura and the skin (Burstein et al. 1998). In this paradigm, the central trigeminovascular neurons develop hypersensitivity in the periorbital skin, manifested as increased responsiveness to mild cutaneous stimuli (brushing, heat, or cold) to which they showed only minimal or no response prior to their sensitization. The induction of central sensitization by intracranial stimulation of the dura and the ensuing extracranial hypersensitivity in this rat study were taken to suggest that a similar process occurs in patients during migraine.

Extracranial hypersensitivity during migraine was first noted in 1873 (Liveing 1873) and later documented in the 1950s (Wolff et al. 1953; Selby and Lance 1960). At that time, extracranial hypersensitivity was ascribed to "hematomas that develop hours after onset of headache as a result of damage to vascular walls of blood vessels such as the temporal artery" (Wolff et al. 1953), or to "widespread distension of extracranial blood vessels or spasm of suboccipital scalp muscles" (Selby and Lance 1960). The current view, however, is that extracranial hypersensitivity is a manifestation of central neuronal sensitization rather than of extracranial vascular pathophysiology. Recent quantitative tests in which stimulation was applied to the surface of the skin showed that pain thresholds to mechanical, heat, and cold cutaneous stimuli decrease significantly during migraine in the majority of patients (Burstein et al. 2000). This skin hypersensitivity, termed cutaneous allodynia, is typically found in the periorbital area on the side of the migraine headache. Patients commonly notice cutaneous allodynia during migraine when they become irritated by innocuous activities such as combing, shaving, taking a shower, wearing eyeglasses or earrings, or resting their head on the pillow on the headache side. Ipsilateral cephalic allodynia is likely to be mediated by sensitization of trigeminovascular neurons in the medullary dorsal horn that process sensory inputs from the dura and periorbital skin. In many patients, increased skin sensitivity during migraine is also felt extracephalically in the arms and legs. Patients experiencing such "extended allodynia" are bothered by wearing tight clothes, a watch, bracelet, necklace, socks, or bra. This extended allodynia is likely to be mediated by higher-order nociceptive neurons that process somatosensory signals from the dura as well as from extracephalic skin.

Central sensitization can be either dependent on or independent of activity (Ji et al. 2003). The induction of sensitization in second-order trigeminovascular neurons, using chemical stimulation of the rat dura, is activity dependent, as evidenced by lidocaine blockade of afferent inputs from the dura. Once established, however, sensitization of the second-order trigeminovascular neurons becomes activity independent, as it can no longer be interrupted by lidocaine on the dura (Burstein et al. 1998). Translating these findings in the context of migraine with allodynia, it appears that central sensitization depends on incoming impulses from the meninges in the early phase of the attack and maintains itself in the absence of such sensory input later on. This view is strongly supported by the effects of the anti-migraine 5-HT$_{1B/1D}$ agonists, known as triptans, on the induction and maintenance of central sensitization in the rat (Burstein and Jakubowski 2004) and by the corresponding effects of early and late triptan therapy on allodynia during migraine (Burstein et al. 2004). In the rat, triptan administration concomitant with chemical irritation of the dura effectively prevents the development of central sensitization. Similarly, treating patients with triptans early, within 60 minutes of the onset of migraine, effectively blocks the development of cutaneous allodynia. However, neither central neuronal sensitization in the rat nor cutaneous allodynia in patients can be reversed by late triptan treatment (2 hours after the application of sensitizing agent to the dura in the animal model, and 4 hours after the onset of migraine in allodynic patients). Most importantly, central sensitization appears to play a critical role in the management of migraine headache in allodynic patients. While non-allodynic patients can be rendered pain-free with triptans at any time during an attack, allodynic patients can be rendered pain-free only if treated with triptans early in the attack, before the establishment of cutaneous allodynia (Burstein et al. 2004).

The findings that triptans cannot block ongoing sensitization in second-order trigeminovascular neurons is consistent with the evidence that these neurons do not posses the 5-HT$_{1D}$ receptor (Potrebic et al. 2003) that mediates the neuronal action of these drugs. If triptans do not abort migraine in the presence of allodynia (i.e., central sensitization), how do they render the patient pain-free in the absence of allodynia? The simple option would be a peripheral action of triptans that suppresses ongoing sensitization in the meningeal nociceptors that bombard the second-order neurons in the dorsal horn. However, the evidence shows that sensitized meningeal nociceptors are not inhibited by triptans (Levy et al. 2004). Thus, it appears that triptans abort migraine by a central, presynaptic action in the dorsal horn that blocks transmission of nociceptive signals between first- and second-order trigeminovascular neurons.

MODULATION OF CENTRAL SENSITIZATION

A growing body of evidence suggests that while migraine patients are mostly non-allodynic during the first years of their migraine experience, they are eventually destined to develop allodynia during their migraine attacks (Burstein et al. 2000, 2004; Mathew et al. 2004). It is therefore possible that repeated migraine attacks over the years have cumulative adverse consequences on the function of the trigeminovascular pathway, one of which is susceptibility to develop central sensitization. The threshold for a central trigeminovascular neuron to enter a state of sensitization depends on the balance between incoming nociceptive signals and their modulation by spinal and supraspinal pathways. Many of the modulatory supraspinal pathways converge on the PAG and rostral ventromedial medulla (RVM) (Fields and Basbaum 1999). Recent imaging studies have shown that the PAG is activated during migraine (Weiller et al. 1995) and that it contains abnormally high levels of iron in patients with a long history of migraine, suggesting an abnormal neuronal functioning (Welch et al. 2001). Abnormal PAG functioning can either *enhance* activity of RVM neurons that *facilitate* pain transmission in the dorsal horn or *suppress* activity of RVM neurons that *inhibit* such transmission (Porreca et al. 2002). This change may enhance excitability and thus promote responses of second-order trigeminovascular neurons to incoming nociceptive signals from the meninges, resulting in a reduced threshold for entering a state of central sensitization. Furthermore, the transition from episodic to chronic migraine that occurs in some patients over the years may involve a shift in the underlying pathophysiology from a transient to chronic state of sensitization. Altered functions of modulatory supraspinal pain pathways can contribute to this progression in migraine pathophysiology.

THE BRAINSTEM GENERATOR THEORY

A rather radical view on migraine pathophysiology originated from a 1987 report suggesting that the PAG constitutes a so-called "headache generator." In that study, 15 out of 175 pain patients (8.5%) developed migraine-like headache immediately after undergoing implantation of electrodes at (or near) the PAG for relieving intractable pain (Raskin et al. 1987). This point of view has promoted an interpretation that activation of the PAG during migraine is the source, rather than the consequence, of migraine pain (Weiller et al. 1995; Bahra et al. 2001). However, numerous studies have yielded overwhelming evidence to disprove the concept of the PAG as a "headache generator." The first line of evidence is that persistent postoperative headache lasting 3 months or longer is routinely observed in 9–38% of patients undergoing craniotomy for a wide variety of procedures, with or without electrode placement (Harner et al. 1993; Gokalp et al. 1995; Kaur et al. 2000; Gee et al. 2003; Schaller and Baumann 2003). This crucial information was not available to Raskin et al. when they made the statement that "comparable headache syndromes have not been seen following craniotomy or burr hole placement performed for a variety of disorders."

The second line of evidence comes from neuroimaging studies in humans (Hsieh et al. 1996; Iadarola et al. 1998; Petrovic et al. 1999; Derbyshire et al. 2002) and from Fos expression studies in animals (Bandler et al. 2000), demonstrating that PAG activation occurs in numerous non-headache pain paradigms. This evidence indicates that PAG activation is a universal consequence of nociceptor activation anywhere in the body, which is perfectly consistent with the multiple input arriving at the PAG from nociceptive neurons through the length of the spinal cord. The third line of evidence is that electrical stimulation of the PAG produces general pain relief throughout the body (Hosobuchi et al. 1977). This evidence indicates that modulation of pain by the PAG is nonspecific, which is consistent with the anatomical evidence that individual RVM neurons project to multiple segments of the spinal cord and terminate in the dorsal horn (Basbaum et al. 1978; Holstege and Kuypers 1982; Martin et al. 1985; Fields et al. 1995). Finally, the fourth line of evidence is that stimulation of the PAG or RVM cannot generate firing in spinothalamic tract neurons; it can only increase or decrease the firing of these neurons in responses to noxious stimulation of their peripheral receptive fields (Porreca et al. 2002). Accordingly, it is activation of specific dorsal horn neurons by input they receive from peripheral nociceptors that determines where pain modulation is needed. In the case of migraine, it is activation of trigeminovascular neurons in the medullary dorsal horn by inputs from meningeal nociceptors.

ACTIVATION OF MENINGEAL NOCICEPTORS

In spite of extensive research, the endogenous mechanisms by which meningeal nociceptors become activated have not yet been identified. We shall briefly review three hypotheses that attempt to describe endogenous cascades of events in the dura that may lead up to activation of meningeal nociceptors during the headache phase of migraine.

NEUROGENIC INFLAMMATION HYPOTHESIS

According to this hypothesis, meningeal nociceptors are activated by local release of endogenous inflammatory mediators through a process termed *neurogenic inflammation* (Moskowitz 1984; Moskowitz and Macfarlane 1993). The process refers to a host of events, including local increase in blood flow, leakage of plasma protein from blood vessels, mast cell degranulation, and platelet aggregation. Neurogenic inflammation can be evoked experimentally by noxious stimulation of nociceptors that innervate a given tissue and the subsequent release of vasoactive neuropeptides such as substance P, neurokinin A, and CGRP (Holzer 1988). Similar markers of neurogenic inflammation and neuropeptide release have been induced in the rat dura by antidromic activation of meningeal afferents through electrical stimulation of the trigeminal ganglion (Markowitz et al. 1987; Dimitriadou et al. 1991). Support for the role of neurogenic inflammation in migraine comes from evidence that plasma protein extravasation and mast cell degranulation can be blocked in the rat by antimigraine drugs, such as ergot alkaloids and triptans (Markowitz et al. 1987; Buzzi and Moskowitz 1990), and by nonsteroidal anti-inflammatory agents, such as indomethacin and acetylsalicylic acid (Buzzi et al. 1989).

The neurogenic inflammation hypothesis does not explain, however, what causes the initial activation of meningeal nociceptors that triggers neurogenic inflammation in the dura. The next hypothesis has been proposed in an attempt to address this dilemma.

CORTICAL SPREADING DEPRESSION HYPOTHESIS

Cortical spreading depression (CSD) refers to a wave of brief excitation followed by prolonged (15–30-minute) inhibition of neuronal activity that propagates slowly across the cortex at a rate of 2–6 mm/minute. This neural phenomenon was first observed by Leao (1944) in the cortex of anesthetized rabbits and was later correlated with localized changes in blood flow that spread through the cortex at a similar rate (Lauritzen 1994). CSD has been implicated in the pathophysiology of migraine on the basis of neuroimaging studies showing slowly migrating changes in cortical blood flow in patients tested during the visual aura phase of migraine (Lauritzen 1994; Bowyer et al. 2001; Hadjikhani et al. 2001; James et al. 2001). Since aura precedes the onset of headache by 20–30 minutes, it was postulated that CSD may lead up to the initial activation of meningeal nociceptors. But how would abnormal cortical activity produce an impact on dural pain fibers and blood vessels across the pia mater and arachnoids?

Although direct electrophysiological evidence for the activation of trigeminovascular neurons by CSD is still lacking (Ebersberger et al. 2001), the CSD hypothesis relies on two suppositions that are based on two independent sets of observation. One assumption is that molecules such as potassium ions, hydrogen ions, and glutamate that are released extracellularly during CSD in the cortex (Brinley et al. 1960; Rapoport and Marshall 1964; James et al. 2001) diffuse through the overlying meninges and activate meningeal nociceptors. The other assumption is that the induction of neurogenic inflammation in the dura by CSD (Bolay et al. 2002) is mediated by an antidromic axonal reflex that propagates through collateral trigeminal axons that innervate both the pia and dura. This assumption may be consistent with the finding that sensory denervation of the meninges blocks CSD-induced neurogenic inflammation in the dura (Bolay et al. 2002). To date, however, there is no anatomical evidence for the presumed existence of individual trigeminal axons that innervate both the pia and dura.

NITRIC OXIDE HYPOTHESIS

The implication of nitric oxide (NO) in migraine headache comes from evidence that systemic administration of NO donors such as glyceryl trinitrate causes an immediate transient headache in normal subjects and delayed migraine-like headache in migraineurs (Iversen et al. 1989). Three hypotheses have been proposed for NO action in migraine: vasoactive action, inflammatory action, and neuronal action. The first hypothesis proposed that NO induces migraine through dilation of cerebral blood vessels (Iversen et al. 1989). The second hypothesis proposed that NO triggers migraine through induction of meningeal inflammation (Reuter et al. 2001). The third hypothesis proposed that NO triggers migraine by directly activating and sensitizing meningeal nociceptors and central trigeminovascular neurons (Koulchitsky et al. 2004; Levy and Strassman 2004). As with previous hypotheses, there is no evidence for endogenous release of NO in the meninges during migraine.

Research of the past 30 years has yielded significant advances on three major fronts. It triggered the development of animal models that have facilitated our understanding of the pathophysiology of migraine-like headache. It has promoted the view that migraine pain originates intracranially by nonvascular disturbances, thus displacing the long-standing view of extracranial vascular dysfunction. The treatment of migraine has been greatly improved with the development of triptans as antimigraine drugs. In spite of these recent advances, much work is still needed to discover the cascade of events that leads up to activation of meningeal nociceptors and the onset of headache.

ACKNOWLEDGMENTS

Supported by NIH grants DE13347, NS051484, NS35611 to Dr. Burstein.

REFERENCES

Andres KH, von During M, Muszynski K, Schmidt RF. Nerve fibres and their terminals of the dura mater encephali of the rat. *Anat Embryol (Berl)* 1987; 175:289–301.

Anthony M. The treatment of migraine: old methods, new ideas. *Aust Fam Physician* 1993; 22:1434–1435, 1438–1439, 1442–1443.

Armstrong D, Jepson JB, Keele CA, Stewart JW. Pain-producing substances in human inflammatory exudates and plasma. *J Physiol (Lond)* 1957; 135:350–370.

Bahra A, Matharu MS, Buchel C, Frackowiak RS, Goadsby PJ. Brainstem activation specific to migraine headache. *Lancet* 2001; 357:1016–1017.

Bandler R, Keay KA, Floyd N, Price J. Central circuits mediating patterned autonomic activity during active vs. passive emotional coping. *Brain Res Bull* 2000; 53:95–104.

Basbaum AI, Clanton CH, Fields HL. Three bulbospinal pathways from the rostral medulla of the cat: an autoradiographic study of pain modulating systems. *J Comp Neurol* 1978; 178:209–224.

Beck PW, Handwerker HO. Bradykinin and serotonin effects on various types of cutaneous nerve fibers. *Pflugers Arch* 1974; 347:209–222.

Benjamin L, Levy MJ, Lasalandra MP, et al. Hypothalamic activation after stimulation of the superior sagittal sinus in the cat: a Fos study. *Neurobiol Dis* 2004; 16:500–505.

Blau JN, Dexter SL. The site of pain origin during migraine attacks. *Cephalalgia* 1981; 1:143–147.

Bolay H, Reuter U, Dunn AK, et al. Intrinsic brain activity triggers trigeminal meningeal afferents in a migraine model. *Nat Med* 2002; 8:136–142.

Bowyer SM, Aurora KS, Moran JE, Tepley N, Welch KM. Magnetoencephalographic fields from patients with spontaneous and induced migraine aura. *Ann Neurol* 2001; 50:582–587.

Brinley FJ Jr, Kandel ER, Marshall WH. Potassium outflux from rabbit cortex during spreading depression. *J Neurophysiol* 1960; 23:246–256.

Burstein R, Jakubowski M. Analgesic triptan action in an animal model of intracranial pain: a race against the development of central sensitization. *Ann Neurol* 2004; 55:27–36.

Burstein R, Yamamura H, Malick A, Strassman AM. Chemical stimulation of the intracranial dura induces enhanced responses to facial stimulation in brain stem trigeminal neurons. *J Neurophysiol* 1998; 79:964–982.

Burstein R, Yarnitsky D, Goor-Aryeh I, Ransil BJ, Bajwa ZH. An association between migraine and cutaneous allodynia. *Ann Neurol* 2000; 47:614–624.

Burstein R, Jakubowski M, Collins B. Defeating migraine pain with triptans: a race against the development of cutaneous allodynia. *Ann Neurol* 2004; 55:19–26.

Buzzi MG, Moskowitz MA. The antimigraine drug, sumatriptan (GR43175), selectively blocks neurogenic plasma extravasation from blood vessels in dura mater. *Br J Pharmacol* 1990; 99:202–206.

Buzzi MG, Sakas DE, Moskowitz MA. Indomethacin and acetylsalicylic acid block neurogenic plasma protein extravasation in rat dura mater. *Eur J Pharmacol* 1989; 165:251–258.

Davis KD, Dostrovsky JO. Activation of trigeminal brain-stem nociceptive neurons by dural artery stimulation. *Pain* 1986; 25:395–401.

Davis KD, Dostrovsky JO. Responses of feline trigeminal spinal tract nucleus neurons to stimulation of the middle meningeal artery and sagittal sinus. *J Neurophysiol* 1988; 59:648–666.

Davis KD, Meyer RA, Campbell JN. Chemosensitivity and sensitization of nociceptive afferents that innervate the hairy skin of monkey. *J Neurophysiol* 1993; 69:1071–1081.

Derbyshire SW, Jones AK, Creed F, et al. Cerebral responses to noxious thermal stimulation in chronic low back pain patients and normal controls. *Neuroimage* 2002; 16:158–168.

Dimitriadou V, Buzzi MG, Moskowitz MA, Theoharides TC. Trigeminal sensory fiber stimulation induces morphological changes reflecting secretion in rat dura mater mast cells. *Neuroscience* 1991; 44:97–112.

Ebersberger A, Schaible HG, Averbeck B, Richter F. Is there a correlation between spreading depression, neurogenic inflammation, and nociception that might cause migraine headache? *Ann Neurol* 2001; 49:7–13.

Fields HL, Basbaum AI. Central nervous system mechanisms of pain modulation. In: Wall PD, Melzack R (Eds). *Textbook of Pain,* Vol. 4. London: Churchill Livingston, 1999, pp 243–257.

Fields HL, Malick A, Burstein R. Dorsal horn projection targets of ON and OFF cells in the rostral ventromedial medulla. *J Neurophysiol* 1995; 74:1742–1759.

Gee JR, Ishaq Y, Vijayan N. Postcraniotomy headache. *Headache* 2003; 43:276–278.

Goadsby PJ, Hoskin KL. Inhibition of trigeminal neurons by intravenous administration of the serotonin (5HT)1B/D receptor agonist zolmitriptan (311C90): are brain stem sites therapeutic target in migraine? *Pain* 1996; 67:355–359.

Goadsby PJ, Zagami AS. Stimulation of the superior sagittal sinus increases metabolic activity and blood flow in certain regions of the brainstem and upper cervical spinal cord of the cat. *Brain* 1991; 114:1001–1011.

Gokalp HZ, Arasil E, Erdogan A, et al. Tentorial meningiomas. *Neurosurgery* 1995; 36:46–51; discussion 51.

Guzman F, Braun C, Lim RKS. Visceral pain and the pseudoaffective response to intra-arterial injection of bradykinin and other algesic agents. *Arch Int Pharmacodyn Ther* 1962; 136:353–384.

Hadjikhani N, Sanchez Del Rio M, Wu O, et al. Mechanisms of migraine aura revealed by functional MRI in human visual cortex. *Proc Natl Acad Sci USA* 2001; 98:4687–4692.

Harner SG, Beatty CW, Ebersold MJ. Headache after acoustic neuroma excision. *Am J Otol* 1993; 14:552–555.

Hollander W, Michaelson AL, Wilkins RW. Serotonin and antiserotonins. I. Their circulatory respiratory and renal effects in man. *Circulation* 1957; 16:246–255.

Holstege G, Kuypers HG. The anatomy of brain stem pathways to the spinal cord in cat. A labeled amino acid tracing study. *Prog Brain Res* 1982; 57:145–175.

Holzer P. Local effector functions of capsaicin-sensitive sensory nerve endings: involvement of tachykinins, calcitonin gene-related peptide and other neuropeptides. *Neuroscience* 1988; 24:739–768.

Hoskin KL, Kaube H, Goadsby PJ. Central activation of the trigeminovascular pathway in the cat is inhibited by dihydroergotamine. A c-Fos and electrophysiological study. *Brain* 1996; 119:249–256.

Hosobuchi Y, Adams JE, Linchitz R. Pain relief by electrical stimulation of the central gray matter in humans and its reversal by naloxone. *Science* 1977; 197:183–186.

Hsieh JC, Stahle-Backdahl M, Hagermark O, et al. Traumatic nociceptive pain activates the hypothalamus and the periaqueductal gray: a positron emission tomography study. *Pain* 1996; 64:303–314.

Iadarola MJ, Berman KF, Zeffiro TA, et al. Neural activation during acute capsaicin-evoked pain and allodynia assessed with PET. *Brain* 1998; 121(Pt 5):931–947.

Iversen HK, Olesen J, Tfelt-Hansen P. Intravenous nitroglycerin as an experimental model of vascular headache. Basic characteristics. *Pain* 1989; 38:17–24.

James MF, Smith JM, Boniface SJ, Huang CL, Leslie RA. Cortical spreading depression and migraine: new insights from imaging? *Trends Neurosci* 2001; 24:266–271.

Ji RR, Kohno T, Moore KA, Woolf CJ. Central sensitization and LTP: do pain and memory share similar mechanisms? *Trends Neurosci* 2003; 26:696–705.

Kaube H, Keay KA, Hoskin KL, Bandler R, Goadsby PJ. Expression of c-fos-like immunoreactivity in the caudal medulla and upper cervical spinal cord following stimulation of the superior sagittal sinus in the cat. *Brain Res* 1993; 629:95–102.

Kaur A, Selwa L, Fromes G, Ross DA. Persistent headache after supratentorial craniotomy. *Neurosurgery* 2000; 47:633–636.

Keller JT, Marfurt CF. Peptidergic and serotoninergic innervation of the rat dura mater. *J Comp Neurol* 1991; 309:515–534.

Keller JT, Saunders MC, Beduk A, Jollis JG. Innervation of the posterior fossa dura of the cat. *Brain Res Bull* 1985; 14:97–102.

Koulchitsky S, Fischer MJ, De Col R, Schlechtweg PM, Messlinger K. Biphasic response to nitric oxide of spinal trigeminal neurons with meningeal input in rat—possible implications for the pathophysiology of headaches. *J Neurophysiol* 2004; 92:1320–1328.

Lambert GA, Lowy AJ, Boers PM, Angus-Leppan H, Zagami AS. The spinal cord processing of input from the superior sagittal sinus: pathway and modulation by ergot alkaloids. *Brain Res* 1992; 597:321–330.

Lauritzen M. Pathophysiology of the migraine aura. The spreading depression theory. *Brain* 1994; 117:199–210.

Leao A. Spreading depression of activity in cerebral cortex. *J Neurophysiol* 1944; 7:359–390.

Levy D, Jakubowski M, Burstein R. Disruption of communication between peripheral and central trigeminovascular neurons by a 5HT1B1D receptor agonist: implications for migraine therapy with triptans. *Proc Natl Acad Sci USA* 2004; 101(12):4274–4279.

Levy D, Strassman AM. Mechanical response properties of A and C primary afferent neurons innervating the rat intracranial dura. *J Neurophysiol* 2002; 88:3021–3031.

Levy D, Strassman AM. Modulation of dural nociceptor mechanosensitivity by the nitric oxide-cyclic GMP signaling cascade. *J Neurophysiol* 2004; 92(2):766–772.

Liveing E. *On Megrim, Sick Headache.* Nijmegen: Arts & Boeve, 1873.

Malick A, Jakubowski M, Elmquist JK, Saper CB, Burstein R. A neurohistochemical blueprint for pain-induced loss of appetite. *Proc Natl Acad Sci USA* 2001; 98:9930–9935.

Markowitz S, Saito K, Moskowitz MA. Neurogenically mediated leakage of plasma protein occurs from blood vessels in dura mater but not brain. *J Neurosci* 1987; 7:4129–4136.

Martin GF, Vertes RP, Waltzer R. Spinal projections of the gigantocellular reticular formation in the rat. Evidence for projections from different areas to laminae I and II and lamina IX. *Exp Brain Res* 1985; 58:154–162.

Mathew N, Kailasam J, Seifert T. Clinical recognition of allodynia in migraine. *Neurology* 2004; 63(5):848–852.

Mayberg M, Langer RS, Zervas NT, Moskowitz MA. Perivascular meningeal projections from cat trigeminal ganglia: possible pathway for vascular headaches in man. *Science* 1981; 213:228–230.

Mizumura K, Sato J, Kumazawa T. Effects of prostaglandins and other putative chemical intermediaries on the activity of canine testicular polymodal receptors studied in vitro. *Pflugers Arch* 1987; 408:565–572.

Moskowitz MA. The neurobiology of vascular head pain. *Ann Neurol* 1984; 16:157–168.

Moskowitz MA, Macfarlane R. Neurovascular and molecular mechanisms in migraine headaches. *Cerebrovasc Brain Metab* 1993; 5:159–177.

Neugebauer V, Schaible HG, Schmidt RF. Sensitization of articular afferents to mechanical stimuli by bradykinin. *Pflugers Arch* 1989; 15:330–335.

Penfield W, McNaughton F. Dural headache and innervation of the dura mater. *Arch Neurol Psychiatry* 1940; 44:43–75.

Petrovic P, Ingvar M, Stone-Elander S, Petersson KM, Hansson P. A PET activation study of dynamic mechanical allodynia in patients with mononeuropathy. *Pain* 1999; 83:459–470.

Porreca F, Ossipov MH, Gebhart GF. Chronic pain and medullary descending facilitation. *Trends Neurosci* 2002; 25:319–325.

Potrebic S, Ahn AH, Skinner K, Fields HL, Basbaum AI. Peptidergic nociceptors of both trigeminal and dorsal root ganglia express serotonin 1D receptors: implications for the selective antimigraine action of triptans. *J Neurosci* 2003; 23:10988–10997.

Rapoport SI, Marshall WH. Measurement of cortical pH in spreading cortical depression. *Am J Physiol* 1964; 206:1177–1180.

Raskin NH, Hosobuchi Y, Lamb S. Headache may arise from perturbation of brain. *Headache* 1987; 27:416–420.

Rasmussen BK, Jensen R, Olesen J. A population-based analysis of the diagnostic criteria of the International Headache Society. *Cephalalgia* 1991; 11:129–134.

Ray BS, Wolff HG. Experimental studies on headache. Pain-sensitive structures of the head and their significance in headache. *Arch Surg* 1940; 41:813–856.

Reuter U, Bolay H, Jansen-Olesen I, et al. Delayed inflammation in rat meninges: implications for migraine pathophysiology. *Brain* 2001; 124:2490–2502.

Schaller B, Baumann A. Headache after removal of vestibular schwannoma via the retrosigmoid approach: a long-term follow-up-study. *Otolaryngol Head Neck Surg* 2003; 128:387–395.

Selby G, Lance JW. Observations on 500 cases of migraine and allied vascular headache. *J Neurol Neurosurg Psychiatry* 1960; 23–32.

Sicuteri F. Vasoneuractive substances and their implication in vascular pain. *Res Clin Stud Headache* 1967; 1:6–45.

Steen KH, Reeh PW, Anton F, Handwerker HO. Protons selectively induce lasting excitation and sensitization to mechanical stimulation of nociceptors in rat skin, in vitro. *J Neurosci* 1992; 12:86–95.

Strassman AM, Mason P, Moskowitz M, Maciewicz RJ. Response of medullary trigeminal neurons to electrical stimulation of the dura. *Brain Res* 1986; 379:242–250.

Strassman AM, Mineta Y, Vos BP. Distribution of fos-like immunoreactivity in the medullary and upper cervical dorsal horn produced by stimulation of dural blood vessels in the rat. *J Neurosci* 1994; 14:3725–3735.

Strassman AM, Raymond SA, Burstein R. Sensitization of meningeal sensory neurons and the origin of headaches. *Nature* 1996; 384:560–564.

Uddman R, Edvinsson L, Ekman R, Kingman T, McCulloch J. Innervation of the feline cerebral vasculature by nerve fibers containing calcitonin gene-related peptide: trigeminal origin and co-existence with substance P. *Neurosci Lett* 1985; 62:131–136.

Weiller C, May A, Limmroth V, et al. Brain stem activation in spontaneous human migraine attacks. *Nat Med* 1995; 1:658–660.

Welch KM, Nagesh V, Aurora SK, Gelman N. Periaqueductal gray matter dysfunction in migraine: cause or the burden of illness? *Headache* 2001; 41:629–637.

Wolff HG. *Headache and Other Head Pain.* New York: Oxford University Press, 1963.

Wolff HG, Tunis MM, Goodell H. Studies on migraine. *Arch Intern Med* 1953; 92:478–484.

Yamamura H, Malick A, Chamberlin NL, Burstein R. Cardiovascular and neuronal responses to head stimulation reflect central sensitization and cutaneous allodynia in a rat model of migraine. *J Neurophysiol* 1999; 81:479–493.

Zagami AS, Lambert GA. Stimulation of cranial vessels excites nociceptive neurones in several thalamic nuclei of the cat. *Exp Brain Res* 1990; 81:552–566.

Zwetsloot CP, Caekebeke JF, Jansen JC, Odink J, Ferrari MD. Blood flow velocity changes in migraine attacks: a transcranial Doppler study. *Cephalalgia* 1991; 11:103–107.

Correspondence to: Rami Burstein, PhD, Department of Anesthesia and Critical Care, Harvard Institutes of Medicine, Room 830, 77 Avenue Louis Pasteur, Boston, MA 02115, USA. Tel: 617-667-0806; Fax: 617-975-5329; email: rburstei@caregroup.harvard.edu.

The Paths of Pain 1975–2005, edited by
Harold Merskey, John D. Loeser, and Ronald
Dubner, IASP Press, Seattle, © 2005.

11

Glia and Pain: Past, Present, and Future

Linda R. Watkins and Steven F. Maier

*Department of Psychology and Center for Neuroscience,
University of Colorado at Boulder, Boulder, Colorado, USA*

This chapter reviews the history of the discovery of glial involvement in pain facilitation, examines present evidence of the extent to which glia (microglia and astrocytes) participate in pain modulation, and explores the future clinical implications of this body of work. Development of drug therapies aimed at controlling glial activation and glial proinflammatory products is predicted to be an important next step in achieving clinical pain control.

HISTORICAL OVERVIEW

Two independent and distinct lines of research led to the recognition of glial modulation of pain. Intriguingly, neither originally derived from studies of pain. The first line of research, beginning in the mid-1980s, was focused on understanding immune-to-brain communication (Hart 1988). The aim was to understand how peripheral immune challenges such as viruses or bacteria led to the generation by the central nervous system (CNS) of a wide-ranging constellation of changes aimed at enhancing host survival. These evolutionarily old, phylogenetically ubiquitous "sickness responses" include physiological changes (e.g., increased sleep, changes in blood chemistry, and fever), endocrine changes (release of stress hormones), and behavioral changes (e.g., decreased exploration, decreased sexual activity, loss of social dominance, and decreased food/water intake) (Maier and Watkins 1998). Sickness responses are argued to enhance survival by suppressing energy usage by processes unrelated to host defense and by generating energy from bodily stores. In turn, this energy is put toward the service of fever, which hinders pathogen replication while enhancing the proliferation and function of the host's immune cells as well as other aspects of host defense (Maier and Watkins 1998).

It was not until the early 1990s that pain facilitation was recognized as an integral part of this sickness response (Maier et al. 1992; Watkins and Maier 2000). The understanding of sickness-induced hyperalgesia was greatly facilitated by ongoing investigations of mechanisms underlying classical sickness responses. By this time, a large literature had accumulated which documented that CNS proinflammatory cytokines, including tumor necrosis factor (TNF), interleukin (IL)-1, and IL-6, were critically involved in the generation of every sickness response studied (Maier and Watkins 1998). Furthermore, glia were implicated as a major source of these proinflammatory substances. Thus, it seemed that glia and glial proinflammatory cytokines would be central to the generation of sickness-induced hyperalgesia as well. This prediction turned out to be correct, as did the prediction that peripheral inflammation/trauma, more generally, could "tap into" this circuitry, leading to exaggerated pain responses that are created, in part, by glial activation and proinflammatory cytokine release (Watkins and Maier 2000; Watkins et al. 2001).

The second line of research that led to the acceptance of a role of glia in pain again began divorced from pain research. Beginning in the early 1970s (Sjostrand 1971), a literature emerged documenting a fascinating phenomenon, namely that CNS microglia and astrocytes become activated following trauma to peripheral nerves. In animal studies, trauma to pure motor nerves led to glial activation surrounding the axotomized motor neurons, and trauma to sensory nerves led to glial activation in the central region where the sensory terminals were degenerating. It was not until the early-to-mid-1990s that a link between neuropathic pain and glial activation was proposed (Garrison et al. 1991, 1994). Importantly, this work demonstrated that a drug (MK801) that blocked neuropathic pain behaviors blocked glial activation as well. Thus, at the very least, neuropathic pain and glial activation were strongly correlated.

A FEW POINTS ABOUT GLIA

There are four points that bear clarifying about microglia and astrocytes before we proceed with a discussion of their role in pain modulation. The first point is that the existing focus on astrocytes and microglia as a source of proinflammatory mediators is an accident of history. These two cell types caught the attention of researchers because they show distinct alterations in morphology and upregulate their expression of easily visualized activation markers in response to activation. While eye-catching, microglia and astrocytes are not the only cell type in the CNS that can produce the proinflammatory products that will be described below as being associated with pain facilitation. Proinflammatory cytokines, for example, can also be produced by fibroblasts, endothelial cells, other types of glia, and some neurons as well (Tilders et al. 1994). Indeed, while such cells have been implicated in the generation of the sickness responses described above (Tilders et al. 1994), their potential involvement in pain facilitation remains unexplored. Thus, while astrocytes and microglia are clearly involved, it should not be assumed that these are the only non-neuronal sources of pain-enhancing substances.

The second point is that glia are not bothersome cells that should be destroyed in an effort to resolve pain syndromes. Rather, they are each important for the health and homeostasis of the CNS. Normally, microglia are quiescent, having no known basal function other than surveillance for debris, pathogens, and the like (Kreutzberg 1996). Astrocytes, on the other hand, regulate extracellular ions, sequester extracellular neurotransmitters, and perform other "housekeeping" functions. Astrocytes encapsulate synapses and actively participate in synaptic communication, responding to synaptically released neurotransmitters by releasing glial substances into the synapse as well (Barres 1991; Barres and Barde 2000). Under such conditions, astrocytes are "active" but not "activated."

The third point is that microglia and astrocytes can show dramatic changes in function upon activation. Most relevant to pain facilitation, these cells can now produce an array of substances that are neuroexcitatory and neurotoxic. Substances released by activated glia include proinflammatory cytokines (TNF, IL-1, and IL-6), nitric oxide, reactive oxygen species, prostaglandins, excitatory amino acids, and adenosine triphosphate (ATP) (Kreutzberg 1996; Ridet et al. 1997). Whether glia participate in the loss of neurons reported under neuropathic pain conditions (Moore et al. 2002) has not yet been explored, but this possibility is logical given their release profile. Microglia and astrocytes can synergize in their functions, and so products released by one cell type can stimulate the release of proinflammatory substances from the other. In addition, proinflammatory substances released by these glia can synergize in terms of their effects on other cells. Thus, while these glia are distinct cell types, they can act in unison to create a neuroexcitatory state.

The fourth and final point is that glia do not have axons. They cannot relay sensory information from the spinal cord to the brain. Hence, any role they play in pain modulation must be indirect. One can conceptualize glia as "volume controls" where substances released by activated glia cause incoming sensory afferents to increase their release of neurotransmitter, thereby amplifying their "pain" message. Similarly, these proinflammatory substances also cause pain transmission neurons to increase their excitability, further amplifying the "pain" message sent to the brain. Thus, preventing such glial alterations in the functioning of the pain pathway can be conceptualized as "turning down the gain on pain" (Watkins and Maier 2003).

CURRENT CONCEPTS OF GLIA AND PAIN

Research generated in numerous laboratories utilizing diverse animal models can be distilled down to seven key points. First, every animal model of pain facilitation examined causes activation of microglia and astrocytes in the spinal cord dorsal horn, including following inflammation and damage to peripheral tissues, peripheral nerves, spinal nerves, and the spinal cord (for complete citations, see Watkins 2001; Watkins and Maier 2003). Second, pharmacological disruption of glial activation prevents or reverses pain facilitation in every animal model that has been tested (Meller et al. 1994; Watkins et al. 1994; Milligan et al. 2000; Raghavendra et al. 2003a; Chacur et al. 2004; Ledeboer et al. 2005). Disruption has been tested using both a general glial metabolic inhibitor (fluorocitrate) and a compound that selectively disrupts the activation of microglia (minocycline). The fact that minocycline is far more effective at preventing than reversing enhanced pain states suggests that microglia are predominantly involved early in the development of pain facilitation whereas astrocytes gain prominence over time (Raghavendra et al. 2003a; Ledeboer et al. 2005). Third, pharmacological antagonism of substances that are released by activated glia block or reverse pain facilitation (Milligan et al. 2001b, 2003; Sweitzer et al. 2001a). Fourth, of the substances released by activated glia, proinflammatory cytokines (especially IL-1 and TNF) are critical for pain facilitation. Blockade of proinflammatory cytokines can both block the development of, and reverse, enhanced pain states (Sweitzer et al. 2001a; Milligan et al. 2001b, 2003). Indeed, we have observed that proinflammatory cytokines are involved in the long-term maintenance of neuropathic pain, as blockade of proinflammatory cytokine function even 1–2 months after chronic constriction injury (CCI) of the sciatic nerve reverses neuropathic pain behavior (Milligan et al. 2004a). Fifth, activation of spinal cord glia is sufficient to induce pain facilitation (Meller et al. 1994; Milligan et al. 2001b). Strikingly, intrathecal injection of microglia activated in vitro is sufficient to enhance pain (Tsuda et al. 2003). Sixth, blockade of glial activation or glial proinflammatory products does not affect nociceptive thresholds of control animals (Meller et al. 1994; Milligan et al. 2000, 2003; Sweitzer et al. 2001a). Thus, glia do not appear to regulate pain responsivity under basal conditions. And seventh, blockade of glial activation or their proinflammatory products does not make the organism analgesic. Rather, it resolves the amplification of pain and returns the organism to a normal level of pain responsivity (Meller et al. 1994; Milligan et al. 2000, 2003; Sweitzer et al. 2001a). Taken together, these findings create a convincing picture of glial involvement in enhanced pain states.

The evidence reviewed above supports the idea that glia, once activated, contribute to the initiation and maintenance of enhanced pain states. However, this work does not address what causes spinal cord glia to shift from a basal to an activated state. This critical issue is just beginning to be investigated. There are several possible candidates. The first are neurotransmitters and neuromodulators already implicated in pain transmission and pain facilitation, such as substance P, ATP, excitatory amino acids, and nitric oxide; evidence from experiments using glial cultures suggests that such substances can activate glia (Araque et al. 1999). The second are pathogens or spinal trauma, which can activate glia and induce enhanced pain states (Meller et al. 1994; Milligan et al. 2001b). Fractalkine, a protein expressed selectively on the extracellular membrane of neurons (Chapman et al. 2000), is an additional candidate. Neuronal activation can lead to the release of fractalkine from the neuronal surface to form a diffusible signal to nearby microglia, which express fractalkine receptors (Chapman et al. 2000). Hence, this is a putative neuron-to-glia signal. Upon binding of fractalkine to glia, glia release IL-1 and induce enhanced pain responses (Milligan et al. 2004b). Indeed, the administration of a fractalkine receptor antagonist a week after the induction of neuropathic pain attenuated both mechanical allodynia and thermal hyperalgesia, indicating that peripheral nerve damage can lead to a perseverative release of fractalkine within the spinal cord, contributing to neuropathic pain responses (Milligan et al. 2004b).

An additional avenue for glial activation has just recently started to receive attention. This is, that drugs administered with the intent to produce analgesia may also result in glial activation. Thus, glia can act as a counter-regulator of pain suppression. To date, investigations have focused exclusively on morphine, and the results are quite intriguing. It has been shown that intrathecal morphine activates glia, causing them to release proinflammatory cytokines. Moreover, the blockade of spinal IL-1, for example, potentiates the acute effects of intrathecal morphine, delays the development of morphine tolerance, and suppresses the expression of allodynia and hyperalgesia induced by morphine abstinence (Johnston et al. 2004). Parallel results have been reported in response to repeated systemic morphine administration, which causes glial activation and proinflammatory cytokine production (Song and Zhao 2001; Raghavendra et al. 2002, 2003b, 2004). The implications of such studies are profound because they indicate that drugs delivered to induce analgesia may be rendered less effective by the fact that they simultaneously trigger the activation of pronociceptive responses by glia. Whether the results observed with morphine will generalize to other analgesics is as yet unknown. However, it is notable that other compounds used for clinical pain control have been observed to release proinflammatory cytokines from peripheral immune cells (Verrotti et al. 2001; Kubera et al. 2004). This finding raises the possibility that they may exert similar actions on microglia and astrocytes.

IMPLICATIONS FOR THE FUTURE

Taken together, the evidence reviewed here suggests that controlling glial activation and glial proinflammatory products would be effective for ameliorating clinical pain and enhancing the analgesic efficacy of drugs such as morphine. However, human clinical trials on the effect of "glial therapy" do not yet exist. This is a therapeutic strategy awaiting exploration.

From the animal studies reviewed above, several candidate strategies are obvious. Perhaps the most obvious would simply be to prevent glia from becoming activated. While glial metabolic inhibitors, such as fluorocitrate, are useful in animal studies when tested at low doses and at short post-drug intervals, such compounds are not feasible for clinical use because chronic suppression of glial function leads to the accumulation of excitatory amino acids and consequent neuroexcitability and neurotoxicity. As noted previously, glia are important for the health and homeostasis of the CNS, so simply destroying glia is not an option.

A similar, but more selective, strategy would be to prevent microglial activation with a compound such as minocycline. However, based on animal studies to date, this approach does not appear to be clinically feasible because the importance of microglia to pain facilitation appears to wane over time (Raghavendra et al. 2003a; Ledeboer et al. 2005). That is, minocycline can powerfully prevent the creation of enhanced pain states but is far less effective at reversing enhanced pain once it becomes established. From such studies it appears that astrocytes become the dominant glial type involved during persistent pain enhancement. If these results from animal studies translate to humans, it appears unlikely that minocycline is a compound likely to achieve clinical success.

Given that animal models point to glial proinflammatory cytokines as critical mediators, it is tempting to focus on selective cytokine antagonists. Indeed, several antagonists of IL-1 and TNF have been developed, including anakinra, infliximab, and etanercept. However, none of these agents can cross the blood-brain barrier. This drawback would necessitate chronic infusion via an indwelling catheter if such drugs were to be used for clinical pain control. In addition, targeting a single proinflammatory cytokine is unlikely to be an effective long-term strategy. This is because (a) the proinflammatory cytokines are very powerful, so that as few as 10 molecules need to bind to exert a physiological effect (Dinarello 1999); (b) the profiles of proinflammatory cytokine production can shift with time and circumstance (Dinarello 1999); and (c) proinflammatory cytokine function is redundant, and different cytokines can substitute for each other such that, for example, TNF can take over the functions of IL-1 if the latter is absent (Bluthe et al. 2000).

Given these constraints, a broader approach may prove more efficacious clinically. One approach may be to inhibit intracellular signaling cascades activated in response to proinflammatory cytokines binding to their receptors or to block signaling cascades leading to the production of proinflammatory cytokines. p38 mitogen-activated protein (MAP) kinase is a major kinase involved in both of these functions (Watkins et al. 1999). Indeed, p38 MAP kinase inhibitors have been observed to block enhanced pain states in animal models (Milligan et al. 2001a, 2003; Svensson et al. 2003). At least some of these compounds cross the blood-brain barrier, so they can be effective upon systemic administration (Milligan et al. 2001a). However, at least the more selective p38 MAP kinase inhibitors have been reported to fail to reverse established pain states. That finding, when added to the fact that p38 MAP kinase plays as yet unknown roles in neurons (Kim et al. 2002), raises concerns that need to be further explored before considering this approach clinically.

Propentofylline provides another approach for disrupting proinflammatory cytokine production. This compound has been used successfully in animal models to both prevent and reverse enhanced pain states (Sweitzer et al. 2001b). Propentofylline has been reported to reduce glial activation, reduce the production of proinflammatory cytokines and nitric oxide, increase the uptake of extracellular excitatory amino acids, and increase extracellular adenosine. Although this is a complex profile of actions, it is one consistent with reducing pain. Given that propentofylline is approved by the U.S. Food and Drug Administration for other uses, is orally active, and crosses the blood-brain barrier, it seems an attractive compound. However, systemic delivery of this or other similar drugs would alter the functioning of the peripheral immune system and glial function in the brain, in addition to the intended spinal targets. As glia and proinflammatory cytokines in the brain are increasingly recognized as playing physiologically relevant roles in sleep, thermoregulation, learning and memory, and hormone regulation (Maier and

Watkins 1998), the impact of systemic propentofylline on both immune system and brain glial functioning needs to be considered.

Lastly, a very new direction is non-viral gene therapy designed to drive the intrathecal production of the anti-inflammatory cytokine interleukin-10 (IL-10). In collaboration with Avigen, we have been exploring the potential of this powerful anti-inflammatory cytokine for pain control under the auspices of a National Institutes of Health translational research grant (Milligan et al. 2005a,b). IL-10 cannot be administered peripherally because it does not cross the blood-brain barrier and, in addition, would be expected to alter peripheral immune function (Moore et al. 2001). Although it is effective in reversing neuropathic pain upon acute intrathecal delivery, IL-10 has a short half-life (Moore et al. 2001), so infusion of the protein is neither clinically feasible nor cost-effective. However, we have developed a novel *non*viral gene therapy that releases IL-10 into the cerebrospinal fluid following lumbar puncture administration. This approach leads to resolution of neuropathic pain behaviors for over 3 months, at which time treatment is repeated to reinstate the pain-free state (Watkins and Maier 2003). Notable advantages are that: (1) spinally overexpressed IL-10 does not affect normal responsivity to pain in control animals; (2) overexpressed IL-10 both prevents and reverses pathological pain states; (3) spinal cord neurons do not express IL-10 receptors, so this therapy will not alter normal neuronal function; (4) the therapy remains restricted to the spinal cord, leaving brain and body unexposed to IL-10; and (5) given the known intracellular signaling pathways that it activates, IL-10 should selectively suppress the proinflammatory responses of glia while leaving the basal activities of these cells unaltered (Ledeboer et al. 2003; Watkins and Maier 2003). Taken together, this intriguing profile suggests that the overexpression of IL-10 may indeed be an avenue worth evaluation in clinical trials.

CONCLUSIONS

Convincing evidence from multiple laboratories and across diverse animal models clearly demonstrates that spinal cord microglia and astrocytes are important contributors to the creation and maintenance of pain facilitation, including neuropathic pain. Glia do not transmit pain messages to the brain, but rather can be thought of as a "volume control" that regulates pain transmission by neurons in the spinal cord. In addition, they limit the effectiveness of morphine and perhaps other analgesic drugs. Recognition of these key roles of glia is exciting as it provides a novel therapeutic target for clinical pain control.

ACKNOWLEDGMENTS

This work was supported by research grants from NIH (DA018156, DA015642, DA015656, NS40696, NS38020) and Avigen.

REFERENCES

Araque A, Parpura V, Sanzgiri RP, Haydon PG. Tripartite synapses: glia, the unacknowledged partner. *Trends Neurosci* 1999; 22:208–215.

Barres BA. New roles for glia. *J Neurosci* 1991; 11:3685–3694.

Barres BA, Barde Y. Neuronal and glial cell biology. *Curr Opin Neurobiol* 2000; 10:642–648.

Bluthe RM, Laye S, Michaud B, et al. Role of interleukin-1-beta and tumour necrosis factor-alpha in lipopolysaccharide-induced sickness behavior: a study with interleukin-1 type I receptor-deficient mice. *Eur J Neurosci* 2000; 12:4447–4456.

Chacur M, Milligan ED, Sloane EM, et al. Snake venom phospholipase A2s (Asp49 and Lys49) induce mechanical allodynia upon peri-sciatic administration: involvement of spinal cord glia, proinflammatory cytokines and nitric oxide. *Pain* 2004; 108:180–191.

Chapman GA, Moores K, Harrison D, et al. Fractalkine cleavage from neuronal membranes represents an acute event in the inflammatory response to excitotoxic brain damage. *J Neurosci* 2000; 20:RC87(1–5).

Dinarello CA. Overview of inflammatory cytokines and their role in pain. In: Watkins LR, Maier SF (Eds). *Cytokines and Pain*. Basel: Birkhauser Verlag, 1999, pp 1–19.

Garrison CJ, Dougherty PM, Kajander KC, Carlton SM. Staining of glial fibrillary acidic protein (GFAP) in lumbar spinal cord increases following a sciatic nerve constriction injury. *Brain Res* 1991; 565:1–7.

Garrison CJ, Dougherty PM, Carlton SM. GFAP expression in lumbar spinal cord of naive and neuropathic rats treated with MK-801. *Exp Neurol* 1994; 129:237–243.

Hart BL. Biological basis of the behavior of sick animals. *Neurosci Biobehav Rev* 1988; 12:123–137.

Johnston IN, Milligan ED, Martin D, Maier SF, Watkins LR. Spinal proinflammatory cytokines modulate morphine analgesia and subsequent tolerance, hyperalgesia and allodynia. *Proc Soc Neurosci* 2004; 29.

Kim SY, Bae JC, Kim JY, et al. Activation of p38 MAP kinase in the rat dorsal root ganglia and spinal cord following peripheral inflammation and nerve injury. *Neuroreport* 2002; 13:2483–2486.

Kreutzberg GW. Microglia: a sensor for pathological events in the CNS. *Trends Neurosci* 1996; 19:312–318.

Kubera M, Kenis G, Bosmans E, et al. Stimulatory effect of antidepressants on the production of IL-6. *Int Immunopharmacol* 2004; 4:185–192.

Ledeboer A, Wierinckx A, Bol JGJM, et al. Regional and temporal expression patterns of interleukin-10, interleukin-10 receptor and adhesion molecules in the rat spinal cord during chronic relapsing EAE. *J Neuroimmunol* 2003; 136:94–103.

Ledeboer A, Sloane EM, Milligan ED, et al. Selective inhibition of spinal cord microglial activation attenuates mechanical allodynia and proinflammatory cytokine expression in rat models of pain facilitation. *Pain* 2005; 115:71–83.

Maier SF, Watkins LR. Cytokines for psychologists: implications of bidirectional immune-to-brain communication for understanding behavior, mood, and cognition. *Psychol Rev* 1998; 105:83–107.

Maier SF, Wiertelak EP, Watkins LR. Endogenous pain facilitatory systems: anti-analgesia and hyperalgesia. *Am Pain Soc J* 1992; 1:191–198.

Meller ST, Dykstra C, Grzybycki D, Murphy S, Gebhart GF. The possible role of glia in nociceptive processing and hyperalgesia in the spinal cord of the rat. *Neuropharmacology* 1994; 33:1471–1478.

Milligan ED, Mehmert KK, Hinde JL, et al. Thermal hyperalgesia and mechanical allodynia produced by intrathecal administration of the human immunodeficiency virus-1 (HIV-1) envelope glycoprotein, gp120. *Brain Res* 2000; 861:105–116.

Milligan ED, O'Connor KA, Armstrong CB, et al. Systemic administration of CNI-1493, a p38 MAP kinase inhibitor, blocks HIV-1 gp120-induced enhanced pain states in rats. *J Pain* 2001a; 2:326–333.

Milligan ED, O'Connor KA, Nguyen KT, et al. Intrathecal HIV-1 envelope glycoprotein gp120 induces enhanced pain states mediated by spinal cord proinflammatory cytokines. *J Neurosci* 2001b; 21:2808–2819.

Milligan ED, Twining C, Chacur M, et al. Spinal glia and proinflammatory cytokines mediate mirror-image neuropathic pain. *J Neurosci* 2003; 23:1026–1040.

Milligan ED, Langer SJ, Sloane EM, et al. Gene therapy using naked plasmid DNA coding the anti-inflammatory gene, interleukin-10 (IL10): repeated injections lead to long-term pain control in chronic constriction injury (CCI) rats. *Proc Am Pain Soc* 2004a; 5(Suppl 1):16.

Milligan ED, Zapata V, Chacur M, et al. Evidence that exogenous and endogenous fractalkine can induce spinal nociceptive facilitation. *Eur J Neurosci* 2004b; 20:2294–2302.

Milligan ED, Sloane EM, Langer SJ, et al. Controlling neuropathic pain by adeno-associated virus driven production of the anti-inflammatory cytokine, interleukin-10. *Mol Pain* 2005a; 1(9). Available at: www.molecularpain.com/content/.

Milligan ED, Langer SJ, Sloane EM, et al. Controlling pathological pain by adenovirally driven spinal production of the anti-inflammatory cytokine, interleukin-10. *Eur J Neurosci* 2005b; in press.

Moore KA, Kohno T, Karchewski LA, et al. Partial peripheral nerve injury promotes a selective loss of GABAergic inhibition in the superficial dorsal horn of the spinal cord. *J Neurosci* 2002; 22:6724–6731.

Moore KW, deWaal Malefyt R, Coffman RL, O'Garra A. Interleukin-10 and the interleukin-10 receptor. *Annu Rev Immunol* 2001; 19:683–765.

Raghavendra V, Rutkowski MD, DeLeo JA. The role of spinal neuroimmune activation in morphine tolerance/hyperalgesia in neuropathic and sham-operated rats. *J Neurosci* 2002; 22:9980–9989.

Raghavendra V, Tanga F, DeLeo JA. Inhibition of microglial activation attenuates the development but not existing hypersensitivity in a rat model of neuropathy. *J Pharmacol Exp Ther* 2003a; 306:624–630.

Raghavendra V, Tanga F, Rutkowski MD, DeLeo JA. Anti-hyperalgesic and morphine-sparing actions of propentofylline following peripheral nerve injury in rats: mechanistic implications of spinal glia and proinflammatory cytokines. *Pain* 2003b; 104:655–664.

Raghavendra V, Tanga FY, DeLeo JA. Attenuation of morphine tolerance, withdrawal-induced hyperalgesia, and associated spinal inflammatory immune responses by propentofylline in rats. *Neuropsychopharmacology* 2004; 29:327–334.

Ridet JL, Malhotra SK, Privat A, Gage FH. Reactive astrocytes: cellular and molecular cues to biological function. *Trends Neurosci* 1997; 20:570–577.

Sjostrand J. Neuroglial proliferation in the hypoglossal nucleus after nerve injury. *Exp Neurol* 1971; 30:178–189.

Song P, Zhao ZQ. The involvement of glial cells in the development of morphine tolerance. *Neurosci Res* 2001; 39:281–286.

Svensson CI, Marsala M, Westerlund A, et al. Activation of p38 MAP kinase in spinal microglia is a critical link in inflammation induced spinal pain processing. *J Neurochem* 2003; 86:1534–1544.

Sweitzer SM, Martin D, DeLeo JA. Intrathecal interleukin-1 receptor antagonist in combination with soluble tumor necrosis factor receptor exhibits an anti-allodynic action in a rat model of neuropathic pain. *Neuroscience* 2001a; 103:529–539.

Sweitzer SM, Schubert P, DeLeo JA. Propentofylline, a glial modulating agent, exhibits antiallodynic properties in a rat model of neuropathic pain. *J Pharmacol Exp Ther* 2001b; 297:1210–1217.

Tilders FJ, DeRijk RH, Van Dam AM, et al. Activation of the hypothalamus-pituitary-adrenal axis by bacterial endotoxins: routes and intermediate signals. *Psychoneuroendocrinology* 1994; 19:209–232.

Tsuda M, Shigemoto-Mogami Y, Koizumi S, et al. P2X4 receptors induced in spinal microglia gate tactile allodynia after nerve injury. *Nature* 2003; 424:778–783.

Verrotti A, Basciani F, Trotta D, et al. Effect of anticonvulsant drugs on interleukins-1, -2 and -6 and monocyte chemoattractant protein-1. *Clin Exp Med* 2001; 1:133–136.

Watkins LR, Maier SF. The pain of being sick: implications of immune-to-brain communication for understanding pain. *Annu Rev Psychol* 2000; 51:29–57.

Watkins LR, Maier SF. Glia: a novel drug discovery target for clinical pain. *Nat Rev Drug Discov* 2003; 2:973–985.

Watkins LR, Wiertelak EP, Furness LE, Maier SF. Illness-induced hyperalgesia is mediated by spinal neuropeptides and excitatory amino acids. *Brain Res* 1994; 664:17–24.

Watkins LR, Hansen MK, Nguyen KT, Lee JE, Maier SF. Dynamic regulation of the proinflammatory cytokine, interleukin-1-beta: molecular biology for non-molecular biologists. *Life Sci* 1999:449–481.

Watkins LR, Milligan ED, Maier SF. Glial activation: a driving force for pathological pain. *Trends Neurosci* 2001; 24:450–455.

Correspondence to: Linda R. Watkins, PhD, Department of Psychology and Center for Neuroscience, University of Colorado at Boulder, Boulder, CO 80309-0345, USA. Tel: 303-492-7034; Fax: 303-492-2967; email: lwatkins@psych.colorado.edu.

The Paths of Pain 1975–2005, edited by
Harold Merskey, John D. Loeser, and Ronald
Dubner, IASP Press, Seattle, © 2005.

12

Pharmacology of Inflammatory Pain

Andy Dray

AstraZeneca Research and Development, Montreal, Canada

Inflammation is a complex set of interactions among tissue factors in response to a variety of perturbations ranging from infection to tissue trauma. This process leads to targeted destruction of foreign bodies and damaged tissues, followed by assisted repair. If these aspects are not properly balanced, inflammation leads to persistent tissue damage caused by leukocytes, lymphocytes, and macrophages (Nathan 2002). The key elements involved in inflammatory pain are a variety of immune cells (macrophages and neutrophils) and resident cells (Schwann cells and mast cells) that produce an orchestrated array of mediators. These mediators recruit peripheral autonomic and sensory systems and cause the activation and sensitization of peripheral nociceptors, thus inducing pain (Hunt and Mantyh 2001; Scholz and Woolf 2002).

Inflammatory mediators include acids, proteases, chemoattractants, and a variety of prostanoids, cytokines, and chemokines. Most act locally to modulate nerve excitability, but some mediators, such as nitric oxide and tumor necrosis factor-α (TNF-α), can damage nerves and may induce elements of neuropathic pain. Cytokines can also enter the circulation to produce distant inflammatory changes. Peripheral inflammation and nerve injury produce secondary changes in the central nervous system (CNS), particularly in the spinal cord, where secondary hyperexcitability arises and neuroglial cells become active to release inflammatory mediators and cell regulators (Hunt and Mantyh 2001; Watkins and Maier 2002).

Inflammatory pain therapy continues to be dominated by opioids and nonsteroidal anti-inflammatory drugs (NSAIDs), but both drug classes have major limitations with respect to efficacy or side effects, and there is a clear need for improved therapies. This chapter provides an account of the current and emerging concepts of inflammatory pain pharmacology and identifies molecular substrates that will guide new therapeutic approaches.

SENSITIZATION AND HYPEREXCITABILITY
OF PERIPHERAL NOCICEPTORS

Sensitization of nociceptors (C and Aδ fibers) and the induction of hyperexcitability are separate key processes occurring in inflammatory pain that underlie the clinical signs of hyperalgesia, allodynia, and ongoing pain. A number of cellular mechanisms can drive each process, and several overlapping processes may be responsible for the same symptom. An additional complexity is that patients may show a multiplicity of symptoms through stages of chronic pain. Sensitization to exogenous stimuli, such as mechanical or thermal stimuli, is produced by the actions of a variety of inflammatory mediators via an equally large variety of specific membrane receptors located on nociceptor terminals (Scholz and Woolf 2002). Many of these receptors are G-protein-coupled receptors (GPCRs), which signal via the production of the second messengers cyclic adenosine monophosphate (cAMP), cyclic guanosine monophosphate (cGMP), diacylglycerol, and phospholipase C, coupled with intracellular protein kinases (PKA and several isotypes of PKC). In their turn, these kinases phosphorylate specific cellular proteins, including ligand-gated (TRPV1) and voltage-gated ($Na_V1.8$) membrane ion channels, which appear to be pivotal determinants of peripheral nerve excitability. These processes cause nociceptors to be activated at a threshold that is lower than the physiological threshold and induce sustained neural firing. In addition, excitability in afferent pathways can be altered by changes in the synthesis of receptors, ion channels, and enzymes, controlled by retrograde signaling to the sensory neuron cell body, which alters gene transcription and sensory cell phenotype (Woolf and Salter 2000).

Symptoms of hyperalgesia and dysesthesia may also be caused by stimulation of low-threshold sensory fibers as a result of local inflammatory damage, as well as by alterations in the way in which sensory signals are processed by the CNS. Secondary hyperexcitability of the CNS (central sensitization) occurs through a number of cellular mechanisms, including activity-dependent phosphorylation of synaptic proteins, gene transcription changes, and increased trafficking of receptors and channels (Woolf and Salter 2000).

MEDIATORS AND TARGETS FOR PERIPHERAL
INFLAMMATORY PAIN

Kinins. Bradykinin is an important early mediator of inflammatory pain, causing nociceptor activation and sensitization via constitutively expressed bradykinin B2 receptors on peripheral nociceptors. The abundant metabolite, des-Arg^9 bradykinin (kallidin), activates B1 receptors, which also occur constitutively in low abundance, but are dramatically upregulated in many tissues following tissue injury by mediators such as interleukin (IL)-1-β (Fox et al. 2003). These kinins cause a cascade of secondary changes, including prostanoid production and phosphorylation of signaling proteins, thus sensitizing sensory transduction elements such as the capsaicin (TRPV1) receptor and causing heat hyperalgesia (Liang et al. 2001).

An abundance of evidence from animal models supports the therapeutic potential for bradykinin receptor antagonists (Stewart 2004). For example, B2 and B1 antagonists (Burgess et al. 2000; Fox et al. 2003) produce robust antihyperalgesic effects in a variety of animal models of inflammatory hyperalgesia. However, these antagonists have not been evaluated in clinical pain, although they inhibit other kinin-mediated changes in humans, such as cancer, allergies, and vasodilatation.

Protease-activated receptors. Several proteases from circulating inflammatory cells and the vascular epithelium cleave a variety of protease-activated receptors (PARs) associated with sensory neurons (Vergnolle et al. 2001). This reaction exposes tethered ligand domains that bind and activate PARs. PAR2, in particular, has been highlighted as a regulator of sensory nerve excitability; it plays an important role in inflammatory hyperalgesia. PAR2 agonists contribute to "neurogenic inflammation" through stimulating the release of peripheral substance P and calcitonin gene-related peptide (CGRP). Peripheral nerve activation in turn contributes to spinal hyperexcitability via activation of neurokinin-1 (NK1) and CGRP receptors. PAR2-receptor activation directly increases dorsal root ganglion (DRG) excitability and sensitizes them to capsaicin-induced activation of TRPV1 receptors via a PKC mechanism (Amadesi et al. 2004). In keeping with this mechanism, deletion of the TRPV1-receptor gene or pretreatment with the TRPV1 antagonist capsazepine abolished PAR2-induced thermal hyperalgesia (Amadesi et al 2004). These data suggest that TRPV1 is required for PAR2-induced hyperalgesia. On the other hand, PAR1 is also co-expressed on peptide-containing DRG. PAR1 agonists induce neurogenic inflammation, although they do not sensitize TRPV1 receptors, nor do they induce hyperalgesia; rather, they reduce mechanical hyperalgesia.

Cannabinoid receptors (CB1 and CB2) are widely distributed in the nervous system. They modulate pain via CB1 receptors located in the CNS and on peripheral nerves and via CB2 receptors, found mainly in peripheral immune tissues (Rice et al. 2002). Several fatty acids such as anandamide, 2-arachidonylglycerol, and palmitoylethanolamide are endogenous ligands for these receptors. Specific antagonists for CB1 and CB2 have been used to characterize receptor functions.

Several clinical studies have supported the therapeutic efficacy of cannabinoids in pain, but improvements in efficacy as well as reduction of CNS side effects are needed. Agonists at the peripheral cannabinoid receptors may address this latter issue. Several CB2-selective ligands show antinociceptive effects in a variety of inflammatory and neuropathic pain models (Malan et al. 2003), without CNS side effects such as catalepsy or motor impairments. This analgesic effect is most likely due to an indirect effect on the release of neuroactive substances from inflamed or surrounding tissues. On the other hand, peripherally restricted CB1 agonists can directly reduce inflammatory hyperalgesia by reducing nociceptor excitability, also without deleterious side effects (Richardson et al. 1998).

Other approaches to exploit the endogenous cannabinoid systems have targeted fatty acid amide hydrolysis, the major degradation pathway for endogenous cannabinoids. In mice lacking the fatty acid amide hydrolase (FAAH) enzyme (Cravatt et al. 2001) or in mice treated with novel FAAH inhibitors (Lichtman et al. 2004), the analgesic efficacy of anandamide is greater, and the pain threshold is higher, in acute pain tests. However, we lack convincing evidence that FAAH inhibition produces antihyperalgesic effects in inflammatory pain models.

Sensory-neuron-specific receptors. Other exploratory approaches involve targeting a family of DRG-specific GPCRs, the sensory-neuron-specific receptors (SNSRs). These receptors are related to a larger and phylogenetically diverse family of Mas-related genes. They are selectively expressed in subsets of small sensory neurons and are co-localized with TRPV1 (Lembo et al. 2002). The endogenous ligand for SNSRs is unconfirmed, but several mammalian peptide ligands have been identified, including the proenkephalin-derived bovine adrenal medullary peptide 22 (BAM22) and its fragment BAM8-22, as well as unrelated peptides such as γ_2-melanocyte-stimulating hormone. These substances do not activate opioid receptors; rather, they increase peripheral and spinal excitability and potentiate thermal and mechanical nociception (Grazzini et al. 2004). Such findings suggest that a receptor antagonist should be sought to inhibit hyperalgesia.

Prostanoids. A variety of prostanoid cyclooxygenase (COX) enzyme products (PGE_2, PGD_2, PGF_2-α, thromboxane, and PGI_2) occur during inflammation, but prostaglandin E_2 (PGE_2) is considered to be the major contributor to inflammatory pain. Blocking the major synthetic enzymes, COX-1 (constitutive) and COX-2 (inducible), and inhibiting prostanoid receptors continue to be important approaches for reducing inflammatory pain (Flower 2003). Experience with selective inhibitors of COX-2 (e.g., celecoxib and rofecoxib) shows improved safety but little improvement in analgesia, suggesting that it may be necessary to block all COX isoforms so as to maximize analgesic efficacy. An alternative approach for clinical improvement is to combine COX inhibition with nitric oxide donation. Molecules created by this technique (NO-naproxen and NO-ibuprofen) show improved efficacy and safety over the parent NSAID due to actions of cleaved nitric oxide (Fiorucci et al. 2001).

Recently a splice variant of COX-1 has been identified, COX-3 (Chandrasekharan et al. 2002), but it has lower enzymic capability. Its distribution and low abundance in the central and peripheral nervous system does not make it a compelling target for analgesia. However, the NSAIDs acetaminophen (paracetamol), diclofenac, and phenacetin have some degree of selectivity for COX-3. Furthermore, gene deletion studies suggest that COX-3 inhibition may be linked with the antipyretic and analgesic properties of NSAIDs (Chandrasekharan et al. 2002). Clearly, further studies are needed to link this enzyme to inflammatory pain pathophysiology.

Another route of inhibiting PGE_2 synthesis is via the blockade of prostaglandin E synthase (PGES), a major route of conversion of prostaglandin H_2 to PGE_2. Two isoforms of the enzyme have been identified, a membrane- or microsomal-associated enzyme (mPGES-1) and a cytosolic enzyme (cPGES/p23), which are linked with COX-2- and COX-1-dependent PGE_2 production, respectively (Jakobsson et al. 1999). Both isoforms are upregulated by inflammatory mediators. Gene deletion studies in mice indicate an important role for mPGES in acute and chronic inflammation and in inflammatory pain (Trebino et al. 2003).

Prostaglandin E receptors. PGE_2 exerts its effects via a variety of EP receptors (EP1, 2, 3, and 4), present both in peripheral sensory neurons and in the spinal cord. Activation of these receptors produces complex effects ranging from Ca influx to cAMP activation or inhibition. In the periphery, sensitization by PGE_2 has been shown to be cAMP mediated with enhancement of TTX-r sodium currents via channel phosphorylation (England et al. 1996). However, in the spinal cord, excitability was enhanced by EP1 receptors but reduced by an EP3-α agonist, suggesting complex prostanoid regulation of inflammatory pain (Bar et al. 2004).

Cytokines are produced by a variety of immune cells and by brain neuroglial cells in response to injury and inflammation. Probably the best characterized of these powerful mediators of hyperalgesia are IL1-β and TNF-α, which act via specific receptors on sensory neurons. Their effects can be attenuated by endogenous receptor antagonists that sequester the ligand as well as by neutralizing antibodies. Indeed, the TNF-α antibody etanercept has been developed to treat chronic inflammation, and the presence of TNF-α has been correlated with a number of painful inflammatory clinical conditions (Lindenlaub and Sommer 2003). Cytokines induce hyperalgesia by several direct and indirect actions. IL1-β activates nociceptors directly and produces heat sensitization via intracellular kinase activation, but it may also indirectly cause nociceptor sensitization via the production of kinins and prostanoids (Sommer and Kress 2004). TNF-α also activates sensory neurons directly and initiates a cascade of inflammatory reactions through the production of IL1, IL6, and IL8. It is significant that direct TNF-α application in the periphery induces neuropathic pain behavior that is blocked by ibuprofen and celecoxib (Schäfers et al. 2004), while nerve ligation causes increased TNF-α in damaged as well as adjacent axons (Schäfers et al. 2003).

Chemokines are important peripheral and central mediators of inflammation. The major chemokines and their respective receptors are MDC (macrophage-derived chemokine)/CCR4, RANTES (regulated upon activation, normal T-cell expressed and secreted)/CCR5, fractalkine/CX3CR1, and SDF-1-α (stromal cell-derived factor-1-α)/CXCR4. Receptors are located on leukocytes, on central neurons, and on neuroglial cells (Watkins and Maier 2002). Apart from their major chemoattractant effects, chemokines contribute directly to inflammatory hyperalgesia through G-protein-coupled activation and through sensitization of sensory neurons (Oh et al. 2001).

Ion channels are major regulators of nerve excitability, influenced by chemical modulators (ligand-gated channels) or by membrane polarization (voltage-gated channels). The capsaicin receptor, formerly called VR1 for vanilloid receptor 1 and now called TRPV1, has long been an attractive target for novel analgesia therapy. TRPV1 is a ligand-gated ion channel whose activation by capsaicin increases intracellular Ca^{2+}. It is a member of the transient receptor potential (TRP) channel family, some members of which are involved in other forms of signal transduction in sensory nerves. TRPV1 has the properties of a noxious heat transducer; accordingly, deletion of the TRPV1 gene prevents inflammatory heat hyperalgesia in mice (Caterina et al. 2000).

The TRPV1 receptor has assumed an increasingly prominent role in regulating sensory neuronal excitability in inflammatory pain. A variety of inflammatory agents including protons, bradykinin, adenosine triphosphate (ATP), PGE_2, 12-lipoxygenase products, PAR2, anandamide, and nerve growth factor indirectly sensitize TRPV1, or regulate its expression, to cause thermal hyperalgesia. A common mechanism appears to be GPCR-mediated stimulation of phospholipase C, the formation of the intermediate molecules inositol trisphosphate and diacylglycerol, and the activation and mobilization of protein kinase C (Vellani et al. 2001), which can phosphorylate the TRPV1 receptor.

Earlier analgesia strategies targeting TRPV1 focused on capsaicin-like agonists that induced functional inactivation of sensory fibers by causing reversible subepidermal degeneration. This method has been successfully translated into the clinic with the introduction of a number of topical capsaicin therapies for inflammatory pain (see Watson, this volume). Currently, there is a focus on TRPV1 channel blockers or selective antagonists of the TRPV1 receptor. Supporting these approaches, it has been found that competitive and noncompetitive TRPV1 antagonists (Sachez-Baez et al. 2002) block chemical and thermal pain sensitivity, heralding the emergence of a novel therapy.

Other TRP channels (TRPA1, TRPV3, and TRPV4) have been suggested to be involved in pain transduction. For example, TRPA1 (formerly ANKTM1) is co-localized with TRPV1 and is activated by capsaicin and mustard oil, but can also be sensitized by inflammatory mediators including bradykinin to produce cold-induced burning pain (Bandell et al. 2004). In addition, TRPV1 can oligomerize with other TRP family members including TRPV3. TRPV3 is also a heat transducer that is sensitive in the physiological temperature range; it responds to noxious heat, but is insensitive to capsaicin. So far, there are few chemical tools to help characterize the functions of these TRP receptors.

Other ligand-gated ion channels are also important for regulating peripheral excitability. The Na/K repolarizing "pacemaker current," Ih, which is activated during membrane hyperpolarization, is important for generation of rhythmic and spontaneous action potentials in sensory neurons following nerve injury. Ih currents are controlled by cyclic nucleotides (cAMP and cGMP) via a family of ligand-gated ion channels, the hyperpolarization-activated, cyclic nucleotide-gated (HCN) "pacemaker" channels, which are constitutively expressed in sensory nerves and are differentially distributed after crush or inflammatory nerve injuries (Chaplan et al. 2003). Nerve injury enhances the Ih current, which can be blocked pharmacologically with the specific inhibitor ZD7288. This prevents repetitive firing in damaged sensory neurons and reverses touch hypersensitivity in neuropathic pain models (Chaplan et al. 2003).

The unique localization of the purinergic $P2X_3$ receptor associate channel to small sensory fibers has highlighted its importance in pain. Large amounts of the endogenous ligand ATP are released after tissue injury and during inflammatory injuries, while ATP and its stable analogue $\alpha\beta$-Me ATP induce pain and are pronociceptive when administered intradermally in volunteers.

In chronic inflammatory pain, $P2X_3$-mediated excitability is enhanced, while reduction of $P2X_3$ receptors, by antisense oligonucleotide administration, reduces hyperalgesia evoked by inflammation as well as by administration of $\alpha\beta$-Me ATP (Honore et al. 2002). Several $P2X_3$ antagonists have been shown to reduce pain in a number of acute and chronic pain models (e.g., Jarvis et al. 2002).

A variety of voltage-gated sodium channels, characterized by their primary structure and by their sensitivity to tetrodotoxin (TTX), are involved in regulating sensory neural excitability (Eglen et al. 1999). For example, the TTX-resistant sodium channel $Na_V1.8$ is uniquely expressed in small sensory neurons; it is downregulated in small injured axons but upregulated in adjacent uninjured C fibers (Gold et al. 2003) and in DRG neurons following inflammation. $Na_V1.8$ appears to be important for the generation of abnormal excitability in sensory axons. Knockdown of $Na_V1.8$ in pain models markedly reduces abnormal pain responsiveness (Lai et al. 2003). Inflammation also causes the overexpression of TTX-sensitive channels such as $Na_V1.7$ in several types of sensory neurons in models of inflammatory pain (Gould et al. 2004), and knockdown of $Na_V1.7$ channels abolished inflammatory pain (Nassar et al. 2004). In humans, $Na_V1.7$ gene defects are associated with peripheral nerve hyperexcitability and with the pain of erythromelalgia (Cummins et al. 2004). Interestingly, overexpression of $Na_V1.7$ could be prevented by pretreatment with COX-1 and COX-2 inhibitors, including ibuprofen. Novel sodium channel blockers (e.g., NW-1029) produce activity-dependent block of peripheral nerves and antihyperalgesia in models of inflammatory and neuropathic pain (Veneroni et al. 2003). Overall, however, channel blockers still appear insufficiently selective to avoid cardiac and CNS side effects. An alternative approach to selective channel inactivation may be to block the injury-induced overexpression of TTX-sensitive channels such as $Na_V1.8$ by preventing interaction with p-11, an annexin II-related protein that tethers the channel to the nerve membrane (Okuse et al. 2002).

Finally, with respect to calcium channels, N-type $Ca_V2.2$ channels are unique to neurons and are critical for pain neurotransmission. Thus, deletion of the N-channel gene reduces inflammatory and neuropathic pain while selective blockers such as ziconotide reportedly have efficacy across a range of chronic pain conditions. Another and possibly more validated approach targets the $\alpha_2\delta_1$ calcium channel subunit, the substrate for the antiallodynic drug gabapentin. This subunit is important for channel assembly and is expressed in small DRG and spinal neurons; its overexpression has been associated with allodynia in a number of specific pain models (Luo et al. 2002).

Neurotrophins represent an important family of regulatory proteins essential for sensory nerve development, survival, and determination of chemical phenotype. Nerve growth factor (NGF) has been most studied with respect to inflammatory hyperalgesia because its production is upregulated by inflammation in macrophages, fibroblasts, and Schwann cells. NGF acts via two membrane receptors, TrkA and p75, to activate a number of kinase pathways, leading to altered gene transcription and the increased synthesis of sensory neuropeptides (substance P and CGRP) and ion channels (TRPV1 and $Na_V1.8$). Administration of exogenous NGF induces thermal and mechanical hyperalgesia via mast cell degranulation and by directly increasing sensory neuronal excitability (Sah et al. 2003). Small-molecule NGF antagonists are not available, although TrK-A-IgG and NGF antisera have confirmed the importance of NGF in hyperalgesia. NGF also induces the synthesis of another neurotrophin, brain-derived neurotrophic factor (BDNF), from sensory neurons. Release of BDNF onto spinal dorsal horn cells acts via TrK-B receptors to initiate a signaling cascade that contributes, via the phosphorylation of NMDA receptors, to increasing spinal excitability. Administration of TrK-B IgG reduced inflammatory hyperalgesia in a number of animal models. Finally, glial cell-line-derived neurotrophic factor (GDNF) represents an extensive family of ligands and membrane receptor complexes that have an important role in regulating peripheral and central neural phenotypes. Although it does not appear to play a specific role in inflammation, GDNF has been shown to have neuroprotective and restorative properties in a number of neurodegenerative and neuropathic pain states (Sah et al. 2003). Unfortunately, clinical observations using GDNF have shown unacceptable side effects, which has discouraged therapeutic developments.

CENTRAL MEDIATORS OF INFLAMMATORY PAIN

A variety of studies have demonstrated an important role for spinal inflammatory and neuroimmune processes triggered by peripheral inflammation and nerve injuries. These processes involve the regulation of a variety of receptors, channels, and enzymes with patterns that may differentiate one pain state from another (Honore et al. 2000). In addition, activation of spinal neuroglial cells (microglia, astrocytes, and satellite cells) stimulates a cascade of secondary excitability changes (Watkins and Maier 2002). Neuroglia make close-junctional connections with other cells, providing a means of spreading excitability changes beyond the boundaries of spinal segmental input. Neuroglia also secrete a number of mediators such as nitric oxide, neurotrophins, IL1-β, TNF-α, free radicals, and glutamate. In addition, neuroglial mediators may contribute to spinal excitability by causing dysfunction or degeneration of inhibitory spinal neurons (Moore et al. 2002). In keeping with an important role for neuroglial mediators, treatments with anti-inflammatory agents or modulators of neuroglial activity such as propentofylline and minocycline inhibit glial activation, slow the release of glial products, and reduce behavioral signs of hyperexcitability (Watkins and Maier 2002; Raghavendra et al. 2003).

The release of inflammatory mediators from neuroglial cells is controlled by specific receptors, such as various purinergic and chemokine receptors. $P2X_7$ receptors are expressed in CNS tissues including neurons and neuroglia (Deuchars et al. 2001). They are upregulated in chronic pain patients. Deletion of the $P2X_7$-receptor gene abolished mechanical and thermal pain in mice (Chessell et al. 2005). Other studies have shown that increased spinal microglial $P2X_4$ expression occurs after peripheral nerve lesions and is related to mechanical allodynia. The development of allodynia was blocked by the selective $P2X_3$ antagonist trinitrophenyl (TNP)-ATP (Tsuda et al. 2003). Remarkably, spinal administration of activated microglia reproduced TNP-ATP-sensitive mechanical allodynia in naive animals. With respect to chemokine receptors, CXCR4, CCR4, and CX3CR1 are expressed in microglia and in sensory neurons, and block of CX3CR1 by a fractalkine-receptor-neutralizing antibody induced antiallodynic effects in a model of peripheral nerve inflammation (Milligan et al. 2004).

COX-1 (in the glia) and COX-2 (in the ventral horn cells) are constitutively present in the spinal cord and are increased by inflammation, by peripheral nerve injury, and by administration of cytokines, leading to increased production of PGE_2. Several NSAIDs have been shown to reduce inflammatory hyperalgesia via inhibition of spinal COX activity (Yaksh et al. 2001). Several mechanisms have been proposed for PGE_2-induced changes in spinal excitability via specific receptors and via the release of glutamate. Recently, the spinal effects of PGE_2 have been further linked with a glycine receptor. Accordingly, deletion of the GlyR3-α subunit gene reduced pain sensitivity caused by PGE_2 administration and inflammation (Harvey et al. 2004).

A peripheral increase in the expression of opioid peptides (from immune cells) and receptors (on sensory and sympathetic nerves) also occurs after inflammation. Indeed, it has long been known that direct peripheral administration of opioids reduces inflammatory pain (Stein et al. 2003). Inflammation also induces opioid changes in the CNS and spinal cord (Hurley and Hammond 2000), including increased synthesis and release of opioid peptides such as dynorphin and enkephalin, along with increased trafficking of opioid receptors. For example, increased opioid-receptor trafficking occurs from the endoplasmic reticulum to the cell membrane, with a concomitant increase in the analgesic potency of μ and δ opioids (Cahill et al. 2001).

As mentioned earlier, inflammatory mediators also activate a number of protein kinases in sensory neurons and in the spinal cord. These kinases, including PKA, PKC, and mitogen-activated protein kinases (MAPKs), are considered to be important downstream regulators of excitability through alteration of gene transcription and through post-translational modification of target proteins (Woolf and Salter 2000). Several types of MAPKs, including extracellular signal-regulated kinases, cJun kinase, N-terminal kinase, and p38 kinase, are considered as targets for inflammatory pain. For example, several inhibitors of p38 kinase exhibit anti-inflammatory and anti-hyperalgesic properties in a variety of animal models (Schäfers et al. 2003).

CONCLUSIONS

Effective pain therapy remains enormously challenging despite increases in our knowledge of pain etiology and mechanisms drawn from animal studies. Detailed clinical knowledge is still lacking, particularly with respect to the complexity of overlapping mechanisms and time-related changes that underlie the initiation and progression of pain. Investigations of pain phenomena (e.g., sensitization) and specific mechanisms- (e.g., TRPV1 regulation) have highlighted key molecular approaches toward reducing peripheral and central sensitization and hyperexcitability. For inflammatory pain, among the most comprehensively studied drug targets are mediators (ATP, prostanoids, kinins, cytokines, chemokines, and neurotrophins) that sensitize nociceptors or increase their excitability, often converging on the regulation of voltage-gated ($Na_V1.8$, $Na_V1.7$, $Ca_V2.2$) and ligand-gated (TRPV1, $P2X_3$) ion channels. An important emerging feature of these families of mediators is their ability to produce localized cytotoxic changes, including neurodegeneration, thus introducing elements of neuropathic pain that compound chronic, unresolved inflammation. Secondary changes in central excitability are further driven by phenotypic changes and by peripheral inputs that enhance neurotransmission through the phosphorylation (e.g., MAPK) of membrane receptors and channels. Among these secondary CNS changes, the activation of neuroglial cells has emerged most prominently. Neuroglia release many inflammatory mediators ($IL1\beta$, TNF-α, nitric oxide, and glutamate) that cause further cascades of chemical signaling and possible neurodegeneration. Control of neuroglial activity may be attained through antagonism of purinergic receptors ($P2X_4$, $P2X_7$) and through inhibition of chemokine control (CCR2, CXCR3). At present, most molecular targets are poorly validated. Translating these approaches into the pain clinic remains a significant, but surmountable, drug development challenge.

REFERENCES

Amadesi S, Nie J, Vergnolle N, et al. Protease-activated receptor 2 sensitizes the capsaicin receptor transient receptor potential vanilloid receptor 1 to induce hyperalgesia. *J Neurosci* 2004; 24:4300–4312.

Bandell M, Story GM, Hwang SW, et al. A noxious cold ion channel TRPA1 is activated by pungent compounds and bradykinin. *Neuron* 2004; 41:849–853.

Bar K-J, Natura G, Telleria-Diaz A, et al. Changes in the effect of spinal prostaglandin E2 during inflammation: prostaglandin EP1-EP4 receptors in spinal nociceptive processing of input from the normal and inflamed knee joint. *J Neurosci* 2004; 24:642–651.

Burgess GM, Perkins MN, Rang HP, et al. Bradyzide, a potent nonpeptide B2 bradykinin receptor antagonist with long-lasting oral activity in animal models of inflammatory hyperalgesia. *Br J Pharmacol* 2000; 129:77–86.

Cahill CM, Morinville A, Lee M-C, et al. Prolonged morphine treatment targets δ opioid receptors to neuronal plasma membranes and enhances δ-mediated antinociception. *J Neurosci* 2001; 21:7598–7607.

Caterina MJ, Leffer A, Malmberg AB, et al. Impaired nociception and pain sensation in mice lacking the capsaicin receptor. *Science* 2000; 288:306–313.

Chandrasekharan NV, Dai H, Roos KLT, et al. COX-3, a cyclooxygenase-1 variant inhibited by acetaminophen and other analgesic/antipyretic drugs: cloning, structure, and expression. *Proc Natl Acad Sci USA* 2002; 99:13926–13931.

Chaplan SR, Guo H-Q, Lee DH, et al. Neuronal hyperpolarization-activated pacemaker channels drive neuropathic pain. *J Neurosci* 2003, 23:1169–1178.

Chessell IP, Hatcher JP, Davey PT, et al. Disruption of the P2X7 purinoceptor gene abolishes chronic inflammatory and neuropathic pain. *Pain* 2005; 114:386–396.

Cravatt BJ, Demarest K, Patricelli MP, et al. Supersensitivity to anandamide and enhanced endogenous cannabinoid signalling in mice lacking fatty acid amide hydrolyse. *Proc Natl Acad Sci USA* 2001; 98:9371–9376.

Cummins TR, Dib-Hajj SD, Waxman SG. Electrophysiological properties of mutant $Na_V1.7$ sodium channels in a painful inherited neuropathy. *J Neurosci* 2004; 24:8232–8236.

Deuchars SA, Atkinson L, Brooke RE, et al. Neuronal P2X7 receptors are targeted to presynaptic terminals in the central and peripheral nervous systems. *J Neurosci* 2001; 21:7143–7152.

Eglen RM, Hunter JC, Dray A. Ions in the fire: recent ion-channel research and approaches to pain therapy. *Trends Pharmacol Sci* 1999; 8:337–342.

England S, Bevan S, Dougherty RJ. PGE2 modulates the tetrodotoxin-resistant sodium current in neonatal dorsal root ganglion neurons via the cyclic AMP-protein kinase A cascade. *J Physiol* 1996; 495:429–440.

Fiorucci S, Antonelli E, Burgand J-L, et al. Nitric-oxide releasing NSAIDs: a review of their current status. *Drug Saf* 2001; 24:801–811.

Flower RJ. The development of COX2 inhibitors. *Nat Rev* 2003; 2:179–191.

Fox A, Wotherspoon G, McNair K, et al. Regulation and function of spinal and peripheral neuronal B (1) bradykinin receptors in inflammatory mechanical hyperalgesia. *Pain* 2003; 104:683–691.

Gold MS, Weinreich D, Kim CS, et al. Redistribution of Na(V)1.8 in uninjured axons enables neuropathic pain. *J Neurosci* 2003; 23:158–166.

Gould HJ, England JD, Soignier RD, et al. Ibuprofen block changes in $Na_V1.7$ and 1.8 sodium channels associated with complete Freund's adjuvant-induced inflammation in rat. *J Pain* 2004; 5:270–280.

Grazzini E, Puma C, Roy MO, et al. Sensory neuron-specific receptor activation elicits central and peripheral nociceptive effects in rats. *Proc Natl Acad Sci USA* 2004; 101:7171–7180.

Harvey RJ, Depner UB, Wassle H, et al. Glyα3: an essential target for spinal PGE_2-mediated inflammatory pain sensitization. *Science* 2004; 304:884–887.

Honore P, Rogers SD, Schwei MJ, et al. Murine models of inflammatory, neuropathic and cancer pain each generate a unique set of neurochemical changes in the spinal cord and sensory neurons. *J Neurosci* 2000; 98:585–598.

Honore P, Kage K, Mikusa J, et al. Analgesic profile of intrathecal P2X3 antisense oligo-neucleotide treatment in chronic inflammatory and neuropathic pain states in rats. *Pain* 2002; 99:11–19.

Hunt SP, Mantyh P. The molecular dynamics of pain control. *Nat Rev* 2001; 2:83–91.

Hurley RW, Hammond DL. The analgesic effects of supraspinal μ and δ opioid receptor agonists are potentiated during persistent inflammation *J Neurosci* 2000; 20:1249–1259.

Jakobsson PJ, Thoen S, Morgenstern R, et al. Identification of human prostaglandin E synthase: a microsomal, glutathione-dependent, inducible enzyme, constituting a potential novel drug target. *Proc Natl Acad Sci USA* 1999; 96:7220–7225.

Jarvis MF, Burgard EC, McGaraughty S. et al. A-317491, a novel potent and selective non nucleotide antagonist of P2X(3) and P2X(2/3) receptors, reduces chronic inflammatory and neuropathic pain in the rat. *Proc Natl Acad Sci USA* 2002; 99:17179–17184.

Lai J, Hunter JC, Porreca F. The role of voltage-gated sodium channels in neuropathic pain. *Curr Opin Neurobiol* 2003; 13:291–297.

Lembo PMC, Grazzini E, Groblewski T, et al. Proenkephalin A gene products activate a new family of sensory neuron-specific GPCRs. *Nat Neurosci* 2002; 5:201–209.

Liang YF, Haake B, Reeh PW. Sustained sensitization and recruitment of rat cutaneous nociceptors by bradykinin and a novel theory of its excitatory action. *J Physiol* 2001; 532:229–239.

Lichtman AH, Leung D, Shelton CC, et al. Reversible inhibitors of fatty acid amide hydrolase that promote analgesia: evidence for an unprecedented combination of potency and selectivity. *J Pharmacol Exp Ther* 2004; 311(2):441–448.

Lindenlaub T, Sommer C. Cytokines in sural nerve biopsies from inflammatory and non-inflammatory neuropathies. *Acta Neuropathol* 2003; 105:593–602.

Luo ZD, Calcutt NA, Higuera ES, et al. Injury type-specific calcium channel alpha (2) delta-1 subunit up-regulation in rat neuropathic pain models correlates with antiallodynic effects of gabapentin. *J Pharmacol Exp Ther* 2002; 303:1199–1205.

Malan TP, Ibrahim MM, Lai J, et al. CB_2 cannabinoid receptor agonists: pain relief without psychoactive effects? *Curr Opin Pharmacol* 2003; 3:62–67.

Milligan ED, Zapata V, Chacur M, et al. Evidence that exogenous and endogenous fraktalkine can induce spinal nociceptive facilitation in rats. *Eur J Neurosci* 2004; 20:2294–2302.

Moore AK, Kohno T, Karchewski LA, et al. Partial peripheral nerve injury promotes a selective loss of GABAergic inhibition in the superficial dorsal horn of the spinal cord. *J Neurosci* 2002; 22:6724–6731.

Nassar MA, Stirling LC, Forlani G, et al. Nociceptor-specific gene deletion reveals a major role for $Na_v1.7$ (PNI) in acute and inflammatory pain. *Proc Natl Acad Sci USA* 2004; 101:12706–12711.

Nathan C. Points of control in inflammation. *Nature* 2002; 420:846–852.

Oh SB, Tran PB, Gillard SE, et al. Chemokines and glycoprotein 120 produce pain hypersensitivity by directly exciting primary nociceptive neurons. *J Neurosci* 2001; 21:5027–5035.

Okuse K, Malik-Hall M, Baker MD, et al. Annexin II light chain regulates sensory neurone-specific sodium channel expression. *Nature* 2002; 417:653–656.

Raghavendra V, Tanga F, Rutkowski MD, et al. Anti-hyperalgesic and morphine-sparing actions of propentofylline following peripheral nerve injury in rats: mechanistic implications of spinal glia and proinflammatory cytokines. *Pain* 2003; 104:655–664.

Rice ASC, Farquhar-Smith WP, Nagy I. Endocannabinoids and pain: spinal and peripheral analgesia in inflammation and neuropathy. *Prostaglandins Leukot Essent Fatty Acids* 2002; 66:243–256.

Richardson JD, Kilo S, Hargreaves KM. Cannabinoids reduce hyperalgesia and inflammation via interactions with peripheral CB1 receptors. *Pain* 1998; 75:111–119.

Sachez-Baez F, Carbonell T, de Felipe C, et al. Attenuation of thermal nociception and hyperalgesia by VR1 blockers. *Proc Natl Acad Sci USA* 2002; 99:2374–2379.

Sah DWY, Ossipov MH, Porreca F. Neurotrophic factors as novel therapeutics for neuropathic pain. *Nat Rev Drug Discov* 2003; 2:460-472.

Schäfers M, Svensson CI, Sommer C, et al. Tumor necrosis factor-alpha induces mechanical allodynia after spinal nerve ligation by activation of p38 MAPK in primary sensory neurons. *J Neurosci* 2003; 23:2517–2521.

Schäfers M, Marziniak M, Sorkin LS, et al. Cyclooxygenase inhibition in nerve-injury and TNF-induced hyperalgesia in the rat. *Exp Neurol* 2004; 185:160–168.

Scholz J, Woolf CJ. Can we conquer pain? *Nat Neurosci* 2002; 5:1062–1065.

Sommer C, Kress M. Recent findings on how proinflammatory cytokines cause pain: peripheral mechanisms in inflammatory and neuropathic hyperalgesia. *Neurosci Lett* 2004; 361:184–187.

Stein C, Schafer M, Machelska H. Attacking pain at its source: new perspectives on opioids. *Nat Med* 2003; 9:1003–1008.

Stewart JM. Bradykinin antagonists: discovery and development. *Peptides* 2004; 25:527–732.

Trebino CE, Stock JL, Gibbons CP, et al. Impaired inflammatory and pain responses in mice lacking an inducible prostaglandin E synthase. *Proc Natl Acad Sci USA* 2003; 100:9044–9049.

Tsuda M, Shigemoto-Mogami Y, Koizumi S, et al. P2X4 receptors induced in spinal microglia gate tactile allodynia after nerve injury. *Nature* 2003; 424:778–783.

Vellani V, Mappleback S, Moriondo A, et al. Protein kinase C activation gating of the vanilloid receptor VR1 by capsaicin, protons, heat and anandamide. *J Physiol* 2001; 534:813–825.

Veneroni O, Maj R, Calbresi M, et al. Anti-allodynic effect of NW-1029, a novel Na channel blocker, in experimental animal models of inflammatory and neuropathic pain. *Pain* 2003; 102:17–25.

Watkins LR, Maier S. Beyond neurons: evidence that immune and glial cells contribute to pathological pain states. *Physiol Rev* 2002; 82:981–1011.

Woolf CJ, Salter MW. Neuronal plasticity: increasing the gain in pain. *Science* 2000; 288:1765–1769.

Yaksh TL, Dirig DM, Conway CM, et al. The acute hyperalgesic action of non-steroidal, anti-inflammatory drugs and release of spinal prostaglandin E2 is mediated by the inhibition of constitutive spinal cyclooxygenase-2 (COX-2) but not COX-1. *J Neurosci* 2001; 21:5847–5853.

Correspondence to: Andy Dray, PhD, AstraZeneca Research and Development, 7171 Frederick Banting Street, Montreal, PQ, Canada H4S 1Z9. Email: andy.dray@astrazeneca.com.

The Paths of Pain 1975–2005, edited by
Harold Merskey, John D. Loeser, and Ronald
Dubner, IASP Press, Seattle, © 2005.

13

Pharmacological Control of Pain: Non-Opioid Targets

Anthony H. Dickenson[a] and Jean-Marie Besson[b]

[a]Department of Pharmacology, University College London, London,
United Kingdom; [b]INSERM Unit 161, Ambroise Pare Hospital,
Boulogne-Billancourt, France

This chapter considers recent data on targets in pain control. Our aim is not to provide an exhaustive review of the thousands of studies on non-opioid systems in pain and analgesia that have been published over the last 30 years but to consider targets that have led to useful drugs or may lead to drugs of the future (Besson 1999). The literature abounds with contradictions and different interpretations of data, partly because various studies use wide ranges of doses, different routes, different models and tests, and a variety of measures. We present here some of the most important targets based on their novelty and a substantial body of supporting data.

Many different experimental approaches have been used, but it is clear that the role of a particular target can only be fully elucidated in integrated systems. Molecular approaches have been helpful in identifying channels and receptors in pain pathways, and approaches such as genetic deletion of defined receptors and channels in mice have been invaluable in identifying function where drugs do not exist that can selectively act on the particular system (see Wood et al. 2000). However, issues such as compensations, downstream changes, and the background phenotype of the animals can complicate interpretation of data. Use of antisense technology and sRNA (small RNA) can circumvent some of these problems, but studies using these methods are complicated by issues such as delivery to the required site.

It is fair to say that many drug actions may be highly selective but rarely specific and that a number of animal studies will report effects that may be seen in animals at doses that are not tolerable in human volunteers or patients. Whereas basic science can be invaluable in modeling clinical conditions, it will generally provide data on potential efficacy of a drug rather than thera-peutic windows. A major problem is that simple measures of side effects (e.g., sedation and motor effects) can be made in animals, but factors that are key to human tolerability such as drug actions on cognitive and affective function can only be assessed in humans. Many in vitro studies use cells or tissue from immature animals, although many of their receptors and chan-nels have structures, distributions, and functions that differ from those in adults. Also, isolated tissues from adults are likely to have only part of the circuitry intact, and so mechanisms derived from these approaches may not operate in integrated systems. Patients will seek medical assistance with pain syndromes above the threshold; visual analogue pain scores in clinical trials are frequently toward the upper end of the scale (Sindrup and Jensen 1999). On the other hand, behavioral studies in animals in many cases will rely on withdrawal measures, which by definition are threshold responses (Mogil et al. 1999). However, electrophysiological studies (despite the problem of anesthesia) can provide information on suprathreshold responses, as can surrogate measures of activity such as c-fos labeling (Catheline et al. 1999; Hunt and Mantyh 2001; Suzuki et al. 2002). Novel approaches such as the study of gene array data in various pathological states will also shed light on changes in systems, but verification of targets will be difficult (see Wang et al. 2002).

PERIPHERAL MECHANISMS AFTER TISSUE DAMAGE

It has now become very clear that the polymodal nature of the nocicep-tor is due to the fact that it is not a single entity but is composed of a number of proteins that can sense many sensory and chemical stimuli (Millan 1999; Cummins et al. 2000; Wood et al. 2000; Julius 2003). Due to the inaccessi-bility of receptors on the fine C fibers, molecular techniques have been very useful in identifying the channels and receptors that contribute to the polymodal nature of nociceptive sensory neurons. Knockout studies have been instrumental in defining the potential roles of channels where selective drugs do not yet exist. The important roles of the novel sodium channels $Na_V1.8$ and 1.9 in generating activity in various pain models, along with their selective location in fine fibers, make these channels an attractive target (Cummins et al. 2000; Wood et al. 2000; Lai et al. 2004). Further-more, drugs acting on these channels should avoid cardiac and central ner-vous system (CNS) side effects and could also be given by oral routes. Interest is also moving toward understanding the function of particular po-tassium channels in small sensory fibers (Passmore et al. 2003).

The number of receptors that are responsive to chemical mediators is almost overwhelming. Many proteins that at first appeared to have selective activation parameters now appear to have several physical and chemical modes of activation. In a sense, a receptor or channel with the ability to integrate a number of stimuli may provide a far better target than a highly selective receptor. However, how can one define the most important receptor in a family? There are many receptors for adenosine triphosphate (ATP) and hydrogen ions (acid pH) (Burnstock et al. 2000; Wood et al. 2000). Among physical stimuli, it is well known that thermal stimuli act on a defined family, the capsaicin-activated vanilloid receptor family now known as the transient receptor potential vanilloid (TRPV) receptors; however, the more pressing clinical problem of unavoidable mechanical stimuli is at present without a molecular target. In the case of TRPV1, selective drugs are needed because knockouts reveal highly selective deficits at defined temperatures, although how this finding may translate to therapeutic effects is still unclear. Not only do the TRPV receptors include warm and cold receptors, but the TRPV1 channel is not simply gated by noxious temperatures but can also be activated by acid, ATP, and endocannabinoids. Thus, blocking this channel could have various effects other than simply attenuating responses to thermal stimuli (Julius 2003), although protons and ATP have many other receptors that would still operate.

Chemical mediators such as ATP, prostanoids, bradykinin, serotonin, histamine, and hydrogen ions can act on nociceptors through activation of their receptors located on the fine afferent fibers (Eglen et al. 1999; Millan 1999). In the case of mediators such as ATP, which acts on a large family of purinergic receptors, transgenic approaches have been very useful in defining roles of the various receptors, revealing that the $P2X_3$ and $P2X_7$ receptors may have important roles in pain and other functions. The therapeutic actions of drugs that block the $P2X_3$ receptor may have to be balanced against this receptor's roles in bladder function (Dray and Perkins 1993; Dray et al. 1997; Burnstock et al. 2000). There is an important distinction between activation and sensitization of the peripheral terminals of primary afferent nociceptors, yet bradykinin can achieve both effects. Despite knockouts and a number of experimental drugs that selectively block the constitutive B2 and the inducible B1 bradykinin receptors, together with many years of research, no related drugs have reached the clinic. Other mediators have actions that are primarily sensitizing, such as prostaglandins. It is notable that sensitization reduces the threshold for activation of nociceptors so that other chemical and natural stimuli can more easily activate them. One consequence could be that the threshold for the TRPV1 receptor, normally 42°C, could fall into the range of body temperature, so that ongoing burning pain could result.

Further to the activation of C-fibers, both substance P and calcitonin-gene-related peptide (CGRP) are released through the axon reflex and alter blood vessel tone. Both neuropeptides also liberate prostaglandins, which have receptors on the vascular elements around a site of injury. The resulting vasodilation not only is the cause of edema but also facilitates the access of bradykinin and serotonin (5HT) from plasma. These events are key to headaches, and the triptans, drugs that activate the inhibitory $5HT_{1B/D}$ receptors, have proved highly successful in reducing migraines. It is unclear why the participation of this receptor in attenuating the peripheral events leading to changes in blood flow and promoting hyperresponsiveness of nociceptors is restricted to cranial tissues (Millan 1999; Landy et al. 2004). Interestingly, emphasis is moving toward the participation of central events in the provocation of headache (Landy et al. 2004).

Another therapeutic advance was based on the identification of two isoforms of cyclooxygenase (COX), the key enzyme for the synthesis of prostaglandins in inflammatory exudates. The realization that COX exists in two forms led to the manufacture of inhibitors of the inducible COX-2 isoform (coxibs), including several that have reached the clinic (Chen et al. 2004; Hinz and Brune 2004). The coxibs appear to have efficacy similar to the older, nonselective COX inhibitors (nonsteroidal anti-inflammatory drugs) in terms of pain reduction, but they have reduced gastrointestinal side effects and lack the vascular actions of the older drugs. This latter effect means that bleeding is reduced, but the cardioprotective effects are lost (Appleton 1997); this has recently led to warnings and withdrawals. The original idea that COX-2 was the inducible form of the enzyme has been challenged by the finding that the spinal cord contains appreciable amounts of the enzyme and that both in animals and humans, acute effects can be seen in response to non-tissue-damaging stimuli (Koppert et al. 2004).

There have been major advances in the understanding of the roles of growth factors, for example nerve growth factor, glial-cell-line-derived neurotrophic factor, and brain-derived neurotrophic factor, which are produced by neural and non-neural tissue. A body of evidence suggests that the levels of these factors influence the responsiveness, phenotype, and regrowth of sensory neurons. Thus, growth factors are likely to be important in states of both inflammation and nerve injury, although attempts to manipulate these factors for clinical indications has yet to be realized and could be fraught with problems due to their ubiquitous roles in support of neuronal and non-neuronal functions (McMahon at al. 1993; Millan 1999; Boucher et al. 2000).

In a similar way, many studies have revealed that cytokines can influence sensory neurons and so relate to the processes of inflammation and neuropathy, although again, manipulation of large molecules such as these is not without problems (Sommer 2001). Cytokine research with an emphasis on spinal events has led to interest in glial and astrocyte function based on central changes in non-neuronal cells in different pain states (see Watkins and Maier, this volume). New research suggests further studies on how glia and astrocytes, originally thought to be passive supporting cells, may be fruitful targets (Watkins and Maier 2003).

Finally, many physiological and clinical studies have focused on the involvement of the sympathetic nervous system in certain pain states including nerve injury, but the role of sympathectomy remains a matter of debate (Jänig and Baron 2001).

PERIPHERAL MECHANISMS AFTER NERVE INJURY

Neuropathic pain involves a number of changes in the periphery that seem to affect central systems of transmission and modulation (Sindrup and Jensen 1999; Cummins et al. 2000; Suzuki and Dickenson 2000; Wood et al. 2000; Lai et al. 2004). The initial events of neuropathic pain are thought to be generated in damaged peripheral sensory neurons within the nerve itself, and so some of the pain symptoms can be independent of peripheral nociceptor activation. Because some fibers will be destroyed or may become non-functional, numbness and sensory loss are common. Thus, both stimulus-dependent and stimulus-independent symptoms can occur, so that allodynia, hyperalgesia, and sensory loss can coexist. Following damage to peripheral nerves, various changes can occur in nerves, altering their activity, properties, and transmitter content. The recent advent of a number of animal models of neuropathic pain states has facilitated understanding of the peripheral mechanisms involved. Damaged nerves may start to generate ongoing ectopic activity due to the accumulation and clustering of sodium channels around the damaged axons. Evidence also indicates that mechanoreceptors become highly sensitive to applied stimuli. This aberrant activity can spread rapidly to the cell body in the dorsal root ganglia. In addition to changes within the nerve, sympathetic efferents become able to activate sensory afferents. These peripheral ectopic impulses can cause spontaneous pain and prime the spinal cord to exhibit enhanced evoked responses to stimuli, which themselves have greater effects due to increased sensitivity of the peripheral nerves. The positive symptoms strongly suggest changes within the nervous system that are excessive attempts to compensate for sensory loss, since nerve damage should equate with deficits.

This peripheral activity may be a rational basis for the use of systemic local anesthetics in neuropathic states, given that damaged nerves are highly sensitive to systemic sodium channel blockers. It is also probably part of the basis for the effects of established effective anticonvulsants, such as carbamazepine, that block sodium channels. The ability of C fibers to generate action potentials, via both classical and unique sodium channels with very low tetrodotoxin sensitivity, suggests that these could be important targets for drugs, as discussed above. However, the observed downregulation of these channels in neuropathic models may indicate a potential place for such drugs in the control of pain after tissue damage rather than neuropathy, although this is still unclear (Waxman 1999; Suzuki and Dickenson 2000; Wood et al. 2000; Lai et al. 2004). However, the re-emergence of the embryonic sodium channel $Na_V1.3$ after nerve injury points toward a contribution of this channel in the peripheral events of nerve injury pain. Antagonists for all these channels are still awaited (Cummins et al. 2000).

THE PROBLEM OF CANCER PAIN

In the past, models of cancer-induced pain used systemic injection of carcinoma cells, resulting in systemically unwell animals with multiple randomly sited bone metastases. This methodology made the investigation of specific neuronal and pharmacological alterations that occur in cancer-induced bone pain almost impossible. In 1999, Schwei et al. reported a mouse model of cancer-induced bone pain that paralleled the clinical condition in terms of pain development and bone destruction, but was confined to the mouse femur. This model has been now taken into rats, while others have used different cancer cells and different bones (Honore et al. 2000; Medhurst et al. 2002). Following injection of the cancer cells to the defined bone, the ability to seal the site has lead to a huge step forward in understanding mechanisms. This model induces progressive bone destruction, with elevated osteoclast activity and likely involvement of prostaglandins and protons in the periphery. However, the progressive bone destruction leads to a denervation of bone afferent fibers so that the nocifensive behaviors, which include ongoing, spontaneous, and movement-induced hyperalgesia/allodynia, are likely to result from components of tissue damage and neuropathic states (Honore et al. 2000; Medhurst et al. 2002).

There are marked changes in the neurochemical status of the dorsal horn of the spinal cord receiving nociceptive input from the injected bone. These changes involve an increased expression of the prohyperalgesic peptide dynorphin and a remarkable astrocyte hypertrophy. However, many neurotransmitters that undergo alterations in neuropathy or inflammation do not change in this model (Schwei et al. 1999; Honore et al. 2000). The progressive nocifensive behavior, the bone destruction, and the dorsal horn neurochemical markers all suggest that cancer-induced bone pain is a unique pain state. Further support for this proposal comes from studies on spinal neurons where changes in excitability that parallel the behavioral changes are also very different from those seen in other animal models of pain (Urch et al. 2003). These models will be invaluable both in determining the mechanisms of cancer pain and in assessing novel treatments in preclinical settings.

CENTRAL EXCITATORY SYSTEMS

The very different peripheral events that accompany inflammation, neuropathy, and cancer all generate action potentials in different ways. These action potentials propagate to the dorsal horn of the spinal cord, carrying the sensory information generated from nociceptors (in the case of inflammation) or generated both from nociceptors and from intrinsic ectopic and other activities (in the case of nerve damage). With the arrival of the peripheral signals at the first synapse, not only are excitatory mechanisms of prime importance in transmission through to the higher centers, but inhibitory transmitter systems start to play a major role in balancing incoming excitations with inhibitions (see Dickenson et al. 1997).

As peripheral neurons become more active, action potentials arrive in their central terminals, and calcium channels open in the membrane. These channels are critical for transmitter release and are important in neuronal excitability. Results with agents that block neuronal voltage-sensitive calcium channels suggest an increase in central neuronal excitability after both inflammation and nerve damage that involves the N-, P-, and T-type calcium channels (Vanegas and Schaible 2000). N-type channels show the most marked expression and functional changes after nerve injury (Matthews and Dickenson 2001; Cizkova et al. 2002).

Gabapentin is an antiepileptic drug that has analgesic activity in neuropathic pain states from varying origins. Recent randomized controlled trials in patients concluded that gabapentin can be an effective treatment for these pain states (Sindrup and Jensen 1999). The mechanism of action of gabapentin and the new drug, pregabalin, is not clearly established, but both drugs must interact with calcium channels because they bind to the $\alpha_2\delta$ subunit of these channels (Gee et al. 1996). How this mechanism translates into its clinical effects is unclear because the subunit is found in all calcium channels, although selective actions on the $\alpha_2\delta$ subunit only interfere with abnormal activity. In models of neuropathy, upregulation of the $\alpha_2\delta$ subunit has been observed in correlation with the action of gabapentin (Luo et al. 2002), but the drug also shows efficacy in short-term inflammatory models such as that caused by formalin. The nature of these state-dependent effects is unknown. Agents that block transmitter release as the afferents enter the spinal cord will attenuate transmission at the first step in the multiple polysynaptic pathways from the periphery to the highest centers.

Synaptic transmission in the dorsal horn starts with activation of these voltage-dependent calcium channels (VDCCs) so that C fibers release their transmitters. Most fibers contain and release glutamate, whereas a proportion also contains substance P and CGRP, and yet others are nonpeptide (the IB4 population). The peptide content and phenotype are altered by tissue and nerve damage such that increases and decreases in substance P content have been reported. The major transmitter is glutamate, an excitatory amino acid (EAA) that has been implicated in transmission from primary afferent nociceptors to dorsal horn neurons through various combinations of receptors on neurons in various laminae of the dorsal horn. These receptors include α-amino-3-hydroxy-5-methyl-4-isoxazole propionate (AMPA), kainate, N-methyl-D-aspartate (NMDA), and metabotropic receptors. The degree and duration of spinal neuronal activation is determined by these receptors acting in concert with those for peptides (Dickenson 1995; Millan 1999). The AMPA receptor is an unlikely target because it is implicated in most of the fast synaptic transmission in the CNS, and the large number of metabotropic receptors and a lack of good tools have made their function hard to gauge.

Thus, in recent years, attention has focused on the actions of glutamate acting on the NMDA receptor as a pivotal event in the transmission of persistent pain. NMDA-receptor antagonists have been tested as potential therapies for neuropathic pain states, based on earlier results from animal studies showing important roles of this receptor in spinal activity that follows short- and long-term inflammation and nerve damage as well as a number of other peripheral insults (Dickenson 1995; Millan 1999; Petrenko et al. 2003). NMDA receptors have been implicated in "wind-up" and related changes such as spinal hyperexcitability and long-term potentiation, events that enhance and prolong sensory transmission (Svendsen 1999; Sandkuhler 2000; Willis 2002). Persistent injury states such as neuropathy may produce a prolonged activation of the NMDA receptor subsequent to a sustained afferent input, producing an enhanced evoked release of the amino acid. Ectopic impulse generation in peripheral nerves and dorsal root ganglia, alterations in the phenotype of damaged nerves, and loss of inhibitory γ-aminobutyric acid (GABA) controls may all contribute to greater activation of the NMDA-receptor-channel complex (Dickenson et al. 2001). In fact, observed increases in receptive field size after nerve injury could arise from hyperexcitable spinal neurons now responding to weak inputs that are unable to excite the neuron under normal conditions. There is evidence to suggest that NMDA receptors are involved in the induction and maintenance of certain pathological pain states, possibly via the sensitization of dorsal horn neurons.

Several studies clearly show that central sensitization and wind-up can be observed in laboratory models of inflammation and neuropathic pain and can be demonstrated in human psychophysical studies. The degree of wind-up induced in patients appears to relate to the pain condition in groups of patients with musculoskeletal pains, fibromyalgia, and neuropathic pains (Price et al. 1994a,b; Gottrup et al. 2000; Jorum et al. 2003; Staud et al. 2003; Banic et al. 2004). Numerous clinical studies have reported the use of NMDA-receptor antagonists in various neuropathic pain states and surrogate models, including phantom limb pain, postamputation stump pain, and postherpetic neuralgia (Gottrup et al. 2000; Jorum et al. 2003). The main drawback of most NMDA-receptor antagonists such as ketamine, however, is the severe side-effect profile seen at therapeutic doses. Other blockers such as memantine and dextromethorphan seem to lack the efficacy of ketamine in humans, which is predictable from the animal data. NMDA receptors are ubiquitous and are implicated in sensory perception, cognition, and consciousness, so that nonselective antagonism will inevitably result in unwanted psychotropic effects.

A final approach to the modulation of NMDA-receptor-mediated activity would rely on the synthesis of subtype-selective drugs that target certain NMDA receptors. Antagonists of the NR2B receptor appear promising from animal studies, with a reduced side-effect profile compared to existing NMDA receptor antagonists, probably due to the restricted location of the receptor, which does include the spinal cord (see Petrenko et al. 2003; Smith 2003).

A lot of interest has centered on events downstream from the NMDA receptor. It is well established that the influx of calcium through the receptor channels is a key event in the links between pain signaling and the expression of certain genes that may contribute to central sensitization and other aspects of nociception (Hunt and Mantyh 2001). Furthermore, NMDA-mediated wind-up-like mechanisms lead to intracellular changes, such as the generation of nitric oxide and prostanoids, highly diffusible mediators that are important downstream mechanisms. The block of the actions of nitric oxide reduced many of the manifestations of central hypersensitivity (Meller and Gebhart 1993), but the wide role of this mediator, in common with many other intracellular targets (Petersen-Zeitz and Basbaum 1999), means that manipulation is highly unlikely to selectively alter pain without changing other functions, even if one were to target the neuronal forms of enzymes with wide distributions.

CENTRAL MODULATION OF PAIN

Whereas the majority of the early studies on the mechanisms of pain concentrated on modulatory systems such as opioids, the previous sections illustrate to what extent interest in excitatory events has overtaken research on the roles of inhibitions. Despite the fact that a number of receptor systems can be activated by transmitters and drugs to produce analgesic effects—opioid receptors, α_2 adrenoceptors, some of the 5HT receptors (5HT$_1$ in particular), the adenosine A1 receptor, and cannabinoids—the efficacy and therapeutic range of the gold standard, morphine, has been almost impossible to beat (Yaksh and Noueihed 1985; Dickenson 1995; Millan 1999; Chapman and Iversen 2002). Whereas the 5HT$_{1B/D}$-receptor agonists, the triptans, are highly effective in migraine, recent advances in opioid therapy have been based on routes and formulations of the drugs rather than novel agents, Thus, although many years have elapsed since the discovery of the opioid receptors and the detailed knowledge of their four main types, μ, δ, κ, and opioid-receptor-like 1 (ORL1) and of the various opioid peptides that act on these receptors, no non-μ drugs have reached the clinic. This lack of novel opioids is not due to a lack of research because molecular studies of the opioid receptors have revealed detailed knowledge of their structure, their mechanisms, and their precise location in the nervous system. Emphasis has therefore moved toward trying to improve opioid actions through combination therapies. For example, subtypes, interactions, and changes in expression of the opioid receptors have been shown in animals, but as yet the basic findings have been difficult to relate to the use of opioids in patients (Dickenson and Suzuki 1999). An impressive list of conditions and mechanisms, including nerve injury and inflammation, can reduce or enhance opioid analgesia (Dickenson and Suzuki 1999; Rowbotham 2001), and other receptor systems can interact with the analgesic and pro-tolerance effects of morphine, including levels of excitability via NMDA receptors, cholecystokinin (CCK), and dynorphin (Basbaum 1995; Nichols et al. 1995; Rygh et al. 2000). In the case of the NMDA receptor and CCK, there is proof of this concept in the clinic.

It is also interesting to note the way in which opinions change on the pharmacotherapy of pain. The first studies on neuropathic pain reported this pain state to be resistant to the analgesic effects of morphine, but after a decade, consensus is shifting toward another view. It is now generally acknowledged that neuropathic pain is not insensitive, but rather patients can have a reduced sensitivity to systemic opioid drugs. A large body of data on animals shows that opioids can reduce some neuronal and behavioral responses that may be related to symptoms of neuropathic pain. The extent to which morphine can induce pain relief now appears be related to the route of administration and perhaps also to the symptoms and the duration of the neuropathy (see Dickenson and Suzuki 1999; Field et al. 1999; Le Guen et al. 2001).

Several neurotransmitters are involved in descending pain modulation and facilitation from brainstem and midbrain centers (e.g., norepinephrine, serotonin, glutamate, and GABA) (Basbaum and Fields 1978; Yaksh and Noueihed 1985; Besson and Chaouch 1987; Basbaum and Besson 1991; Fields et al. 1991; Dickenson 1994; Urban and Gebhart 1999; Hunt and Mantyh 2001; Porreca et al. 2002; Ren and Dubner 2002). This field of research, which initially emphasized the ways in which the supraspinal sites could inhibit pain, has now moved toward studying descending facilitations. Different neurotransmitters acting on their receptor classes in different areas will interact synergistically, and others will interact antagonistically. Thus, the balance between the activity in these various systems will determine the final level of pain (Millan 2002).

Importantly, supraspinal monoamine systems are also controlled by opioid receptors, and this mechanism forms an important component of opioid analgesia (Millan 1999) and influences the ways in which antidepressants, α_2-adrenoceptor agonists such as clonidine, and the triptans interact with norepinephrine and serotonin transmission. The profile of α_2-adrenoceptor agonists is interesting because animal data have shown that the analgesia and sedation are likely to be inseparable. Thus, drugs acting on these receptors may not be useful other than in the perioperative period in humans, but these dual properties in animals have proved valuable in veterinary practice.

An example of the ways in which systems interact is the finding that substance P-responsive neurons in the dorsal horn are at the origin of a spinobulbospinal loop that has a major bearing on spinal cord neuronal excitability. These pain-specific neurons project to areas of the brain important in affective responses to pain such as autonomic changes, fear, and anxiety. Changes in this circuit may underlie the plasticity induced by neuropathy and other pain states. Lamina I projection neurons that express neurokinin-1 (NK1) ascend to brainstem regions including the parabrachial area (PB), the periaqueductal gray (PAG), and the thalamus, thus supplying parts of the brain associated with affective and cognitive functions (Bester et al. 2000; Todd 2002). It is clear that this is a parallel processing pathway to the classical spinothalamic tract; while the latter may underlie the sensory-discriminative aspects of pain, the lamina I pathway is more likely to play a role in the affective components (Fig. 1). Interestingly, these areas can be imaged in humans with functional magnetic resonance imaging and other techniques, allowing comparison of human and rodent data. Selective targeting of lamina I/III NK1-expressing neurons through the use of substance P-saporin (SP-SAP), a remarkable modern technique for the ablation of specific neurons in defined areas (Mantyh et al. 1997), reveals marked deficits in behavioral hyperalgesia, in parallel with reduced excitability of deep dorsal horn neurons in the spinal cord (Nichols et al. 1999; Khasabov et al. 2002). The ability to reproduce many of the electrophysiological changes through pharmacological block of spinal $5HT_3$ receptors led to the hypothesis that NK1-expressing lamina I/III neurons are at the origin of a spinobulbospinal loop that drives serotonergic excitatory influences from the brainstem (Suzuki et al. 2002). These findings contribute to the recent body of evidence demonstrating important roles of descending facilitations in the control of pain states including neuropathy (Urban and Gebhart 1999; Porreca et

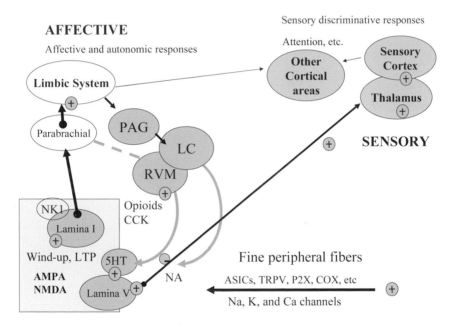

Fig. 1. A schematic diagram of the pathways of pain from peripheral sites to the spinal cord and on to higher centers. Peripheral receptors and channels such as acid-sensitive ion channels (ASICs), TRPV, P2X, sodium and potassium ion channels, and enzymes such as cyclooxygenase (COX) play key roles in generating activity in afferents, which in turn releases glutamate and peptides into the spinal cord. Here these transmitters act on their receptors such as the neurokinin-1 (NK1) and N-methyl-D-aspartate (NMDA) receptors to activate ascending pathways to the affective areas (LC = locus ceruleus; PAG = periaqueductal gray; RVM = rostroventral medial medulla) and sensory-discriminative areas of the brain. States of spinal hyperexcitability can be induced such as wind-up and long-term potentiation (LTP). Modulatory influences at spinal and supraspinal sites such as norepinephrine (NA), serotonin (5HT), cholecystokinin (CCK), and opioids can alter this activity.

al. 2002). Higher centers play key roles in cognition, memory, attention, and punishment, and so research on the ways in which centers involved in the higher processing of pain interact with sensory transmission may well yield further targets for therapy. One circuit may well be this type of loop whereby areas important in anxiety and attention that are likely to change in chronic pain patients can facilitate spinal events (see Hunt and Mantyh 2001; Rahman et al. 2003). The ability not simply to image pain but to examine drug effects in humans will be a powerful tool for understanding the ways in which analgesics alter CNS function (Rogers et al. 2004). Furthermore, these techniques will allow the effects of pain and drugs on higher processes to be quantified and will lead to a better understanding of the pharmacology of the brain in relation to pain.

Substance P was the first pain transmitter to be studied, and its investigation has a long and varied history. Much of the early work supported the idea that it played an important excitatory role in pain transmission, although this concept was not without controversy. Further support came from studies in knockout animals, but its potential role as a human pain transmitter was not supported by the failure of NK1-receptor antagonists to provide pain relief in patients (Hill 2003). Whether this was due to inappropriate testing of symptoms or patient groups or a genuine mismatch between animals and patients is still debated.

CONCLUSIONS

Attempts have been made to relate symptoms of pain to mechanisms in order to provide a rational approach to treatment (Woolf et al. 1998). This approach has been most relevant to neuropathy, where sensory testing can be used to provide detail of particular symptoms in patients (Hansson 2003). However, mechanism-based treatment is far from practical on the basis of current knowledge, and it is clear that what is measured in animals in terms of allodynia may not always relate to the human symptom, nor may the mechanisms coincide. In addition, where the mechanisms of allodynia described in the literature have counterparts in humans, they range from changes in particular peripheral sodium channels to central hyperexcitability of spinal circuits; furthermore, they are convincingly linked to superficial spinal neuronal function as well as to wind-up-like events in deep neurons of the spinal cord. Descending facilitations from the brainstem to spinal cord are also critical. Thus. it would appear that multiple mechanisms can elicit a single symptom, which would fit with ideas based on the causes of neuropathy in humans and the various models used in animals. Disparate causes ranging from diabetes to viral infections to trauma may cause pain symptoms and allodynias that appear identical and are not predictive of the syndrome (Rasmussen et al. 2004). The issue may therefore be that effective drugs in pain are able to act on common targets that modulate aberrant activity caused by multiple mechanisms, rather than necessarily acting on the causal mechanisms.

Overall, the marked complexity of pain transmission in terms of multiple mechanisms acting at peripheral and central sites and multiple pain-engaging pathways that interact with sensory, affective, and autonomic regions of the brain is a logical rationale for combination therapy. The common clinical approach of using multiple drugs to treat difficult pains thus has strong support from what we know about basic mechanisms of pain and analgesia. In common with other CNS therapies, the principle that drugs can either increase inhibitions or decrease excitations makes the use of combinations of appropriate agents logical when single agents are insufficient (Dickenson and Sullivan 1993; Yaksh and Malmberg 1994). Furthermore, the use of adjuncts to enhance opioid analgesia or reduce side effects has a long history, and this approach is now being applied to other agents.

Thus, the 30 years, since the 1st World Congress of the IASP have seen huge advances in the understanding of pain mechanisms. These advances not only have translated into novel drugs but just as importantly, have lead to an understanding of the multiple mechanisms of pain and how and why analgesic treatments work. A rational basis for treatment, close links between scientists and clinicians, and better information for pain patients are just some of the benefits that have resulted from this work.

REFERENCES

Appleton I. Non-steroidal anti-inflammatory drugs and pain. In: Dickenson AH, Besson JM (Eds). *The Pharmacology of Pain,* Handbook of Experimental Pharmacology, Vol. 130. Springer-Verlag, 1997, pp 43–60.

Banic B, Petersen-Felix S, Andersen OK, et al. Evidence for spinal cord hypersensitivity in chronic pain after whiplash injury and in fibromyalgia. *Pain* 2004; 107:7–15.

Basbaum AI. Insights into the development of opioid tolerance. *Pain* 1995; 61:349–353.

Basbaum AI, Fields HL. Endogenous pain control mechanisms: review and hypothesis. *Ann Neurol* 1978; 4:451–462.

Basbaum AI, Besson JM. *Towards a New Pharmacotherapy of Pain: Report of the Dahlem Workshop on Towards a New Pharmacotherapy of Pain: Beyond Morphine.* Chichester: Wiley, 1991.

Besson JM. The neurobiology of pain. *Lancet* 1999; 353:1610–1615.

Besson JM, Chaouch A. Peripheral and spinal mechanisms of nociception. *Physiol Rev* 1987; 67:67–186.

Bester H, Chapman V, Besson JM, Bernard JF. Physiological properties of the lamina I spinoparabrachial neurons in the rat. *J Neurophysiol* 2000; 83:2239–2259.

Boucher T, Kerr BJ, Ramer MS, Thompson SWN, McMahon SB. Neurotrophic factor effects on pain-signaling systems. In: Devor M, Rowbotham MC, Wiesenfeld-Hallin Z (Eds). *Proceedings of the 9th World Congress on Pain,* Progress in Pain Research and Management, Vol. 16. Seattle: IASP Press, 2000, pp 175–189.

Burnstock G, McMahon SB, Humphrey PPA, Hamilton SG. ATP (P2X) receptors and pain. In: Devor M, Rowbotham MC, Wiesenfeld-Hallin Z (Eds). *Proceedings of the 9th World Congress on Pain,* Progress in Pain Research and Management, Vol. 16. Seattle: IASP Press, 2000, pp 63–76.

Catheline G, Le Guen S, Honore P, Besson JM. Are there long-term changes in the basal or evoked Fos expression in the dorsal horn of the spinal cord of the mononeuropathic rat? *Pain* 1999; 80:347–357.

Chapman V, Iversen L. Cannabinoids: a real prospect for pain relief. *Curr Opin Pharmacol* 2002; 2:50–55.

Chen LC, Elliott RA, Ashcroft DM. Systematic review of the analgesic efficacy and tolerability of COX-2 inhibitors in post-operative pain control. *J Clin Pharm Ther* 2004; 29:215–229.

Cizkova D, Marsala J, Lukacova N, et al. Localization of N-type Ca^{2+} channels in the rat spinal cord following chronic constrictive nerve injury. *Exp Brain Res* 2002; 147:456–463.

Cummins TR, Dib-Hajj SD, Black JA, Waxman SG. Sodium channels as molecular targets in pain. In: Devor M, Rowbotham MC, Wiesenfeld-Hallin Z (Eds). *Proceedings of the 9th World Congress on Pain,* Progress in Pain Research and Management, Vol. 16. Seattle: IASP Press, 2000, pp 77–91.

Dickenson AH. NMDA receptor antagonists as analgesics. In: Fields HL, Liebeskind JC (Eds). *Pharmacological Approaches to the Treatment of Pain: New Concepts and Critical Issues,* Progress in Pain Research and Management, Vol. 1. Seattle: IASP Press, 1994, pp 173–187.

Dickenson AH. Spinal cord pharmacology of pain. *Br J Anaesth* 1995; 75:193–200.

Dickenson AH, Sullivan AF. Combination therapy in analgesia: seeking synergy. *Curr Opin Anaesthesiol* 1993; 6:861–865.

Dickenson AH, Suzuki R. Function and dysfunction of opioid receptors in the spinal cord. In: Kalso E, McQuay HJ, Wiesenfeld-Hallin Z (Eds). *Opioid Sensitivity of Chronic Noncancer Pain,* Progress in Pain Research and Management, Vol. 14. Seattle: IASP Press, 1999, pp 77–74.

Dickenson AH, Chapman V, Green GM. The pharmacology of excitatory and inhibitory amino acid-mediated events in the transmission and modulation of pain in the spinal cord. *Gen Pharmacol* 1997; 28:633–638.

Dickenson AH, Matthews EA, Suzuki R. Central nervous system mechanisms of pain in peripheral neuropathy. In: Hansson PT, Fields HL, Hill RG, Marchettini P (Eds). *Neuropathic Pain: Pathophysiology and Treatment,* Progress in Pain Research and Management, Vol. 21. Seattle: IASP Press, 2001, pp 85–106.

Dickenson AH, Matthews EA, Suzuki R. Neurobiology of neuropathic pain: mode of action of anticonvulsants. *Eur J Pain* 2002; 6(Suppl A):51–60.

Dray A. Peripheral mediators of pain. In: Dickenson AH, Besson JM (Eds). *The Pharmacology of Pain,* Handbook of Experimental Pharmacology, Vol. 130. Springer-Verlag, 1997, pp 21–42.

Dray A, Perkins MN. Bradykinin and inflammatory pain. *Trends Neurosci* 1993; 16:99–104.

Eglen RM, Hunter JC, Dray A. Ions in the fire: recent ion-channel research and approaches to pain therapy. *Trends Pharmacol Sci* 1999; 20:337–342.

Field MJ, McCleary S, Hughes J, Singh L. Gabapentin and pregabalin, but not morphine and amitriptyline, block both static and dynamic components of mechanical allodynia induced by streptozocin in the rat. *Pain* 1999; 80:391–398.

Fields HL, Heinricher MM, Mason P. Neurotransmitters in nociceptive modulatory circuits. *Annu Rev Neurosci* 1991; 14:219–245.

Hansson P. Difficulties in stratifying neuropathic pain by mechanisms. *Eur J Pain* 2003; 7:353–357.

Gee NS, Brown JP, Dissanayake VU, et al. The novel anticonvulsant drug, gabapentin (Neurontin), binds to the alpha 2 delta subunit of a calcium channel. *J Biol Chem* 1996; 271:5768–5776.

Gottrup H, Hansen PO, Arendt-Nielsen L, Jensen TS. Differential effects of systemically administered ketamine and lidocaine on dynamic and static hyperalgesia induced by intradermal capsaicin in humans. *Br J Anaesth* 2000; 84:155–162.

Honore P, Rogers SD, Schwei MJ, et al. Murine models of inflammatory, neuropathic and cancer pain each generates a unique set of neurochemical changes in the spinal cord and sensory neurones. *Neurosci* 2000; 98:585–598.

Hill R. New targets for analgesic drugs In: Dostrovsky JO, Carr DB, Koltzenburg (Eds). *Proceedings of the 10th World Congress on Pain,* Progress in Pain Research and Management, Vol. 24. Seattle: IASP Press, 2003, pp 419–436.

Hinz B, Brune K. Pain and osteoarthritis: new drugs and mechanisms. *Curr Opin Rheumatol* 2004; 16:628–633.

Hunt SP, Mantyh PW. Molecular basis of pain control. *Nat Rev* 2001; 2:83–91.

Jänig W, Baron R. The role of the sympathetic nervous system in neuropathic pain: clinical observations and animal models. In: Hansson PT, Fields HL, Hill RG, Marchettini P (Eds). *Neuropathic Pain: Pathophysiology and Treatment,* Progress in Pain Research and Management, Vol. 21. Seattle: IASP Press, 2001, pp 125–149.

Jorum E, Warncke T, Stubhaug A. Cold allodynia and hyperalgesia in neuropathic pain: the effect of *N*-methyl-D-aspartate (NMDA) receptor antagonist ketamine: a double-blind, cross-over comparison with alfentanil and placebo. *Pain* 2003; 101:229–235.

Julius D. The molecular biology of thermosensation. In: Dostrovsky JO, Carr DB, Koltzenburg M (Eds). *Proceedings of the 10th World Congress on Pain,* Progress in Pain Research and Management, Vol. 24. Seattle: IASP Press, 2003, pp 63–70.

Khasabov SG, Rogers SD, Ghilardi JR, et al. Spinal neurons that possess the substance P receptor are required for the development of central sensitization. *J Neurosci* 2002; 22:9086–9098.

Koppert W, Wehrfritz A, Körber N, et al. The cyclooxygenase isozyme inhibitors parecoxib and paracetamol reduce central hyperalgesia in humans. *Pain* 2004; 108:148–153.

Lai J, Porreca F, Hunter JC, Gold MS. Voltage-gated sodium channels and hyperalgesia. *Annu Rev Pharmacol Toxicol* 2004; 44:371–397.

Landy S, Rice K, Lobo B. Central sensitisation and cutaneous allodynia in migraine: implications for treatment. *CNS Drugs* 2004; 18:337–342.

Le Guen S, Besson JM. Intravenous morphine does not modify dorsal horn touch-evoked allodynia in the mononeuropathic rat: a Fos study. *Pain* 2001; 92:389–398.

Luo ZD, Calcutt NA, Higuera ES, et al. Injury type-specific calcium channel alpha 2 delta-1 subunit up-regulation in rat neuropathic pain models correlates with antiallodynic effects of gabapentin. *J Pharmacol Exp Ther* 2002; 303:1199–1205.

Mantyh P, Rogers S, Honore P, et al. Inhibition of hyperalgesia by ablation of lamina I spinal neurons expressing the substance P receptor. *Science* 1997; 27:275–279.

Matthews EA, Dickenson AH. Effects of spinally delivered N- and P-type voltage-dependent calcium channel antagonists on dorsal horn neuronal responses in a rat model of neuropathy. *Pain* 2001; 92:235–246.

Medhurst SJ, Walker K, Bowes M, et al. A rat model of bone cancer pain. *Pain* 2002; 96:129–140.

Meller ST, Gebhart GF. Nitric oxide (NO) and nociceptive processing in the spinal cord. *Pain* 1993; 52:127–136.

Millan MJ. The induction of pain: an integrative review. *Prog Neurobiol* 1999; 57:1–164.

Millan MJ. Descending control of pain. *Prog Neurobiol* 2002; 66:354–474.

Mogil JS, Wilson SG, Bon K, et al. Heritability of nociception I: responses of 11 inbred mouse strains on 12 measures of nociception. *Pain* 1999; 80:67–82.

Nichols ML, Bian D, Ossipov MH, Lai J, Porreca F. Regulation of antiallodynic efficacy by CCK in a model of neuropathic pain in rats. *J Pharmacol Exp Ther* 1995; 275:1339–1345.

Nichols M, Allen B, Rogers S, et al. Transmission of chronic nociception by spinal neurons expressing the substance P receptor. *Science* 1999; 286:1558–1561.

Passmore GM, Selyanko AA, Mistry M, et al. KCNQ/M currents in sensory neurons: significance for pain therapy. *J Neurosci* 2003; 23:7227–7236.

Petersen-Zeitz KR, Basbaum AI. Second messengers, the substantia gelatinosa and injury-induced persistent pain. *Pain* 1999; 6(Suppl):S5–S12.

Petrenko AB, Yamakura T, Baba H, Shimoji K. The role of *N*-methyl-D-aspartate (NMDA) receptors in pain: a review. *Anesth Analg* 2003; 97:1108–1116.

Porreca F, Ossipov MH, Gebhart GF. Chronic pain and medullary descending facilitation. *Trends Neurosci* 2002; 25:319–325.

Price DD, Mao J, Mayer D1. Central neural mechanisms of normal and abnormal pain states. In: Fields HL, Liebeskind JC (Eds). *Pharmacological Approaches to the Treatment of Pain: New Concepts and Critical Issues,* Progress in Pain Research and Management, Vol. 1. Seattle: IASP Press, 1994, pp 61–84.

Price DD, Mao J, Frenk H, Mayer DJ. The *N*-methyl-D-aspartate receptor antagonist dextromethorphan selectively reduces temporal summation of second pain in man. *Pain* 1994; 59:165–174.

Rahman W, Suzuki R, Dickenson AH. Pains, brains and spinal gains: facilitatory mechanisms underlying altered pain states. *J Palliat Med Palliat Care* 2003; 2:82–89.

Rasmussen P, Sindrup S, Jensen TS, Bach FW. Therapeutic outcome in neuropathic pain: relationship to evidence of nervous system lesion. *Eur J Neurol* 2004; 11:545–553.

Ren K, Dubner R. Descending modulation in persistent pain: an update. *Pain* 2002; 100:1–6.

Rogers R, Wise RG, Painter DJ, Longe SE, Traccy I. An investigation to dissociate the analgesic and anesthetic properties of ketamine using functional magnetic resonance imaging. *Anesthesiology* 2004; 100(2):292–301.

Rowbotham MC. Efficacy of opioids in neuropathic pain. In: Hansson PT, Fields HL, Hill RG, Marchettini P (Eds). *Neuropathic Pain: Pathophysiology and Treatment,* Progress in Pain Research and Management, Vol. 21. Seattle: IASP Press, 2001, pp 203–213.

Sommer C. Cytokines and neuropathic pain. In: Hansson PT, Fields HL, Hill RG, Marchettini P (Eds). *Neuropathic Pain: Pathophysiology and Treatment,* Progress in Pain Research and Management, Vol. 21. Seattle: IASP Press, 2001, pp 37–62.

Rygh LJ, Green M, Athauda N, et al. Effect of spinal morphine after long-term potentiation of wide dynamic range neurones in the rat. *Anesthesiology* 2000; 92:140–146.

Sandkuhler J. Learning and memory in pain pathways. *Pain* 2000; 88:113–118.

Schwei MJ, Honore P, Rogers SD, et al. Neurochemical and cellular reorganization of the spinal cord in a murine model of bone cancer pain. *J Neurosci* 1999; 10886–10897.

Sindrup SH, Jensen TS. Efficacy of pharmacological treatments of neuropathic pain: an update and effect related to mechanism of drug action. *Pain* 1999; 83:389–400.

Smith PF. Therapeutic *N*-methyl-D-aspartate receptor antagonists: will reality meet expectation? *Curr Opin Investig Drugs* 2003; 4(7):826–832.

Staud R, Robinson ME, Vierck CJ, et al. Ratings of experimental pain and pain-related negative affect predict clinical pain in patients with fibromyalgia syndrome. *Pain* 2003; 105:215–222.

Suzuki R, Dickenson AH. Neuropathic pain: nerves bursting with excitement. *Neuroreport* 2000; 11:R17–21.

Suzuki R, Morcuende S, Webber M, et al. Superficial NK1 expressing neurones control spinal excitability by activation of descending pathways. *Nat Neurosci* 2002; 5:1319–1326.

Todd AJ. Anatomy of primary afferents and projection neurones in the rat spinal dorsal horn with particular emphasis on substance P and the neurokinin 1 receptor. *Exp Physiol* 2002; 87:245–249.

Urban MO, Gebhart GF. Supraspinal contributions to hyperalgesia. *Proc Natl Acad Sci USA* 1999; 96:7687–7692.

Urch CE, Donovan-Rodríguez T, Dickenson AH. Alterations in dorsal horn neurones in a rat model of cancer-induced bone pain. *Pain* 2003; 106:347–356.

Vanegas H, Schaible H. Effects of antagonists to high-threshold calcium channels upon spinal mechanisms of pain, hyperalgesia and allodynia. *Pain* 2000; 85:9–18

Wang H, Sun H, Della Penna K, et al. Chronic neuropathic pain is accompanied by global changes in gene expression and shares pathobiology with neurodegenerative diseases. *Neuroscience* 2002; 114:529–546.

Watkins LR, Maier SF. Glia: a novel drug discovery target for clinical pain. *Nat Rev Drug Discov* 2003; 2:973–985.

Waxman S. The molecular pathophysiology of pain: abnormal expression of sodium channel genes and its contribution to hyperexcitability of primary sensory neurons. *Pain* 1999; 6:S133–140.

Willis WD. Long-term potentiation in spinothalamic neurons. *Brain Res Brain Res Rev* 2002; 40:202–214.

Wood LN, Akopian AN, Cesare P, et al. The primary nociceptor: special functions, special receptors. In: Devor M, Rowbotham MC, Wiesenfeld-Hallin Z (Eds). *Proceedings of the 9th World Congress on Pain,* Progress in Pain Research and Management, Vol. 16. Seattle: IASP Press, 2000, pp 47–62.

Woolf C, Bennett GJ, Doherty M, et al. Towards a mechanism-based classification of pain. *Pain* 1998; 77:227–229.

Yaksh TL, Malmberg AB. Interaction of spinal modulatory systems. In: Fields HL, Liebeskind JC (Eds). *Pharmacological Approaches to the Treatment of Pain: New Concepts and Critical Issues,* Progress in Pain Research and Management, Vol. 1. Seattle: IASP Press, 1994, pp 151–171.

Yaksh TL, Noueihed R. The physiology and pharmacology of spinal opiates. *Annu Rev Pharmacol Toxicol* 1985; 25:433–462.

Correspondence to: Anthony H. Dickenson, PhD, Department of Pharmacology, University College London, London WC1E 6BT, United Kingdom. Email: anthony.dickenson@ucl.ac.uk.

The Paths of Pain 1975–2005, edited by
Harold Merskey, John D. Loeser, and Ronald
Dubner, IASP Press, Seattle, © 2005.

14

Opiate Analgesia: The Last 40 Years

Tony L. Yaksh

*Department of Anesthesiology, University of California,
San Diego, California, USA*

*And here I cannot but break out in praise of the Great God, the Giver of all
good things, who has granted to the human race, as a comfort in their
afflictions, no medicine of the value of opium.*

Thomas Sydenham (1666)

The ability of opiates to attenuate the response to stimuli that would
otherwise initiate pain behavior has had a profound effect upon medicine.
Aside from the therapeutic virtue of opiates, the insights provided by investigations of their actions have provided a unifying theme for advances in our
understanding of the neurobiology of nociception that came to fruition during the latter part of the 20th century. This chapter reviews the landmarks of
our current understanding.

MEMBRANE ACTIONS OF OPIATES

Sertürner demonstrated in 1803 that the analgesic actions of laudanum
(the alcoholic extract of the poppy resin) could be found in a single component, morphine (Jaffe 1968). This profound observation emphasized the role
of a single compound in mediating the therapeutic effect. Over the first part
of the 20th century, pharmaceutical chemists produced a variety of modifications of the opium-derived alkaloids that varied considerably in activity,
emphasizing the need for a specific structural motif (Braenden et al. 1955).
As early as 1914, it was appreciated that some structures (e.g., n-allylnorcodeine) lacked activity, but blocked the sedative and respiratory-depres-
sant effects of morphine (and not those of barbiturates), i.e., they were morphine
antagonists (Pohl 1915). This distinction suggested a notion of mechanistic

specificity as compared to a nonspecific stimulant. The literature through
the early 1950s, particularly with ex vivo bioassays, emphasized, by virtue
of the definitive pharmacology, that opiates and their antagonists were com-
petitively interacting with a specific site (c.f. Gyand and Kosterlitz 1966).
The notion of multiple opioid receptors was explicitly asserted by Martin
and colleagues (1976), who defined the distinct pharmacological profiles
representing the μ- and κ-opioid receptors based on behavioral bioassays in
dogs and humans. Kosterlitz postulated the δ-opioid receptor based on ex
vivo bioassays (Lord et al. 1977). Work with radioligand binding sought to
identify such a site based on the differential affinity of behaviorally active
and inactive stereoisomers of opiate agonists (Pert and Snyder 1973). The
hypotheses of multiple receptors based on the pharmacological analyses
were completely confirmed some 20 years later with the cloning and expression of three principal classes of opioid receptors (c.f. Knapp et al. 1995).
Current work suggests a number of subtypes that at present appear to be
splice variants or perhaps receptor dimers (Law et al. 2000).

Early work emphasized that these receptors were members of the super-
family of G-protein-coupled receptors (Christie 1991). Specifically, the observed effects were typically inhibited by pertussis toxin, emphasizing a role
for Gi/o protein. As is the case for many G-protein-coupled receptors, the
intracellular coupling though β-arrestin and activation of protein kinases
leads to an internalization of the receptor (Sternini et al. 1996). Electrophysiologically, μ, δ (North et al. 1987), and κ (Grudt 1993) receptors
induce a membrane hyperpolarization through an inwardly rectifying K^+
channel activated by a membrane G protein. In addition, there is a concurrent inhibition by μ/δ (Piros et al. 1995) and κ (Kaneko et al. 1994) opioid
agonists of the opening of voltage-sensitive Ca^{2+} channels, an action that
attenuates terminal release of neurotransmitters. The joint effect of this activity would be to reduce the excitability of the neuron and terminal transmitter realease. While the principal effects of the μ receptor appear inhibitory, some work suggests that this receptor may also couple though a Gs
protein and exert a direct stimulatory effect (Crain and Shen 1996). Convergence of the pharmacology (structure-activity relationships, antagonist activity), defined in vitro and in vivo in animal and human models of
nociception, emphasized the likely role of such receptors in mediating the
analgesic actions of the many opioid structural homologues. Again, the importance of these receptors has been completely confirmed after 20 years by
in vivo studies using animals with diminished expression of the respective
receptor protein (Kieffer and Gaveriaux-Ruff 2002).

DEFINING SYSTEMS THAT MEDIATE OPIOID ANTINOCICEPTION

The essential issue, as first addressed in the early 1960s, is to ask where in the organism are there opioid receptors through which the opiates act to alter pain behavior? Giving the drug systemically means that all opioid sites are probably affected. As shown later, using receptor autoradiography, opioid binding occurs heterogeneously throughout the brain (see Atweh and Kuhar 1977). It was not likely that all sites contribute to the behaviorally defined "analgesic" effect of opiates. Accordingly, the principal strategy to define sites of opiate action for analgesia employed targeted neuraxial delivery using chronically implanted stereotactically guided microinjection cannulae for the delivery of submicroliter quantities of drugs into specific brain sites or through intrathecal catheters for spinal delivery. The use of such focal delivery systems in unanesthetized animals along with assessment of their behavioral response to noxious stimuli has provided fundamental insights into opioid-receptor-linked systems that regulate pain behavior. There is insufficient space here to address the entire complexity of these actions, so we will focus on three principal sites: supraspinal sites (the brainstem and forebrain), the spinal cord, and the periphery.

SUPRASPINAL OPIOID ACTIONS

BRAINSTEM

Site of action. The elegant studies of Tsou and Jang (1964) first revealed that the local action of morphine in the periventricular gray would block thermally evoked hindlimb reflexes in the unanesthetized rabbit. Subsequent work almost 10 years later confirmed the medial distribution for such sites, particularly in the more caudal mesencephalic periaqueductal gray (PAG) in a variety of animals including mice (Criswell 1976), rats (Sharpe et al. 1974), cats (Ossipov et al. 1984), and primates (Pert and Yaksh 1975) (Fig. 1). Local delivery of microgram quantities of morphine produced a potent antinociception. While the primary focus has typically been the PAG, systematic mapping studies as first conducted in primates emphasized a relatively continuous distribution of medial sites coursing rostrocaudally adjacent to the mesencephalic aqueduct and third ventricle and a more lateral distribution that traveled from the medulla up through the mesencephalon (Fig. 1). These observations in primates were confirmed by focused studies in rats. Microinjection of morphine into the following sites yielded potent antinociceptive effects: the mesencephalic reticular formation (Haigler

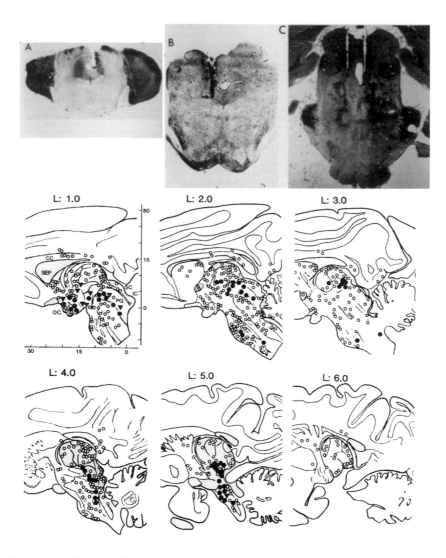

Fig. 1. Top: Histology from the mouse, rat, and monkey showing the location of microinjection sites wherein morphine yielded a significant elevation in the nociceptive threshold. (A) Coronal section taken though mouse brain indicating the locus of the microinjection site in the mesencephalic central gray. (B) Coronal section taken through the rat brain indicating the locus of two microinjection sites (upper and lower arrows) in the dorsal and ventral quadrant of the mesencephalic central gray. The upper arrow indicates an inactive site and the lower arrow an active site. (C) Coronal section taken through primate mesencephalic central gray indicating the locus of two microinjection sites (left and right). Both sites were equally active, indicating lack of contribution of ventricular access (adapted from Yaksh and Rudy 1978). Bottom: Schematic plates taken from sagittal histology (1–6 mm of midline) of the rhesus monkey. Each dot displays the effects of a single injection of morphine sulfate given through chronically implanted guide cannulae. Symbols indicate magnitude of change in shock titration threshold: O = <25%; ▼ = 25–50%; ● = >50%. (Redrawn from Pert and Yaksh 1974.)

and Spring 1978), the caudal medulla with medial sites overlapping the region of the cell bodies of the nucleus raphe (Levy and Proudfit 1979), and lateral sites that correspond grossly to the region of the nucleus giganto-cellularis (Takagi et al. 1977).

Pharmacology. The opiate pharmacology of these local actions was defined by demonstrating the relative activity of multiple agonists, their stereospecificity, and the routine reversal of these effects by the opioid antagonist naloxone given systemically or into the microinjection site. Based on the relative activity of several receptor agonists and antagonists in the PAG, these effects appeared to be mediated primarily by μ receptors. Opioid agents yield a powerful, dose-dependent antinociception, with μ receptors being much more potent than δ receptors, whereas in the medulla both μ and δ sites have been associated with antinociception (Jensen and Yaksh 1986).

Mechanisms of antinociception following brainstem opioid action. Systematic microinjection investigations showed that opiates exert an antinociceptive effect by acting at several discrete brainstem sites. Through what mechanisms do brainstem opiate receptors coupled to these systems act to alter nociceptive processing?

Bulbospinal projections. Evidence for brainstem regulation of spinal nociceptive function came from the demonstration of inhibition of afferent-evoked flexor reflex activity in the ventral roots through enhanced activity at spinal monoamine terminals (Anden et al. 1966). Early work with systemically delivered morphine introduced the concept that opiates served to enhance this descending modulation (Sato and Takagi 1971). In the studies with opiate microinjection, a common observation was an increased latency of spinal nociceptive reflexes (tail flick, skin twitch), which occurred at doses that did not alter normal motor function; these injections significantly reduced dorsal horn neuronal activity otherwise evoked by noxious stimuli (Gebhart and Jones 1988). These effects suggested that brainstem opiates were activating a bulbospinally mediated suppression of spinal nociceptive processing. Direct experimental support for the assertion of a functional role of brainstem opiate regulation of spinal nociceptive processing by bulbospinal outflow is firmly based on three sets of observations: (1) Spinal delivery of α_2-adrenergic antagonists reversed the PAG-morphine inhibition of spinal nociceptive reflexes (Camarata and Yaksh 1985). The antagonist pharmacology is similar for the spinal reflex inhibition evoked by morphine within the PAG as well as by direct stimulation of the PAG with focal electrical stimulation (Hammond and Yaksh 1984) or with excitatory amino acids (Satoh et al. 1983). (2) Direct evidence of increased bulbospinal outflow is provided by spinal release of amines secondary to brainstem morphine injection (Yaksh and Tyce 1979) or electrical stimulation (Takagi et al. 1979). (3) If bulbospinal pathway activation regulates spinal nociceptive processing, the direct activation of receptors postsynaptic to the bulbospinal projections by intrathecal delivery of the respective agonists should mimic the supraspinal action of morphine. Indeed, intrathecal α_2-adrenoceptor agonists produce a powerful regulation of pain behavior across various species (Yaksh and Reddy 1981), including humans (Eisenach et al. 1989).

Given the importance of the activation of bulbospinal projections to brainstem opiate actions, an important issue relates to the mechanisms through which local opioids initiate the descending control. While direct naloxone-sensitive excitatory links of opiates have been reported (Crain and Shen 1990), opioids have been considered to exert mainly a suppressive effect upon neuronal excitability (Duggan and North 1983). As initially proposed by Yaksh et al. (1976), it was reasonable to consider that the net outflow evoked by morphine from any given region must reflect an inhibition of an inhibition.

The antinociceptive effects generated by injection of GABA antagonists into the PAG (Moreau and Fields 1986) supported this "inhibition of an inhibition" thesis. The complexity of the organization of these descending pathways has been emphasized by the work of Fields and colleagues (Fields and Heinricher 1985). They emphasized the existence of a dual projection system: (1) "off-cells" exert an inhibitory effect on spinal nociceptive processing and are indirectly activated by opioids, and (2) "on-cells" serve to facilitate nociceptive transmission and are directly inhibited by opioids (Heinricher et al. 1992). Importantly, "on-cells" show significant activation during opiate withdrawal, suggesting that these cells play a role in opiate withdrawal hyperalgesia.

Bulbo-diencephalic/cortical projections. While intrathecal antagonism of the bulbospinal systems diminishes the anti-reflexive effects of PAG morphine, concurrent examination of rat behavior (e.g., using the hot-plate test) revealed only a transient attenuation of supraspinally mediated pain responses (Yaksh 1979). Similarly, lesions made just caudal to the PAG significantly diminished the effects of PAG electrical stimulation on the tail-flick response (a spinal reflex), but not on responses to the hot-plate test (Morgan et al. 1989). Such observations emphasize that other PAG-opiate systems must be superimposed on the descending modulation to account for the effects of supraspinal opiates on the organized response to a strong stimulus. As discussed below, the action of opioid agonists at several fore-brain sites may contribute to the overall opiate effect. In addition to other opioid sites, local circuitry connects the PAG with forebrain systems known to influence motivational and affective components of behavior. Thus, the raphe dorsalis, lying in proximity to the ventral medial PAG, sends serotonergic projections rostrally to a variety of sites, including the nucleus accumbens, amygdala, and lateral thalamus (Westlund et al. 1990). Similarly, the locus ceruleus has ample projections into the limbic forebrain and thalamus (Amaral and Sinnamon 1977). Dialysis studies showed that morphine, probably by an action in or near the dorsal raphe, enhances serotonin release from a variety of forebrain structures (Tao and Auerbach 1995). Both serotonergic and noradrenergic forebrain projections have been implicated in emotionality and maintenance of consciousness, suggesing potential links for the influence of brainstem opiates on higher-order functions (see Byrum et al. 1999).

Direct inhibition of brainstem afferent input. In contrast to indirect inhibition of afferent processing, opiates in the brainstem may directly alter excitatory input into the brainstem core. Many spinobulbar neurons are directly inhibited by opioids delivered in the spinal cord. Based on the likelihood that receptors synthesized in the cell body will be transported to the distal terminals (e.g., Laduron 1984), opioid sites would be presynaptic on the brainstem terminals of spinobulbar neurons. In this regard, cervical hemisection resulted in a significant reduction in opiate binding in the medulla and PAG/mesencephalic reticular formation ipsilateral to the cord hemisection (Ramberg and Yaksh 1989). Significantly, many of the regions in which opioids exert their effects, particularly within the mesencephalon and medulla, receive input from direct spinobulbar projections or collaterals from spinodiencephalic projections (e.g., Lippman and Kerr 1972). These observations suggest that locally administered opiates may alter nociceptive processing through a presynaptic action on the spinofugal terminals, reducing excitatory input into brainstem systems relevant to the organization of the pain response.

FOREBRAIN ACTIONS

Sites. Opiates given into the basolateral amygdala were reported to alter tail-flick and/or hot-plate response latencies (Yaksh et al. 1976; Rodgers 1977). Pharmacological studies with specific agonists have indicated that the actions are mediated by μ, but not κ or δ receptors (Helmstetter et al. 1995). In rats and rabbits, the injection of morphine into the ventral forebrain, notably the nucleus accumbens and preoptic and arcuate nuclei, is able to block spinal nociceptive reflexes (Tseng and Wang 1992).

Forebrain mechanisms. Forebrain circuits that can alter the response to nociceptive stimuli are doubtless complex. The ability of forebrain opiate injections to alter spinal reflexes suggests that one component reflects linkages that alter ascending traffic. Thus, blockade of spinal reflexes by microinjection of opioids into the amygdala is mediated by a serial circuit through the PAG and rostral ventromedial medulla (Helmstetter et al. 1998). Alternately, microinjection of morphine into the nucleus accumbens can attenuate spinal reflexes, an effect that is blocked by lesions of the arcuate nucleus (Yu and Han 1989). The organization of these caudally projecting systems is unclear. Glutamate microinjected into the lateral hypothalamus will increase firing in the PAG and elevate spinal reflex latencies (Behbehani et al. 1988). The injection of NMDA into the arcuate nucleus significantly increases the release of β-endorphin-like immunoreactivity into ventriculocisternal perfusates (Bach and Yaksh 1995). These two examples suggest a picture in which a variety of forebrain structures mediating higher-order functions may feed back through the mesencephalic core.

Supraspinal opiate analgesic actions in humans. Intracerebroventricular opioids have been used for pain relief in cancer patients (Lazorthes 1988). The time of onset for such opioids is relatively rapid, suggesting a proximity of the active site to the ventricular lumen, a finding confirmed by gamma scans of human brain after injection of I^{123}-morphine (Tafani et al. 1989). In this regard, the preclinical studies in species such as the primate have emphasized the importance of the periaqueductal sites. Such a site of action would in fact lie in close proximity to the ventricles and would permit relatively rapid access of a slowly moving drug from the ventricular lumen.

SPINAL OPIOID ACTIONS

Early work showed that systemic opiates inhibited spinal nociceptive reflexes in animals that had undergone spinal transection (Bodo and Brooks 1937; Wikler 1950; Martin et al. 1964). The role of this spinal action in mediating a behaviorally defined analgesia was unclear, however. Studies in transected animals supported a direct effect of opiates on spinal output, although the relevance of this effect to analgesia, if not a general depression of spinal function, was not evident.

Intrathecal delivery. The initial systematic studies on the local spinal effect of morphine failed to observe any effect on pain behavior (Tsou and Jang 1964), and based on diffusion-exclusion studies it was argued that the analgesic effects of opiates were limited to the brain (Herz and Teschemacher 1971). However, with the development of a robust chronic spinal delivery system (Fig. 2), it was demonstrated that intrathecal administration of opiates to the unanesthetized animal yielded a potent and reliable inhibition of the animal's response to strong mechanical and thermal stimuli but not to innocuous tactile stimulation (Yaksh and Rudy 1976, 1977; Yaksh 1981), with no effect upon motor or autonomic function. The lack of motor effects

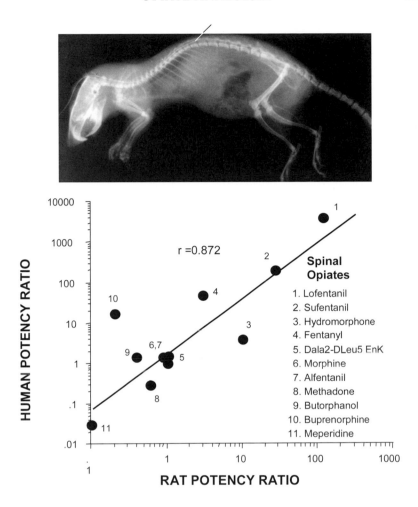

Fig. 2. Top: X-ray showing an intrathecal catheter located on the dorsum of the spinal cord at L2 (see Yaksh and Rudy 1976). Bottom: Relative ordering of activity for clinically effective analgesic doses of spinal opiates in humans relative to the activity of morphine (e.g., morphine = 1) plotted versus the ordering of activity relative to morphine after spinal delivery in the rat on the 52°C hot-plate test (see Yaksh 1997).

in these studies was unexpected, given the early work showing potent hyper-polarizing effects of opiates on ventral horn cells (Jurna et al. 1973). Early work showed this profile of effect in species ranging from amphibia (Stevens and Pezalla 1983) and rodents though cats, dogs, and primates (Yaksh 1987), and, as will be discussed below, in humans.

Pharmacology. Of particular importance, these initial studies displayed the agonist and antagonist structure-activity relationships expected of specific μ-, δ-, and to a lesser degree κ-opioid-receptor-mediated phenomena (Yaksh 1987).

Mechanisms of spinal opiate action. Single-unit recordings of the activity of dorsal horn neurons reveal populations activated by both large (low-threshold) and small (higher-threshold) primary afferents. Opioid agonists administered systemically in transected animals (Kitahata et al. 1974; Le Bars et al. 1975), iontophoretically into the dorsal horn (Calvillo et al. 1974; Zieglgansberger and Bayerl 1976), or topically upon the spinal cord (Homma et al. 1983) produce a selective suppression of the activity initiated by small-fiber, but not large-fiber afferent input in dorsal horn neurons.

Populations of the these opiate-sensitive neurons were shown to project spinofugally in the contralateral-ventrolateral tract (Jurna and Grossman 1976). With regard to opioid receptor binding, prior to the demonstration of the effects of intrathecal morphine in 1976, it was asserted that there was little if any opiate binding in the cord, based on spinal homogenates (Kuhar et al. 1973). Subsequent receptor autoradiography indicated that such binding, though low overall, was localized in the outermost spinal dorsal horn laminae (Atweh and Kuhar 1977). Convergent evidence indicated specifically that μ/δ receptors were present on the spinal terminals of small primary afferents (Gouardères 1985), as well as on intrinsic dorsal horn neurons. The evidence included opioid receptor protein and mRNA in small dorsal root ganglion (DRG) cells and in the superficial dorsal horn; a reduction in opioid binding following application of capsaicin, a C-fiber neurotoxin; and opiate receptor binding in the superficial laminae, where small afferents terminate (Gamse et al. 1979; Fields et al. 1980). Residual receptor binding after rhizotomy and the presence of opioid message observed in the spinal dorsal horn following dorsal root section also supported the presence of opioid receptors postsynaptic to the primary afferent (Gamse et al. 1979; Fields et al. 1980). The presynaptic localization on small primary afferents was consistent with the ability of local opiates to block the opening of voltage-sensitive calcium channels in the DRG (Rusin and Moises 1995). The first demonstration by Jessell and Iversen (1977) of a naloxone-reversible inhibition of substance P release from spinal slices was followed by demonstration in vivo of an inhibition by opiates of evoked substance P release into spinal superfusates (Yaksh et al. 1980). Although studies with antibody-coated microelectrodes showed only a minor effect upon endogenous substance P release (Morton et al. 1990), the ability of intrathecal μ and δ opiates at analgesic doses to prevent stimulus-evoked neurokinin 1 (NK1) receptor internalization (a marker of substance P release) confirms the spinal effect on terminal C-fiber release in the unanesthetized animal (Kondo et al. 2005). Accordingly, current data strongly support the assertion that the presynaptic effects of opiates diminish small-afferent terminal excitability. These assertions are consistent with intracellular recordings from lamina I cells activated by primary afferent stimulation though NK1 receptors, which have demonstrated a presynaptic inhibition by μ-opioid agonists (Cheunsuang et al. 2002).

As noted, opioid receptor sites postsynaptic to the primary afferent have also been indicated. Such receptors most likely mediate the inhibition of dorsal horn excitation evoked by iontophoretically applied glutamate (Zieglgansberger and Bayerl 1976). These receptors are also likely to mediate the hyperpolarization observed in dorsal horn neurons secondary to opiates (Yoshimura and North 1983). Localization of μ-opioid receptor protein has emphasized the heterogeneity of distribution of postsynaptic receptors. Thus, much of the non-afferent μ-receptor protein is present on neurons that typically do not display neurokinin receptors (Spike et al 2002). Accordingly, the opioid regulation of afferent-evoked excitation of NK1-receptor-bearing cells such as marginal neurons, which are activated by small primary afferents, most likely occurs by a presynaptic action. Thus, it appears likely that the selective effects of spinally administered opioids on activity evoked by small-fiber afferents and the correlated effects on behavior (antinociception) depend on both the presynaptic inhibition of small-afferent terminal excitability and postsynaptic hyperpolarization.

In addition to the systems outlined above, evidence has evolved to suggest that opiates may act through a number of neurochemical systems to alter pain behavior. One example is the proposed role of adenosine in various spinal and supraspinal systems that modulate nociceptive processing (see Sawynok and Sweeney 1989).

Spinal actions of opioids in humans. The initial demonstration of the activity of spinal opiates in animals led directly to the delivery of intrathecal and epidural morphine in humans (Behar et al. 1979; Wang et al. 1979). The use of the implantable pump and intrathecal or epidural catheters led to the demonstration of long-term efficacy in cancer pain (Coombs et al. 1981; Onofrio et al. 1981). Subsequent experience has demonstrated analgesic efficacy in a variety of clinical pain states ranging from acute postoperative pain to a variety of chronic malignant and nonmalignant pain states (Wallace and Yaksh 2000). The comparability of the spinal analgesic pharmacology in animals clearly reflects effects comparable to those reported in humans. Thus, the relative ordering of activity of a wide variety of μ-, δ-, and κ-receptor-preferring spinal opioids in human clinical pain states clearly covary with those activities predicted after intrathecal delivery in the rat (see Fig. 2). The effects of spinal opiates are reversed by low doses of systemic naloxone (Rawal et al. 1983). These observations emphasize the comparability of the spinal actions of opiates in humans and in animal models.

PERIPHERAL OPIOID ACTIONS

Peripheral effects. Early work showed that the use of methylated mor-phine, with its reduced central bioavailability, had little effect upon acute nociception, but would reduce behavior initiated by inflammatory stimuli (Smith et al. 1985). Subsequent work employing injection into peripheral sites demonstrated that opiates could, by a local action, attenuate inflamma-tion-induced hyperalgesia (Stein et al. 1989). These effects are naloxone reversible and have a pharmacological profile that emphasizes the likely role of μ and κ, and perhaps less importantly, δ sites (see Stein et al. 1989; Nagasaka and Yaksh 1995).

Mechanisms of peripheral action. Opiate "binding" sites are trans-ported from the DRG to the peripheral terminals of the sensory axon (Laduron 1984). There is no evidence that these sites are coupled to mechanisms governing the normal excitability of the axon. Thus, while high doses of lipid-soluble agents can block the compound action potential, this block is not naloxone reversible and is thought to reflect a "local anesthetic" action (Gissen et al. 1987). Of particular importance, following tissue inflamma-tion, small axons show significant spontaneous activity, which is diminished by local opiates in a naloxone-reversible fashion (Russell et al. 1987; Andreev et al. 1994). The antihyperalgesic effects of opiates applied to the inflamed regions probably occur locally on the terminal itself, as well as through an effect upon inflammatory cells that are present and releasing cytokines that activate or sensitize the nerve terminal (see Pol and Puig 2004).

Peripheral actions of opioids in humans. The antihyperalgesic actions of peripherally injected opiates led to clinical work showing that injection of morphine into the knee joint after knee surgery or adjacent to the wound margins of an incision has a mild antihyperalgesic effect (Stein et al. 1991; Kalso et al. 1997).

INTERACTIONS AMONG OPIATE-REGULATED SYSTEMS

Even with a cursory consideration, it is evident that opiates with an action limited to any of several spinal or supraspinal specific regions can induce potent analgesia. With systemic opiates, it is reasonable to presume that the net behavioral effect of the agent reflects the concurrent action of opiates at each of the brain and spinal sites. In early studies, delivery of opioid antagonists into the cerebral ventricles (Tsou 1963; Vigouret et al. 1973) or into the lumbar intrathecal space (Yaksh and Rudy 1978) could unexpectedly produce a *complete* antagonism of the effects of the systemic opioid agonist. These findings led to the formal proposal that the effects of opiate receptor occupancy in the brain synergize with the effects produced by the concurrent occupancy of spinal receptors (Yaksh and Rudy 1978). With high receptor occupancy (as produced when the drugs are delivered locally), each system was able to independently produce significant antinociception. Yeung and Rudy (1980) first demonstrated the validity of this hypothesis by showing that the concurrent spinal and supraspinal administration of morphine led to a prominent synergy, as indicated by hyperbolic isobolograms. Since then, studies on the interactions between different sites of opiate actions, for example amygdala-PAG (Pavlovic and Bodnar 1998) or locus ceruleus-PAG (Bodnar et al. 1991), have typically demonstrated at least an "effects-additive" interaction if not an outright synergy. An interesting expansion of these interactions arises from consideration of interactions among different components of the opiate-sensitive system. Thus, if spinal and supraspinal opiates display a synergistic interaction, it was hypothesized that intrathecal opiates and α_2-adrenoceptor agonists would similarly interact, and this early hypothesis was confirmed (Yaksh and Reddy 1981). As noted above, the probable role of synergy with systemic opiates is suggested by the ability of spinal or supraspinal receptor antagonism to virtually abolish the analgesic effects of systemic opiates. This assertion is further supported by the observation at the spinal level that stimulation-evoked NK1 internalization is readily blocked by the lumbar intrathecal delivery of an analgesic dose of morphine. In contrast, an equianalgesic dose of systemic morphine has only a modest effect upon that internalization, although a significant block of internalization indeed occurs at higher systemic doses. These observations suggest that the analgesia produced by systemic morphine must reflect actions at non-afferent terminal sites in the spinal cord and elsewhere in the brain (Kondo et al. 2005).

ONGOING COMPLEXITIES

The specific actions of opiates in regulating pain behavior reflect two principal events. First, at sites linked from the forebrain caudally though the PAG and medulla, opiates alter the rostrad flow of afferent information to the brainstem and thalamus by directly reducing terminal excitability or by initiating an indirect modulatory control over afferent transmission. This mechanism acts at virtually every level of the neuraxis but particularly at the spinal level, most likely as early as the first-order synapse. Such selective regulation of afferent traffic provides strong support for the mechanisms underlying selective changes in the acute response to a high-intensity afferent stimulus. Second, there is little doubt that opiates can influence the emotional content of the pain experience. The comment that opiates are the pharmacological equivalent of a prefrontal lobotomy (Jaffe 1968) is an expression of the scope of their impact upon emotionality. It is clear that opiates have direct effects upon supratentorial systems that are known to play a role in affective behavior, such as the PAG and limbic brain. They also exert indirect actions, for example by activating ascending monoamine systems from the brainstem. Interestingly, we might speculate that even the direct spinal effects may play out specifically in these issues of emotionality. Thus, superficial marginal cells project variously into nonsomatosensory thalamic sites and thence into the limbic forebrain (Craig 2003). Current work has emphasized the potential role of regions such as the anterior cingulate as a corollary for the emotional components of pain. It is interesting to note that destruction of these spinal NK1-bearing marginal cells has little effect upon acute pain behavior, but diminishes the behavioral components of persistent pain states (Nichols et al. 1999). In this fashion, we might anticipate that even spinal opiates might, by blocking specific spinal output, have a potent and specific effect upon the afferent drive that contributes to the affective component of pain.

CONCLUDING COMMENTS

This chapter began by noting that development over the past 40 years of our understanding of the mechanisms of opiates in altering pain behavior has provided an important substrate for advancing our understanding of the role of systems in pain processing. First, the importance of bulbospinal modulation of spinal pain nociceptive processing was reviewed. The ability of opiates administered at discrete sites to block spinal reflexes, in conjunction with the parallel effects of brainstem electrical stimulation to inhibit pain behavior (Reynolds 1969) and spinal reflexes (Mayer et al. 1971), and the reversal of these effects with intrathecal aminergic antagonists provided a complex model for a behaviorally relevant interplay between ascending input and the regulation of afferent input at the level of the first-order synapse. Second, development of a simple and robust local delivery system in rodents permitted the demonstration that opiates with an action limited to the spinal cord served to alter supraspinally organized pain behavior. Much as the work of Gower (1888) with ventrolateral cord injury revealed the functional significance of the information carried in the ventrolateral tract, the spinal analgesic work provided the initial assertion that afferent processing of noxious stimuli possessed a distinct modulatory pharmacology and that this encoding had behavioral significance. Thus, the afferent message generated by a tissue-injuring stimulus was distinctively encoded at the level of the spinal dorsal horn, and the pharmacology was such that specific modulation of components of this sensory message to higher centers would alter the functional significance of the peripheral stimulus so that it was not longer painful. These observations were additionally important because they rapidly led to the broad appreciation of the role played in pain processing by a variety of non-opioids. Finally, the spinal action of opioids has had a prominent impact on clinical practice. Thus, 2 years after the preclinical reports, clinical reports using morphine intrathecally (Wang et al. 1979) and epidurally (Behar et al. 1979) appeared and multiplied rapidly. Peer-reviewed reports of neuraxial opiate use began to appear, rising from 296 for the period 1978–1982 to 669 for 1983–87 and on to 1057 for 1998–2003. In short, it is clear that research into the mechanisms of opioid analgesia has contributed substantively to the advances we have made in our understanding of the mechanisms by which pain is processed at all levels of the neuraxis.

REFERENCES

Amaral DG, Sinnamon HM. The locus ceruleus: neurobiology of a central noradrenergic nucleus. *Prog Neurobiol* 1977; 9:147–196.

Anden NE, Jukes MG, Lundberg A, Vyklicky L. The effect of DOPA on the spinal cord. 1. Influence on transmission from primary afferents. *Acta Physiol Scand* 1966; 67:373–386.

Andreev N, Urban L, Dray A. Opioids suppress spontaneous activity of polymodal nociceptors in rat paw skin induced by ultraviolet irradiation. *Neuroscience* 1994; 58:793–798.

Atweh SF, Kuhar MJ. Autoradiographic localization of opiate receptors in rat brain. I. Spinal cord and lower medulla. *Brain Res* 1977; 124:53–67.

Bach FW, Yaksh TL. Release of beta-endorphin immunoreactivity into ventriculo-cisternal perfusate by lumbar intrathecal capsaicin in the rat. *Brain Res* 1995; 701:192–200.

Behar M, Magora F, Olshwang D, Davidson JT. Epidural morphine in treatment of pain. *Lancet* 1979; 1:527–529.

Behbehani MM, Park MR, Clement ME. Interactions between the lateral hypothalamus and the periaqueductal gray. *J Neurosci* 1988; 8:2780–2787.

Bodnar R, Paul D, Pasternak GW. Synergistic analgesic interactions between the periaqueductal gray and the locus coeruleus. *Brain Res* 1991; 558:224–230.

Bodo RC, Brooks CM. The effects of morphine on blood sugar and reflex activity in the chronic spinal cat. *J Pharmacol Exp Ther* 1937; 61:82–88.

Braenden OJ, Eddy NB, Halbach H. Synthetic substances with morphine like effects. Relationship between chemical structure and analgesic action. *Bull World Health Organ* 1955; 13:937–998.

Byrum CE, Ahearn EP, Krishman KR. A neuroanatomic model for depression. *Prog Neuropsychopharmacol Biol Psychiatry* 1999; 23:175–193.

Calvillo O, Henry JL, Neuman RS. Effects of morphine and naloxone on dorsal horn neurones in the cat. *Can J Physiol Pharmacol* 1974; 52:1207–1211.

Camarata PJ, Yaksh TL. Characterization of the spinal adrenergic receptors mediating the spinal effects produced by the microinjection of morphine into the periaqueductal gray. *Brain Res* 1985; 336:133–142.

Cheunsuang O, Maxwell D, Morris R. Spinal lamina I neurones that express neurokinin 1 receptors: II. Electrophysiological characteristics, responses to primary afferent stimulation and effects of a selective mu-opioid receptor agonist. *Neuroscience* 2002; 111:423–434.

Christie MJ. Mechanisms of opioid actions on neurons of the locus coeruleus. *Prog Brain Res* 1991; 88:197–205.

Coombs DW, Saunders RL, Gaylor MS, et al. Continuous epidural analgesia via implanted morphine reservoir. *Lancet* 1981; 2:425–426.

Craig AD. Distribution of trigeminothalamic and spinothalamic lamina I terminations in the cat. *Somatosens Mot Res* 2003; 20:209–222.

Crain SM, Shen KF. Opioids can evoke direct receptor-mediated excitatory effects on sensory neurons. *Trends Pharmacol Sci* 1990; 11:77–81.

Crain SM, Shen KF. Modulatory effects of Gs-coupled excitatory opioid receptor functions on opioid analgesia, tolerance, and dependence. *Neurochem Res* 1996; 21:1347–1351.

Criswell HD. Analgesia and hyperreactivity following morphine microinjections into mouse brain. *Pharmacol Biochem Behav* 1976; 4:23–26.

Duggan AW, North RA. Electrophysiology of opioids. *Pharmacol Rev* 1983; 35:219–281.

Eisenach JC, Lysak SZ, Viscomi CM. Epidural clonidine analgesia following surgery: phase I. *Anesthesiology* 1989; 71:640–646.

Fields HL, Heinricher MM. Anatomy and physiology of a nociceptive modulatory system. *Philos Trans R Soc Lond B Biol Sci* 1985; 308:361–374.

Fields HL, Emson PC, Leigh BK, Gilbert RFT, Iversen LL. Multiple opiate receptor sites on primary afferent fibres. *Nature (Lond)* 1980; 284:351–353.

Gamse R, Holzer P, Lembeck F. Indirect evidence for presynaptic location of opiate receptors on chemosensitive primary sensory neurones. *Naunyn Schmiedebergs Arch Pharmacol* 1979; 308:281–285.

Gebhart GF, Jones SL. Effects of morphine given in the brainstem on the activity of dorsal horn nociceptive neurons. *Prog Brain Res* 1988; 77:229–243.

Gissen AJ, Gugino LD, Datta S, Miller J, Covino BG. Effects of fentanyl and sufentanil on peripheral mammalian nerves. *Anesth Analg* 1987; 66:1272–1276.

Gouardères C, Cros J, Quirion R. Autoradiographic localization of μ, δ and κ opioid receptor binding sites in rat and guinea pig spinal cord. *Neuropeptides* 1985; 5:331–342.

Gower WR. *Manual of the Diseases of the Nervous System.* Philadelphia, 1888.

Grudt TJ, Williams JT. Kappa-Opioid receptors also increase potassium conductance. *Proc Natl Acad Sci USA* 1993; 90:11429–11432.

Gyand EA, Kosterlitz HW. Agonist and antagonist actions of morphine-like drugs on the guinea-pig isolated ileum. *Br J Pharmacol* 1966; 27:514–527.

Haigler HJ, Spring DD. A comparison of the analgesic and behavioral effects of [D-Ala²] met-enkephalinamide and morphine in the mesencephalic reticular formation of rats. *Life Sci* 1978; 23:1229–1240.

Hammond DL, Yaksh TL. Antagonism of stimulation-produced antinociception by intrathecal administration of methysergide or phentolamine. *Brain Res* 1984; 298:329–337.

Heinricher MM, Morgan MM, Fields HL. Direct and indirect actions of morphine on medullary neurons that modulate nociception. *Neuroscience* 1992; 48:533–543.

Helmstetter FJ, Bellgowan PS, Poore LH. Microinfusion of mu but not delta or kappa opioid agonists into the basolateral amygdala results in inhibition of the tail flick reflex in pentobarbital-anesthetized rats. *J Pharmacol Exp Ther* 1995; 275:381–388.

Helmstetter FJ, Tershner SA, Poore LH, Bellgowan PS. Antinociception following opioid stimulation of the basolateral amygdala is expressed through the periaqueductal gray and rostral ventromedial medulla. *Brain Res* 1998; 779:104–118.

Herz A, Teschemacher H. Activities and sites of antinociceptive action of morphine-like analgesics and kinetics of redistribution following intravenous, intracerebral and intraventricular application. *Adv Drug Res* 1971; 6:79–119.

Homma E, Collins JG, Kitahata LM, Matsumoto M, Kawahara M. Suppression of noxiously evoked WDR dorsal horn neuronal activity by spinally administered morphine. *Anesthesiology* 1983; 58:232–236.

Jaffe JH. Narcotic analgesics. In: Goodman LS, Gilman A (Eds). *The Pharmacological Basis of Therapeutics,* 3rd ed. New York: MacMillan, 1968, pp 247–284.

Jensen TS, Yaksh TL III. Comparison of the antinociceptive action of mu and delta opioid receptor ligands in the periaqueductal gray matter, medial and paramedial ventral medulla in the rat as studied by the microinjection technique. *Brain Res* 1986; 372:301–312.

Jessell TM, Iversen LL. Opiate analgesics inhibit substance P release from rat trigeminal nucleus. *Nature* 1977; 268:549–551.

Jurna I, Grossman W. The effect of morphine on the activity evoked in ventrolateral tract axons of the cat spinal cord. *Exp Brain Res* 1976; 24:473–484.

Jurna I, Grossmann W, Theres C. Inhibition by morphine of repetitive activation of cat spinal motoneurones. *Neuropharmacology* 1973; 12:983–993.

Kaneko S, Fukuda K, Yada N, et al. Ca^{2+} channel inhibition by kappa opioid receptors expressed in *Xenopus* oocytes. *Neuroreport* 1994; 5:2506–2508.

Kalso E, Tramer MR, Carroll D, McQuay HJ, Moore RA. Pain relief from intra-articular morphine after knee surgery: a qualitative systematic review. *Pain* 1997; 71:127–134.

Kieffer BL, Gaveriaux-Ruff C. Exploring the opioid system by gene knockout. *Prog Neurobiol* 2002; 66:285–306.

Kitahata LM, Kosaka Y, Taub A, et al. Lamina-specific suppression of dorsal-horn unit activity by morphine sulfate. *Anesthesiology* 1974; 41:39–48.

Knapp RJ, Malatynska E, Collins N, et al. Molecular biology and pharmacology of cloned opioid receptors. *FASEB J* 1995; 9:516–525.

Kondo I, Marvizon JC, Song B, et al. Inhibition by spinal mu- and delta-opioid agonists of afferent-evoked substance P release. *J Neurosci* 2005; 25:3651–3660.

Kuhar MJ, Pert CB, Snyder SH. Regional distribution of opiate receptor binding in monkey and human brain. *Nature* 1973; 245:447–450.

Laduron PM. Axonal transport of opiate receptors in capsaicin-sensitive neurones. *Brain Res* 1984; 294:157–160

Law PY, Wong YH, Loh HH. Molecular mechanisms and regulation of opioid receptor signaling. *Annu Rev Pharmacol Toxicol* 2000; 40:389–430.

Lazorthes Y. Intracerebroventricular administration of morphine for control of irreducible cancer pain. *Ann NY Acad Sci* 1988; 531:123–132.

Le Bars D, Menétrey D, Conseiller C, Besson JM. Depressive effects of morphine upon lamina V cells activities in the dorsal horn of the spinal cat. *Brain Res* 1975; 98:261–277.

Levy RA, Proudfit HK. Analgesia produced by microinjection of baclofen and morphine at brain stem sites. *Eur J Pharmacol* 1979; 57:43–55.

Lippman HH, Kerr FW. Light and electron microscopic study of crossed ascending pathways in the anterolateral funiculus in monkey. *Brain Res* 1972; 40:496–499.

Lord JA, Waterfield AA, Hughes J, Kosterlitz HW. Endogenous opioid peptides: multiple agonists and receptors. *Nature* 1977; 267:495–499.

Martin WR, Eades CG, Fraser HF, Wikler A. Use of hindlimb reflexes of the chronic spinal dog for comparing analgesics. *J Pharmacol Exp Ther* 1964; 144:8–11.

Martin WR, Eades CG, Thompson JA, Huppler RE, Gilbert PE. The effects of morphine- and nalorphine- like drugs in the nondependent and morphine-dependent chronic spinal dog. *J Pharmacol Exp Ther* 1976; 197:517–532.

Mayer DJ, Wolfle TL, Akil H, Carder B, Liebeskind JC. Analgesia from electrical stimulation in the brainstem of the rat. *Science* 1971; 174:1351–1354.

Moreau JL, Fields HL. Evidence for GABA involvement in midbrain control of medullary neurons that modulate nociceptive transmission. *Brain Res* 1986; 397:37–46.

Morgan MM, Sohn JH, Liebeskind JC. Stimulation of the periaqueductal gray matter inhibits nociception at the supraspinal as well as spinal level. *Brain Res* 1989; 502:61–66.

Morton CR, Hutchison WD, Duggan AW, Hendry IA. Morphine and substance P release in the spinal cord. *Exp Brain Res* 1990; 82:89–96.

Nagasaka H, Yaksh TL. Effects of intrathecal μ, δ, and κ agonists on thermally evoked cardiovascular and nociceptive reflexes in halothane-anesthetized rats. *Anesth Analg* 1995; 80:437–443.

Nichols ML, Allen BJ, Rogers SD. Transmission of chronic nociception by spinal neurons expressing the substance P receptor. *Science* 1999; 286:1558–1561.

North RA, Williams JT, Surprenant A, Christie MJ. Mu and delta receptors belong to a family of receptors that are coupled to potassium channels. *Proc Natl Acad Sci USA* 1987; 84:5487–5491.

Onofrio BM, Yaksh TL, Arnold PG. Continuous low-dose intrathecal morphine administration in the treatment of chronic pain of malignant origin. *Mayo Clin Proc* 1981; 56:516–520.

Ossipov MH, Goldstein FJ, Malseed RT. Feline analgesia following central administration of opioids. *Neuropharmacology* 1984; 23:925–929.

Pavlovic ZW, Bodnar RJ. Opioid supraspinal analgesic synergy between the amygdala and periaqueductal gray in rats. *Brain Res* 1998; 779:158–169.

Pert A, Yaksh TL. Localization of the antinociceptive action of morphine in primate brain. *Pharmacol Biochem Behav* 1975; 3:133–138.

Pert CB, Snyder SH. Opiate receptor: demonstration in nervous tissue. *Science* 1973; 179:1011–1014.

Piros ET, Prather PL, Loh HH, et al. Ca^{2+} channel and adenylyl cyclase modulation by cloned mu-opioid receptors in GH3 cells. *Mol Pharmacol* 1995; 47:1041–1049.

Pohl J. Ueber das N-allylnorcodeine, einen antagonisten des morphins. *Z Exp Path Ther* 1915; 17:370–378.

Pol O, Puig MM. Expression of opioid receptors during peripheral inflammation. *Curr Top Med Chem* 2004; 4:51–61.

Ramberg DA, Yaksh TL. Effects of cervical spinal hemisection of dihydromorphine binding in brainstem and spinal cord in cat. *Brain Res* 1989; 483:61–67.

Rawal N, Mollefors K, Axelsson K, Lingardh G, Widman B. An experimental study of urodynamic effects of epidural morphine and of naloxone reversal. *Anesth Analg* 1983; 62:641–647.

Reynolds DV. Surgery in the rat during electrical analgesia induced by focal brain stimulation. *Science* 1969; 164:444–445.

Rodgers RJ. Elevation of aversive threshold in rats by intra-amygdaloid injection of morphine sulphate. *Pharmacol Biochem Behav* 1977; 6:385–390.

Russell NJW, Schaible H-G, Schmidt RF. Opiates inhibit the discharges of fine afferent units from inflamed knee joint of the cat. *Neurosci Lett* 1987; 76:107–112.

Rusin KI, Moises HC. Mu-opioid receptor activation reduces multiple components of high-threshold calcium current in rat sensory neurons. *J Neurosci* 1995; 15:4315–4327.

Sato M, Takagi H. Further observation on the enhancement by morphine of the central descending inhibitory influence on spinal sensory transmission. *Jpn J Pharmacol* 1971; 21:671–672.

Satoh M, Oku R, Akaike A. Analgesia produced by microinjection of L-glutamate into the rostral ventromedial bulbar nuclei of the rat and its inhibition by intrathecal α-adrenergic blocking agents. *Brain Res* 1983; 261:361–364.

Sawynok J, Sweeney MI. The role of purines in nociception. *Neuroscience* 1989; 32:557–569.

Sharpe LG, Garnett JE, Cicero TJ. Analgesia and hyperreactivity produced by intracranial microinjections of morphine into the periaqueductal gray matter of the rat. *Behav Biol* 1974; 11:303–313.

Smith TW, Follenfant RL, Ferreira SH. Antinociceptive models displaying peripheral opioid activity. *Int J Tissue React* 1985; 7:61–67.

Spike RC, Puskar Z, Sakamoto H. MOR-1-immunoreactive neurons in the dorsal horn of the rat spinal cord: evidence for nonsynaptic innervation by substance P-containing primary afferents and for selective activation by noxious thermal stimuli. *Eur J Neurosci* 2002; 15:1306–1316.

Stein C, Millan MJ, Shippenberg TS, Peter K, Herz A. Peripheral opioid receptors mediating antinociception in inflammation. Evidence for involvement of mu, delta and kappa receptors. *J Pharmacol Exp Ther* 1989; 248:1269–1275.

Stein C, Comisel K, Haimerl E, et al. Analgesic effect of intra-articular morphine after arthroscopic knee surgery. *N Engl J Med* 1991; 325:1123–1126.

Sternini C, Spann M, Anton B, et al. Agonist-selective endocytosis of mu opioid receptor by neurons *in vivo*. *Proc Natl Acad Sci USA* 1996; 93:9241–9246.

Stevens CW, Pezalla PD. A spinal site mediates opiate analgesia in frogs. *Life Sci* 1983; 33:2097–2103.

Sydenham T. Medical Observations Concerning the History and Care of Acute Diseases (1666). In: Latham RG (Ed). *The Works of Thomas Sydenham, MD,* Vol. 1. London: Sydenham Society, 1848, pp 172–173.

Tafani JA, Lazorthes Y, Danet B, et al. Human brain and spinal cord scan after intracerebroventricular administration of iodine-123 morphine. *Int J Rad Appl Instrum B* 1989; 16:505–509.

Takagi H, Satoh M, Akaike A, Shibata T, Kuraishi Y. The nucleus reticularis gigantocellularis of the medulla oblongata is a highly sensitive site in the production of morphine analgesia in the rat. *Eur J Pharmacol* 1977; 45:91–92.

Takagi H, Shiomi H, Kuraishi Y, Fukui K, Ueda H. Pain and the bulbospinal noradrenergic system: pain-induced increase in normetanephrine content in the spinal cord and its modification by morphine. *Eur J Pharmacol* 1979; 54:99–107

Tao R, Auerbach SB. Involvement of the dorsal raphe but not median raphe nucleus in morphine-induced increases in serotonin release in the rat forebrain. *Neuroscience* 1995; 68:553–561.

Tseng LF, Wang Q. Forebrain sites differentially sensitive to beta-endorphin and morphine for analgesia and release of Met-enkephalin in the pentobarbital-anesthetized rat. *J Pharmacol Exp Ther* 1992; 261:1028–1036.

Tsou K. Antagonism of morphine analgesia by the intracerebral microinjection of nalorphine. *Acta Physiol Sin* 1963; 26:332–337.

Tsou K, Jang CS. Studies on the site of analgesic action of morphine by intracerebral microinjection. *Scient Sin* 1964; 13:1099–1109.

Vigouret J, Teshemacher H, Albus K, Herz A. Differentiation between spinal and supraspinal sites of action of morphine when inhibiting the hind limb flexor reflex in rabbits. *Neuropharmacology* 1973; 12:111–121.

Wallace M, Yaksh TL. Long-term spinal analgesic delivery: a review of the preclinical and clinical literature. *Reg Anesth Pain Med* 2000; 25:117–157.

Wang JK, Nauss LA, Thomas JE. Pain relief by intrathecally applied morphine in man. *Anesthesiology* 1979; 50:149–151.

Westlund KN, Sorkin LS, Ferrington DG, et al. Serotoninergic and noradrenergic projections to the ventral posterolateral nucleus of the monkey thalamus. *J Comp Neurol* 1990; 295:197–207.

Wikler A. Sites and mechanisms of action of morphine and related drugs in the central nervous system *Pharmacol Rev* 1950; 2:435–506.

Yaksh TL. Direct evidence that spinal serotonin and noradrenaline terminals mediate the spinal antinociceptive effects of morphine in the periaqueductal gray. *Brain Res* 1979; 160:180–185.

Yaksh TL. Spinal opiate analgesia: characteristics and principles of action. *Pain* 1981; 11:293–346.

Yaksh TL. Spinal opiates: a review of their effect on spinal function with emphasis on pain processing. *Acta Anaesthesiol Scand* 1987; 31:25–37.

Yaksh TL. Pharmacology and mechanisms of opioid analgesic activity. *Acta Anaesthesiol Scand* 1997; 41:94–111.

Yaksh TL, Reddy SVR. Studies in the primate on the analgetic effects associated with intrathecal actions of opiates, α-adrenergic agonists and baclofen. *Anesthesiology* 1981; 54:451–467.

Yaksh TL, Rudy TA. Analgesia mediated by a direct spinal action of narcotics. *Science* 1976; 192:1357–1358.

Yaksh TL, Rudy TA. Studies on the direct spinal action of narcotics in the production of analgesia in the rat. *J Pharmacol Exp Ther* 1977; 202:411–428.

Yaksh TL, Rudy TA. Narcotic analgesics: CNS sites and mechanisms of action as revealed by intracerebral injection techniques. *Pain* 1978; 4:299–359.

Yaksh TL, Tyce GM. Microinjection of morphine into the periaqueductal gray evokes the release of serotonin from spinal cord. *Brain Res* 1979; 171:176–181.

Yaksh TL, Wilson PR. Spinal serotonin terminal system mediates antinociception. *J Pharmacol Exp Ther* 1979; 208:446–453.

Yaksh TL, Yeung JC, Rudy TA. Systematic examination in the rat of brain sites sensitive to the direct application of morphine: observation of differential effect within the periaqueductal gray. *Brain Res* 1976; 114:83–103.

Yaksh TL, Jessell TM, Gamse R, Mudge AW, Leeman SE. Intrathecal morphine inhibits substance P release from mammalian spinal cord *in vivo*. *Nature* 1980; 286:155–156.

Yeung JC, Rudy TA. Multiplicative interaction between narcotic agonism expressed at spinal and supraspinal sites of antinociceptive action as revealed by concurrent intrathecal and intracerebroventricular injections of morphine. *J Pharmacol Exp Ther* 1980; 215:633–642.

Yoshimura M, North RA. Substantia gelatinosa neurones in vitro hyperpolarised by enkephalin. *Nature (Lond)* 1983; 305:529–530.

Yu LC, Han JS. Involvement of arcuate nucleus of hypothalamus in the descending pathway from nucleus accumbens to periaqueductal grey subserving an antinociceptive effect. *Int J Neurosci* 1989; 48:71–78.

Zieglgansberger W, Bayerl H. The mechanism of inhibition of neuronal activity by opiates in the spinal cord of cat. *Brain Res* 1976; 115:111–128.

Correspondence to: Tony L. Yaksh, PhD, Department of Anesthesiology, University of California, San Diego, 9500 Gilman Drive, La Jolla, CA 92093, USA. Tel: 619-543-3597; Fax: 619-543-6070; email: tyaksh@ucsd.edu.

The Paths of Pain 1975–2005, edited by
Harold Merskey, John D. Loeser, and Ronald
Dubner, IASP Press, Seattle, © 2005.

15

Neuropathic Pain:
From the Nociceptor to the Patient

James N. Campbell and Richard A. Meyer

*Department of Neurosurgery and Applied Physics Laboratory, Johns Hopkins
University, Baltimore, Maryland, USA*

When Harold Merskey initially contacted us regarding the project of taking a look at our field of pain over a 30-year span as a commemoration of the first IASP World Congress on Pain, we took a particular interest. It was in 1975, the same year as that first Congress, that the two authors met and the seeds for a sustained scientific collaboration were sown. This chapter will reconstruct our understanding of the field of pain, particularly neuropathic pain, in 1975 and trace our journey to the present, making note of some important insights pertinent to our areas of study over what seems a very short period of time.

The late 1960s and early 1970s marked an awakening of interest in the field of pain. Several historical forces caught the imagination of investigators and clinicians. The Western world learned about the Chinese art of acupuncture, being told that it could be safely used to replace traditional Western anesthesia. The opiate receptor was discovered (Pert and Snyder 1973). The gate control theory was published by Ronald Melzack and Patrick Wall (1965). Ainsley Iggo and Edward Perl "discovered" the nociceptor by performing the first recordings of individual nociceptive afferents in the skin (Bessou and Perl 1969; Iggo and Ogawa 1971). And John Bonica formed the IASP, the first professional organization dedicated to the study of pain.

Our focus was to understand the patient that Silas Weir Mitchell so elegantly described (see Zimmermann, this volume)—the patient with injury to the nervous system that develops severe burning in the area innervated by the injured nerve. We recognized the paradox that has puzzled many great minds in the basic and clinical neurosciences. This paradox concerns the question of how disruption of the signaling system leads to heightened pain. We, along with many others, were puzzled and fascinated that patients with disrupted afferent inputs to the brain presented with heightened pain sensibility (hyperalgesia).

TWO SCHOOLS OF THOUGHT

A healthy tension pervaded scientific meetings and writings about pain in 1975. One school of thought can be traced to the influence of Henry Head (1920). Patrick Wall was its eloquent spokesman. While this school of thought is difficult to articulate in brief, its proponents disavowed any simple relationship between nociceptors and pain sensation (Wall maintained, at least at times, that C fibers had no direct sensory function). The caricature Wall routinely portrayed as a "straw man" for his arguments was Descartes' drawing showing fire at a person's foot leading to direct activation of the brain. Wall had clearly come under the influence of Head, who in turn must have been strongly influenced by works of his predecessor Hughlings Jackson. Jackson had observed that lesions of the motor system lead to positive signs and symptoms. Cutting the corticospinal tract not only led to the inability to contract muscles volitionally, but also led to increased activation of muscle by the cells of the anterior horn (spasticity, increased tone). This was viewed as a release phenomenon. Head was fascinated by postherpetic zoster (Oaklander 1999), and observed the startling coexistence of loss of sensibility with pain and hyperalgesia. The logic of considering this pain as a "release" phenomenon was clearly compelling. Hence, Head conceived the notion of "protopathic" (in essence, pain) sensibility, which he reasoned was under tonic control from epicritic sensibility. Epicritic sensibility corresponded to the ability to locate and discriminate between tactile stimuli. Melzack and Wall (1965) in their gate control model took this a step further and proposed that large-fiber (epicritic) input suppressed the inputs of small fibers and thereby suppressed pain. Neuropathic pain was basically a failure of this suppression mechanism and represented a release phenomenon.

The alternative view, articulated with equal erudition by Edward Perl and Ainsley Iggo (among several others), advocated for a primal role of the nociceptor in accounting for all pain phenomena. This view is often referred to as the theory of specificity. The thesis is that nociceptors have the capability to convey pain sensation independently (one would suspect that Perl and Iggo would disavow this characterization as being overly simplistic—but this was a dialogue of the times). Activation of nociceptors equals pain—hence a labeled line. To understand neuropathic pain, one needed to look no further than the nociceptor. Nerve injury leads to abnormal activity in the nociceptive pathways—hence pain.

PSYCHOPHYSICAL AND NEUROPHYSIOLOGICAL STUDIES

Our work over many years has probed this relationship between pain and activities in primary afferents. The basic and simple essence of our approach is to perform psychophysical studies in tandem with neurophysiological studies. Cause is inferred from a correlative analysis. To the extent possible, one applies the same stimuli in each approach. In studying peripheral neural mechanisms of painful stimuli, we measure the signals that enter the central nervous system (CNS) from the peripheral nerves and calculate the painfulness of the stimuli using psychophysical techniques; this method allows us to draw conclusions about the CNS processing. We performed the primary afferent studies in anesthetized monkey and the psychophysical studies in humans. Cross-species applicability was a tacit assumption. Similar correlational analyses have been performed by others in the Mountcastle group to establish that, within the tactile system, the capacity to detect and discriminate between cutaneous stimuli is nearly identical for monkeys and humans (Talbot et al. 1968; LaMotte and Mountcastle 1975).

Human microneurography was and is an important technique to consider as an alternative to recordings in the anesthetized monkey. Although we recognize the great importance of microneurography, we rejected this approach for our work for several reasons: (1) The recording quality of C fibers in human microneurography experiments is poor, thus requiring the use of indirect techniques to determine levels of response. In comparison, recordings in the monkey can be done with elegance and can be maintained for many hours. (2) Certain classes of afferents are somehow excluded by the microneurography technique. Aδ afferents are notoriously difficult to find in the human recordings, although psychophysical experiments point to their ubiquity (Campbell and LaMotte 1983). In contrast, Aδ nociceptors may be found routinely in the teased-fiber primate studies (Treede et al. 1998). (3) Pentobarbital anesthesia has no influence on the response properties of nociceptors (in contrast to inhalation anesthetics) (Campbell et al. 1984). (4) What has been gleaned from human studies has indicated no major differences in the response properties of nociceptors in humans and monkeys. What human microneurography studies do allow uniquely is microelectrical stimulation of identified afferents combined with recordings of evoked sensations. Not only can we record afferents, but we can determine the outcome of electrical stimulation of these afferents in terms of evoked sensation. Whether it is possible to selectively stimulate single afferents is disputed (Wall and McMahon 1985), but this technique has been helpful in learning about the role of nociceptors in signaling pain (Torebjörk and Ochoa 1983).

The specific role of nociceptors in signaling pain was buttressed by the finding that the stimulus-response function of nociceptors to heat stimuli closely parallels that of human pain ratings to the same stimuli (Meyer and Campbell 1981b). A major deficiency in this specificity construct, however, is the lack of a similar correspondence when mechanical stimuli are considered. The stimulus-response functions of conventional nociceptors become saturated well below the pain threshold (this statement may not hold for "mechanically insensitive" nociceptors). A potential resolution of this dilemma is the recent finding that nociceptor responses to mechanical stimuli may not reach saturation if one considers the population response (Slugg et al. 2004). Typically, nociceptors have been studied based on the responses to stimuli applied to the most sensitive part of the receptive field. However, as stimulus forces increase, nociceptors begin responding to forces delivered away from these punctate areas of sensitivity. To determine how the population of nociceptors responds to mechanical stimuli, it is necessary to determine their response to stimuli at any position within the receptive field. When this analysis is performed, we find that the population-response function of nociceptors does not reach saturation at higher forces (Slugg et al. 2004). The following question now arises: If nociceptor discharge can account for normal pain sensation, is neuropathic pain merely a matter of having increased nociceptor sensitivity and spontaneous discharge?

PRIMARY AND SECONDARY HYPERALGESIA

Studying the hyperalgesia that accompanies tissue injury can help us understand many things about neuropathic pain. Thomas Lewis (1942) determined that hyperalgesia occurred not only in the area of tissue injury (the zone of primary hyperalgesia), but also in the adjacent region (the zone of secondary hyperalgesia). Contemporary psychophysical studies have looked in detail at the characteristics of these two forms of hyperalgesia. After heat injury of the glabrous skin with a 30-second 53°C burn, hyperalgesia to heat and mechanical stimuli is readily apparent in the zone of primary hyperalgesia. Interestingly, however, in the zone of secondary hyperalgesia, there is enhancement of pain to mechanical stimuli, but no heat hyperalgesia. If injuries are applied near one another, the zone between them becomes hyperalgesic to mechanical stimuli and, for a time, *hypo*algesic to heat (Raja et al. 1984).

In an initial series of studies to investigate the peripheral mechanisms of primary hyperalgesia, we applied a heat injury and looked for changes in the properties of nociceptors in the glabrous skin of the hand. *The C-fiber nociceptors did not become sensitized* (whereas in hairy skin they do). Rather, a particular class of A-fiber nociceptors responsive to heat and mechanical stimuli, termed Type I A-fiber mechano-heat-sensitive nociceptors (AMHs), became sensitized and accounted for the hyperalgesia to heat (Meyer and Campbell 1981a). *Neither type of nociceptor became sensitized to mechanical stimuli* after the heat injury, despite the readily apparent hyperalgesia to mechanical stimuli.

A solution to this dilemma comes from the finding that there exists a class of nociceptors that are initially insensitive to mechanical stimuli but that develop mechanical sensitivity after inflammation. These nociceptors are called mechanically-insensitive afferents or "silent" nociceptors and have been identified in multiple tissues including the skin (Meyer et al. 1991), knee joint (Schaible and Schmidt 1985), viscera (Häbler et al. 1988), and cornea (Tanelian 1991).

Using intradermal injection of capsaicin as a technique to produce secondary hyperalgesia, LaMotte et al. (1991) discovered two forms of mechanical hypersensitivity. One was pain to light stroking of the skin (allodynia), and the other was heightened pain to punctate stimuli (punctate hyperalgesia).

From his work decades ago, Lewis believed that changes in the properties of nociceptors accounted for both primary and secondary hyperalgesia. Lewis noted that a distinctive reddening (flare response) occurred in the region of secondary hyperalgesia, and he was able to show that this phenomenon was neurogenic and peripheral in origin. For example, if an injury was applied to a region deprived of innervation by a post-ganglionic injury (i.e., a lesion distal to the dorsal root ganglion), the flare response could not be evoked. If the lesion was preganglionic, the flare response could still be evoked. The flare response appears to result from antidromic spread of action potentials to the branches of the nociceptors. The depolarization in these terminals leads to a release of vasoactive substances that cause vasodilation and thus reddening. Lewis suggested that these vasoactive compounds also sensitized the adjoining nociceptors, producing what he termed "spreading sensitization": a spread of sensitization from the directly injured nociceptors to those in adjacent uninjured regions.

To study whether spreading sensitization occurs in primates, we performed both psychophysical and neurophysiological studies of heat injury to the skin. We had already determined that C- and A-fiber mechano-heat-sensitive nociceptors in the primary zone did not become sensitized to mechanical stimuli after a burn injury. To study this phenomenon further, we applied burn injuries and cuts to the region around the receptive field of nociceptors. We also injured part of the receptive field and tested for changes in responsiveness in the other part of the receptive field (Campbell et al. 1988a). Finally, because spreading sensitization was presumed to result from antidromic activation of nociceptors, we electrically stimulated the nerve proximally and looked for evidence of sensitization (Meyer et al. 1988). None of these experiments yielded positive findings—sensitization was not evident. Thus, spreading sensitization was discounted as a potential mechanism for secondary hyperalgesia and neuropathic pain (Schmelz et al. 1996).

If the mechanism for secondary hyperalgesia is not peripheral, it must be central. The leading candidate is central sensitization, whereby central pain-signaling neurons of the dorsal horn develop enhanced sensitivity to stimuli. Data support the hypotheses that touch-provoked pain results from central sensitization to the input of tactile afferents (Simone et al. 1991) and that punctate hyperalgesia results from central sensitization to the input of nociceptors (Raja et al. 1999).

A fascinating aspect of central sensitization, and one that has not been fully appreciated in studies of CNS mechanisms, is that the sensitization to nociceptor input appears to apply to only one class of nociceptors. This finding was demonstrated in experiments where the skin in the zone of secondary hyperalgesia was desensitized with capsaicin. Capsaicin destroys the terminals of the fibers that contain the TRPV1 (capsaicin) receptor. Heat sensibility was eliminated, indicating that the mechano-heat-sensitive nociceptors were nonfunctional. Nevertheless, punctate hyperalgesia was preserved (Fuchs et al. 2000). Moreover, punctate hyperalgesia was shown by pressure block experiments to be served by Aδ fibers (Magerl et al. 2001). Thus, it appears that punctate hyperalgesia represents a central sensitization to the input of mechanically (but not thermally) sensitive Aδ nociceptors. Whether this finding applies to neuropathic pain is not yet clear.

The zone of secondary hyperalgesia depends on what is happening at the zone of primary hyperalgesia. If the area of injury is iced, or if local anesthesia is applied to the zone of primary hyperalgesia, the zone of secondary hyperalgesia reduces. This observation suggests that central mechanisms might play a pivotal role in explaining neuropathic pain, but that this pain is dependent on the dynamic input of nociceptors. Thus, peripheral sensitization has a dynamic effect on central sensitization. This understanding has a substantial impact on approaches to neuropathic pain. The suggestion is that the ongoing input of nociceptive afferents may dictate whether central sensitization is present. Therapeutic targeting of this peripheral input may still have efficacy even if central sensitization is operative.

CAN AFFERENTS OTHER THAN NOCICEPTORS SIGNAL PAIN?

In studying hyperalgesia associated with tissue injury, one of the clear psychophysical phenomena is touch-provoked pain (allodynia). Stroking pain is a frequent finding in neuropathic pain states as well. One of the tenets of the so-called "labeled line" theory is that nociceptors signal pain. One of the tenets of Melzack and Wall's gate control theory is that large fibers (those concerned with tactile sense) suppress the input of nociceptive afferents. In elegant experiments by Torebjörk and colleagues (1992), a microelectrode was inserted into the superficial peroneal nerve and was stimulated at a fixed frequency and intensity to produce tactile paresthesia referred to a small area on the top of the foot. Capsaicin was then injected beside this area to produce a zone of secondary hyperalgesia that encompassed the region of referred sensation. Electrical stimulation at the same intensity and frequency then evoked pain. Thus, large fibers normally responsible for innocuous sensations acquire the capacity to signal pain.

We examined this question in patients with touch-provoked pain in the context of nerve injury and also complex regional pain syndrome. Ischemia induced by inflation of a sphygmomanometer was used to produce an orderly loss of afferent function. Touch sensibility goes away early in the block. We showed that as tactile sensation disappeared, touch-provoked pain disappeared as well (Campbell et al. 1988b). Thus, tactile afferents may acquire the capacity to evoke pain, and provocation of pain is not exclusively served by nociceptive fibers. At the same time, this finding argues against a tenet of the gate control hypothesis by suggesting that tactile fibers do not necessarily have an inhibitory effect on the inputs of nociceptive fibers.

This suggestion raises an issue with regard to the mechanism for pain relief with dorsal column stimulation. This therapy was based on the prediction of the gate control hypothesis that activation of large fibers should suppress pain. However, many patients who obtain relief of pain with dorsal column stimulation have touch-provoked pain. As an explanation of this dilemma, we hypothesized that pain relief with dorsal column stimulation is dependent on frequency of stimulation and that the connections between large-diameter afferents and central pain-signaling neurons are subject to conduction block. Alternatively, stimulation at a sufficient frequency may lead to a sustained (and renewable) refractory period by blocking the activation of these central pain-signaling neurons by both nociceptive and large-diameter afferents. Whatever the mechanism, it is most likely that pain relief from dorsal column stimulation is mediated by a jamming effect blocking the processing of central pain-signaling neurons. These hypotheses have yet to be tested.

ROLE OF NOCICEPTORS IN NEUROPATHIC PAIN

Studies of primary and secondary hyperalgesia teach us that ongoing input from nociceptive afferents may account for aspects of behavioral signs of neuropathic pain. The finding in animals that axotomy by itself is sufficient to evoke a behavioral state that shares characteristics with neuropathic pain in humans has provided ways to investigate the mechanisms of neuropathic pain in detail. One issue is whether signaling from the nerve injury zone by itself can drive the neuropathic pain state, given a role for central sensitization. Cases that corroborate this possibility have been reported (Gracely et al. 1992). Indeed, we have seen cases where patients had widespread touch-provoked pain due to a discrete nerve injury. The hyperalgesia clearly exceeded the boundaries of the injured nerve. Yet, anesthetizing the nerve injury site was sufficient to remove all evidence of hyperalgesia.

Many investigators have recorded from the neuroma created by the nerve injury. We used this technique in a baboon model involving a superficial radial nerve, a nerve frequently implicated in traumatic neuropathic pain states (Meyer et al. 1985). There is indeed a low rate of spontaneous activity in the C fibers that innervate the neuroma. High rates of spontaneous activity in A fibers have been reported following injuries to mixed nerves that contain motor fibers (Proske et al. 1995; Michaelis et al. 2000). It is likely that much of this spontaneous activity arises from fibers that normally would innervate muscle spindles. The relevance to neuropathic pain is unclear.

Spontaneous activity is one way for nociceptive afferents to cause pain in the case of traumatic nerve injury. Neuromas also develop ectopic mechanical sensitivity, and thus the location of the nerve may be of some importance as well. Operations to remove a neuroma (a euphemism for what is really neuroma relocation) may be effective in relieving pain. Clinical experience suggests that removing injured nerves from pressure points and from points of tethering may be helpful in relieving pain in many cases (Burchiel et al. 1993).

THE INTACT NOCICEPTOR HYPOTHESIS

Many authors have advocated that spontaneous activity arising in the dorsal root ganglion (DRG) may account for aspects of neuropathic pain (Boucher et al. 2000; Liu et al. 2000, 2001). They have shown that large (presumably Aβ) DRG cells develop increased activity after distal spinal nerve axotomy. Anesthetizing the DRG or performing a dorsal rhizotomy of an injured spinal nerve removed mechanical hyperalgesia. This finding suggests that inputs of the injured spinal nerve play a dynamic role in causing the hyperalgesia to manifest in the partly denervated foot. However, how increased Aβ input could cause central sensitization is unclear. In normal subjects, touching the skin leads to a barrage of Aβ-fiber activity but does not cause hyperalgesia, suggesting that a phenotype switch is needed. Prior data raised the idea that central sprouting of Aβ fibers into denervated pain-signaling cells in the dorsal horn might occur, but more recent data bring this observation into question (Woolf et al. 1995; Bao et al. 2002). Prior studies have not indicated the presence of increased spontaneous activity in injured C-fiber afferents of the lesioned spinal nerve, but these studies may have overlooked low-level spontaneous activity because of the high-frequency activity in larger fibers.

Quite different results were obtained in our studies at Johns Hopkins University regarding the effects of L5 dorsal rhizotomy on pain from L5 spinal nerve transection. Hyperalgesia to mechanical stimuli was unaffected whether the rhizotomy was done before or after the nerve injury (Li et al. 2000). In addition, recordings of intact afferents from the L4 nerve root revealed spontaneous activity in unmyelinated fibers (Wu et al. 2001). Although the discharge frequency was low (median: 7 action potentials/5 minutes), about half of the C fibers exhibited spontaneous activity 1 day after the lesion. In some cases this spontaneous activity could be stopped by anesthetic injected in the receptive field of the nociceptive fiber. Thus, uninjured nociceptive afferents may play an important role in the development of neuropathic pain.

THE SYMPATHETIC NERVOUS SYSTEM AND PAIN

The concept of a role for the intact nociceptor received an impetus from previous work aimed at understanding the phenomenon of sympathetically maintained pain (SMP). SMP refers to pain that is dependent on the function of the sympathetic nervous system. This condition may be seen after nerve injury or soft tissue injury. SMP by definition is that pain which is relieved by a sympathetic block. The effects are known to be mediated by α-adrenergic receptors because phentolamine given intravenously replicates the effects of the sympathetic block (Raja et al. 1991).

The sympathetic nerve fibers release norepinephrine in the skin. One of the initial thoughts was that SMP involved abnormalities within the sympathetic nervous system. However, it was found that injection of norepinephrine into the skin produced pain in patients with SMP (but not in normal controls), suggesting the development of an enhanced adrenergic sensitivity

(Torebjörk et al. 1995; Ali et al. 2000). Patients with postherpetic neuralgia also reported pain with injection of epinephrine into the skin (Choi and Rowbotham 1997). Walker and Nulson in 1948 noted that stimulation of the distal side of a severed sympathetic trunk recreated pain in nerve-injury patients with apparent SMP.

Sato and Perl (1991) conducted the pivotal experiments that point to the underlying mechanism of SMP. In the presence (but not in the absence) of a partial nerve injury, sympathetic stimulation activated the nociceptors that shared the innervation territory of the injured nerve. We examined this effect in a primate model (Ali et al. 1999). The L6 nerve root was severed in the monkey. In electrophysiological studies, a skin flap from the top of the foot was dissected out and placed into an in vitro preparation that allowed recordings to be made in response to pharmacological agents. Two striking abnormalities were noted in the recordings from the partly denervated skin flaps. First, about half of the C-fiber nociceptors were sensitive to α_1-adrenergic agonists. Secondly, spontaneous activity was also prominent in the C-fiber nociceptors. The findings of spontaneous activity were also confirmed in a rat model. Moreover, other diseases (with no clear nerve pathology) may induce catechol sensitization of nociceptors (Sato et al. 1993).

That nociceptors acquire functional α_1-adrenergic receptors is supported further by work of Drummond et al. (1996). A radioligand for α_1 adrenergic receptors was administered to skin biopsies from patients with complex regional pain syndrome. Quantitative autoradiography demonstrated higher concentrations of these receptors in the epidermal and dermal layers in the painful limb as opposed to the nonpainful limb and the limbs of normal controls.

A further link is provided by Ruocco et al. (2000). Somatic innervation to the lower lip is provided through the mental nerve, whereas sympathetic innervation is provided through the superior cervical ganglion. These investigators lesioned the mental nerve and observed sprouting of sympathetic fibers to the upper dermis, an area normally devoid of sympathetic innervation. This sprouting would increase the likelihood of nociceptor/sympathetic coupling.

The importance of this work is that it points to a fourth site that may play a role in neuropathic pain. The four sites are (1) the injured axon at the point of axotomy; (2) the DRG cell of the injured axon; (3) the CNS, via central sensitization (unjustly considered here as being only one mechanism); and (4) the intact nociceptor. The latter provides a biological rationale for distal therapies, such as topical lidocaine and capsaicin. It is also possible that the intact nociceptor is activated along the nerve as well. The mechanisms for abnormalities in the intact nociceptor are undergoing intense scrutiny at present. A possibility is that neurotrophic molecules released from the regions of partial denervation (such as keratinocytes and Schwann cells) may sensitize the nociceptors.

LOSS OF INHIBITION

A concept that has in some ways lost its popularity for the moment goes back to the old idea of Head that the epicritic sensibility suppresses protopathic sensibility. Although the terms *epicritic* and *protopathic* are no longer appropriate, the idea that "innocuous" channels of sensory information suppress "noxious" channels of information merits consideration. A pressure block or ischemic block of a peripheral nerve leads to a somewhat orderly loss of sensation. At the point that the innocuous sense of cooling is lost, cooling stimuli induce a burning pain sensation (Wahren et al. 1989; Yarnitsky and Ochoa 1990). The most likely explanation is that under normal circumstances, cold-sensitive fibers suppress the input of cold-sensitive nociceptors. Work is under way to test these findings with regard to other modalities of sensation.

CONCLUSIONS

Thirty years ago we wondered whether we would ever figure out why patients sometimes developed devastating pain after soft tissue and nerve injury. We sometimes wondered whether the pain described by these patients in reaction to light stroking of the skin might be due to problems in the psychiatric realm. We had little to offer these patients.

Very substantial progress has been made. We have been able to unearth a rich complexity of nociceptor biology and relate the functions of these receptors to various aspects of pain sensibility. The neurophysiological and psychophysical studies of secondary hyperalgesia have suggested mechanisms relevant to understanding neuropathic pain. We understand in some detail how the sympathetic nervous system can mediate pain. Several candidate peripheral and central mechanisms have been identified. We understand why lightly touching the skin may cause pain and see this as an indication of central sensitization. The list goes on, and clearly in this short chapter we have only touched on a few of the many insights acquired over a 30-year period.

A paradox is evident as well. Neuropathic pain can be largely understood as the effects of enhanced input of nociceptive afferents—a simple concept. Yet in the clinic we are still besieged by miserable patients suffering with severe pain that we cannot control adequately. Morphine helps, but it has a high side-effect profile. Occasionally we see patients who are candidates for the dorsal root entry zone (DREZ) surgical procedure, a new development within the past 30 years. This procedure can work wonders in patients with plexus avulsion, for example. But there are few examples such as this. How is it that we control pain so poorly if all we have to do is reduce the input of a single class of afferents? If the past 30 years is any measure, we will have overcome this challenge 30 years from today.

ACKNOWLEDGMENTS

We are extremely grateful to the many students and post-doctoral fellows who have collaborated with us over the years. We also appreciate funding that has been provided mainly from the National Institutes of Health.

REFERENCES

Ali Z, Ringkamp M, Hartke TV, et al. Uninjured C-fiber nociceptors develop spontaneous activity and alpha adrenergic sensitivity following L6 spinal nerve ligation in the monkey. *J Neurophysiol* 1999; 81:455–466.

Ali Z, Raja SN, Wesselmann U, et al. Intradermal injection of norepinephrine evokes pain in patients with sympathetically maintained pain. *Pain* 2000; 88:161–168.

Bao L, Wang HF, Cai HJ, et al. Peripheral axotomy induces only very limited sprouting of coarse myelinated afferents into inner lamina II of rat spinal cord. *Eur J Neurosci* 2002; 16:175–185.

Bessou P, Perl ER. Response of cutaneous sensory units with unmyelinated fibers to noxious stimuli. *J Neurophysiol* 1969; 32:1025–1043.

Boucher TJ, Okuse K, Bennett DL, et al. Potent analgesic effects of GDNF in neuropathic pain states. *Science* 2000; 290:124–127.

Burchiel KJ, Johans TJ, Ochoa J. The surgical treatment of painful traumatic neuromas. *J Neurosurg* 1993; 78:714–719.

Campbell JN, LaMotte RH. Latency to detection of first pain. *Brain Res* 1983; 266:203–208.

Campbell JN, Raja SN, Meyer RA. Halothane sensitizes cutaneous nociceptors in monkeys. *J Neurophysiol* 1984; 52:762–770.

Campbell JN, Khan AA, Meyer RA, Raja SN. Responses to heat of C-fiber nociceptors in monkey are altered by injury in the receptive field but not by adjacent injury. *Pain* 1988a; 32:327–332.

Campbell JN, Raja SN, Meyer RA, Mackinnon SE. Myelinated afferents signal the hyperalgesia associated with nerve injury. *Pain* 1988b; 32:89–94.

Choi B, Rowbotham MC. Effect of adrenergic receptor activation on post-herpetic neuralgia pain and sensory disturbances. *Pain* 1997; 69:55–63.

Drummond PD, Skipworth S, Finch PM. alpha 1-adrenoceptors in normal and hyperalgesic human skin. *Clin Sci (Colch)* 1996; 91:73–77.

Fuchs PN, Campbell JN, Meyer RA. Secondary hyperalgesia persists in capsaicin desensitized skin. *Pain* 2000; 84:141–149.

Gracely RH, Lynch SA, Bennett GJ. Painful neuropathy: altered central processing maintained dynamically by peripheral input. *Pain* 1992; 51:175–194.

Häbler H-J, Jänig W, Koltzenburg M. A novel type of unmyelinated chemosensitive nociceptor in the acutely inflamed urinary bladder. *Agents Actions* 1988; 25:219–21.

Head H. *Studies in Neurology*. London: H. Frowde; Hooder & Stoughton, 1920.

Iggo A, Ogawa H. Primate cutaneous thermal nociceptors. *J Physiol* 1971; 216:77P–78P.

LaMotte RH, Mountcastle VB. Capacities of humans and monkeys to discriminate between vibratory stimuli of different frequency and amplitude: a correlation between neural events and psychophysical measurements. *J Neurophysiol* 1975; 37:539–559.

LaMotte RH, Shain CN, Simone DA, Tsai E-FP. Neurogenic hyperalgesia: Psychophysical studies of underlying mechanisms. *J Neurophysiol* 1991; 66:190–211.

Lewis T. In: *Pain*. New York: Macmillan, 1942.

Li Y, Dorsi MJ, Meyer RA, Belzberg AJ. Mechanical hyperalgesia after an L5 spinal nerve lesion in the rat is not dependent on input from injured nerve fibers. *Pain* 2000; 85:493–502.

Liu C-N, Wall PD, Ben Dor E, et al. Tactile allodynia in the absence of C-fiber activation: altered firing properties of DRG neurons following spinal nerve injury. *Pain* 2000; 85:503–521.

Liu X, Zhou JL, Chung K, Chung JM. Ion channels associated with the ectopic discharges generated after segmental spinal nerve injury in the rat. *Brain Res* 2001; 900:119–127.

Magerl W, Fuchs PN, Meyer RA, Treede R-D. Roles of capsaicin-insensitive nociceptors in cutaneous pain and secondary hyperalgesia. *Brain* 2001; 124:1754–1764.

Melzack R, Wall PD. Pain mechanisms: a new theory. *Science* 1965; 150:971–979.

Meyer RA, Campbell JN. Myelinated nociceptive afferents account for the hyperalgesia that follows a burn to the hand. *Science* 1981a; 213:1527–1529.

Meyer RA, Campbell JN. Peripheral neural coding of pain sensation. *Johns Hopkins APL Technical Digest* 1981b; 2:164–171.

Meyer RA, Raja SN, Campbell JN, Mackinnon SE, Dellon AL. Neural activity originating from a neuroma in the baboon. *Brain Res* 1985; 325:255–260.

Meyer RA, Campbell JN, Raja SN. Antidromic nerve stimulation in monkey does not sensitize unmyelinated nociceptors to heat. *Brain Res* 1988; 441:168–172.

Meyer RA, Davis KD, Cohen RH, Treede R-D, Campbell JN. Mechanically insensitive afferents (MIAs) in cutaneous nerves of monkey. *Brain Res* 1991; 561:252–261.

Michaelis M, Liu X, Jänig W. Axotomized and intact muscle afferents but not skin afferents develop ongoing discharges of dorsal root ganglion origin after peripheral nerve lesion. *J Neurosci* 2000; 20:2742–2748.

Oaklander AL. The pathology of shingles: Head and Campbell's 1900 monograph. *Arch Neurol* 1999; 56:1292–1294.

Pert CB, Snyder SH. Opiate receptor: demonstration in nervous tissue. *Science* 1973; 179:1011–1014.

Proske U, Iggo A, Luff AR. Mechanical sensitivity of regenerating myelinated skin and muscle afferents in the cat. *Exp Brain Res* 1995; 104:89–98.

Raja SN, Campbell JN, Meyer RA. Evidence for different mechanisms of primary and secondary hyperalgesia following heat injury to the glabrous skin. *Brain* 1984; 107:1179–1188.

Raja SN, Treede R-D, Davis KD, Campbell JN. Systemic alpha-adrenergic blockade with phentolamine: a diagnostic test for sympathetically maintained pain. *Anesthesiology* 1991; 74:691–698.

Raja SN, Meyer RA, Ringkamp M, Campbell JN. Peripheral neural mechanisms of nociception. In: Wall PD, Melzack P (Eds). *Textbook of Pain*. Edinburgh: Churchill Livingstone, 1999, pp 11–57.

Ruocco I, Cuello AC, Ribeiro-da-Silva A. Peripheral nerve injury leads to the establishment of a novel pattern of sympathetic fibre innervation in the rat skin. *J Comp Neurol* 2000; 422:287–296.

Sato J, Perl ER. Adrenergic excitation of cutaneous pain receptors induced by peripheral nerve injury. *Science* 1991; 251:1608–1610.

Sato J, Suzuki S, Iseki T, Kumazawa T. Adrenergic excitation of cutaneous nociceptors in chronically inflamed rats. *Neurosci Lett* 1993; 164:225–228.

Schaible HG, Schmidt RF. Effects of an experimental arthritis on the sensory properties of fine articular afferent units. *J Neurophysiol* 1985; 54:1109–1122.

Schmelz M, Schmidt R, Ringkamp M, et al. Limitation of sensitization to injured parts of receptive fields in human skin C-nociceptors. *Exp Brain Res* 1996; 109:141–147.

Simone DA, Sorkin LS, Oh U, et al. Neurogenic hyperalgesia: central neural correlates in responses of spinothalamic tract neurons. *J Neurophysiol* 1991; 66:228–246.

Slugg RM, Campbell JN, Meyer RA. The population response of A- and C-fiber nociceptors in monkey encodes high-intensity mechanical stimuli. *J Neurosci* 2004; 24:4649–4656.

Talbot WH, Darian-Smith I, Kornhuber HH, Mountcastle VB. The sense of flutter-vibration: comparison of the human capacity with response patterns of mechanoreceptive afferents from the monkey hand. *J Neurophysiol* 1968; 31:301–334.

Tanelian DL. Cholinergic activation of a population of corneal afferent nerves. *Exp Brain Res* 1991; 86:414–420.

Torebjörk E, Ochoa J. Selective stimulation of sensory units in man. *Adv Pain Res Ther* 1983; 5:99–104.

Torebjörk HE, Lundberg LER, LaMotte RH. Central changes in processing of mechanoreceptive input in capsaicin-induced secondary hyperalgesia in humans. *J Physiol* 1992; 448:765–780.

Torebjörk E, Wahren LK, Wallin G, Hallin R, Koltzenburg M. Noradrenaline-evoked pain in neuralgia. *Pain* 1995; 63:11–20.

Treede R-D, Meyer RA, Campbell JN. Myelinated mechanically insensitive afferents from monkey hairy skin: heat-response properties. *J Neurophysiol* 1998; 80:1082–1093.

Wahren LK, Torebjörk E, Jorum E. Central suppression of cold-induced C fibre pain by myelinated fibre input. *Pain* 1989; 38:313–319.

Walker AE, Nulson F. Electrical stimulation of the upper thoracic portion of the sympathetic chain in man. *Arch Neurol Psychiatry* 1948; 59:559–560.

Wall PD, McMahon SB. Microneuronography and its relation to perceived sensation. A critical review. *Pain* 1985; 21:209–229.

Woolf CJ, Shortland P, Reynolds M, et al. Reorganization of central terminals of myelinated primary afferents in the rat dorsal horn following peripheral axotomy. *J Comp Neurol* 1995; 360:121–134.

Wu G, Ringkamp M, Hartke TV, et al. Early onset of spontaneous activity in uninjured C-fiber nociceptors after injury to neighboring nerve fibers. *J Neurosci* 2001; 21:RC140.

Yarnitsky D, Ochoa JL. Release of cold–induced burning pain by block of cold-specific afferent input. *Brain* 1990; 113:893–902.

Correspondence to: James N. Campbell, MD, Department of Neurosurgery, Johns Hopkins Hospital, 600 N. Wolfe Street, Meyer 5-109, Baltimore, MD 21287-7509, USA. Email: jcampbel@jhmi.edu.

The Paths of Pain 1975–2005, edited by
Harold Merskey, John D. Loeser, and Ronald
Dubner, IASP Press, Seattle, © 2005.

16

Animal Models and Their Clinical Implications

Gary J. Bennett

Department of Anesthesia, Faculty of Dentistry, and Centre for Research on Pain, McGill University, Montreal, Quebec, Canada

We had very few animal models of pain 30 years ago. The tail-flick assay for mice and rats had been in use for a long time (D'Amour and Smith 1941). The key to its success was its elegant simplicity: the animal is wrapped in a towel and its tail is placed in a shallow groove, with a radiant heat source (the light bulb from a 35-mm slide projector) positioned above the tip of the tail and a photocell situated beneath it. The tail-flick activates the photocell circuit, which turns off a clock and the heat source. The tail-flick latency measured in this way is an objective, non-biased measure of the animal's pain threshold. Cognoscenti of the tail-flick test knew that the tail should be blackened with a Magic Marker to reduce reflectance and thus standardize heat absorption, and that a cut-off time was necessary to prevent accidentally burning the tail. This simple procedure was the mainstay of pharmacological experiments for many years. We have learned a great deal about the tail-flick assay since then. We have the anatomical details of the input and output circuits (Grossman et al. 1982). We know that it is not, as originally thought by many, a simple spinal reflex; the spinal circuit is under powerful descending modulating influences from several brainstem nuclei (reviewed in Fields 2004). The reflex is now known to be triggered by different primary afferent fiber inputs, depending on the rate of heating: very rapid heating activates Aδ-fiber nociceptors and yields short withdrawal latencies, while slower heating activates mainly C-fiber nociceptors and yields distinctly longer latencies (Yeomans and Proudfit 1996; Yeomans et al. 1996). Drugs that increase or decrease blood flow to the tail are now known to produce an artifact—they shorten or lengthen the reflex's latency due to a simple change in the starting temperature of the tail skin (Hole and

Tjolsen 1993). Nevertheless, the tail-flick assay is still one of our most reliable tests of acute nociception in animals.

A simple modification of the tail-flick apparatus yielded the paw-flick assay, which has also proven to be remarkably useful (Hargreaves et al. 1988). The animal stands on a plate of window glass, and a radiant heat source (the same projector bulb) is directed through an aperture from below. The heat source and a timer are controlled by the same photocell circuit, which in this case is activated by light reflected from the bottom of the hindpaw and switches off when the paw-withdrawal reflex interrupts the reflected light. The paw-flick assay has several advantages, including an easily obtained doubling of the amount of data available per animal (they have two hindpaws but only one tail) and the elimination of the need to restrain the animal, which can walk about while confined beneath an up-turned plastic cage. As with even the simplest methods, there are "tricks to the trade," most importantly, keeping the glass floor warm and being certain to test only when the skin of the hindpaw is in contact with the glass (Bennett and Hargreaves 1990; Hirata et al. 1990).

The tail-flick assay could not be criticized on practical grounds, but there was always a pervasive air of dissatisfaction around it. Three arguments were made. First, concern was raised that an apparent analgesic response might represent a purely motor inhibition—the animal still felt pain but could not move. The objection is logical, but it has never been shown to lead to error (no investigator would take a tail-flick measure on an animal that was paralyzed or too sedated to stand). The second argument, a more sophisticated version of the first, was the possibility that the neural circuits that controlled the reflex might be parallel to, and largely independent of, those that mediate the experience of pain, and thus one might be blocked by a drug while the other was not. In a trivial sense, this is what is observed with general anesthesia—the awareness of pain is absent while the reflex is still present. But the reverse, a drug effect that blocks only the pain-evoked reflex (and not other motor reflexes) while sparing pain sensation, has never been found. The third objection is related to the second, but goes beyond it. I do not recall if it was ever made explicitly, but I believe that there was a sense that a mouse's tail-flick was just not "human" enough. Human pain was certainly somewhere in the brain, and the rodent's tail-flick response remained after transecting the spinal cord.

The desire for a more "integrated" pain-evoked behavior was usually thought to be satisfied by using the hot-plate test, which had also been introduced many years previously (Woolfe and MacDonald 1944). The mouse or rat was confined within a tall cylinder of transparent plastic that was placed on a hot metal floor (usually made of copper and heated uniformly to around 55°C via water circulated beneath it; the "correct" temperature was hotly debated). A stopwatch measured the latency to the animal's "escape behavior." This model has never been very satisfactory. There has never been agreement on what constitutes the behavior to be measured; lifting a paw off the plate, rearing up on the side of the cylinder or trying to jump out, or hopping from one paw to another? Moreover, it was easy to see that the exposure to the heat varied in an uncontrollable way: the exposure was greatest if the animal stood still, and decreased if it walked about.

The debate over pain-evoked reflexes versus "integrated" pain behaviors was part of a larger philosophical debate over the clinical relevance of animal models of pain. The controversy took place largely in the context of semantics, but simply put, the issue was whether or not animal pain was the same as human pain. The words "painful" and "pain" were banished from the animal literature and replaced by "noxious" and "nociception." There was, perhaps, a good reason to banish "painful." It was commonplace to read of a "painful stimulus." This is sloppy language. A stimulus may cause pain, but pain is not a property of the stimulus—it is a property of the organism that responds to the stimulus. "Noxious" is a useful word in that in emphasizes the usual (but not simple or invariant) relationship between tissue damage and the sensation of pain. On the other hand, in my opinion, the insistence on the use of "nociception" is pernicious: it substitutes a fancy neologism that few understand for a simple word understood by all, and it grants an unearned victory to those who maintain that there is a fundamental difference between pain in animals and pain in human beings. As argued elsewhere (Bennett 2001), the evidence that animals feel pain is of precisely the same kind as the evidence that you feel pain; of course, the evidence that I feel pain is of an essentially different kind. We can have no direct knowledge of the subjective sensations of others, neither of another person nor of any other kind of animal. We assume that other people have subjective experiences like ours. We know, of course, that this is not always true (the other person may be colorblind, or tone-deaf, or congenitally insensitive to pain), but it is approximately true and hence useful (how could driving on the highway be possible if it were not?). It is reasonable to make the same assumption about an animal that is sufficiently like us. From the Darwinian perspective, we may say the same for any animal with a nervous system. The sense of pain has obvious evolutionary value and is surely highly conserved. It is not a mere coincidence that one can evoke a withdrawal reflex by pinching a worm or a college sophomore. From a practical perspective, the strongest argument that animal pain models are relevant to the clinic comes from pharmacology. For example, Fig. 1 shows rank orderings of the analgesic potencies, relative to morphine, of 10 opioids in humans relative

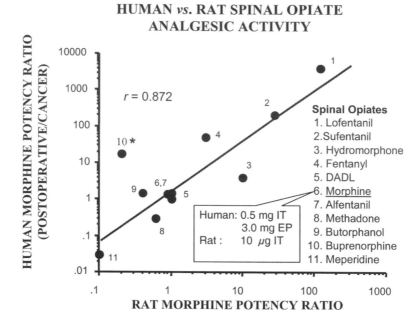

Fig. 1. The relative potencies of various opioids relative to morphine for intrathecal administration to rats tested on the hot-plate (abscissa) versus intrathecal (IT) or epidural (EP) administration to human patients with postoperative or cancer pain (ordinate). In the rat hot-plate assay, buprenorphine has the properties of a partial agonist. Reprinted from Yaksh (1997), with permission.

to their respective potencies in rats tested with the hot-plate assay. It is difficult to imagine that the extraordinary correspondence is a coincidence; the drugs must be working on neural circuits that are highly similar. One could also point to the non-obvious efficacy of some anti-epileptic drugs, such as gabapentin, in the control of neuropathic pain in both rats and humans. In summary, the debate can be settled (or at least avoided) by saying that the subjective sensation of pain in humans and animals may or may not be identical—we will never know for certain—but that the neural mechanisms that produce them are sufficiently similar for experiments on one to be relevant to the other.

Another problem arose with the use of the tail-flick and hot-plate assays: they were useless in testing the nonsteroidal anti-inflammatory drugs (NSAIDs) that were then under development. Anti-inflammatory drugs have no effect on acute normal pain. The significance of this discrepancy was, I think, not fully appreciated at the time. It hinted that there were different kinds of pain that responded differently to drugs, and of course this possibility implies that their neural mechanisms might be at least partly different. In any case, the need for an assay for NSAIDs prompted the development of several animal models of inflammatory pain. The most important of these evoked hindpaw swelling via a subcutaneous injection of the immune stimuli, complete Freund's adjuvant (a mineral oil emulsion of heat-killed tuberculosis bacilli) or carrageenan (a colloid extracted from red algae). The Randall-Siletto (1957) device was developed to test the pressure-pain thresholds of these animals. The rat is wrapped in a towel, and its hindpaw placed between an underlying support and a conical stylus. The motor-driven stylus is slowly advanced to squeeze the paw until the animal pulls its paw away (or, in a variant method, until it squeaks). The inflammatory pain models were not in the mainstream of pain research until fairly recently. They were used primarily in experiments examining anti-inflammatory drugs, where the primary end-point was more often the reduction of swelling, rather than the reversal of hyperalgesia. An exception to this practice was the development of the formalin test (Dubuisson and Dennis 1977). A small volume of dilute formalin (usually 10–20 µL of a 4% solution) is injected subcutaneously in the hindpaw. Within a few seconds the animal begins to vigorously shake ("flick") the paw and continues to do so for several minutes. Paw-flicking then ceases for several minutes, only to resume for a second, longer period of flicking. This two-phase response has continued to fascinate researchers. Interest in the phenomenon was rekindled when it was proposed that the first phase of responding represented acute nociceptive pain, while the second phase reflected central sensitization-like processes (Yamamoto and Yaksh 1992).

The tail-flick and hot-plate assays test acute, threshold-level pain in the context of a healthy animal. For many years, clinicians had been telling basic researchers (indeed, they still do) that there is something about clinical pain that is fundamentally different from the pain being studied in the laboratory. On the basic research side, there was, perhaps, a naive hope that the pain measured by the tail-flick was clinical pain in essence, with magnitude and duration the only real differences. A separate but related issue affected electrophysiologists who were trying to characterize pain-responsive neurons and their interconnections. The discovery of nociceptor sensitization (Bessou and Perl 1969) introduced a sort of biological Heisenberg Uncertainty Principle—the act of measurement changed the system that was being measured. The use of anything but the mildest and briefest pain stimulus changed the response characteristics of the cells being studied, making repeated measurements from the same animal meaningless (one would be averaging apples and oranges). For many years, electrophysiological analyses of pain all but ignored anything but brief, threshold-level pain stimuli in normal animals.

The field of animal models of pain is vastly different today. Of course, the clinicians were right, and what we now call acute nociceptive pain is indeed fundamentally different from the clinical pain seen in the presence of inflammation, and even more different than the clinical pain seen after damage to certain regions of the nervous system. Experimentally, this became crystal clear with Woolf's (1983) demonstration that inflammation evoked changes in the excitability of pain-processing pathways in the spinal cord. Subsequent work showed that this effect, known as central sensitization, is mediated (at least in part) by the release of glutamate from C-nociceptor terminals onto N-methyl-D-aspartate (NMDA) receptors (Woolf and Thompson 1991). The hippocampal NMDA receptor was well known to be a key player in learning, and thus the neural circuits that mediated pain were understood to be inherently "plastic." Models of the pain produced by inflammation are now a significant part of pain research.

Interest in the plasticity of the neural mechanisms mediating pain was reinforced by the introduction of animal models of neuropathic pain. Wall's description of an experimental anesthesia dolorosa (Wall et al. 1979) brought neuropathic pain to the forefront of the field. Denervating the rat's hindpaw caused the animal to bite and chew the insensate appendage. This self-mutilation, termed "autotomy," was interpreted as the animal's response to a spontaneously painful paw—the equivalent of a phantom foot. This interpretation was challenged, and defended, forcefully (Rodin and Kruger 1984; Devor 1991). There were two fundamental problems with the autotomy model. First, its clinical relevance was suspect because self-mutilation is a very rare phenomenon in patients. Second, autotomy is spontaneous behavior, and if it is indeed related to pain, then the relation must always be inferred, never proven. Thus, the second important impetus to the study of neuropathic pain required a model of partial denervation that permitted stimulus-evoked pain to be studied. The first such model, the chronic constriction injury, was reported by Bennett and Xie in 1988. Related models of post-traumatic painful peripheral neuropathy soon followed (Seltzer et al. 1990; Kim and Chung 1992), as did models of painful diabetic neuropathy (Courteix et al. 1993), of the central pain syndrome seen after spinal cord injury (Hao et al. 1992), and recently, of pain due to an acute herpes zoster infection (Fleetwood-Walker et al. 1999), as well as a similar model that uses the herpes simplex virus (Andoh et al. 1995).

It seems as if a new animal model of pain is announced every month. There is a clear trend toward tissue- and disease-specificity. It is generally understood that, for example, a model of inflammatory cutaneous pain may not teach us everything about all inflammatory pain conditions, and thus we must analyze separately the pain that arises from an inflamed bladder or inflamed muscle (see the reviews by Kehl and Fairbanks 2003 and Joshi and Gebhart 2000). This is not an issue of cognitive style, of "splitters" versus "lumpers." They really are different. For example, there is evidence of a unique pharmacological responsiveness for the pain arising from inflamed gut (Joshi et al. 2000). We also see a more concentrated effort toward developing models of specific human conditions, and this effort is not splitting hairs either. For example, it is now clearly established that unique pain mechanisms are associated with bone cancer, and that these mechanisms may even differ with different kinds of tumor cells (Sabino et al. 2003). Clinically relevant heterogeneity of neuropathic pain mechanisms is also becoming clear via experiments on models of the pain conditions produced by anti-HIV false nucleoside therapy, and by chemotherapy with taxanes, vinca alkaloids, and platinum-complex drugs (Aley et al. 1996; Polomano et al. 2001; Authier et al. 2003; Joseph et al. 2004).

The animal models have taught us a lot. Thirty years ago, one might have had a discussion of "What are the neural mechanisms of pain?" Today, that question seems hopelessly naive. We now know that pain is not one thing, but many things, and that it is wonderfully (woefully?) complex. We know that the pain one feels when stepping on a tack is a far different thing than the pain from an arthritic toe, and a very far different thing than the diabetic's painful feet. There are still questions about the clinical relevance of all this work, and impatience with the slow journey from benchside to bedside is widespread. Nevertheless, we are on the right track.

REFERENCES

Aley KO, Reichling DB, Levine JD. Vincristine hyperalgesia in the rat: a model of painful vincristine neuropathy in humans. *Neuroscience* 1996; 73:259–265.

Andoh T, Shiraki K, Kurokawa M, Kuraishi Y. Paresthesia induced by cutaneous infection with herpes simplex virus in rats. *Neurosci Lett* 1995; 190:101–104.

Authier N, Gillet JP, Fialip J, Eschalier A, Coudore F. An animal model of nociceptive peripheral neuropathy following repeated cisplatin injections. *Exp Neurol* 2003; 182:12–20.

Bennett GJ. Animal models of pain. In: Kruger L (Ed). *Methods in Pain Research*. Boca Raton, FL: CRC Press, 2001, pp 67–99.

Bennett GJ, Hargreaves KM. Reply to Hirata and his colleagues. *Pain* 1990; 42:255.

Bennett GJ, Xie Y-K. A peripheral mononeuropathy in rat that produces disorders of pain sensation like those seen in man. *Pain* 1988; 33:87–107.

Bessou P, Perl ER. Response of cutaneous sensory units with unmyelinated fibers to noxious stimuli. *J Neurophysiol* 1969; 32:1025–1043.

Courteix C, Eschalier A, Lavarenne J. Streptozocin-induced diabetic rats: behavioural evidence for a model of chronic pain. *Pain* 1993; 53:81–88.

D'Amour FE, Smith DL. A method for determining loss of pain sensation. *J Pharmacol Exp Ther* 1941; 72:74–79.

Devor M. Sensory basis of autotomy in rats. *Pain* 1991; 45:109–110.

Dubuisson D, Dennis SG. The formalin test: a quantitative study of the analgesic effects of morphine, meperidine, and brain stem stimulation in rats and cats. *Pain* 1977; 4:161–174.

Fields H. State-dependent opioid control of pain. *Nat Rev Neurosci* 2004; 5:565–575.

Fleetwood-Walker SM, Quinn JP, Wallace C, et al. Behavioural changes in the rat following infection with varicella-zoster virus. *J Gen Virol* 1999; 80:2433–2436.

Grossman ML, Basbaum AI, Fields HL. Afferent and efferent connections of the rat tail flick reflex (a model used to analyze pain control mechanisms). *J Comp Neurol* 1982; 206:9–16.

Hao JX, Xu XJ, Aldskogius H, Seiger A, Wiesenfeld-Hallin Z. Photochemically induced transient spinal ischemia induces behavioral hypersensitivity to mechanical and cold stimuli, but not to noxious-heat stimuli, in the rat. *Exp Neurol* 1992; 118:187–194.

Hargreaves K, Dubner R, Brown F, Flores C, Joris J. A new and sensitive method for measuring thermal nociception in cutaneous hyperalgesia. *Pain* 1988; 32:77–88.

Hirata H, Pataky A, Kajander K, LaMotte RH, Collins JG. A model of peripheral mononeuropathy in the rat. *Pain* 1990; 42:253–255.

Hole K, Tjolsen A. The tail-flick and formalin tests in rodents: changes in skin temperature as a confounding factor. *Pain* 1993; 53:247–254.

Joseph EK, Chen X, Khasar SG, Levine JD. Novel mechanism of enhanced nociception in a model of AIDS therapy-induced painful peripheral neuropathy in the rat. *Pain* 2004; 107:147–158.

Joshi SK, Gebhart GF. Visceral pain. *Curr Rev Pain* 2000; 4:499–506.

Joshi SK, Su X, Porreca F, Gebhart GF. Kappa-opioid receptor agonists modulate visceral nociception at a novel, peripheral site of action. *J Neurosci* 2000; 20:5874–5879.

Kehl LJ, Fairbanks CA. Experimental animal models of muscle pain and analgesia. *Exerc Sport Sci Rev* 2003; 31:188–194.

Kim SH, Chung JM. An experimental model for peripheral neuropathy produced by segmental spinal nerve ligation in the rat. *Pain* 1992; 50:355–363.

Polomano RC, Mannes AJ, Clark US, Bennett GJ. A painful peripheral neuropathy in the rat produced by the chemotherapeutic drug, paclitaxel. *Pain* 2001; 94:293–304.

Randall LO, Selitto JJ. A method for measurement of analgesic activity on inflamed tissue. *Arch Int Pharmacodyn* 1957; 4:409–414.

Rodin BE, Kruger L. Deafferentation in animals as a model for the study of pain: an alternative hypothesis. *Brain Res* 1984; 319:213–228.

Sabino MA, Luger NM, Mach DB, et al. Different tumors in bone each give rise to a distinct pattern of skeletal destruction, bone cancer-related pain behaviors and neurochemical changes in the central nervous system. *Int J Cancer* 2003; 104:550–558.

Seltzer Z, Dubner R, Shir Y. A novel behavioral model of neuropathic pain disorders produced in rats by partial sciatic nerve injury. *Pain* 1990; 43:205–218.

Wall PD, Scadding JW, Tomkiewicz MM. The production and prevention of experimental anesthesia dolorosa. *Pain* 1979; 6:175–182.

Woolf CJ. Evidence for a central component of post-injury pain hypersensitivity. *Nature* 1983; 306:686–688.

Woolf CJ, Thompson SW. The induction and maintenance of central sensitization is dependent on *N*-methyl-D-aspartic acid receptor activation; implications for the treatment of post-injury pain hypersensitivity states. *Pain* 1991; 44:293–299.

Woolfe G, MacDonald AD. The evaluation of the analgesic action of pethidine hydrochloride (Demerol). *J Pharmacol Exp Ther* 1944; 80:300–307.

Yaksh TL. Pharmacology and mechanisms of opioid analgesic activity. *Acta Anaesthesiol Scand* 1997; 41:94–111.

Yamamoto T, Yaksh TL. Comparison of the antinociceptive effects of pre- and posttreatment with intrathecal morphine and MK801, an NMDA antagonist, on the formalin test in the rat. *Anesthesiol* 1992; 77:757–763.

Yeomans DC, Proudfit HK. Nociceptive responses to high and low rates of noxious cutaneous heating are mediated by different nociceptors in the rat: electrophysiological evidence. *Pain* 1996; 68:141–150.

Yeomans DC, Pirec V, Proudfit HK. Nociceptive responses to high and low rates of noxious cutaneous heating are mediated by different nociceptors in the rat: behavioral evidence. *Pain* 1996; 68:133–140.

Correspondence to: Gary J. Bennett, PhD, Anesthesia Research Unit, 3655 Promenade Sir William Osler, McIntyre Building, Room 1202, Montreal, Quebec, Canada H3G 1Y6. Tel: 514-398-3432; Fax: 514-398-8241; email: gary. bennett@mcgill.ca.

The Paths of Pain 1975–2005, edited by
Harold Merskey, John D. Loeser, and Ronald
Dubner, IASP Press, Seattle, © 2005.

17

Sensory Quantification and Pain

Ulf Lindblom

*Department of Clinical Neurosciences, Section of Neurology, Karolinska
Institute and Gösta Ekman Laboratory for Sensory Research, Department
of Psychology, Stockholm University, Stockholm, Sweden*

Quantitative somatosensory testing (QST) developed from a background of existing techniques for measuring functions of the special senses of vision and hearing. More recently, psychophysicists have provided validated methods for the scaling of perceptions in general (Ekman and Sjöberg 1965; Berglund 1991; Borg 1994). The psychophysics of pain, including quantification of experimental pain in normal subjects and of clinical pain in some patient groups, was explored in pioneering studies by Wolff et al. (1943), Hardy et al. (1952), and Beecher (1959). Studies both in animal models and in pain patients have been widely extended during the ensuing decades.

Validated methods for quantifying the magnitude of suprathreshold pain in neurologically healthy individuals were developed by leading psychologists such as Gracely et al. (1994), while neurophysiologists and clinical neuroscientists studied patients with neuropathic pain. A detailed review of the state of the art of somatosensation and pain as of 1993 is presented in the proceedings from a multidisciplinary international symposium organized at the Wenner-Gren Center in Stockholm and published by IASP Press (Boivie et al. 1994). The 31 presentations at this meeting were organized into the following five sections: basic and applied psychophysics, quantitative sensory testing in health and disease, peripheral and central mechanisms of sensitization, models of sensory alterations and their assessment, and central processing. At the same time, a consensus report on quantitative sensory testing was published in *Neurology* by the Peripheral Neuropathy Association (Dyck et al. 1993).

This chapter reviews physiological and clinical aspects of sensory quantification as initiated and developed by myself and many coworkers in the Department of Neurology of the Karolinska Institute, in close collaboration with Björn Meyerson of the Department of Neurosurgery and Staffan Arnér of the Department of Anesthesiology. Increasing focus has centered on the application of sensory quantification in pain patients and particularly on its use in evaluating the somatosensory profiles of neuropathic pain. I myself witnessed an increasing majority of pain patients among the referrals to the Somatosensory Laboratory at the Department of Neurology, and after my retirement Per Hansson took over as head of the now independent Neurogenic Pain Unit. The various clinical and basic scientists involved in pain management and research at "Karolinska" initiated the Karolinska Institute Center for Pain Research in 1993.

In pain research and management it is important to record not only *quantitative* but also *qualitative* aberrations of evoked perceptions. In neuropathic pain, such aberrations may constitute a significant part of the patients' symptomatology and can be assessed in statistical terms. An early description of the often painful dysesthesias in neuropathic pain was presented by Mitchell in 1872, followed by an account by Foerster (1927), who termed these symptoms "hyperpathia." In addition to abnormal quality and magnitude of evoked perceptions, neuropathic patients report abnormal spread or dislocation of pain, as well as a temporal distortion with abnormal latency, summation of repeated stimuli, and aftersensation (Noordenbos 1959; Lindblom 1979, 1985; Lindblom and Verrillo 1979). Any research protocol for application in pain patients should include scaling and recording of ongoing pain before, during, and after testing, such as by means of the most commonly used visual analogue technique.

MECHANORECEPTION

TOUCH

Mechanical exteroreceptors sensitive to touch typically require deformation at a minimum speed, "critical slope," for evocation of impulse discharge, and are rapidly adapting (Lindblom 1958, 1965, 1974). The perception of touch is thus tested with dynamic stimuli such as a superficial stroke on the skin with a pencil, soft brush, or finger. Stimulus quantification is ascertained in terms of width and bending pressure of the brush moved at a standardized rate and distance on the skin. Hypo- or hyperesthesia can be quantified by numerical scaling, for example, on a 0–10-point scale, or by free magnitude estimation (Berglund and Harju 2003). Identical testing of unaffected skin, often performed contralaterally, should routinely be done for comparison. The validity of contralateral testing is usually acceptable in the clinical routine, but it may be scientifically invalid because of systemic dysnociception in patients with conditions such as fibromyalgia (Berglund et al. 2002) or in connection with subacute musculoskeletal nociception (Kosek and Ordeberg 2000b). Berglund et al. (1997) used the individual power functions for the unaffected thenar to transform the perceived intensity scales to a common unit of measurement. Qualitative perceptual aberrations of affected skin (paresthesias and dysesthesias) should be recorded by selecting from a list of common perceptual abnormalities or from a list of the patient's freely chosen descriptors.

The first clinical study I conducted after receiving my doctorate in physiology was in patients with classical trigeminal neuralgia and constitutes an early example of sensory quantification and clinical pain. The study was performed in collaboration with Professor Eric Kugelberg, who was then head of the Department of Neurology at the Royal Serafimer Hospital in Stockholm (Kugelberg and Lindblom 1959). The aim was to study the mechanisms of the pain attacks by applying quantified mechanical stimuli at the patients' pain trigger zones. These zones, found by careful probing with a fingertip or von Frey filament, were most often located in the nasolabial furrow. The patients' pain attacks were typically evoked by dynamic mechanical stimuli such as touch, chewing, and talking, but not by slowly pinching the skin, by maintaining pressure, or by applying warmth or cold, even at normally painful temperatures.

Stimulus quantification was ascertained by means of finger strokes with standardized repetition rates (Fig. 1, top) or by pulses from a mechanical stimulator with variable amplitude, frequency, and duration (Fig. 1, bottom). The stimulator had been developed in my thesis work on excitability and functional organization within a peripheral tactile unit (Lindblom 1958). Stimulus quantification enabled us to characterize the pathophysiology of trigeminal pain attacks in terms of critical rate and amplitude of pain provoking skin displacement, spatiotemporal summation, and post-attack refractoriness. The latter was a consequence of the pain rather than of the provoking stimulus. During the first part of the refractory state, not even strong stimuli could provoke pain, which some patients had discovered and used to their advantage, such as by using the temporary respite as an opportunity to chew vigorously without pain. Thereafter, the refractoriness gradually faded, as illustrated by the relation of stimulus frequency to the attack interval in Fig. 1 (top). Fig. 1 (bottom panel) illustrates the successive prolongation of temporal summation of the vibratory stimulus required to elicit a pain attack during intravenous (i.v.) lidocaine infusion until the final block occurred. A molecular biologist might interpret these induced excitability changes in terms of abnormal sodium channels as a possible basis of tic douloureux (Black et al. 2001).

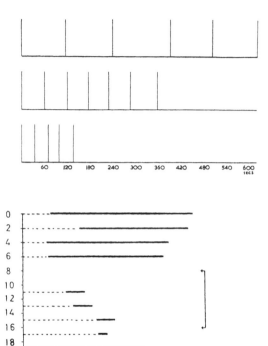

Fig 1. The top panel displays three series of trigeminal pain attacks illustrating relative refractoriness in a patient resting horizontally: upper row, "spontaneous" attacks every second minute, i.e., without apparent external stimulus; middle row, doubling of attack frequency during finger stroking of trigger area at the rate of three strokes per second; further increase of attack frequency during finger stroking at the rate of 6 strokes per second. The bottom panel shows successive blockade of trigeminal neuralgia during i.v. lidocaine 2 mg/kg (between arrows). Top records before injection: minute-long pain attacks evoked every other minute by vibratory stimulation in the trigger zone. Note successive prolongation of stimulation for evoking pain during the infusion and shortening of attack length until total blockade. (From Kugelberg and Lindblom 1959.)

Pain evoked by touch or by other innocuous stimulation of uninflamed skin, as in patients with trigeminal neuralgia, was later termed "allodynia" in the IASP taxonomy (Merskey 1979; Merskey and Bogduk 1994). Tic douloureux may thus be classified as a special case of allodynic pain. However, the term "allodynia" was adopted to cover more common situations such as mechanical allodynia (to touch or light pressure) or thermal allodynia (most often to cold) in cases of peripheral neuralgia, spinal cord injury pain, and post-stroke pain.

POINTED TOUCH: VON FREY FILAMENTS
OR MECHANICAL STIMULATORS

Von Frey's classical means of quantifying touch by means of a series of hairs or, nowadays, nylon filaments of different calibers and preferably with logarithmically spaced bending pressures, are still widely used for quantification of sensitivity to touch and pressure. The perception threshold is the most commonly assessed parameter in human subjects; in animal studies the equivalent is the threshold for withdrawal or other specified reactions. Nylon filaments have the disadvantage of variable bending pressures due to variations in air moisture or temperature; the use of glass fibers can eliminate this source of error (Fruhstorfer et al. 2001).

Suprathreshold testing of touch and pressure perception is feasible with von Frey filaments with bending pressures up to about 15 g, with variations depending upon the softness and innervation density of various body regions and on the shape of the particular filament ends, which may be sharply cut or rounded. Coactivation of nociceptors may occur with as little as 5 g of pressure in soft skin regions; thus, the stimulation may elicit not only touch but a pricking component. This situation implies that psychophysical functions may not be strictly tactile and underlines the importance of recording the perceptual character of each stimulation. It becomes particularly important in neuropathic pain patients, in whom perceptual distortions are common constituents of the typical sensory abnormalities (Lindblom and Verrillo 1979; Lindblom 1985). The most common intraindividual reference when testing with von Frey filaments is provided by stimulation at the corresponding contralateral and supposedly unaffected location.

Electromagnetic devices producing mechanical pulses of a particular wave form may also be used to quantify perception threshold and determine the suprathreshold intensity function of touch and pressure (Lindblom 1976).

TACTILE DISCRIMINATION

Studies on human subjects enable assessment of discriminative touch by testing two-point discrimination or figure writing.

VIBRATION

The vibratory sense, predominantly mediated by Pacinian corpuscles (and to some extent by Meissner's end organs and hair follicle endings), is a sensitive and useful parameter for the quantitative neurological assessment of neuropathic conditions, including mono- and polyneuropathies, and sometimes of central nervous system (CNS) lesions. Quantitative testing of the vibratory sense does not appear to have been widely applied in clinical pain contexts. However, a potentially interesting application might be to test, in pain patients with mechanical allodynia to touch or pressure, whether the allodynia involves the Pacinian corpuscle large-fiber system.

PRESSURE

Electromagnetic devices with blunt-ended probes, or forceps with flat surfaces, are used to record pressure applied to soft tissues. This established technique is now used worldwide to quantify threshold or suprathreshold functions of pressure and pain sensitivity. In order to reduce variability of response, a number of standard regional application sites have been selected for which normative values are available (Jensen 1990). In pain patients, various additional test sites may have to be selected depending upon the regional distribution of the particular painful disorder under study.

I was involved in the development of the Swedish algometer technique, which started with an investigation of the pressure pain threshold in the temporal region of headache patients (Jensen et al. 1986). We used a cylindric plastic probe of 0.5 cm^2 contact area and a slightly rounded circular edge to avoid incisive tissue damage. Fig. 2 shows records from a patient with painful sciatic neuropathy to whom the blunt probe was applied to the sole of the foot. Note the slightly raised threshold of the right bottom trace,

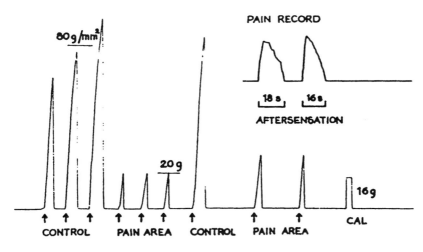

Fig. 2. Potentiometric recordings of pain thresholds and aftersensations in a patient with sciatic nerve causalgia. A blunt-ended pressure algometer was applied in the pain area (foot sole), where pain was elicited at an abnormally low pressure, 20 g/mm^2, compared with 80 g/mm^2 contralaterally. About 30 g/mm^2 pressure in the pain area evoked intense pain, with 16 to 18 seconds of aftersensation. (From Lindblom 1985.)

indicating neuropathic hypoesthesia but with allodynia, and the top record showing an abnormally prolonged painful response to slightly suprathreshold stimulation.

As an alternative to the blunt probe, a forceps with a flat grip may be used for pinching fingers, toes, ear flaps, or cutaneous folds in areas with suitably loose skin. Fig. 3 illustrates allodynia to pinching the skin in a patient with ulnar nerve neuropathy. This allodynia was blocked by dorsal column stimulation, after which the pain threshold was increased compared to that on the radial side as an expression of neuropathic hypoalgesia (from Hansson and Lindblom 1992).

The Swedish pressure algometer is commercially available, and the technique has been widely tested and is used internationally (Jensen 1990). Swedish researcher Eva Kosek has published several papers including her doctoral thesis (Kosek 1996), presenting pioneering findings on pressure pain thresholds as well as selected suprathreshold functions in fibromyalgia patients and in healthy control subjects. The enhanced pressure pain sensitivity in fibromyalgia patients was shown to be located deep to the skin and not restricted to muscle tissue. These findings indicated a dysfunction of endogenous modulation of nociceptive input rather than muscle pathology as the cause of the tenderness in fibromyalgia (Kosek et al. 1995). Furthermore, the fibromyalgia patients exhibited a generalized increase in deep and cutaneous pain sensitivity. This increased sensitivity was unrelated to spontaneously

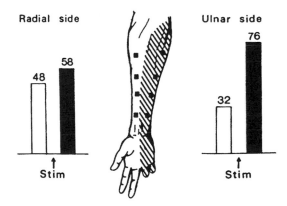

Fig. 3. In this patient with ulnar nerve neuralgia, examination with pinch algometry at sites indicated by filled squares and averaged (open bars, before treatment) revealed a lower pain threshold (32 g/mm^2) on the affected medial volar surface of the lower arm compared to the unaffected lateral volar part and corresponding sites of the contralateral arm, where it was 40–60 g/mm^2. After a 30-minute period of dorsal column stimulation, the ongoing pain was abolished and the pain threshold to pinch (filled bars) was significantly increased to 76 g/mm^2 in the pain area, reflecting a neuropathic loss, but it was not significantly altered in unaffected skin. (From Hansson and Lindblom 1992.)

ongoing pain and was most likely due to a CNS dysfunction (Kosek et al. 1996). Pressure pain sensitivity in fibromyalgia patients increased during and following isometric contraction, while it decreased in healthy subjects (Kosek and Ekholm 1995; Kosek et al. 1996a). On the other hand, no modulation of pressure pain sensitivity was found during the tourniquet test in fibromyalgia patients as opposed to healthy controls (Kosek et al. 1996b).

Further studies by Kosek and coworkers revealed how endogenous pain-regulating mechanisms such as heterotopic noxious conditioning stimulation (HNCS; Kosek and Hansson 1997) and diffuse noxious inhibitory control (DNIC) could be studied in clinical conditions such as fibromyalgia, rheumatoid arthritis, and painful osteoarthritis. These kinds of studies, based upon techniques of sensory quantification, can lead to useful findings and discussion of basic physiological relevance, provided that adequate protocols are applied.

For further reading on pressure algometry, see the publications by Jensen (1990) and Treede et al. (2002), as well as the recent discussion paper by Gracely et al. (2003). The latter includes the interesting suggestion that aborted DNIC may be one of the consequences of the apparently generic central dysnociception in fibromyalgia, as was demonstrated by Kosek and Ordeberg (2000a,b) and by Kosek and Lundberg (2003). In patients with systemically (and bilaterally) altered nociception, the usual easy technique of comparing sensory tests in a painful area with contralateral controls may not be valid, at least as far as nociceptive tests are concerned. Reference data on different unaffected body parts from healthy subjects of different ages (Harju 2002) are thus essential for the evaluation of patients who cannot be assumed to have unaffected body parts.

THERMOSENSIBILITY

THRESHOLDS

During the early 1970s it became progressively apparent, from a clinical neurological perspective, and particularly in the area of somatosensation and pain, that it is important to asses the thermal senses quantitatively as well as qualitatively.

Normally, in the resting stage, there is a neutral zone from about 30°C to about 32°C of skin temperature without ongoing thermal perception. The comfortably (hedonic) warm and cold perception zones are at skin temperatures up to 40°–45°C and down to 20°C, but above or below these zones, thermoreceptors signal heat pain or cold pain, respectively. For the clinical research setting it was apparent that a graded, more versatile, and less cumbersome and time-consuming methodology was needed than the commonly used application of radiant heat or heated or chilled objects.

At the meeting on sensory reception organized by the Academy of Sciences of the USSR in Leningrad in October of 1974, I met Heinrich Fruhstorfer from the Institute of Physiology of the University of Marburg. He was using the Peltier technique according to Kenshalo (1970) for cutaneous heating and cooling and a round, flat, metallic, water-circulated probe to measure reaction times to hot or cold stimuli applied to the skin. I described the Karolinska clinical sensory research laboratory designed for investigation of neurological patients, and we agreed to a joint project. A month later, Fruhstorfer arrived with his car packed with equipment. Our first clinical studies were conducted in patients with peripheral neuropathies such as uremic polyneuropathy or with central neuropathic conditions such as multiple sclerosis. These early studies convinced us that what we called the "Marstock technique" (from *Mar*burg and *Stock*holm), built on the Peltier principle, was a handy and versatile tool for the assessment of thermal sensitivity (Fruhstorfer et al. 1976a,b).

Several studies with the Marstock technique revealed important diagnostic uses in neurology, such as the previously undiagnosed small-fiber neuropathy in patients with Welander's hereditary myopathy (Borg et al. 1987). In polyneuropathies previously diagnosed as large-fiber neuropathy, or with other diagnoses such as inclusion body myositis, C-fiber sensory dysfunction was discovered (Arnardóttir et al. 2003). Ericson and Borg (1999) demonstrated sensory C-fiber loss in Charcot Marie Tooth disease type 2, which contradicted general belief (since type 1 is the demyelinative variant). The recovery of sensory functions after skin transplantation in patients with burn injuries could be studied more precisely with the Marstock technique than with other methods (Hermanson et al. 1986).

The Marstock technique successively spread internationally and was described by Verdugo and Ochoa (1992) as a key method for functional evaluation of small-caliber afferent channels. It is applicable in elderly patients as well as in juveniles and children (Hilz et al. 1998). The technique has further been successfully applied in multisymptomatic patients, such as the fraction of patients who demonstrate a positive neurological response to antiviral therapy in HIV (Martin et al. 2000) and to enzyme replacement therapy in Fabry's disease (Schiffmann et al. 2001).

In neuralgia patients, the functions of C and Aδ fibers could be evaluated and specified in terms of hypo- or hyperfunction as an important complement to the quantification of the large-fiber submodalities of touch and pressure. The functions of cold, warmth, and nociception could be recorded in terms of hypo- and hyperfunction as well as of qualitative dysfunction

(Lindblom and Verrillo 1979; Lindblom 1985, 1994). The Marstock record-ing in Fig. 4 is an illustrative example of the sensitivity of the method in neuropathic pain patients. In this patient with meralgia paresthetica, sensory dysfunction was dominated by pronounced cold allodynia (Lindblom 1985).

Fruhstorfer's thermal pulse stimulator was of interest to those dealing with pain patients with regard to the reaction time measurements and the possibility of differential diagnosis of neuralgic mechanisms as having a peripheral or cerebral location. Six neuralgia patients with hyperalgesia who were assessed by Lindblom and Verrillo (1979) by means of cold or warm pulses, and also by Lindblom (1974) using tactile pulses from the mechani-cal pulse stimulator, participated in a third trial using the thermal pulse stimulator (Fruhstorfer and Lindblom 1984). The patients reported all stimuli in the non-noxious ranges as painful, i.e., as allodynic. From the reaction time measurements, we concluded that the painful tactile stimuli had been

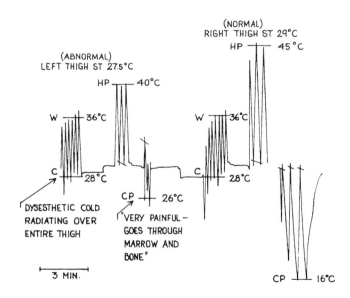

Fig. 4. Records of cutaneous thermal sensitivity in a patient with a common type of neuralgia (meralgia paresthetica). The trace shows the interface temperature between the thermode and the skin during stimulation. The current, which drives the temperature from the resting skin temperature where there is no stimulus-evoked sensation, is switched by the patient several successive times, first at the perception for warmth (W) and cold (C). The ensuing peaks at W and C thus indicate the perception thresholds of warmth and cold, 36° and 28°C, respectively, equal on both sides. The patient is then instructed to switch at the perception of pain on warm stimulation, which occurred at 45°C on the right side (normal) and 40°C on the pain side (hyperalgesia); with cold stimulation, pain was felt on the affected side at 26°C (allodynia) and on the control side at 16°C (normal). Note hyperpathic signs on the affected side, with dysesthetic perception with radiation at the cold threshold, and allodynic, radiating cold pain. (From Lindblom 1985.)

conducted in sensory A fibers and the painful cold stimuli in Aδ fibers. We determined that the painful nature of the responses in these patients were probably due to CNS processes, i.e., "central sensitization." The exciting topic of possible mechanisms of central sensitization cannot be presented in this brief chapter, but has been discussed in full in the recent IASP publication *Neuropathic Pain: Pathophysiology and Treatment* by Hansson et al. (2001).

The basis for the discussion of the CNS pathophysiology of somatosensory dysfunctions, such as the much-discussed role of thalamic lesions, has naturally improved significantly with new imaging techniques. Boivie et al. (1989) found that the extent and distribution of the lesion responsible for somatosensory dysfunction was quite varied, reporting that only two of nine cases with thalamic involvement had the lesion restricted to the thalamus. In the larger study on central post-stroke pain, Bowsher (1996), who was also one of the pioneers of quantitative sensory testing, and his colleagues (Bowsher et al. 1998) found the incidence of thalamic lesions to be as high as 60% in central post-stroke pain (CPSP). Different investigators agree that the crucial pathophysiology of CPSP is a more or less severe dysfunction of the somatosensory system, practically always due to an anatomical lesion. The different symptomatic expressions and clinical entities of central pain are comprehensively described in Boivie's review in the *Textbook of Pain* (1999), as well as in his recent personal tribute to quantitative sensory testing (Boivie 2003); see also his chapter in this volume for an overview.

SUPRATHRESHOLD TESTING

Modality-specific perception *thresholds* are easy to assess quantitatively once a versatile and suitably controlled stimulation technology has been established. The data can be statistically handled and easily related to normative data. From a clinical point of view, however, the threshold represents only one end of the sensory spectrum, whereas patients usually first notice *suprathreshold* sensory dysfunctions as constituents of daily life.

Suprathreshold screening of cutaneous sensibility is mandatory for proper neurological evaluation, both for clinical management and for assessing study criteria, as in the study by Berglund et al. (1997). The screening can be performed with time-saving and easily protocoled bedside techniques and is usually less time-consuming and often more informative than one particular sensory quantification procedure. For the patient, the screening serves as a rational introduction to the concept of diagnostic somatosensory testing. The screening procedure has been described with examples of protocols (Lindblom 1986), and may be summarized as follows. Bedside testing preferably starts with tactile stimulation by means of a soft pencil or the examiner's finger in the painful area, alternating with stimulation of unaffected skin for comparison and marking the area distribution of abnormal sensibility on a body scheme. Sensitivity to pinprick is tested by means of disposable needles or with a pricking pain-testing roller (unfortunately no longer commercially available). Thermal perception is best screened by means of two stainless steel rollers (Marchettini et al. 2003), one for warmth kept at about 43°C and the other kept at room temperature for cold stimulation.

Quantification of suprathreshold somatosensation presupposes a psychophysical protocol with a graded stimulation technique using the subject's magnitude estimation of the evoked perceptions. In my study with Ron Verrillo on patients with neuropathic pain (Lindblom and Verrillo 1979), we applied free magnitude estimation (with numbers) of the perception of mechanical stimulation of cutaneous low-threshold mechanoreceptors in the painful area. Graded intensity functions were obtained in all patients from both the painful area and the contralateral pain-free skin. Abnormally steep magnitude functions were revealed in the painful area of all patients. The slope of the subjective intensity functions averaged 0.80 for the pain areas compared to 0.51 for the control areas. The steepness was unrelated to the threshold magnitudes, but it demonstrated that the suprathreshold domain was also hyperpathic in addition to the threshold allodynia. This result had been anticipated based on the patients' anamnestic data and was further elucidated by the results with supraliminal heat pain stimuli and by the discussion by Hansson and Lindblom (1992).

Fig. 5 (reproduced from Lindblom and Ochoa 1992) illustrates schematically the principal suprathreshold abnormalities of common sensation, as can be assessed separately for each modality by means of selective mechanical, thermal, or nociceptive stimulation. Suprathreshold hypo- and hyperfunctions may both exist combined with normal threshold (thin line in panel A and thick line in panel C), with increased threshold (A), or with lowered threshold (thin line in panel C).

A systematic study with free magnitude estimation and master scaling according to Berglund (1991) was initiated in patients with neuropathic pain, and the results in the first 10 patients were described by Berglund et al. (1997). Fig. 6 reproduces the psychophysical functions for von Frey filament stimulation in two of the patients. Fig. 6A is from a 41-year-old man with neuralgia in the right hand after traumatic amputation of digits two through four. Stimulation was performed on the distal palm outside but adjacent to the territory of the injured digital nerves. The psychophysical function shows an increased sensation magnitude with tactile allodynia (filled diamonds), apparently inhibited by the stimulation with the thicker filaments.

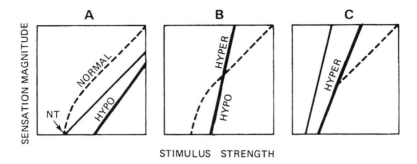

Fig. 5. Diagrammatic illustration of principal suprathreshold quantitative abnormalities, as can be assessed separately for each somatosensory modality by means of selective mechanical, thermal, or painful stimulation. Stimulus strength is plotted against subjective magnitude of sensation quantified by magnitude estimation. Normal intensity functions (hatched lines) are typically power functions. NT on the abscissa indicates normal threshold. Thick solid lines represent observed functions of hypoalgesia, mixed hypo- and hyperalgesia, and hyperalgesia, respectively. Thin solid lines represent hypothetical functions of hypoalgesia with retained threshold in part A, and hyperalgesia with lowered threshold in part C. (From Lindblom and Ochoa 1992.)

Fig. 6B is from a 52-year-old woman with left-sided postoperative intercostal neuralgia. The psychophysical function shows an increased sensation magnitude with tactile allodynia for all stimulations in the pain-affected area. The frequency of various descriptors chosen by the 10 patients was significantly abnormal for all tactile stimulation at the painful area (these results were confirmed in 21 patients by Berglund et al. 2001).

A more recent study by Berglund et al. (2002) was concerned with perceptual analysis of cold dysesthesia and hyperalgesia in fibromyalgia. Fibromyalgia patients displayed a characteristic distortion of their sensory processing of cold, including paradoxical burning sensations, while perceived quality for warmth was unaffected. It was speculated that dysfunctions in cold perception in fibromyalgia and post-stroke pain patients may be indicative of centrally induced pain conditions (Berglund et al. 1999).

CONCLUDING REMARKS

Although the IASP was not involved in the early development of sensory quantification, it rapidly became active in promoting the methodology for clinical application and studies as well as for animal experimentation on pain mechanisms.

The founding members of IASP appointed a taxonomy task force under the chairmanship of Harold Merskey, and the *Classification of Chronic Pain*

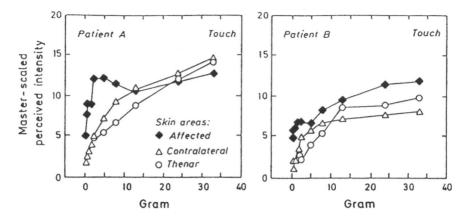

Fig. 6. Psychophysical functions for von Frey filament stimulations. Patient A was a 41-year-old man with neuralgia in the right hand after traumatic amputation of digits two through four. Stimulations were applied to the distal palm "extraterritorially" of the injured digital nerves. The psychophysical function shows an increased sensation magnitude with tactile allodynia (filled diamonds), apparently inhibited by the thicker filaments, with normal sensitivity at the contralateral side (open triangles) and at the thenar (open circles). Patient B was a 52-year-old woman with left-sided postoperative intercostal neuralgia. The psychophysical function shows an increased sensation magnitude with tactile allodynia for all stimulations in the pain-affected area (filled diamonds), with normal sensitivity contralaterally (open triangles) and at the thenar (open circles). The verbal descriptors "pricking" and "pain" were chosen by both patients for all stimulations in the pain area. (From Berglund et al. 1997.)

(with descriptions of chronic pain syndromes and definitions of pain terms) was published in 1986. This effort inspired the world-wide community of pain researchers and clinicians to use standardized terminology as an obligatory basis for the mutual understanding of clinical diagnoses and pain mechanisms, forming the foundations of the common language that is used today at most pain clinics.

With the application of the IASP taxonomy, pain-related somatosensory dysfunctions came into focus as well. In particular, data were forthcoming on abnormal pain evoked by low grades of touch, pressure, and thermal stimulation, now known as allodynia (Merskey 1979, 1986; Merskey and Bogduk 1994). The term "dysesthesia," which formerly could include painful perceptions, is now recommended for qualitatively abnormal threshold or suprathreshold perceptions that are not painful.

ACKNOWLEDGMENTS

This work was supported by funds from the Karolinska Institutet and by a grant from the Swedish Foundation for Health Care Sciences and Allergy Research.

REFERENCES

Arnardóttir S, Svanborg E, Borg K. Inclusion body myositis—sensory dysfunction revealed with quantitative determination of somatosensory thresholds. *Acta Neurol Scand* 2003; 107:1–6.

Beecher K (Ed). *Measurement of Subjective Responses.* New York: Oxford University Press, 1959.

Berglund B. Quality assurance in environmental psychophysics. In: Bolanowski SJ, Gescheider GA (Eds). *Ratio Scaling of Psychological Magnitudes—A Tribute to the Memory of S.S. Stevens.* Hillsdale, NJ: Erlbaum, 1991, pp 140–161.

Berglund B, Harju E.-L. Master scaling of perceived intensity of touch, cold and warmth. *Eur J Pain* 2003; 7:323–334.

Berglund B, Harju E-L, Lindblom U. Psychophysical testing of somatosensory functions in neuropathic pain patients. In: Jensen TS, Turner JA, Wiesenfeld-Hallin Z (Eds). *Proceedings of the 8th World Congress on Pain,* Progress in Pain Research and Management, Vol. 8. Seattle: IASP Press, 1997, pp 435–447.

Berglund B, Harju E-L, Kosek E, Lindblom U. Are dysfunctions in cold perception in fibromyalgia and post-stroke pain patients indicative of centrally induced pain conditions? In: Killen PR, Uttal WR (Eds). *Proceedings of the International Association for Applied Psychophysics.* Tempe, AZ: International Society for Psychophysics, 1999, pp 130–135.

Berglund B, Harju E-L, Lindblom U. Peripheral and central neuropathic pain characterized by perceived quality and magnitude of touch, cold and warmth. *Arch Center Sensory Res* 2001; 6:(2)31–53.

Berglund B, Harju E-L, Kosek E, Lindblom U. Quantitative and qualitative perceptual analysis of cold dysesthesia and hyperalgesia in fibromyalgia. *Pain* 2002; 96:177–187.

Black JA, Dib-Hajj S, Cummins TR, et al. Sodium channels as therapeutic targets in neuropathic Pain. In: Hansson PT, Fields HL, Hill RG, Marchettini (Eds). *Neuropathic Pain: Pathophysiology and Treatment,* Progress in Pain Research and Management, Vol. 21. Seattle: IASP Press, 2001, pp 19–36.

Boivie J. Central pain. In: Wall PD, Melzack R (Eds). *Textbook of Pain,* 4th ed. Edinburgh: Churchill Livingstone, 1999, pp 879–914.

Boivie J. Central pain and the role of quantitative sensory testing (QST) in research and diagnosis. *Eur J Pain* 2003; 7:339–343.

Boivie J, Leijon G, Johansson I. Central post-stroke pain—a study of the mechanisms through analyses of the sensory abnormalities. *Pain* 1989; 37(2):173–185.

Boivie J, Hansson P, Lindblom U (Eds). *Touch, Temperature, and Pain in Health and Disease: Mechanisms and Assessments,* Progress in Pain Research and Management, Vol. 3. Seattle: IASP Press, 1994.

Borg G. Psychophysical scaling: an overview. In: Boivie J, Hansson P, Lindblom U (Eds). *Touch, Temperature, and Pain in Health and Disease: Mechanisms and Assessments,* Progress in Pain Research and Management, Vol. 3. Seattle: IASP Press, 1994, pp 27–39.

Borg K, Borg J, Lindblom U. Sensory involvement in distal myopathy (Welander). *J Neurol Sci* 1987; 80:323–332.

Bowsher D. Central pain: clinical and physiological characteristics. *J Neurol Neurosurg Psychiatry* 1996; 61:62–69.

Bowsher D, Leijon G, Thuomas K-Å. Central post-stroke pain: correlation of magnetic resonance imaging with clinical pain characteristics and sensory abnormalities. *Neurology* 1998; 51:1352–1358.

Dyck PJ, et al. Quantitative sensory testing: a consensus report from the Peripheral Neuropathy Association. *Neurology* 1993; 43:1050–1052.

Ekman G, Sjöberg L. Scaling. *Ann Rev Psychol* 1965; 16:451–474.

Ericson U, Borg K. Analysis of sensory function in Charcot-Marie-Tooth disease. *Acta Neurol Scand* 1999; 99:291–296.

Foerster O. *Die Leitungsbanen des Schmerzgefühls.* Vienna: Urban & Schwarzenberg, 1927.

Fruhstorfer H, Lindblom U. Sensory abnormalities in neuralgic patients studied by thermal and tactile pulse stimulation. In: von Euler C, Franzén O, Lindblom U, Ottoson D (Eds). *Somatosensory Mechanisms,* Wenner-Gren International Symposium Series, Vol. 41. London: Macmillan Press, 1984, pp 353–361.

Fruhstorfer H, Lindblom U, Schmidt WG. Method for quantitative estimation of thermal thresholds in patients. *J Neurol Neurosurg Psychiatry* 1976a; 39:1071–1075.

Fruhstorfer H, Goldberg JM, Lindblom U, Schmidt WG. Temperature sensitivity and pain thresholds in patients with peripheral neuropathy. In: Zotterman Y (Ed). *Sensory Functions of the Skin,* Wenner-Gren International Symposium Series, Vol. 27. Stockholm: Pergamon Press, 1976b, pp 507–519.

Fruhstorfer H, Gross W, Selbmann O. von Frey hairs: new materials for a new design. *Eur J Pain* 2001; 5(3):341–342.

Gracely RH. Studies of pain in normal man. In: Wall PD, Melzack R (Eds). *Textbook of Pain,* 3rd ed. Edinburgh: Churchill Livingstone, 1994, pp 315–336.

Gracely RH, Grant MAB, Giesecke T. Evoked pain measures in fibromyalgia. *Best Pract Res Clin Rheumatol* 2003; 17:593–609.

Hansson P, Lindblom U. Hyperalgesia assessed with quantitative sensory testing (QST) in patients with neurogenic pain. In: Willis WD Jr (Ed). *Hyperalgesia and Allodynia.* New York: Raven Press, 1992, pp 335–343.

Hansson P, Fields H, Hill R, Marchettini P (Eds). *Neuropathic Pain: Pathophysiology and Treatment,* Progress in Pain Research and Management, Vol. 21. Seattle: IASP Press, 2001, pp 1–277.

Hardy JD, Wolff HG, Goodell H. *Pain Sensations and Reactions.* Baltimore: Williams and Wilkins, 1952.

Harju E-L. Quantitative and qualitative analysis of touch, cold and warmth in health, neuropathic pain and fibromyalgia. Dissertation. Stockholm: Department of Psychology, Stockholm University, 2001.

Harju E-L. Cold and warmth perception mapped for age, gender, and body area. *Somatosens Mot Res* 2002; 19(1):61–75.

Hermanson A, Jonsson C-E, Lindblom U. Sensibility after burn injury. *Clin Physiol* 1986; 6:507–521.

Hilz MJ, Stemper B, Schweibold G, et al. Quantitative thermal perception testing in 225 children and juveniles. *J Clin Neurophysiol* 1991; 15:529–534.

Jensen K. Quantification of tenderness by palpation and use of pressure algometers. In: Friction JR, Award A (Eds). *Myofascial Pain and Fibromyalgia,* Advances in Pain Research and Therapy, Vol. 17. New York: Raven Press, 1990, pp 167–181.

Jensen K, Orbeak-Andersen H, Olesen J, Lindblom U. Pressure-pain-threshold in human temporal region. Evaluation of a new pressure-algometer. *Pain* 1986; 25:313–323.

Kenshalo DR. Psychophysical studies of temperature sensitivity. In: Neff WD (Ed). *Contributions to Sensory Physiology,* Vol. 4. New York: Academic Press, 1970, pp 17–74.

Kosek E. Somatosensory dysfunction in fibromyalgia. Doctoral thesis. Stockholm, 1996.

Kosek E, Ekholm J. Modulation of pressure pain thresholds during and following isometric contraction. *Pain* 1995; 61:481–486.

Kosek E, Ordeberg G. Lack of pressure pain modulation by heterotopic noxious conditioning stimulation in patients with painful osteoarthritis before, but not following, surgical pain relief. *Pain* 2000a; 88:69–78.

Kosek E, Ordeberg G. Abnormalities of sensory perception in patients with painful osteoarthritis normalize following successful treatment. *Eur J Pain* 2000b; 4:229–238.

Kosek E, Hansson P. Modulatory influence on somatosensory perception from vibration and heterotopic noxious conditioning stimulation (HNCS) in fibromyalgia patients and healthy subjects. *Pain* 1997; 70:41–51.

Kosek E, Lundberg L. Segmental and plurisegmental modulation of pressure pain thresholds during static muscle contractions in healthy individuals. *Eur J Pain* 2003; 7:251–258.

Kosek E, Ekholm J, Hansson P. Increased pressure pain sensibility in fibromyalgia patients is located deep to the skin but not restricted to muscle tissue. *Pain* 1995; 63:335–339.

Kosek E, Ekholm J, Hansson P. Sensory dysfunction in fibromyalgia patients with implications for pathogenetic mechanisms. *Pain* 1996; 68:375–383.

Kugelberg E, Lindblom U. The mechanism of the pain in trigeminal neuralgia. *J Neurol Neurosurg Psychiatry* 1959; 22:36–43.

Lindblom U. Excitability and functional organization within a peripheral tactile unit. *Acta Physiol Scand* 1958; 44(Suppl 153):1–84.

Lindblom U. Properties of touch receptors in distal glabrous skin of the monkey. *J Neurophysiol* 1965; 28:966–985.

Lindblom U. Touch perception threshold in human glabrous skin in terms of displacement amplitude on stimulation with single mechanical pulses. *Brain Res* 1974; 82:205–210.

Lindblom U. Touch perception threshold in terms of amplitude and rate of skin deformation. In: Iggo, Ilyinsky (Eds). *Somatosensory and Visceral Receptor Mechanisms,* Progress in Brain Research, Vol. 43. Amsterdam: Elsevier, 1976, pp 233–236.

Lindblom U. Sensory abnormalities in neuralgia. In: Bonica JJ, Liebeskind JC, Albe-Fessard DG (Eds). *Proceedings of the Second World Congress on Pain, Advances in Pain Research and Therapy,* Vol. 3. New York: Raven Press, 1979, pp 111–120.

Lindblom U. Assessment of abnormal evoked pain in neurological pain patients and its relation to spontaneous pain: a descriptive and conceptual model with some analytical results. In: Fields HL, et al. (Eds). *Proceedings of the Fourth World Congress on Pain,* Advances in Pain Research and Therapy, Vol. 9. New York: Raven Press, 1985, pp 409–423.

Lindblom U. Clinical and instrumental diagnostic approaches to sensory disturbances in diabetic peripheral neuropathy. In: Asal et al. (Eds). *Diabetes Research and Clinical Practice,* Vol. 2. 1986, pp 213–225.

Lindblom U. Analysis of abnormal touch, pain and temperature sensation in patients. In: Boivie J, Hansson P, Lindblom U (Eds). *Touch, Temperature, and Pain in Health and Disease: Mechanisms and Assessments,* Progress in Pain Research and Management, Vol. 3. Seattle: IASP Press, 1994, pp 63–84.

Lindblom U, Ochoa J. Somatosensory function and dysfunction. In: Asbury AK, McKhann GM, McDonald WI (Eds). *Clinical Neurobiology,* 2nd ed, Diseases of the Nervous System, Vol. 1. Philadelphia: WB Saunders, 1992, pp 213–228.

Lindblom U, Verrillo RT. Sensory functions in chronic neuralgia. *J Neurol Neurosurg Psychiatry* 1979; 42:422–435.

Marchettini P, Maranboni C, Lacerenza M, Formaglio F. The Lindblom roller. *Eur J Pain* 2003; 7:359–364.

Martin C, Solders G, Sönnerborg A, Hansson P. Antiretroviral therapy may improve sensory function in HIV-infected patients. *Neurology* 2000; 54:2120–2127.

Merskey H. Pain terms: a current list with definitions and notes on usage. *Pain* 1979; 6:249–252.

Merskey H. Pain terms: a supplementary note. *Pain* 1982; 14:205–206.

Merskey H (Ed). Classification of chronic pain. *Pain* 1986; (Suppl 3):1–225.

Merskey H, Bogduk N. *Classification of Chronic Pain: Descriptions of Chronic Pain Syndromes and Definitions of Pain Terms,* 2nd ed. Seattle: IASP Press, 1994.

Mitchell SW. *Injuries of Nerves and Their Consequences.* Philadelphia: Lippincott, 1872.

Noordenbos W. *Pain.* Amsterdam: Elsevier, 1959.

Schiffmann R, Kopp JB, Austin HA, et al. Enzyme replacement therapy in Fabry disease: a randomized controlled trial. *JAMA* 2001; 285:2743–2749.

Treede R-D, Rolke R, Andrews K, Magerl W. Topical review: pain elicited by blunt pressure: neurobiological basis and clinical relevance. *Pain* 2002; 98:235–240.

Verdugo R, Ochoa JL. Quantitative somatosensory thermotest. A key method for functional evaluation of small calibre afferent channels. *Brain* 1992; 115:893–913.

Wolff HG, Gasser HS, Hinsey JC (Eds). *Pain*, Association for Research in Nervous and Mental Diseases, Vol. 23. Baltimore: Williams & Wilkins, 1943.

Correspondence to: Ulf Lindblom, MD, DMSc, Department of Clinical Neurosciences, Karolinska Institutet, Djursholmsvaegen 90, SE-18357 Taeby, Sweden. Tel: 46-8-756-6040; Fax: 46-8-756-8028; email: ulf.lindblom@knv.ki.se.

The Paths of Pain 1975–2005, edited by
Harold Merskey, John D. Loeser, and Ronald
Dubner, IASP Press, Seattle, © 2005.

18

Evaluation of Pain Sensations

Richard H. Gracely

*Chronic Pain and Fatigue Research Center, Departments of Internal Medicine,
Rheumatology and Neurology, University of Michigan
and VA Medical Center, Ann Arbor, Michigan, USA*

The history of the assessment of pain sensation can be divided into clinical and laboratory studies. Clinical pioneers investigated the neural ramifications of disease with tools that still find use in conventional neurological examinations: a pin, a cotton swab, a tuning fork, and cooled and heated objects. In the laboratory, psychophysicists collected data on the relation between physical stimulus intensity and the magnitude of stimulus-evoked sensations. The methods used in the clinic and laboratory defined two ends of a continuum. The clinical measures by necessity must be brief, since an evaluation usually includes multiple modalities and many areas of the body. Laboratory methods enjoy the luxury of focusing on a single area and may deliver hundreds, if not thousands, of trials in the quest for stability and accuracy. As described below, this distinction between the methods has been the impetus for many studies and spawned the methods of quantitative sensory assessment (QST).

IASP'S FIRST DECADE: THE APPLICATION OF SENSORY DECISION THEORY TO PAIN ASSESSMENT

Regarding the laboratory psychophysical methods of his day, William James considered the protocol utterly tedious: "This method taxes patience to the utmost" (Boring 1950). For anyone observing the development of pain measurement methods in the late 1970s and early 1980s, the field of pain psychophysics was far from boring. Investigators argued passionately about their viewpoints, and heated debates often approached personal attacks. Meetings were very exciting, and the nuances of measuring pain were major topics of the day. I remember fondly an evening in an entertainment

271

suite at IASP's 1978 World Congress in Montreal. The sponsors had left, leaving myself, another pain psychophysicist (Gary Rollman), and a future president of IASP (Barry Sessle) alone with a full bar. A lively discussion of sensory decision theory and pain measurement continued until dawn.

Sensory decision theory, or signal detection theory (SDT), is concerned with a persistent problem in the analysis of stimulus-evoked sensations (Swets 1964). Although it is often conveniently assumed that ratings of sensory intensity indicate the magnitude of the sensations, SDT recognizes that the path from stimulation to response represents at least two processes. One is the intensity of the stimulus-evoked sensation, and the other is the magnitude of the response chosen to indicate this intensity. Thus, in a pain experiment, a rating of pain reflects both the experience of pain and the particular label used to describe this experience. Investigators are interested in the first, sensory, variable, while the second, labeling, variable is considered to be a nuisance factor that must be carefully controlled by experimental design in order to assess the important sensory factor. If not controlled, the response can be biased by this second factor, referred to as response bias. In a study of pain analgesics, for example, the experience of drug side effects may suggest to subjects that they have received the active drug and not a placebo, and this knowledge may lead to both conscious or unconscious changes in the response to an otherwise unaltered stimulus-evoked sensation.

In SDT theory, this second variable is not a nuisance but rather an important variable that describes a component of a judgment process. In this context, this variable is called the response criterion (and changes in it may be referred to as response bias), representing labeling behavior that is assumed to be independent of the first variable. This first variable is termed discrimination sensitivity and is often symbolized by a parametric parameter represented as d'.

The role of response bias in pain assessment in particular and in psychophysical assessment in general is a major problem in sensory assessment. The methodology of modern psychophysical procedures is designed to control for the effects of common factors that can bias the result. This is especially true for pain assessment, in which a determination of pain can be influenced by a wide variety of situational factors in the experimental situation and by both trait and state characteristics of the individual.

It is conceivable that this emphasis on the malleability of pain response contributed to the widespread distrust of subjective pain reports, and in the 1970s, to attitudes that pain was a minor, "second-class" problem, paling in comparison to "real" medical problems such as cancer and heart disease. How can one believe a person's report of pain when this report is so easily modified by so many factors?

SDT stepped in with the answer. One could apply the method of SDT assessment to a psychophysical study and be able to separate out the wheat from the chaff, the true pain sensation from the bothersome effects of response bias. A group of studies reported effects entirely consistent with this concept. SDT was used to evaluate both the influence of placebo and the influence of a number of active interventions including nitrous oxide, diazepam, morphine, acupuncture, and transcutaneous electrical nerve stimulation (Chapman and Feather 1973; Chapman et al. 1973, 1975, 1976; Clark and Yang 1974; Yang et al. 1979). Placebo produced only a shift in the response criterion, while the active drugs and interventions reduced d' with variable effects on the response criterion.

This methodology made sense, and it seemed that the thorny problem of response bias had been solved. Indeed, my own (first) dissertation project was designed to apply SDT to electrical-stimulation-induced responses in patients with low back pain before and after a behavioral treatment program. However, as with all innovative theories, opposing views quickly emerged.

The major criticism was provided by Rollman (1977), who spent a sabbatical semester writing a critique of the SDT approach. Chapman (1977) provided a detailed reply. Rollman and Chapman agreed about the power of the SDT approach and about the body of evidence provided by this method. The main issue was one of interpretation; Rollman argued that the parameters of discriminability and response criterion could not be equated with pain sensitivity and response bias. This lively exchange generated a good deal of discussion, with the criticism boiling down to a few points (Gracely and Naliboff 1996; Gracely et al. 2004). First, discrimination of pain sensations involves both sensory magnitude and a number of other factors (Rollman 1977; Coppola and Gracely 1983). Discrimination is based on sensory magnitude, variability ("noise") in the sensory system, and variability in choosing labels to describe sensation.

Second, pain is not a simple, pure sensation varying only in intensity. The McGill Pain Questionnaire (Melzack 1975) is based on the concept that pain has many qualities and both evaluative and affective components. The discrimination between sensations could be based on any of these dimensions, such as radiation or temporal characteristics, in addition to pain magnitude (Gracely 1994).

Third, instead of indicating response bias, a change in the response criterion could indicate actual analgesia. The IASP definition of analgesia is an elimination of pain, while anesthesia represents a change in sensitivity to nonpainful sensation. Since pain is defined as a feeling of hurt (with both sensory and affective components), an intervention that reduces the affective, unpleasant aspect of a pain sensation could conceivably result in a change in the response criterion without a change in the discrimination of pain sensations evoked by different levels of painful stimulation.

SDT methodology has resulted in a body of psychophysical evidence in studies ranging from analyses of placebo, acupuncture, and morphine analgesia to comparisons of experimental pain sensitivity between chronic pain patients and healthy control subjects (see references above). The debate focuses attention on issues of pain assessment with beneficial results. Occasionally the issues resurface, as in the recent exchange of letters by Clark (2004) and Gracely et al. (2004). Further clarification will come from future studies that objectively assess these issues rather than advocate a particular position (Gracely et al. 2004).

SCALING CONFUSION

SDT measures of pain sensitivity are based on confusion. Given two different intensities of a painful stimulus, a more sensitive person will confuse them less. Similarly, a person in a state of increased sensitivity will confuse them less than when in a state of decreased sensitivity such as analgesia or cognitive impairment. This concept is not new. It formed the basis of a number of scaling methods before the advent of SDT. Confusion is intimately associated with one of the fundamental properties of perception. This property was identified and refined by the very psychophysicists that William James associated with boredom (Boring 1950). Weber developed the concept that the amount of energy in a stimulus needed to produce a noticeable increase in the stimulus-evoked sensation was some proportion of the stimulus intensity. He termed this difference the "just noticeable difference" (JND) and proposed Weber's law, which states that the percentage increase in a stimulus needed to notice a difference is a constant independent of stimulus intensity. Fechner essentially integrated this formula to provide the logarithmic law (i.e., perceived intensity is related to the logarithm of the stimulus intensity), which forms the basis of ratio scaling methods described below.

Borrowing directly from the work of Weber, Hardy et al. (1948) devised a scale of pain that was based on the JND of pain sensations evoked by radiant heat. The basic concept of this type of scale is that the amount of increased stimulus energy needed to produce a noticeable change in the evoked sensation is proportional to the level of the stimulus. To use an example from vision, a relatively small increase is needed for the observer to notice an increase in the light from the flame of a candle, while a considerable increase is needed for the observer to notice a change in the light from a car headlight. Hardy et al. (1948) defined the "dol" as 2 JNDs, and determined that the range of human perception for painful radiant heat was about 11 dols. The use of discrimination/confusion to form a unit of measurement underlies the SDT methods described above; it is directly related to older discrimination-based scaling procedures developed by Thurstone (1959), such as the paired comparisons and successive categories methods. These methods determine the psychological closeness between stimuli by the amount that they are confused. These methods, which have been rarely used in pain assessment (LaMotte and Campbell 1978), are also related to the more modern item response theory. Item response theory can be used to examine the discriminative capacity of specific items in a pain measurement questionnaire, either for elimination of poor items in subsequent scale development or for weighting the responses to more discriminative items (McArthur et al. 1989).

One of the major problems with confusion scales is an operational problem. There must be some confusion between stimuli to assess the difference between them. Increased sensitivity, defined as less confusion, must still have some confusion for the scaling system to work. Stimuli that are never confused cannot be directly compared by these methods. Confusion scales can measure the difference between the equivalent brightness of one or two candles at some distance but cannot be used to distinguish between a candle and an ordinary room lamp, or between moonlight and sunlight. This problem is solved by direct scaling methods that can theoretically evaluate the effects of stimuli regardless of whether they are confused. One of the most influential methods was championed by S.S. Stevens (1975), who used a direct scaling method that he claimed produced true ratio scales of measurement. According to Stevens, ratio-level measurement was the highest of four classes: (1) nominal, identifying names with no metric information, such as football jersey numbers; (2) ordinal, identifying ranks with no information about distances between values, as finishing first, second, and third in a race; (3) interval, a scale with equal units with no meaningful zero point, such as the Fahrenheit temperature scale; and (4) ratio scales, which have both a true zero point and a defined interval, corresponding to physical scales such as length and mass. To achieve ratio scaling measurement, Stevens's method instructed subjects to make ratio or proportional judgments, using a true unbounded response modality such as assignment of numbers, or a response modality that is pragmatically unlimited such as drawing lines of different length (given enough paper!) or the duration of a button press.

In contrast to the Stevens method, both many previous scales and current pain rating scales are constrained or bounded. Common scales such as category or visual analogue scales are constrained at the bottom by the absence of pain and at the top by a verbal category, number, or end of a line. Bounded scales have a number of potential disadvantages, although the effects of these disadvantages on pain measurement have not been evaluated in detail.

So what do ratio scales and power functions have to do with pain assessment? In developing verbal scales of pain, Gracely and colleagues used a modification of the ratio scaling methods of Tursky (1976) to determine the amount of pain associated with words or short phrases such as mild pain or slightly intense pain. After publication of a few such studies (Gracely et al. 1978a,b, 1979) followed by a brief lull in controversy, a report in *Pain* harshly criticized these studies and the overall approach of ratio scaling. This article (Hall 1981) and the rebuttal (Gracely et al. 1981) revived the fighting spirit of the SDT debates. As with the SDT controversy, this exchange enumerated important issues in pain assessment and brought attention to a number of issues that have improved pain evaluation. Today, most current studies use ratio techniques, including the use of quantified verbal descriptors and the numerous studies using the visual analogue scale, a bounded 10-cm line that possesses ratio scale properties (Price et al. 1983). Only these techniques allow statements of proportional effects such as "the pain was reduced by 50%," and these methods also allow proportional criteria for a clinical effect, such as a 30% reduction in reported pain. This debate also pointed out the danger of being wedded to only one technique, a characteristic especially true of investigators who develop pain assessment methods. Pain assessment can have many goals, from the evaluation of short-term postoperative analgesia to medicolegal determinations of disability. It is unlikely that a single tool is optimal for the breadth of measurement applications.

Pain psychophysics is a growing discipline pursued by an increasing group of talented investigators, many not cited here, who recognize that many of the goals of pain research can only be achieved through verbal descriptions of personal experience.

PAIN INTENSITY AND UNPLEASANTNESS

The discussion up to this point treats pain as a unidimensional variable, much like the loudness of a sound. This is not unusual, since most past and current studies focus on pain in this manner. However, this single dimension has been referred to by various names, the foremost being in terms of intensity or discomfort. Like sound, pain can be expressed in terms of a sensation, and also by a feeling of negative hedonic tone or aversiveness. Pain can be unpleasant, disagreeable, uncomfortable, distressing, or unbearable. Prior to the formation of the IASP in 1975, H.K. Beecher (1957) had emphasized the distinction between pain sensation and the "reaction component" in terms of response to analgesic drugs. This particular point was driven home by an experimental study of opioid action on pain evoked by electrical tooth-pulp stimulation in healthy control subjects (Gracely et al. 1979). Different groups of subjects rated either the intensity or unpleasantness of the stimulus-evoked sensations before and after an intravenous infusion of the potent opioid fentanyl or saline placebo. The venipuncture and infusion were performed in a different room, thus subjects had to be helped as they walked back to the testing room. The ambulation probably contributed to the frequent reports of nausea, which was regarded as a common occurrence after administering opioids to persons not in pain. The results were strikingly different. In comparison to placebo, the opioid significantly decreased the intensity of the pain sensations, while simultaneously increasing the unpleasantness of these sensations. The main result was that in an experiment optimized to discriminate between intensity and unpleasantness, these dimensions of pain, used commonly and almost interchangeably in previous studies, provided opposite results. Although the nausea evoked in the healthy controls may not reflect clinical situations of acute or chronic pain, this result suggested that these dimensions of pain are independent and that the choice of dimension can make a difference. The significant reduction in only the sensory intensity of the pain sensations was in stark contrast to the prevalent notion of the time. Beecher (1957) championed the position that opioids produce analgesia by reducing the unpleasant reaction component, leading to statements such as, "I still feel the pain but it does not bother me any more." No matter what the effects of opioids are on unpleasantness, this study with fentanyl contributed to the growing anatomical and physiological evidence that opioid analgesia includes a significant attenuation of the sensory discriminative aspects of pain (Gracely et al. 1979).

This study employed two strategies to maximize discrimination between the dimensions of intensity and unpleasantness. First, it used separate groups that rated only a single dimension. This aspect of the study was considered to be helpful because methods that assess both dimensions with one group could be vulnerable to a simple tactic in which subjects pair a sensory intensity response with an unpleasantness response (e.g., to be consistent, I will describe all mildly intense sensations as unpleasant, and intense sensations as slightly distressing). In this scenario, subjects rate the stimulus-evoked sensations by one dimension, then use an internal table to provide a rating for the other dimension. This internal table provides an artifactually increased correlation between the dimensions.

The second strategy to maximize discrimination between pain intensity and unpleasantness was to use verbal descriptor scales of each dimension, presented in randomized lists. The use of words describing a particular pain dimension were assumed to facilitate discrimination of that dimension, and the use of randomly ordered lists of words forced choices based on the meaning of words rather than on other irrelevant factors such as the position of the word in an ordered list. The reader can appreciate that, in the latter case, subjects do not even have to read the words, because they could simply remove their glasses if they wear glasses (or put some on if they do not) and just treat the scale as a visual analogue scale, picking a position along the spatial continuum provided by the list of items.

SCALING MULTIPLE DIMENSIONS OF PAIN EXPERIENCE: A DEDICATION TO WARREN S. TORGERSON

The modern era of using words to describe pain began with the work of Warren S. Torgerson, who authored a classic text on psychological scaling, published in 1958. I am grateful that, through the connection of one his students who worked in my laboratory, I had the opportunity to become acquainted with Warren and his thoughts about pain scaling. We often met on his farm, from which I would return with a head full of ideas and shopping bags full of apples and other Torgerson-grown produce. He passed away in 1999, but his ideas continue to influence pain assessment. Warren recognized the immense value of language in describing something as nefarious as pain. He and Ronald Melzack published a classic paper, "On the language of pain" (1971). This work not only acknowledged that pain included unpleasantness components in addition to intensity, but also included a rich variety of qualities, as well as variations in space and time. In this study, Melzack and Torgerson developed a list of 102 pain descriptors gathered from the clinical literature. Both physician and non-physician groups were instructed to classify these descriptors based on similarity of meaning in terms of pain quality. The adjectives were grouped into 16 subclasses under three general classes. The general classes were: "sensory" words, describing pain in terms of temporal, spatial, pressure, and thermal features; "affective" words, describing tension, fear, and autonomic qualities; and "evaluative" words, describing the general intensity of the pain experience. Each subclass contained two to six words that were rated as similar in quality but differing in the magnitude or amount of the quality (e.g., tapping and pounding). The words of each subclass were then scaled for intensity.

After the initial analysis, four new or "miscellaneous" categories were added to include descriptors that did not fit in any of the three general categories.

In the very first volume of the IASP journal *Pain*, Melzack (1975) used this classification scheme as the backbone of the McGill Pain Questionnaire (MPQ). By far the most widely used and studied instrument for multidimensional analysis of pain responses, the MPQ is a descriptor checklist consisting of 78 pain-related adjectives grouped in 20 categories, and other components such as a pain drawing and a simple rating scale of pain intensity. The main descriptor section allows an experience of pain to be scaled in terms of 20 pain qualities or pain dimensions, although in practice the MPQ is typically scored for only the three general dimensions (sensory, affective, and evaluative) by summing the scores of the respective subclasses.

While Melzack developed the MPQ and the subsequent short form of this instrument, Torgerson continued to work on the best method of classifying and quantifying pain descriptors. In the MPQ, each word was assumed to represent the single quality defined by the class or category in which the word was placed, and the different words represented different amounts of this class or category. If the words were colors, each class would be defined by a primary color, and the words would represent different amounts of saturation of that color. Torgerson took a new approach that recognized that particular words most likely do not define a single quality, but rather are likely composites of multiple qualities. In terms of color, the quality of each word represents a mixture of multiple primary colors. The primary qualities are referred to as "ideal types," and each descriptor (or pain described by that descriptor) represents a particular color mix that can be placed on a color wheel according to its distance from each of the primary colors. As with paints, the distances are analogous to the percentage of each primary color in the mix (e.g., green is a mixture of blue and yellow). In the initial studies using this approach, Torgerson quantified 17 pain descriptors and identified four ideal types: bright, slow/rhythmic, thermal, and vibratory-arrhythmic. In multivariate methods such as factor analysis, the meaning of a particular ideal type or factor is determined by stimuli that are close to a particular ideal type, or in visual terms are a short distance from a primary color on a color wheel. If no stimulus is close to an ideal type, the meaning of that particular type may not be obvious.

Torgerson and colleagues (1988) expanded their evaluation to a larger group of words, although the method required that they quantify only small sets of descriptors in each experiment. They performed multiple studies that shared common words so as to anchor the results to a common overall scale. Judges rated the similarity of pairs of descriptors, which formed the basis of an analysis of the underlying structure of how these descriptors are used. The results revealed 19 ideal types as well as an overall quantitative pain intensity scale. These results confirmed the general intensity dimension of the initial MPQ organization while providing an organization of pain descriptors that was more fine-grained than the initial grouping in the MPQ. The results, for example, distinguished between stabbing and drilling by the rotational characteristics of the latter. Of the 19 ideal types, 14 of the qualities appear to be sensory and five affective. Examples of descriptors best indicating the sensory ideal types include sharp, tugging, and pounding. Examples of the affective types included frightful, sickening, and cruel. The use of this approach in back pain patients found a correlation between scores for the sensory qualities and diagnosis, and between the affective qualities and psychological distress (BenDebba et al. 1993).

Torgerson's interests also extended from the evaluation of pain quality to measuring pain quantity. His student Donna Kwilosz focused on pain memory for her doctoral dissertation and helped develop a measure of clinical pain that had three equivalent alternative forms, each with a different set of descriptors (Kwilosz et al. 1984a). This method was based on the descriptor differential scale (DDS; Gracely and Kwilosz 1988), and each of the three forms required subjects to rate their pain four times, each in relation to a different word indicative of pain intensity or unpleasantness. Kwilosz used these measures to solve a thorny problem with pain memory; what is measured—a previous pain or the rating of a previous pain? She found evidence of very good memory for both the intensity and unpleasantness of acute postsurgical pain after a week, as well as an influence of pain magnitude. The results showed a trend for ratings of intensity, but not of unpleasantness, that can be described as "recall spread." More intense pain sensations were recalled as even more intense, while less intense sensations were recalled as even less intense (Kwilosz et al. 1984b).

As Kwilosz worked with the DDS scale, Torgerson became very interested in its properties and designed a model in which the use of the instrument would yield two parameters: a measure of pain magnitude, and a measure of scaling quality or performance of how well patients rated their pain. An unpublished study showed that removing "poor performers" on a blind basis from an analgesic study steadily improved the sensitivity of the study, reaching a peak when about one-third of the subjects were eliminated, then declining as the overall number of subjects became insufficient.

In addition to quantifying pain qualities implied by words, Torgerson was interested in how such words would actually be used to assess pain. Despite the complexities of his methods, he contributed to a simple scale developed by Lenz et al. (1993) to assess pain quality during intra-operative stimulation of the thalamus. Time is of the essence in these studies, and this useful scale characterized the important attributes of evoked pain sensations in a fraction of a minute.

Finally, Torgerson was an international expert on multidimensional scaling and was critical of studies that used patients' responses to questionnaires, such as the MPQ, to make statements about the organization of the questionnaire. I clearly remember sitting in his kitchen, munching an apple just off the tree, when I asked him to explain his problem with this approach. He said that these studies confused associative and semantic meaning. I looked at him blankly. He reiterated: "These studies confuse associative and semantic meaning." Clearly, my puzzled expression indicated that I needed a little explanation. He added, "It's simple, what does butter go with, bread or margarine? Scales are organized by semantic meaning, placing margarine and butter together, while the use of these scales provides associative organizations of a pain syndrome, such as pairing bread with butter." He went on to explain how the analysis of responses to a scale indicates something about the constellations of symptoms within a particular pain syndrome, while analysis of items (see Clark et al. 2001) provides information about the organization of the scale (Gracely 1992; Gracely and Naliboff 1996).

Pain is defined by verbal report, and verbal judgments of pain are the critical dependent measure in basic and clinical studies of human mechanisms of pain and pain control. This brief history highlights some of the issues in evaluating pain as a single dimension or as dual or multiple dimensions. The science of pain measurement continues to be a lively marriage of the sciences of human introspection and pain anatomy, physiology, and behavior. These methods provide the crucial link between human report and human suffering due to pain and other disorders of the afferent nervous system.

ACKNOWLEDGMENT

Butter, margarine, and bread; a toast to the late Warren S. Torgerson.

REFERENCES

Beecher HK. The measurement of pain: prototype for the quantitative study of subjective responses. *Pharmacol Rev* 1957; 9:59–209.

BenDebba M, Torgerson WS, Long DM. Measurement of affective and sensory qualities of back pain. *Abstracts: 7th World Congress on Pain.* Seattle: IASP, 1993, p. 587.

Boring EG. *A History of Experimental Psychology,* 2nd ed. New York: Appleton-Century-Crofts, 1950.

Chapman CR. Sensory decision theory methods in pain research: a reply to Rollman. *Pain* 1977; 3:295–305.

Chapman CR, Feather BW. Effects of diazepam on human pain tolerance and sensitivity. *Psychosom Med* 1973; 35:330–340.

Chapman CR, Murphy TM, Butler SH. Analgesic strength of 33 percent nitrous oxide: a signal detection evaluation. *Science* 1973; 179:1246–1248.

Chapman CR, Gehrig JD,Wilson ME. Acupuncture compared with 33 percent nitrous oxide for dental analgesia: a sensory decision theory evaluation. *Anesthesiology* 1975; 42:532–537.

Chapman CR, Wilson ME, Gehrig JD. Comparative effects of acupuncture and transcutaneous stimulation on the perception of painful dental stimuli. *Pain* 1976; 2:265–283.

Clark WC. Comment on: increased pain sensitivity in fibromyalgia: effects of stimulus type and mode of presentation. *Pain* 2004; 109:524–525.

Clark WC, Yang JC. Acupunctural analgesia? Evaluation by signal detection theory. *Science* 1974; 184:1096–1098.

Clark WC, Janal MN, Hoben EK, Carroll JD. How separate are the sensory, emotional and motivational dimensions of pain? A multidimensional scaling analysis. *Somatosens Mot Res* 2001; 18:31–39.

Coppola R, Gracely RH. Where is the noise in SDT pain assessment? *Pain* 1983; 17:257–266.

Gracely RH. Evaluation of multidimensional pain scales. *Pain* 1992; 48:297–300.

Gracely RH. Methods of testing pain mechanisms in normal man. In: Wall PD, Melzack R (Eds). *Textbook of Pain,* 3rd ed. London: Churchill Livingstone, 1994, pp 315–336.

Gracely RH, Kwilosz DM. The Descriptor Differential Scale: applying psychophysical principles to clinical pain assessment. *Pain* 1988; 35:279–288.

Gracely RH, Naliboff BD. Measurement of pain sensation. In: Kruger L (Ed). *Handbook of Perception and Cognition: Somatosensory Systems.* New York: Raven Press, 1996, pp 243–313.

Gracely RH, McGrath PA, Dubner R. Ratio scales of sensory and affective verbal pain descriptors. *Pain* 1978a; 5:5–18.

Gracely RH, McGrath PA, Dubner R. Validity and sensitivity of ratio scales of sensory and affective verbal pain descriptors. *Pain* 1978b; 5:19–29.

Gracely RH, Dubner R, McGrath PA. Narcotic analgesia: fentanyl reduces the intensity but not the unpleasantness of painful tooth pulp sensations. *Science* 1979; 203:1261–1263.

Gracely RH, Dubner R, McGrath PA. Pain assessment in humans—a reply to Hall. *Pain* 1981; 11:109–120.

Gracely RH, Clauw DJ, Ambrose K, Petzke F. Reply to Clark's letter. *Pain* 2004; 109:525–526.

Hall W. On ratio scales of sensory and affective pain descriptors. *Pain* 1981; 11:101–107.

Hardy JD, Wolff HG, Goodell H. Studies on pain: an investigation of some quantitative aspects of the dol scale of pain intensity. *J Clin Invest* 1948; 27:380–386.

Kwilosz DM, Torgerson WS, Gracely RH. Assessment of clinical pain: parallel forms of the descriptor differential scale. Paper presented at: Annual Meeting of the Eastern Psychological Association, Baltimore, Maryland, April 1984a.

Kwilosz DM, Gracely RH, Torgerson WS. Memory for post-surgical dental pain. *Pain* 1984b; (Suppl 2):426.

LaMotte RH, Cambell JN. Comparison of responses of warm and nociceptive C-fiber afferents in monkey with human judgments of thermal pain. *J Neurophysiol* 1978; 41:509–528.

Lenz FA, Seike M, Richardson RT, et al. Thermal and pain sensations evoked by microstimulation in the area of human ventrocaudal nucleus (Vc). *J Neurophysiol* 1993; 70:200–213.

McArthur DL, Cohen MJ, Schandler SL. A philosophy for measurement of pain. In: Chapman CR, Loeser JD (Eds). *Issues in Pain Measurement.* New York: Raven Press, 1989.

Melzack R. The McGill Pain Questionnaire: major properties and scoring methods. *Pain* 1975; 1:277–299.

Melzack R, Torgerson WS. On the language of pain. *Anesthesiology* 1971; 34:50–59.

Price DD, McGrath PA, Rafii A, Buckingham B. The validation of visual analogue scales as ratio scale measures in for chronic and experimental pain. *Pain* 1983; 17:45–56.

Rollman GB. Signal detection theory measurement of pain: a review and critique. *Pain* 1977; 3:187–211.

Stevens SS. *Psychophysics: Introduction to Its Perceptual, Neural and Social Prospects.* New York: Wiley, 1975.

Swets JA. *Signal Detection and Recognition by Human Observers.* New York: Wiley, 1964.

Thurstone LI. *The Measurement of Values.* Chicago: University of Chicago Press, 1959.

Torgerson WS. *Theory and Methods of Scaling.* New York: John Wiley and Sons, 1958.

Torgerson WS, BenDebba M, Mason KJ. Varieties of pain. In: Dubner R et al. (Eds). Proceedings of the Vth World Congress on Pain. Amsterdam: Elsevier, 1988, pp 368–374.

Tursky B. The development of a pain perception profile: a psychophysical approach. In: Weisenberg M, Tursky B (Eds.) *Pain: New Perspectives in Therapy and Research.* New York: Plenum Press, 1976, pp 171–194.

Yang JC, Clark WC, Ngai SH, Berkowitz BA, Spector S. Analgesic action and pharmacokinetics of morphine and diazepam in man: an evaluation by sensory decision theory. *Anesthesiology* 1979; 51:495–502.

Correspondence to: Richard H. Gracely, PhD, Chronic Pain and Fatigue Research Center, 24 Frank Lloyd Wright Drive, P.O. Box 385, Ann Arbor, MI 48106, USA. Tel: 734-998-6901; Fax: 734-998-6900; email: rgracely@umich.edu.

The Paths of Pain 1975–2005, edited by
Harold Merskey, John D. Loeser, and Ronald
Dubner, IASP Press, Seattle, © 2005.

19

Brain Imaging of Pain:
A Thirty-Year Perspective

M. Catherine Bushnell

Centre for Research on Pain, McGill University, Montreal, Quebec, Canada

In the 1970s, when the IASP was just being formed, Lassen and colleagues (1978) injected the radioisotope Xenon[133] into human volunteers and produced the first images of cerebral hemodynamic changes related to pain. This technique provided little spatial resolution, but suggested that there was an increased blood flow to the frontal lobes during pain. Although these results were very exciting, the technique was difficult to apply to the study of pain because prolonged stimulation periods were required. Then, in the late 1980s, new radiotracers with short half-lives and more sensitive scanning techniques were developed, and the imaging of pain in the human brain was begun in earnest.

Today, we have numerous methods for examining pain-related activity in human brains, and these techniques are applied to the study of both normal and pathological pain processing. These techniques include positron emission tomography (PET), single photon emission computed tomography (SPECT), functional magnetic resonance imaging (fMRI), electroencephalographic (EEG) dipole source analysis, and magnetoencephalographic analysis (MEG). Each of these techniques has advantages and disadvantages in terms of spatial and temporal resolution, sensitivity, and cost. However, all provide measures that can be used as indirect indices of neural activity, and some can be used as measures of neurochemical activity. Despite the many differences among these techniques, results derived from each are generally congruous. Because of space limitations, this chapter will concentrate on data obtained using PET and MRI methodology.

The first three human brain-imaging studies of pain using more sensitive techniques were published in the early 1990s by Talbot et al. (1991) and Jones et al. (1991), using PET, and by Apkarian et al. (1992), using SPECT. All three studies used painful cutaneous heat in normal subjects, and although there were differences in the results, together they indicated that multiple cortical and subcortical brain areas are activated during short-duration heat pain. There have now been dozens of human brain-imaging studies examining cortical and subcortical brain regions involved in acute pain processing in normal subjects. Although there are many differences in activation patterns across studies, a consistent cortical and subcortical network has emerged that includes sensory, limbic, associative, and motor areas. The most commonly activated regions include parts of the primary and secondary somatosensory cortices (S1 and S2), the anterior cingulate cortex (ACC), insular cortex (IC), prefrontal cortex (PFC), thalamus (Th), and cerebellum (CB) (Fig. 1). Pain-evoked activity in these areas is frequently observed using either PET or fMRI techniques, and the activation in these regions is

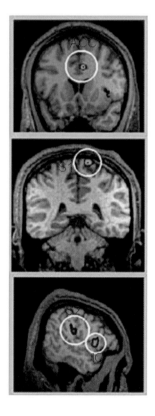

Fig. 1. Functional and anatomical MRI of four subjects exposed to repetitive 9-second painful heat stimuli on the leg (46°C) compared to repetitive warm stimuli (36°C). The circled areas represent regions showing a significantly greater activation during the noxious heat than during the warm stimuli. These areas include the somatosensory cortices S1 and S2, the anterior cingulate cortex (ACC), and the insular cortex (IC). For all images, the right hemisphere is shown at right.

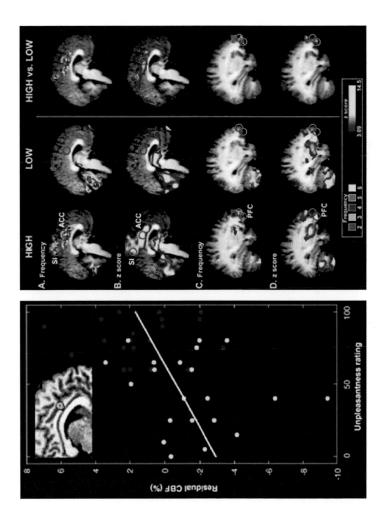

Fig. 2. Left: Activation levels in the anterior cingulate cortex (ACC) during h gh (red) and low (yellow) unpleasantness conditions are significantly correlated with ratings of pain unpleasantness (ANCOVA: $r = 0.42$, $P = 0.005$). CBF = cerebral blood flow. (From Rainville et al. 1997, Fig. 2.) Right: Brain regions showing different activations between high- and low-sensitivity subjects. Circles are centered on regions where the peak differences between groups were located. (From Coghill et al. 2003, Fig. 2.)

consistent with anatomical studies that show probable nociceptive connectivity to these regions.

Now that imaging has provided us with basic information about how the
human brain processes pain, can it be used to clarify functional mechanisms
of normal and pathological pain states? Detractors of the methodology call it
"the new phrenology." Is that all it can be? Can we do more than just
identify pain "spots" in the brain? Below I present some of the directions
that human brain imaging of pain has taken and some of the important
knowledge that it has provided. I believe that we have learned much from
the methodology and that there is still much more that it can provide.

IMAGING TO DETERMINE NEURAL BASIS
OF PERCEPTUAL FEATURES OF PAIN

Whereas the earliest human imaging studies revealed brain regions that
were activated during the presentation of a noxious stimulus, studies now
use more sophisticated analytical techniques that provide a correlation between neural activations and individual perceptual features. In 1997, Rainville
and colleagues used hypnotic suggestions to alter the perception of pain
unpleasantness while the individual continued to feel the same intensity of a
burning sensation produced by emerging the hand in circulating hot water.
Subjects rated pain intensity and unpleasantness after each stimulus presentation. The results showed that pain-evoked activation in the ACC correlated
with the perceived unpleasantness of the noxious stimulus, but not with
either the actual or perceived intensity of the hot water (Fig. 2A). The use of
regression analysis to correlate brain activity with perceptual features of
pain has gained popularity and has been used in a number of studies. For
example, Tölle et al. (1999) used a regression analysis in normal subjects to
show that pain-evoked activation in ACC is more related to affective than to
sensory components of the pain experience. Coghill et al. (1999) showed
that pain-evoked activity in the S1, S2, ACC, and IC regions correlated with
the intensity of a painful stimulus, while that in the dorsolateral PFC did not.
Using similar analytical techniques, Coghill et al. (2003) have now shown
that individual differences in pain sensitivity correlate with neural activity,
as measured using fMRI. That is, people who rate a painful stimulus as more
intense also show more pain-evoked activity in the S1, ACC, and PFC
regions (Fig. 2B). Thus, regression analyses provide a means to understand
circuitry underlying multiple perceptual features, as well as the relationship
between stimulus intensity and neural activity. Such insight can only be
gained through studying pain processing in human subjects.

A related analytical technique involves network analysis of neuroimaging data. In this analysis, cross-correlations are determined among pain-related activations in the brain in order to show which activations may be part of a related circuit. A recent pair of studies by Lorenz and colleagues (2002, 2003) used network analyses to shed light on the specific role of subregions of the frontal cortex in pain perception. The authors compared brain activity evoked during capsaicin-produced thermal allodynia and normal heat pain of equal intensity. The contrast showed considerable activity in the case of allodynia that included multiple frontal regions as well as the medial thalamus, nucleus accumbens, and midbrain. A network analysis of this brain activity demonstrated that dorsal frontal and orbital frontal cortical activities were antagonistic to each other, with the dorsal region limiting the activity of the orbital region and the latter acting in concert with other regions. This antagonistic activity led the authors to hypothesize that the orbital frontal-accumbens-medial thalamus network is engaged in affective perception of pain, while the dorsal frontal cortex acts as a "top-down" controller that modulates pain and thus limits the extent of suffering.

IMAGING ABNORMAL PAIN PROCESSING

Whereas the earliest human pain-imaging studies focused on normal pain processing, many studies are now addressing how the brain is involved in pathological pain states. Data now suggest that there are similarities and differences between normal and pathological pain processing. When patients have damage to the peripheral or central nervous system that leads to a normally innocuous stimulus causing pain (allodynia), brain-imaging studies reveal activation in at least some cortical pain-related regions (Hsieh et al. 1999a; Petrovic et al. 1999; Peyron et al. 2000, 1998; Hofbauer et al. 2001a; Olausson et al. 2001), and such activation most likely underlies the pain experience.

Cortical pain-related activity has also been shown in response to mild pressure stimuli in fibromyalgia patients (Gracely et al. 2002). The experimenters compared stimulus intensities and perception intensities between patients and normal subjects and found that weaker stimuli were needed in fibromyalgia patients to produce the same pain as in normal control subjects. When perceived stimulus intensity was equated, similar regions were activated for patients and controls, but when the physical stimulus intensity was equated, fibromyalgia patients showed greater activation in pain-related brain regions (Fig. 3).

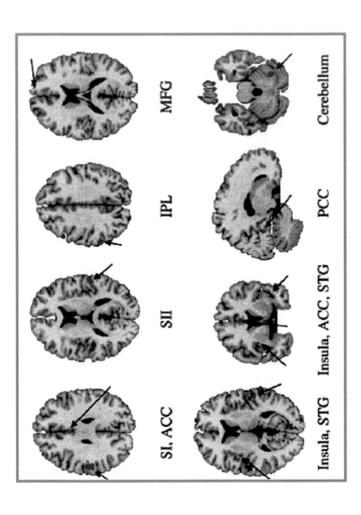

Fig. 3. Comparison of the effects of similar stimulus pressures in fibromyalgia patients and controls. Results of unpaired *t*-test of the mean difference in signal between painful pressure and innocuous touch for each group are shown in standard space superimposed on an anatomic image of a standard brain. Regions in which the response in patients was significantly greater than the response in controls are shown red; regions in which the response in controls was significantly greater than that in patients are shown in green. ACC = anterior cingulate cortex; MFG = middle frontal gyrus; PCC = posterior cingulate cortex; SI = primary somatosensory cortex; SII = secondary somatosensory cortex; STG = superior temporal gyrus (From Gracely et al. 2002, Fig. 3.)

Other studies show that unique aspects of forebrain functioning may be associated with pathological pain states. One example is the evidence of decreased thalamic activity in patients with aberrant pain states (Iadarola et al. 1995; Fukumoto et al. 1999). A SPECT blood flow study in patients with complex regional pain syndrome by Fukumoto et al. (1999) showed a positive relationship between time of symptom onset and reductions in thalamic activity. The ratio between contralateral to ipsilateral thalamic perfusion was larger than 1.0, indicating hyperperfusion, for patients with symptoms for only 3–7 months, and smaller than 1.0, indicating hypoperfusion, for patients with longer-term symptoms (24–36 months).

ANATOMICAL IMAGING—VOXEL-BASED MORPHOMETRY

The study of anatomical changes in the human brain related to disease is becoming an important area of investigation. Voxel-based morphometry (VBM) is a method used to compare local concentrations of gray matter between two groups of individuals. The procedure involves spatially normalizing high-resolution anatomical MRI images from all the subjects in the study into the same stereotactic space and then segmenting the gray matter

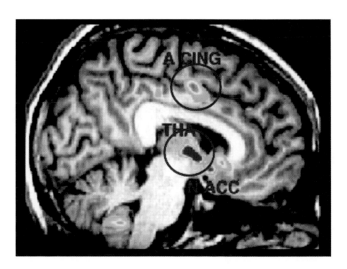

Fig. 4. Negative correlations between pain-specific affective scores on the McGill Pain Questionnaire and μ-opioid-receptor system activation. Brain areas in which significant negative correlations were found between affective pain scores and μ-opioid receptor system activation are superimposed on an anatomically standardized MRI. A CING = anterior cingulate cortex; N ACC = nucleus accumbens; THA = thalamus. (From Zubieta et al. 2001, Fig. 3.)

from the spatially normalized images. The technique has been used to study anatomical differences between patients with various psychiatric disorders and control subjects (Lyoo et al. 2004; Moorhead et al. 2004; Wilke et al. 2004). Apkarian and colleagues (2004) recently applied this technique to the study of chronic low-back pain patients and found that such patients show reduced gray matter density in bilateral dorsolateral prefrontal cortex and right thalamus. The reduced cortical and thalamic density either could be the result of long-term pain or could be a pre-disposing factor for pain becoming chronic. VBM would only be able to differentiate these interpretations if longitudinal data were collected, but it at least provides intriguing information that can be followed up using other techniques.

IMAGING PHARMACOLOGICAL ANALGESIA

Another use of human brain imaging is to examine analgesia mechanisms in the brain. Opioids have been studied the most extensively, using two approaches. The first involves the examination of the brain metabolic function in response to pharmacological agents, and the latter is the direct measurement of receptor activity with and without a pharmacological challenge. Using the first approach, several investigators have tested the effect of μ-opioid agonists on regional cerebral blood flow responses to painful stimuli (Casey et al. 2000; Petrovic et al. 2002; Wise et al. 2004). These studies showed that pain-evoked activation in the ACC, an area rich in opioid receptors, was reduced during opiate analgesia. The second approach involves examining differences in binding of an exogenously applied radiolabeled opiate in the presence and absence of pain. The hypothesis is that when a painful stimulus is applied, endogenous opioids will be released in regions important for analgesia. If an exogenous radiolabeled opiate is administered at the same time as the pain, there will be reduced uptake in regions important for analgesia, since the receptors will be occupied by the endogenously released opioids. In opioid-rich regions that are not important for analgesia, there should be no difference in uptake of the exogenous opiate in the presence or absence of pain. This approach has revealed dynamic changes in the activity of μ-opioid receptors (Zubieta et al. 2001, 2003; Bencherif et al. 2002). Reductions in the in vivo availability of μ-opioid receptors, reflecting the activation of this neurotransmitter system, were observed in the ACC, PFC, IC, thalamus, basal ganglia, amygdala, and periaqueductal gray matter (PAG), suggesting that opioid receptors in these regions are involved in the production of analgesia (Fig. 4).

IMAGING NONPHARMACOLOGICAL ANALGESIA

Psychological factors are known to modulate pain perception in the clinic and in the laboratory (Beydoun et al. 1993; Villemure and Bushnell 2002). Since the mechanisms underlying such modulation are difficult to address in animal studies, human brain imaging has provided an important tool for examining the neural basis of psychological modulation of pain. Human studies examining the effects of attention and distraction show modulation of pain-evoked activity in the thalamus and in several cortical regions, including S1, ACC, and IC (Bushnell et al. 1999; Longe et al. 2001; Bantick et al. 2002). Other regions, including the PAG and parts of the ACC and PFC, are activated when subjects are distracted from pain, suggesting that these regions may be involved in the modulatory circuitry related to attention (Petrovic et al. 2000; Frankenstein et al. 2001; Tracey et al. 2002; Valet et al. 2004).

Hypnotic suggestions also alter pain-evoked activity, and the regions showing modulation depend on the nature of the suggestions (Rainville et al. 1997; Faymonville et al. 2000; Hofbauer et al. 2001b). When subjects are given suggestions to interpret a burning sensation as extremely unpleasant in one condition and as not at all unpleasant in another condition, pain-evoked activity in the ACC is modulated (Rainville et al. 1997). In contrast, when subjects are given suggestions leading them to feel the burning sensation as more or less intense, the most pronounced modulation is in S1 (Hofbauer et al. 2001b). These finding suggest that hypnotic suggestions directed toward altering the affective dimension of pain preferentially modulate activity in limbic regions, whereas those directed toward altering pain sensation modulate activity in sensory regions. When hypnotic suggestions require subjects to continuously attend to the painful stimulus, it is unlikely that modulation of pain-evoked activity is an indirect effect of distraction. It is more likely that hypnotic suggestions invoke modulatory systems other than those involved in selective attention, and these systems most likely involve frontal cortical areas (Rainville et al. 1999).

Other studies have examined the effect of anticipation on pain-evoked activity in the brain. Regions such as S1, ACC, PAG, IC, PFC, and the cerebellum have all been shown to be activated during periods of expectation of pain, before the painful stimulus is presented (Hsieh et al. 1999b; Ploghaus et al. 1999; Sawamoto et al. 2000; Porro et al. 2002).

Investigators have now begun to explore the neural basis of placebo analgesia, which can involve expectation, attention, and conditioning (Petrovic et al. 2002; Wager et al. 2004). Wager and colleagues (2004) performed fMRI experiments involving two types of experimental pain (heat and electric)

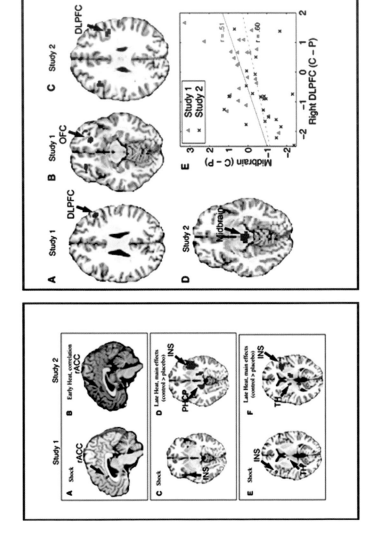

Fig. 5. Left: Pain regions showing more activation during the control condition than during the placebo condition. The pain stimulus in Study 1 was electric shock and that in Study 2 was contact heat. Parts A, C, and E show data during electric shock and B, D, and F show data during heat pain. Right: Prefrontal regions activated with placebo during the anticipation period. Part E is a scatterplot showing the correlation between midbrain placebo effects and right DLPFC placebo effects. rACC = rostral anterior cingulate cortex, INS = insula, PHCP = parahippocampal cortex, TH = thalamus, DLPFC = dorsolateral prefrontal cortex, OFC = orbitofrontal cortex. (From Wager et al. 2004, Figs. 2 and 3.)

and expectation-induced placebo analgesia. They found that placebo analgesia was related to decreased brain activity in pain-sensitive brain regions, including the thalamus, IC, and ACC. Furthermore, the placebo analgesia was associated with increased activity during anticipation of pain in the prefrontal cortex (Fig. 5). Thus, it appears that endogenous modulatory circuits are activated during placebo analgesia and lead to reduced pain transmission to cortical pain-processing areas.

CONCLUSION

There are now scores of brain-imaging studies related to pain or pain modulation. The vast majority of these studies have been published in the last 5 years, and the output continues to grow at an exponential rate. Detractors say that these studies do little to advance our knowledge of brain function. Advocates say that human brain imaging is human functional neuroanatomy and tells us much about where and how pain is processed in the brain. It is certain that we knew little about cortical mechanisms of pain processing before the advent of modern human neuroimaging techniques. These studies showed clearly that regions such as the insular and cingulate cortices, as well as sensory processing areas, are involved in pain perception. The challenge today is to go beyond mapping, to create intelligent experiments that will uncover how different regions participate in normal and aberrant pain processing. In a final cautionary note, we must all remember to integrate multiple lines of evidence in our hypotheses and interpretations. If human brain imaging, monkey neuroanatomy, human and monkey single neuronal recordings, and human lesion studies all implicate a region in pain processing (as is the case for ACC and IC), then we can have much more confidence than could be gained from a single significant activation in a brain-imaging study.

REFERENCES

Apkarian AV, Stea RA, Manglos SH, et al. Persistent pain inhibits contralateral somatosensory cortical activity in humans. *Neurosci Lett* 1992; 140:141–147.

Apkarian AV, Sosa Y, Sonty S, et al. Chronic back pain is associated with decreased prefrontal and thalamic gray matter density. *J Neurosci* 2004; 24(46):10410–10415.

Bantick SJ, Wise RG, Ploghaus A, et al. Imaging how attention modulates pain in humans using functional MRI. *Brain* 2002;125:310–319.

Bencherif B, Fuchs PN, Sheth R, et al. Pain activation of human supraspinal opioid pathways as demonstrated by [¹¹C]-carfentanil and positron emission tomography (PET). *Pain* 2002; 99:589–598.

Beydoun A, Morrow TJ, Shen JF, Casey KL. Variability of laser-evoked potentials: attention, arousal and lateralized differences. *Electroencephalogr Clin Neurophysiol* 1993; 88:173–181.

Bushnell MC, Duncan GH, Hofbauer RK, et al. Pain perception: is there a role for primary somatosensory cortex? *Proc Natl Acad Sci USA* 1999; 96:7705–7709.

Casey KL, Svensson P, Morrow TJ, et al. Selective opiate modulation of nociceptive processing in the human brain. *J Neurophysiol* 2000; 84:525–533.

Coghill RC, Sang CN, Maisog JM, Iadarola MJ. Pain intensity processing within the human brain: a bilateral, distributed mechanism. *J Neurophysiol* 1999; 82:1934–1943.

Coghill RC, McHaffie JG, Yen YF. Neural correlates of interindividual differences in the subjective experience of pain. *Proc Natl Acad Sci USA* 2003; 100:8538–8542.

Faymonville ME, Laureys S, Degueldre C, et al. Neural mechanisms of antinociceptive effects of hypnosis. *Anesthesiology* 2000; 92:1257–1267.

Frankenstein UN, Richter W, McIntyre MC, Remy F. Distraction modulates anterior cingulate gyrus activations during the cold pressor test. *Neuroimage* 2001; 14:827–836.

Fukumoto M, Ushida T, Zinchuk VS, Yamamoto H, Yoshida S. Contralateral thalamic perfusion in patients with reflex sympathetic dystrophy syndrome. *Lancet* 1999; 354:1790–1791.

Gracely RH, Petzke F, Wolf JM, Clauw DJ. Functional magnetic resonance imaging evidence of augmented pain processing in fibromyalgia. *Arthritis Rheum* 2002; 46:1333–1343.

Hofbauer RK, Olausson H, Vainio A, Bushnell MC. Peripheral and central mechanisms underlying allodynia in a nerve injured patient. *Soc Neurosci Abstr* 2001a; 26:441.

Hofbauer RK, Rainville P, Duncan GH, Bushnell MC. Cortical representation of the sensory dimension of pain. *J Neurophysiol* 2001b; 86:402–411.

Hsieh JC, Meyerson BA, Ingvar M. PET study on central processing of pain in trigeminal neuropathy. *Eur J Pain* 1999a; 3:51–65.

Hsieh JC, Stone-Elander S, Ingvar M. Anticipatory coping of pain expressed in the human anterior cingulate cortex: a positron emission tomography study. *Neurosci Lett* 1999b; 262:61–64.

Iadarola MJ, Max MB, Berman KF, et al. Unilateral decrease in thalamic activity observed with positron emission tomography in patients with chronic neuropathic pain. *Pain* 1995; 63:55–64.

Jones AK, Brown WD, Friston KJ, Qi LY, Frackowiak RS. Cortical and subcortical localization of response to pain in man using positron emission tomography. *Proc R Soc Lond B Biol Sci* 1991; 244:39–44.

Lassen NA, Ingvar DH, Skinhoj E. Brain function and blood flow: changes in the amount of blood flowing in areas of the human cerebral cortex, reflecting changes in the activity of those areas, are graphically revealed with the aid of a radioactive isotope. *Sci Am* 1978; 139:62–71.

Longe SE, Wise R, Bantick S, et al. Counter-stimulatory effects on pain perception and processing are significantly altered by attention: an fMRI study. *Neuroreport* 2001; 12:2021–2025.

Lorenz J, Cross DJ, Minoshima S, et al. A unique representation of heat allodynia in the human brain. *Neuron* 2002; 35:383–393.

Lorenz J, Minoshima S, Casey KL. Keeping pain out of mind: the role of the dorsolateral prefrontal cortex in pain modulation. *Brain* 2003; 126:1079–1091.

Lyoo IK, Kim MJ, Stoll AL, et al. Frontal lobe gray matter density decreases in bipolar I disorder. *Biol Psychiatry* 2004; 55:648–651.

Moorhead TW, Job DE, Whalley HC, et al. Voxel-based morphometry of comorbid schizophrenia and learning disability: analyses in normalized and native spaces using parametric and nonparametric statistical methods. *Neuroimage* 2004; 22:188–202.

Olausson H, Marchand S, Bittar RG, et al. Central pain in a hemispherectomized patient. *Eur J Pain* 2001; 5:209–218.

Petrovic P, Ingvar M, Stone-Elander S, Petersson KM, Hansson P. A PET activation study of dynamic mechanical allodynia in patients with mononeuropathy. *Pain* 1999; 83:459–470.

Petrovic P, Kalso E, Petersson KM, Ingvar M. Placebo and opioid analgesia—imaging a shared neuronal network. *Science* 2002; 295:1737–1740.

Petrovic P, Petersson KM, Ghatan PH, Stone-Elander S, Ingvar M. Pain-related cerebral activation is altered by a distracting cognitive task. *Pain* 2000; 85:19–30.

Peyron R, Garcia-Larrea L, Gregoire MC, et al. Allodynia after lateral-medullary (Wallenberg) infarct. A PET study. *Brain* 1998; 121(Pt 2):345–356.

Peyron R, Garcia-Larrea L, Gregoire MC, et al. Parietal and cingulate processes in central pain. A combined positron emission tomography (PET) and functional magnetic resonance imaging (fMRI) study of an unusual case. *Pain* 2000; 84:77–87.

Ploghaus A, Tracey I, Gati JS, et al. Dissociating pain from its anticipation in the human brain. *Science* 1999; 284:1979–1981.

Porro CA, Baraldi P, Pagnoni G, et al. Does anticipation of pain affect cortical nociceptive systems? *J Neurosci* 2002; 22:3206–3214.

Rainville P, Duncan GH, Price DD, Carrier B, Bushnell MC. Pain affect encoded in human anterior cingulate but not somatosensory cortex. *Science* 1997; 277:968–971.

Rainville P, Hofbauer RK, Paus T, et al. Cerebral mechanisms of hypnotic induction and suggestion. *J Cogn Neurosci* 1999; 11:110–125.

Sawamoto N, Honda M, Okada T, et al. Expectation of pain enhances responses to nonpainful somatosensory stimulation in the anterior cingulate cortex and parietal operculum/posterior insula: an event-related functional magnetic resonance imaging study. *J Neurosci* 2000; 20:7438–7445.

Talbot JD, Marrett S, Evans AC, et al. Multiple representations of pain in human cerebral cortex. *Science* 1991; 251:1355–1358.

Tölle TR, Kaufmann T, Siessmeier T, et al. Region-specific encoding of sensory and affective components of pain in the human brain: a positron emission tomography correlation analysis. *Ann Neurol* 1999; 45:40–47.

Tracey I, Ploghaus A, Gati JS, et al. Imaging attentional modulation of pain in the periaqueductal gray in humans. *J Neurosci* 2002; 22:2748–2752.

Valet M, Sprenger T, Boecker H, et al. Distraction modulates connectivity of the cingulo-frontal cortex and the midbrain during pain—an fMRI analysis. *Pain* 2004;109:399–408.

Villemure C, Bushnell MC. Cognitive modulation of pain: how do attention and emotion influence pain processing? *Pain* 2002; 95:195–199.

Wager TD, Rilling JK, Smith EE, et al. Placebo-induced changes in fMRI in the anticipation and experience of pain. *Science* 2004; 303:1162–1167.

Wilke M, Kowatch RA, DelBello MP, Mills NP, Holland SK. Voxel-based morphometry in adolescents with bipolar disorder: first results. *Psychiatry Res* 2004; 131:57–69.

Wise RG, Williams P, Tracey I. Using fMRI to quantify the time dependence of remifentanil analgesia in the human brain. *Neuropsychopharmacology* 2004; 29:626–635.

Zubieta JK, Smith YR, Bueller JA, et al. Regional mu opioid receptor regulation of sensory and affective dimensions of pain. *Science* 2001; 293:311–315.

Zubieta JK, Heitzeg MM, Smith YR, et al. COMT val158met genotype affects mu-opioid neurotransmitter responses to a pain stressor. *Science* 2003; 299:1240–1243.

Correspondence to: M. Catherine Bushnell, PhD, McGill Centre for Research on Pain, 3640 University Street, Room M19, Montreal, Quebec, Canada H3A 2B2. Tel: 514-398-3493; Fax: 514-398-7464; email: catherine.bushnell@mcgill.ca.

The Paths of Pain 1975–2005, edited by
Harold Merskey, John D. Loeser, and Ronald
Dubner, IASP Press, Seattle, © 2005.

20

Central Pain

Jörgen Boivie

Department of Neurology, University Hospital, Linköping, Sweden

Central pain is puzzling not only for patients and their families, but also for health care professionals including doctors, nurses, and other caregivers. In central pain, an arm or leg that apparently has nothing wrong with it can hurt so much and feel so peculiar that it is difficult for patients to find words to describe how it feels. Central pain is also puzzling for researchers because it is difficult to find a plausible explanation for many of its features. This chapter offers a historical view of the development of our knowledge of central pain and reviews the results from research performed in the last 20 years.

Knowledge about central pain in the late 1930s was summarized in an impressive series of papers by Riddoch (1938), who added observations of his own. Many of Riddoch's ideas about central pain showed considerable foresight in light of today's view of the clinical features of patients with central pain. For instance, he discussed the difference between unpleasant and painful sensations, the presence of both spontaneous and evoked pain, the diversity in the quality of central pain, the overreaction to somatic stimuli ("The only constant feature of the thalamic syndrome is over-response to stimuli with or without spontaneous pain"), the many kinds and locations of central lesions that can cause central pain, the uncertainty of the role of autonomic dysfunction, and the role played by patients' ability to cope with the disability caused by central pain (a patient might be "constitutionally gifted with more emotional control" or may have "learned from experience to bear discomforts with fortitude"). Regarding the pathophysiology of central pain, Riddoch supported Head and Holmes's original idea that the crucial lesion is one of the dorsal column-medial lemniscal pathways, which we now know to be incorrect.

The circumstances surrounding current research on central pain are vastly different from those in 1975, when IASP held its 1st World Congress on

Pain. We now have tools including computed tomography (CT) and magnetic resonance imaging (MRI) to better localize lesions. Techniques such as
quantitative sensory testing (QST) allow us to study details about sensory
abnormalities that are crucial for understanding the underlying mechanisms
of central pain, and functional MRI (fMRI) and positron emission tomography (PET) are sophisticated tools for the investigation of abnormalities in
brain function. In addition, we have better resources with which to study
large groups of patients with similar conditions, many new treatments are
available, and we have recognized methods for conducting controlled clinical trials of such treatments.

These techniques and methods have provided much new knowledge, but
many aspects of central pain remain unknown, the most important being a
lack of knowledge about underlying cellular mechanisms, in part because of
the lack of experimental models for central pain caused by brain lesions.
Experience from laboratory techniques to produce experimental lesions in
the spinal cord gives hope that the use of animal models will lead to new
insights into central pain. Another major field in need of improvement is
treatment. Currently available treatment modalities provide relief for many
patients, but there are many others for whom no effective treatment can be
offered.

HISTORICAL PERSPECTIVE

Greiff (1883) appears to have been the first to describe central pain in
his report of a patient who, following cerebrovascular lesions including the
thalamus, developed lasting pain described as "reissende Schmerzen" (tearing pains). Eight years later, Edinger (1891) presented arguments for the
existence of central pain. By then it was known that sensory pathways
project to the thalamus, which was thus thought to play a crucial role in
central pain. Ever since the description of the thalamic syndrome, including
thalamic pain, by Dejerine and Roussy (1906), this pain has remained the
best-known form of central pain. However, only a minority of central pains
are related to thalamic lesions.

Although interest in central pain focused mostly on thalamic pain for
many years, Edinger had introduced the idea early on that cortical lesions
might also cause pain. He also mentioned that the aura of epileptic seizures
can include the experience of pain, as has since been reported by several
authors. It has now been demonstrated beyond doubt that lesions above the
thalamus, in the brainstem, and in the spinal cord can cause central pain (for
a review, see Boivie 1999).

The older literature offers many fascinating, detailed descriptions of symptoms and signs of central pain, but no systematic studies were done at that time. Many of these accounts show that the character of central pain can vary considerably from patient to patient and that it can be excruciating. Authors vividly describe the pain as a crushed feeling, as a scalding sensation, as a cold, stinging feeling, as if boiling water were being poured down the arm, as if the leg were bursting, like something crawling under the skin, like pain pumping up and down the side, as if the painful region were covered with ulcers, like pulling a dressing from a wound, as if a log were hanging from the shoulder, or like a wheel running over the arm (Head and Holmes 1911). As a result of such descriptions, central pain has commonly been thought of as excruciating pain with bizarre characteristics, covering large areas of the body. However, central pain can appear in many guises. It can have a trivial character and may be restricted to a relatively small area, such as distal pain in one arm or in the face.

EPIDEMIOLOGY

There are considerable differences in the prevalence of central pain among the various disorders associated with its onset (Table I). The highest prevalences are found with traumatic spinal cord injuries (SCI), multiple sclerosis (MS), stroke, and syringomyelia (Table I; Boivie 1999). The latter is a rare disease with a very high incidence of central pain.

Two prospective epidemiological studies have been published, one on central post-stroke pain (CPSP; Andersen et al. 1995) and the other on pain following SCI (Siddall et al. 2003). In the stroke study an incidence of 8.4% was found during the first 12 months, and in the spinal cord study 41% of patients developed at-level pain and 34% developed below-level pain during the five years they were followed. Among the stroke patients with somatosensory deficits (42% of all stroke patients studied), the incidence of central pain was 18%. The corresponding figure in a mainly retrospective study

Table I
Estimated prevalence of major disorders with central
pain and calculated number of patients
per 10 million inhabitants

Disease	Patients with Central Pain	
	No.	%
Spinal cord injury	14,000	30.0
Multiple sclerosis	8,500	28.0
Stroke	34,000	8.4

of central pain in 63 patients with brainstem infarct was 44% (MacGowan et al. 1997), with an overall incidence for CPSP of 25%.

A recent study of the prevalence of central pain in 364 patients with MS found that 28% of patients experience, or have experienced, central pain (Österberg et al. 2005). The prevalence of central pain in MS has not been specifically investigated in previous studies of pain in MS, but details provided in some studies support the conclusion that the prevalence is in the order of 25–30%. Trigeminal neuralgia occurs in 5% of MS patients.

LESIONS THAT CAUSE CENTRAL PAIN

Lesion site. Many etiologically different lesions in the brain and spinal cord can cause central pain (Table II). These lesions and dysfunctions are due to many different disease processes. The macrostructure of the lesion is probably less important than its location regarding the probability that it will induce central pain. While it is conceivable that the microstructure of the lesion may be critical in some instances, we lack research data on this matter. There appears to be no correlation between the rapidity with which lesions develop and their tendency to cause central pain.

The role of thalamic lesions is a recurring question in discussions regarding the location of lesions that cause central pain. In their prospective study, Andersen et al. (1995) reported thalamic involvement in 25% of the 191 CPSP patients studied (as assessed by CT scans), but a recently published study of 70 patients using the more sensitive method of MRI found that about 60% had lesions involving the thalamus (Bowsher et al. 1998).

Table II
Causes of central pain

Vascular lesions in the brain and spinal cord
Infarct
Hemorrhage
Vascular malformation
Multiple sclerosis
Traumatic spinal cord injury
Cordotomy
Traumatic brain injury
Syringomyelia and syringobulbia
Tumors
Abscesses
Inflammatory diseases other than MS
Myelitis caused by viruses, syphilis
Epilepsy
Parkinson's disease

The importance of the location of the lesion within the thalamus was eluci-dated in a study of thalamic infarct. The results showed that only patients with lesions including the ventroposterior thalamic region developed central pain (Bogousslavsky et al. 1988).

Sensory abnormalities. Many studies have shown that for a disease process to produce central pain it must affect structures involved in somatic sensibility, which is not surprising, since pain is part of somesthesia (Leijon et al. 1989; Andersen et al. 1995; Bowsher 1996; Pagni 1998; Tasker 2001). Abnormalities in somatic sensibility are the only symptoms and signs be-sides pain that occur in all patients with central pain.

The main features of the sensory abnormalities seen in central pain patients are abnormal sensitivity to temperature and pain and hyperesthesia (Riddoch 1938; Pagni 1998; Tasker 2001). Studies in patients with central pain following stroke, MS, SCI, and syringomyelia that have used quantita-tive methods to assess sensory abnormalities form the basis for the hypoth-esis that central pain only occurs after lesions affecting the spinothalamic pathways, which are the most important pathways for temperature and pain sensibility (Boivie et al. 1989; Vestergaard et al. 1995; Bowsher 1996; Pagni 1998; Finnerup et al. 2003). If this hypothesis turned out to be correct, it would mean that lesions of the dorsal column-medial lemniscal pathways are not necessary for the occurrence of central pain; however, many patients do have such lesions, which certainly affect sensibility (Finnerup et al. 2003). No studies published to date have described patients with central pain whose lesions are unequivocally restricted to the lemniscal pathways.

There is considerable variation in the spectrum of sensory abnormalities among patients with central pain. They may range from a slightly raised threshold for one of the submodalities to complete loss of all somatic sensi-bility in the painful region. Hyperesthesia to touch, moderate cold, and moderate heat, allodynia to touch and cold, and hyperalgesia to cold, heat, or pinprick are common in many central pain conditions and often coexist (Riddoch 1938; Garcin 1968; Boivie et al. 1989; Bowsher 1996; Pagni 1998; Tasker 2001). For instance, some CPSP patients with severely decreased tactile sensibility, even with total loss of normal sensation, have tactile allodynia (Boivie et al. 1989). Head and Holmes (1911) claimed that overre-action to somatic stimuli was the most typical sign of central pain.

The relationship between a change in threshold for a sensory submodality and hypersensitivity (allodynia or hyperalgesia) is of interest in the discus-sion of the mechanisms of central pain. This issue was specifically studied in a recent report. In a group of 13 patients with CPSP, tactile and cold allodynia occurred in patients with normal thresholds as well as in those with abnormal thresholds for touch and cold, but allodynia was more common in patients with normal detection thresholds (Greenspan et al. 2004).

   Neurophysiological examinations.   Because the sensory disturbances in central pain indicate that the lesions affect the spinothalamic pathways, it is of interest to study somatosensory potentials evoked by peripheral stimulation of afferents that activate the spinothalamic pathways. Studies using lasers to stimulate cutaneous heat receptors in patients with CPSP have shown that abnormalities in the laser-evoked cortical potentials, which have a long latency, correlate well with abnormalities in sensitivity to temperature and pain, but not with those in sensitivity to touch and vibration (Casey et al. 1996). Similar results were reported in MS patients (Spiegel et al. 2003).

PAIN CHARACTERISTICS

   Pain location.   About 70% of CPSP patients have hemipain, which in a minority affects the face (Table III). Central pain in patients with MS occurs predominantly in the lower extremities (87%) and upper extremities (31%); about 5% have trigeminal neuralgia. Central pain is experienced as superficial or deep pain, or as having both superficial and deep components, but the high incidence of cutaneous hyperesthesia contributes to the impression that superficial pain dominates.

   Quality of pain.   No pain quality is pathognomonic for central pain. Central pain is not always burning or dysesthetic. In fact, central pain can have any quality, and the variation among patients is great, although some qualities are more common than others (Table IV).

Table III
Common locations of central pain

Stroke
    All of one side
    All of one side except the face
    Arm and/or leg on one side
    Face on one side, extremities on the other side
    The face

Multiple Sclerosis
    Lower half of the body
    One or both legs
    Arm and leg on one side
    Trigeminal neuralgia

Spinal Cord Injury
    Whole body below the neck
    Lower half of the body
    One leg
    At the level of injury

Another basic feature is the presence of more than one pain quality in most patients. Different types of pain can coexist in a body region, or the type of pain may vary in different parts of the body. One would expect the location of the lesion to be a deciding factor regarding the quality of pain. This appears to be partly true, but it is also apparent that similar lesions can lead to different pain qualities.

Intensity of pain. The intensity of central pain ranges from low to extremely high (for examples, see Table V). However, even if the pain is of low or moderate intensity, patients assess the pain as severe because it causes much suffering due to its irritating character and constant presence.

Central pain usually has a constant intensity, but in some patients the intensity varies. These variations seem to occur spontaneously or under the influence of external somatic or psychological stimuli, or they may be due to internal events such as cutaneous stimuli, body movements, visceral stimuli, emotions, and changes in mood.

It is also common for patients with central pain to experience an immediate increase in pain after sudden fear, joy, loud noise, or bright light (Riddoch 1938; Leijon et al. 1989; Bowsher 1996). Experience from clinical practice indicates that central pain is as aggravated by the same psychological factors as other pain conditions, such as anxiety and depression.

Temporal pattern of pain. Central pain may start almost immediately after occurrence of the lesion, or it may be delayed for up to several years; the time frame is impossible to determine in disseminated or slowly progressive diseases such as MS or syringomyelia. Delays of up to 2–3 years are well known in CPSP, but in most patients the pain starts within a few of weeks of the stroke (Mauguiere and Desmedt 1988; Leijon et al. 1989; Andersen et al. 1995; Bowsher 1996).

Most spontaneous central pain is present constantly, with no pain-free intervals. Unfortunately, central pain is usually permanent, but it may remit completely. CPSP may successively decrease and cease completely, but usually it continues throughout life (Leijon and Boivie 1996). A few cases have

Table IV
Qualities of pain reported by patients
with central pain

Burning*	Squeezing	Cramping
Aching*	Throbbing	Smarting
Lancinating*	Cutting	Pulling
Pricking*	Crushing	Sore
Lacerating*	Splitting	Icy feeling
Pressing*	Stinging	
Shooting	Stabbing	

* Asterisks indicate the most common qualities.

Table V
Pain intensity in patients with central post-
stroke pain, assessed with a 0–100-point
visual analogue scale

Lesion Site	N	Mean	Range
Brainstem	8	61	39–94
Thalamus	9	79	68–98
Extrathalamic	6	50	30–91

Source: Data from Leijon et al. (1989).

been reported in which a new supratentorial stroke abolished the pain (Soria and Fine 1991).

PATHOPHYSIOLOGY

SUMMARY OF THE PATHOPHYSIOLOGY OF CENTRAL PAIN

1) The disease process that causes central pain involves the spinothalamic pathways, including the indirect spinoreticulothalamic and spinomesencephalic projections or their trigeminal equivalents, as indicated by abnormalities in sensitivity to pain and temperature. Thalamocortical lesions are also able to precipitate central pain.

2) The lesion probably does not have to involve the dorsal column-medial lemniscal pathways to elicit central pain.

3) The lesion can be located at any level of the neuraxis, from the dorsal horn to the cerebral cortex.

4) Many etiologically diverse processes may cause central pain, but the probability of central pain occurring varies greatly in these diseases, from being rare to occurring in the majority of patients.

5) As yet no single region has been shown to be crucial in the processes underlying central pain, but three thalamic regions that have been the focus of much attention are the ventroposterior, reticular, and medial/intralaminar regions. The role of the cerebral cortex in central pain is unclear.

6) The pain and hypersensitivity experienced by central pain patients are believed to result from increased neuronal activity and reactivity along the somatosensory pathways, as well as from decreased inhibitory mechanisms.

7) The cellular processes underlying central pain are still unknown, but processes involving excitatory amino acids and, in particular, NMDA receptors have been implicated.

HYPOTHESES CONCERNING THE MECHANISMS INVOLVED

Disinhibition by lesions in the medial lemniscal pathways. The notion that central pain is caused by lesions in the dorsal column-medial lemniscal pathway was one of the most favored hypotheses in the first half of the 20th century. The crucial physiological consequence of the lesions was thought to be a disinhibition of neurons in the pain-signaling system. Head and Holmes (1911) were among the first to embrace this notion, discussing it with regard to corticothalamic connections. Later, Foerster (1927) formulated the hypothesis slightly differently when he argued that "epicritic" sensibility (modalities thought to depend on activity within the lemniscal pathways, i.e., touch, pressure, and vibration) normally exerts control over "protopathic" sensibility (sensitivity to pain and temperature).

Lesions in the spinothalamic pathway. In the last two decades, most investigators have found evidence suggesting that the spinothalamic system is affected in the majority of central pain patients (Beric et al. 1988; Boivie et al. 1989; Vestergaard et al. 1995; Bowsher 1996; Pagni 1998; Tasker 2001). This evidence forms the basis for the currently favored hypothesis that central pain occurs only after lesions affecting the spinothalamic system (Boivie et al. 1989; Bowsher et al. 1998; Pagni 1998).

Disinhibition by removal of cold-activated spinothalamic projections. The most recent hypothesis is that of Craig (1998), who proposed that "central pain is due to the disruption of thermosensory integration and the loss of cold inhibition of burning pain." This disruption, according to the hypothesis, is caused by a lesion somewhere along the spinothalamic projections to the thalamus (to the ventroposterior, posterior and mediodorsal nuclear regions comprising the ventral posterior medial nucleus, the posterior part of the ventral medial nucleus, and the ventral caudal part of the medial dorsal nucleus). These projections are thought to tonically inhibit nociceptive thalamocortical neurons, which after a lesion increase their firing and produce pain. The pathway is activated by cold receptors in the periphery, which in turn activate cold-specific and polymodal cells in lamina I of the spinal cord.

Attention and central pain. An interesting case report raises questions about parietal cortical mechanisms in central pain. The patient developed central pain following an infarct in the right parietal cortical region. In addition to hemihypoesthesia, the patient had pronounced neglect of his left arm, where he had burning central pain (Hoogenraad et al. 1994). However, he only had pain when his arm was touched by someone else, and only when he saw that he was going to be touched. This sensation was not just a matter of tactile allodynia, because touching the arm with his right hand did not evoke pain.

Pain memory. Lenz and his collaborators (2000) showed that electrical stimulation in a ventroposterior zone that was deprived of its peripheral input due to a spinal cord lesion or amputation might evoke pain in the deafferented region. Stimulation at these thalamic sites in patients without pain did not evoke pain. The fact that the stimulation was able to evoke pain in deafferented regions indicates that there remains a representation in the CNS of the somatic sensibility for the deafferented region, a kind of long-term memory, which need not necessarily be located in the thalamus. Hypothetically it is possible that such a memory could be activated long after the appearance of the lesion, which may explain the long delay in the onset of central pain in some patients.

TREATMENT

General aspects. Treating central pain is no easy task because there is no universally effective treatment. Clinicians often must try various treatment modalities to get the best results (Table VI). Treatment usually reduces the pain, rather than giving complete relief, but relatively small decreases in pain intensity are often highly valued by patients.

One of the similarities between central pain and peripheral neuropathic pain is their treatment. In both pain categories, antidepressants and antiepileptic drugs are the most frequently used drugs. These drugs have the best documented effects and are the only ones tested in well-conducted clinical trials. They are the first-line treatments, together with transcutaneous

Table VI
Treatment modalities used for central pain;
among antidepressants and antiepileptics, the
most frequently used are listed

Pharmacological
  Tricyclic antidepressant drugs
  Antiepileptic drugs
  Analgesics
  Antiarrhythmic drugs
  Local anesthetic agents
  Other drugs

Sensory Stimulation
  Transcutaneous electrical stimulation (TENS)
  Spinal cord stimulation (SCS)
  Deep brain stimulation (DBS)
  Motor cortex stimulation (MCS)

Neurosurgery
  Cordotomy
  Dorsal root entry zone (DREZ) lesions

electrical nerve stimulation (TENS). For a more thorough discussion of the treatments of neuropathic pain, see Dickenson and Besson (this volume) and Watson (this volume).

It is conceivable that treatment affects some aspects of central pain but not others. Therefore, it would be desirable to assess the effect of treatment on each pain modality separately, in accordance with current ideas about mechanism-based treatments of pain. Another important, but still largely unanswered, question is whether or not the different central pain conditions respond differently to a particular treatment. This issue has not been systematically studied, but such differences appear to exist. Research literature and clinical experience give the impression that CPSP responds better to antidepressants than does central pain in SCI and MS. Conversely, paroxysmal pain in MS seems to respond much better to antiepileptic drugs than other kinds of central pain.

It is still uncertain to what extent patients with central pain benefit from the use of strong analgesics. Many of the treatments listed in Table VI are experimental, although some of them are used quite frequently. From an experimental point of view, adrenergic drugs such as clonidine, $GABA_B$ agonists such as baclofen, or NMDA antagonists such as ketamine might be expected to relieve central pain, but so far no clinical studies have provided results that justify recommendation of their use in clinical practice. The same is true for local anesthetic agents and antiarrhythmic drugs.

Electrical stimulation of the spinal cord or the brain should be reserved for particularly severe and treatment-resistant pain conditions. The exquisite pain suffered by many central pain patients fulfills these criteria. From a review of the literature and from experience with his own patients, Tasker (2001) concluded that spinal cord stimulation is not effective enough in central pain to be recommended, a view he reported to be shared by Gybels and Sweet, Nashold, and Pagni. Instead, Tasker favors deep brain or motor cortex stimulation. In recent years the focus has been on surface stimulation of the motor cortex, with several groups reporting good effects, particularly for CPSP (Tasker 2001).

Many different surgical lesions have been tried to provide relief of central pain, but no particular lesion reliably results in successful outcome (Pagni 1998; Tasker 2001). Dorsal root entry zone (DREZ) lesions have gained interest over recent years for treatment of central SCI pain, but results so far have not been consistent.

Antidepressants. Controlled trials have been conducted with antidepressants only on CPSP (15 patients) and on the central pain in SCI, with conflicting results. The CPSP study reported a statistically significant reduction in pain as compared to placebo (Leijon and Boivie 1989). The NNT for amitriptyline was 1.7 (1.1–3.0). These results contrast with those from a controlled study of amitriptyline on central pain in 44 patients with SCI (Cardenas et al. 2002). The SCI study found no significant effects compared to active placebo, but the doses were relatively low, judging by the plasma concentrations.

Antiepileptic drugs. An effect on central pain has only been demonstrated for lamotrigine in CPSP (Vestergaard et al. 2001), whereas a trend toward an effect on central pain following incomplete SCI was found in another study (Finnerup et al. 2002). In recent years gabapentin has been recommended for the treatment of neuropathic pain. Several case reports describing successful treatment of central pain have appeared, but so far no high-quality controlled studies on central pain have been published. In clinical practice, the results with gabapentin have differed from good to poor.

Analgesics and cannabinoids. The question of whether central pain responds to analgesics is still controversial. The results from short-term, single-blind tests of opioids (Kalman et al. 2002), as well as a controlled clinical trial with the potent μ-opioid agonist levorphanol on patients with CPSP (Rowbotham et al. 2003), indicate low sensitivity to opioids. These findings are similar to the experience of many patients with central pain who undergo operations and receive opioids postoperatively, namely that opioids have a good effect on the pain related to the operation, but no effect on the central pain.

In a study on five patients with CPSP and 10 with SCI, i.v. morphine did not give significant pain relief, but there was a tendency to better pain suppression in the morphine group compared to placebo (Attal et al. 2002). However, in the open post-trial oral medication period, only three patients (17%) continued with morphine for at least 12 weeks. The others discontinued the drug because of side effects and poor relief. The conclusion was that opioids may be useful for a minority of patients with central pain, and that the effect is modest in most of these. This conclusion is in accordance with common clinical experience.

For many years the use of cannabinoids in neuropathic pain has been discussed. The first controlled clinical trial on central pain has now been reported. A significant pain-relieving effect by oral dronabinol was found in 24 patients with MS, during 3 weeks of treatment (Svendsen et al. 2004).

FUTURE RESEARCH

One can draw up a long list of unanswered questions about central pain that future research may resolve. A few of the more important remaining questions are: (1) What are the basic mechanisms underlying central pain? New experimental models might be necessary for this research to be successful, but modern human imaging techniques might also provide valuable information on this issue. (2) What are the factors that determine whether or not a patient will develop central pain? We know that the location of the lesion is crucial, but among patients with seemingly identical lesions, only some develop central pain. (3) How may patients with a high risk of developing central pain be identified? (4) If patients at risk can be identified, how can the development of pain be prevented? (5) How can we develop better treatments? Many patients obtain relief from current treatment modalities, but too many patients receive insufficient relief.

Even though knowledge about many aspects of central pain is lacking, important efforts can be made to improve the situation for patients. One of the most urgent necessities is to promulgate current information in the medical community so that this kind of pain can be correctly identified and patients can receive the best available treatment.

REFERENCES

Andersen G, Vestergaard K, Ingeman-Nielsen M, Jensen TS. Incidence of central post-stroke pain. *Pain* 1995; 61:187–193.

Attal N, Guirimand F, Brasseur L, et al. Effects of IV morphine in central pain. A randomized placebo-controlled study. *Neurology* 2002; 58:554–563.

Beric A, Dimitrijevic MR, Lindblom U. Central dysesthesia syndrome in spinal cord injury patients. *Pain* 1988; 34:109–116.

Bogousslavsky J, Regli F, Uske A. Thalamic infarcts: clinical syndromes, etiology and prognosis. *Neurology* 1988; 38:837–848.

Boivie J. Central pain. In: Wall PD, Melzack R (Eds). *Textbook of Pain*, 4th ed. Edinburgh: Churchill Livingstone, 1999, pp 879–914.

Boivie J, Leijon G, Johansson I. Central post-stroke pain—a study of the mechanisms through analyses of the sensory abnormalities. *Pain* 1989; 37:173–185.

Bowsher D. Central pain: clinical and physiological characteristics. *J Neurol Neurosurg Psychiatry* 1996; 61:62–69.

Bowsher D, Leijon G, Thuomas K-Å. Central post-stroke pain: correlation of MRI with clinical pain characteristics and sensory abnormalities. *Neurology* 1998; 51:1352–1358.

Cardenas DD, Warms CA, Turner JA, et al. Efficacy of amitriptyline for relief of pain in spinal cord injury: results of a randomized controlled trial. *Pain* 2002; 96:365–373.

Casey KL, Beyoun A, Boivie J, et al. Laser-evoked cerebral potentials and sensory function in patients with central pain. *Pain* 1996; 64:485–491.

Craig AD. A New version of the thalamic disinhibition hypothesis of central pain. *Pain Forum* 1998; 7:1–14.

Dejerine J, Roussy G. Le syndrome thalamique. *Rev Neurol (Paris)* 1906; 14:521–532.

Edinger L. Giebt es central antstehender Schmerzen? *Dtsch Z Nervenheilk* 1891; 1:262–282.

Finnerup N, Sindrup S, Bach F, Johannesen I, Jensen T. Lamotrigine in spinal cord injury pain: a randomized controlled trial. *Pain* 2002; 96:375–383.

Finnerup NB, Johannesen I, Fuglsang-Frederiksen A, Bach F, Jensen T. Sensory function in spinal cord injury patients with and without central pain. *Brain* 2003; 126:57–70.

Foerster O. *Die Leitungsbahnen des Schmerzengefühl und die chirurgisiche Behandlung der Schmerzzustände.* Berlin: Urban & Schwarzenberg, 1927.

Garcin R. Thalamic syndrome and pain of central origin. In: Soulairac A, Cahn J, Charpentier J (Eds). *Pain.* London: Academic Press, 1968, pp 521–541.

Greenspan JD, Ohara S, Sarlani E, Lenz FA. Allodynia in patients with post-stroke central pain (CPSP) studied by statistical quantitative sensory testing within individuals. *Pain* 2004; 109:357–366.

Greiff. Zur Localisation der Hemichorea. *Arch Psychol Nervenkr* 1883; 14:598.

Head H, Holmes G. Sensory disturbances from cerebral lesions. *Brain* 1911; 34:102–254.

Hoogenraad T, Ramos L, van Gijn J. Visually induced central pain and arm withdrawal after right parietal infarction. *J Neurol Neurosurg Psychiatry* 1994; 57:850–852.

Kalman S, Österberg A, Sörensen J, Boivie J, Bertler Å. Morphine responsiveness in a group of well-defined multiple sclerosis patients: a study with i.v. morphine. *Eur J Pain* 2002; 6:69–80.

Leijon G, Boivie J. Central post-stroke pain—a controlled trial of amitriptyline and carbamazepine. *Pain* 1989; 36:27–36.

Leijon G, Boivie J. Central post-stroke pain (CPSP)—a long-term follow up. *Abstracts: 8th World Congress on Pain*, Seattle: IASP Press, 1996, p 380.

Leijon G, Boivie J, Johansson I. Central post-stroke pain—neurological symptoms and pain characteristics. *Pain* 1989; 36:13–25.

Lenz F, Lee J, Garonzik I, et al. Plasticity of pain-related neuronal activity in the human thalamus. *Prog Brain Res* 2000; 129:259–273.

MacGowan DJL, Janal MN, Clark WC, et al. Central post-stroke pain and Wallenberg's lateral medullary infarction: frequency, character, and determinants in 63 patients. *Neurology* 1997; 49:120–125.

Mauguiere F, Desmedt JE. Thalamic pain syndrome of Dejérine-Roussy. Differentiation of four subtypes assisted by somatosensory evoked potentials data. *Arch Neurol* 1988; 45:1312–1320.

Österberg A, Boivie J, Thuomas K-A. Central pain in multiple sclerosis—prevalences, clinical characteristics, and mechanisms. *Eur J Pain* 2005; in press.

Pagni C. *Central Pain: A Neurosurgical Challenge.* Torino: Edizioni Minerva Medica, 1998.

Riddoch G. The clinical features of central pain. *Lancet* 1938; 234:1093–1098, 1150–1156, 1205–1209.

Rowbotham M, Twilling L, Davies P, et al. Oral opioid therapy for chronic peripheral and central neuropathic pain. *N Engl J Med* 2003; 348:1223–1232.

Siddall PJ, McClelland JM, Rutkowski SB, Cousins MJ. A longitudinal study of the prevalence and characteristics of pain in the first 5 years following spinal cord injury. *Pain* 2003; 103:249–257.

Soria ED, Fine EJ. Disappearance of thalamic pain after parietal subcortical stroke. *Pain* 1991; 44:285–288.

Spiegel J, Hansen C, Baumgartner U, Hopf H, Treede R. Sensitivity of laser-evoked potentials versus somatosensory evoked potentials in patients with multiple sclerosis. *Clin Neurophysiol* 2003; 114:992–1002.

Svendsen K, Jensen T, Bach F. Does the cannabinoid dronabinol reduce central pain in multiple sclerosis? Randomised double blind controlled crossover trial. *BMJ* 2004; 329:253.

Tasker RR. Central pain states. In: Loeser JD (Ed). *Bonica's Management of Pain*, 2nd ed. Philadelphia: Lippincott, Williams and Wilkins, 2001, pp 433–457.

Vestergaard K, Nielsen J, Andersen G, et al. Sensory abnormalities in consecutive, unselected patients with central post-stroke pain. *Pain* 1995; 61:177–186.

Vestergaard K, Andersen G, Gottrup H, Kristensen BT, Jensen TS. Lamotrigine for central post-stroke pain—a randomised controlled trial. *Neurology* 2001; 56:184–90.

Correspondence to: Jörgen Boivie, MD, Department of Neurology, University Hospital, S-581 85 Linköping, Sweden. Tel: 46-13-22 20 00; email: jorgen.boivie@lio.se.

The Paths of Pain 1975–2005, edited by
Harold Merskey, John D. Loeser, and Ronald
Dubner, IASP Press, Seattle, © 2005.

21

Therapeutic Electrical Neurostimulation from a Historical Perspective

Björn A. Meyerson and Bengt Linderoth

Department of Clinical Neuroscience, Section of Neurosurgery, Karolinska Institute and Karolinska University Hospital, Stockholm, Sweden

This chapter highlights important milestones in the development of the various modes of nervous stimulation, most of which were first reported at IASP congresses and subsequently published in *Pain*. Advances in different forms of electrical stimulation of the nervous system have been a core feature of clinically relevant pain treatments developed in the history of IASP. The tendency has been to replace older lesional methods with less invasive treatments, later to be labeled "neuromodulation." In 1973, John Bonica organized the first multidisciplinary pain meeting, where it was agreed that a world organization for pain researchers and clinicians was needed. The extensive scientific program at that meeting included a large number of presentations covering all forms of electrical stimulation—cutaneous, peripheral nerve, spinal cord, and brain, as well as acupuncture. The speaker list comprised most of the pioneers in the field—Shealy, Sweet, Liebeskind, Long, Nashold, Adams, Fields, and Hosobuchi. The proceedings from the meeting contain most of these presentations as full papers (Bonica 1974), which in addition to their historical value are still of considerable interest.

The fathers of the gate control theory, Ronald Melzack and Patrick Wall, took part in the meeting. Spinal cord stimulation (SCS; then called dorsal column stimulation, DCS) was the first direct clinical application of the notion of a gating mechanism at the first spinal relay. In fact, in their classical publication in *Science* in 1965, Melzack and Wall explicitly stated that the theory could have therapeutic implications by means of selectively activating large-diameter fiber systems. However, in retrospect it is somewhat paradoxical that the theory still seems to be valid as a basis for understanding the mode of action of SCS, because it was thought to apply to pain in general; at that time there was no awareness of the fundamental differences between nociceptive and neuropathic pain. Only in the early 1980s was it universally recognized that SCS is not directly effective for purely nociceptive forms of pain.

At the first and founding meeting of IASP, the 1st World Congress on Pain in Florence in 1975, one of the plenary lectures focused on peripheral nerve stimulation (PNS) and SCS (Long 1976), and another on experimental "brain-stimulation analgesia" (Liebeskind 1976). There were about 20 abstracts each on transcutaneous electrical nerve stimulation (TENS) and on spinal and intracerebral stimulation. All the abstracts were expanded into chapters in the proceedings from the meeting. Some of them represented early experimental studies aimed at elucidating the physiological mechanisms in pain relief by stimulation. For example, one describes inhibition of spinothalamic tract neurons by SCS (Foreman et al. 1976), and another—from a group in Beirut that has published numerous experimental studies on stimulation—deals with cerebral modulation of cuneate nucleus neurons (Jabbur et al. 1976). There were also basic papers on intracerebral stimulation by some of the pioneers in the field (e.g., Basbaum et al. 1976).

The very first volume of *Pain* (1975) included five papers on stimulation. One of them was the first to document that SCS seemed to have a selective action on clinical signs of neuropathic pain, whereas induced nociceptive pain was unaffected (Lindblom and Meyerson 1975). Another paper reported that SCS, applied in cats, could suppress neuronal activity in the dorsal horn evoked by peripheral noxious stimuli (Handwerker et al. 1975).

Many of these early experimental studies of effects of spinal or intracerebral stimulation provided some valuable information about the possible mechanisms involved, and yet their clinical relevance is questionable because they were performed on intact, anesthetized animals subjected to acute nociceptive pain. It was not until the early 1990s that awareness emerged about the profound central changes following nerve injury, and thus it was realized that such experimental studies should preferably employ animal models of the type of pain that is most likely to respond to therapeutic stimulation.

The advancement of stimulation techniques, in particular SCS, the most commonly used technique, is mainly due to technical improvements in the equipment, which have not been matched by a furthering of our understanding of the mechanisms underlying the pain-relieving effects. Compared to what was surveyed in a plenary lecture at the 3rd IASP Congress in Edinburgh in 1981 (Meyerson 1983), it is obvious that we have only recently gained more solid knowledge in this respect (see Meyerson and Linderoth 2003). The evidence base for stimulation therapies is hampered by their inherently invasive nature (except for TENS) and by the fact that these methods (with the notable exception of motor cortex stimulation) induce paresthesias along with analgesia, thus precluding double-blind study designs.

TRANSCUTANEOUS ELECTRICAL NERVE STIMULATION

Cutaneous stimulation was first used solely to screen and select patients for SCS. After a few years, this mode of nerve stimulation became a therapy by itself. Stimulation was originally applied at a relatively high frequency (50–100 Hz) and with an intensity that evoked mild tingling sensations. In the early 1970s, a time of considerable interest and research in traditional Chinese medicine, electro-acupuncture became the basis for low-frequency acupuncture-like (2-Hz pulse trains) TENS applied with high intensity. This alternative form of treatment (also called "burst-stimulation") was first presented internationally at the IASP meeting in Montreal (Sjölund and Eriksson 1979). These authors had demonstrated that the pain-relieving effect with this form of TENS, in contrast to conventional high-frequency stimulation, is associated with the activation of endogenous opioid systems (Sjölund and Eriksson 1976).

TENS is still extensively practiced, and over the years many new pain diagnoses have been added to the list of indications. In contrast to other types of stimulation, TENS can influence both acute and chronic nociceptive pain. The most common indication is musculoskeletal pain. Many clinical TENS studies are available, but few have attained satisfactory scientific quality. A recent Cochrane survey of TENS applied for "low back pain" identified only six studies that qualified for further analysis (Gadsby and Flowerdew 2000). The authors concluded, with considerable reservations, that some pain relief and improved mobility could be obtained, at least in the short term. The same applies to the use of TENS in postoperative pain, although a few randomized studies have demonstrated its usefulness after abdominal surgery (Carroll et al. 1996). Recent years have seen relatively few publications on TENS.

Refractory angina pectoris as a new indication for TENS was introduced to the pain community at the Seattle IASP meeting in 1984 (Mannheimer et al. 1985). Subsequent studies have presented evidence substantiating the efficacy and clinical value of TENS applied for this type of pain, and it has become a standard treatment in many European countries.

PERIPHERAL NERVE STIMULATION

Wall and Sweet tested the basic idea of gate control in 1965 by stimulating their own infraorbital nerves at low intensity via needle electrodes. The same year they treated a patient suffering from pain due to median nerve injury with stimulation via a temporary percutaneous electrode (Wall and Sweet 1967; White and Sweet 1969). After a few years, more systematic studies appeared on the use of implantable electrodes specially designed for peripheral nerve stimulation (PNS). The prime indication for PNS was pain due to injury to an identified major nerve (mononeuropathy) that was confined to the territory of the same nerve, mostly in the upper extremities. In general, the outcome was favorable, with substantial pain relief in 60–70% of patients (e.g., Sweet 1976; for review, see Gybels and Nuttin 2001). Most of the electrodes then used were of a cuff design that tended to cause fibrosis around the nerve. This problem could be avoided when flat, paddle-type electrodes, placed adjacent to the nerve trunk, were introduced instead. In recent years, neuropathic pain conditions confined to the face and neck have also been successfully managed by PNS (Weiner et al. 1999; Johnson and Burchiel 2004). Stimulation applied to the trigeminal ganglion and its roots is a form of PNS. It can be provided either via a percutaneous electrode introduced though the foramen ovale or via a plate electrode placed onto the dura overlying the trigeminal cistern. This form of stimulation was developed for the management of pain in trigeminal neuropathy (Meyerson and Håkanson 1986).

Several experimental studies were designed to explore the possible mechanisms of pain relief with PNS. It appears that stimulation applied at subthreshold intensity to nociceptive fibers may involve both peripheral and central modes of action. The classical experiments of Wall and Gutnik (1974) demonstrated that the enhanced spontaneous discharge produced by a neuroma can be suppressed by low-intensity stimulation of the nerve. By the time of the Bonica symposium in 1973, two reports already indicated that PNS, and perhaps also TENS, acts by suppressing Aδ-fiber activity (Taub and Campbell 1974; Torebjörk and Hallin 1974; see also Ignelzi and Nyquist 1976). Central mechanisms have also been implicated, and Chung et al. (1984) are often cited in this context. They demonstrated, in spinalized monkeys, that PNS could effectively inhibit spinothalamic tract cells, but the most potent effect was obtained with stimulation applied with Aδ-fiber intensity. However, in these animals the peripheral nervous system was intact and normal, limiting the clinical relevance of these findings. A salient feature of PNS is that it may suppress the tactile and thermal allodynia commonly present in mononeuropathy. It is surprising that the effects of PNS have not been further experimentally explored in view of the intensive research in recent years on the pathophysiology of peripheral nerve injury.

SPINAL CORD STIMULATION

In the early 1970s, SCS was enthusiastically embraced as a result of numerous positive reports. At the 1973 Seattle symposium, Shealy (1974) who introduced the method, claimed a success rate of 80% provided that patients with obvious personality disorders were excluded. However, Sweet, skeptical as always, stated that "our results ... are the worst reported thus far" (Sweet and Wepsic 1974). It appears that the majority of the patients then treated with the method suffered from low back pain. Most papers dealing with selection of patients for SCS focused on psychological factors, while no or little attention was paid to the type of pain most likely to respond. In those days, most pain clinicians only distinguished between cancer pain and "benign" pain. By the early 1970s clinical and experimental observations already suggested that SCS did not influence nociceptive pain (Nashold and Friedman 1972; Lindblom and Meyerson 1975), but it was not until about 10 years later that it was universally recognized that SCS is only effective for some neuropathic forms of pain, as well as for pain in peripheral vascular disease and angina, where pain relief may be secondary to an anti-ischemic effect, as discussed below. More stringent indications for SCS have been defined, and the last decade has seen great interest in its usefulness for the management of complex regional pain syndrome types I and II, and also in the possible relationship between a response to temporary sympathetic blocks and the long-term outcome (e.g., Kumar et al. 1997a; Kemler et al. 2004). However, it appears that the most common indication is still what is now often referred to as "failed back surgery syndrome," which in this context has replaced the term "low back pain." However, this term is a confusing misnomer and definitely not a pain diagnosis—it merely indicates that the patient has been subjected to back surgery. The term is also very much discordant with the current trend toward developing mechanism-based pain diagnoses. It should be noted, though, that in several publications on SCS used to treat "failed back surgery syndrome" it is stated that "pain in the leg," which may stand for any type of pain, including neuropathic or even referred "pain," is more likely to respond than pain confined to the lower, axial part of the back (e.g., North et al. 1993).

The dissemination of SCS as an indispensable part of the management of some forms of neuropathic pain has been much linked to improvements of the hardware. The first commercially available electrode was designed for subdural implantation, and somewhat later it was instead placed endodurally (between the dural layers); implantation thus required open surgery (laminectomy). It was therefore an important advance when the percutaneous implantation technique was introduced. The next step was the development of multipolar, first quadripolar, electrodes with programmable polar couplings (Fig. 1). An important technical breakthrough has been the ability to supply the stimulating current by an implantable, patient-controlled pulse generator ("neuro-pacemaker").

The advancement of electrode designs has to some extent been linked to studies by Holsheimer, who developed a computer model of the spread of electrical current from the epidural space (Holsheimer and Wesselink 1997). This model has also been of paramount value for evaluating which neuronal elements and compartments, i.e., the dorsal roots and dorsal columns, may be activated.

As mentioned above, SCS evolved as a direct clinical application of the gate control concept. The general idea of activation of low-threshold fiber systems as a way of turning on inhibitory controls of nociception has withstood the "test of time" (Dickenson 2002). Although the original theory did not account for the drastic plasticity changes taking place in chronic pain conditions, particularly in neuropathy, the presence of paresthesias as a precondition for the pain-relieving effect of SCS further supports the pivotal role of coarse fiber activation. Several alternative models to explain the mode of action of SCS have been presented: (1) the effect results from a simple collision between impulses generated by a peripheral noxious stimulus and those generated by SCS; (2) it results from direct activation of descending pain-controlling pathways contained in the dorsolateral funiculi; or (3) it is mediated via a supraspinal loop involving brainstem relays. In the 1970s–1980s a number of experimental studies addressed this issue. However, virtually all were performed on normal animals, examining the effect of SCS on neuronal responses to transient, nociceptive stimuli. Such an experimental design is hardly clinically relevant. Not until the last decade have such studies been performed on animal models of what is considered to represent neuropathic pain. SCS in such animals may effectively suppress nerve-injury-induced hypersensitivity, similar to allodynia and hyperalgesia, which corresponds to the inhibition of the abnormal discharge pattern in dorsal horn neurons. It has been concluded that the mode of action of SCS is predominantly dependent on the activation of low-threshold, large fibers. The effects are further associated with a decreased release of excitatory

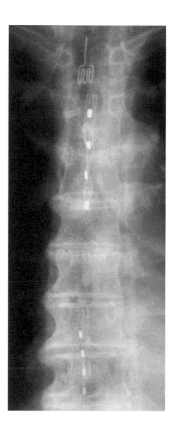
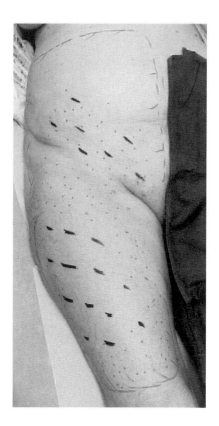

Fig 1. (Left) Radiograph of the thoracic spine of a case illustrating the long-lasting pain-relieving effect of spinal cord stimulation. The patient suffered from postsurgical inguinal neuralgia. She was first treated in 1976 with the uppermost paddle electrode placed endodurally (i.e., between the dura layers). Due to a malfunction of that system, a new strip electrode (middle) was implanted in 1981. This electrode was later, in 1988, replaced by a modern system with a percutaneously implanted electrode (lowest). In 2004 the pulse generator had to be replaced. The patient maintained that she still, 28 years after the first implant, had almost complete pain relief and was dependent on daily stimulation. (Right) Sensitivity changes in the same patient assessed about 50 years after the beginning of pain following lower abdominal surgery. The area within the outlines displayed moderate to marked hyperalgesia. Small dots denote the presence of dynamic and static allodynia and prominent heat hyperalgesia. Black broken lines represent hypoalgesia.

amino acids and with enhancement of GABAergic inhibitory control (for reviews, see Linderoth and Foreman 1999; Meyerson and Linderoth 2003). The debate is unresolved as to whether these effects are mediated at a segmental spinal level or depend on the involvement of a supraspinal loop (El-Khoury et al. 2002).

A large number of clinical reports on the use of SCS have been published over the years. Although only a few of these studies were randomized and controlled, the reported results are concordant, claiming satisfactory outcome (>50% pain relief) in 60–70% of patients with neuropathic pain. In recent years, ischemic pain, both as a result of peripheral vacular disease and in the form of angina pectoris, has emerged as a new indication for SCS. The outcome of SCS used for these indications appears to be even more favorable, with success rates of 70–75% and 80–90%, respectively. In view of the fact that such pain is regarded as nociceptive, for which SCS is otherwise ineffective, it is likely that its alleviation is secondary to a beneficial effect on the ischemia per se (Linderoth and Foreman 1999; Foreman et al. 2004).

The practice of SCS is progressively increasing, and it is now performed mostly by anesthesiologists, while it was previously exclusively in the hands of neurosurgeons. However, considering that SCS remains the only treatment option for many cases of incapacitating neuropathic pain, it is still very much underused.

INTRACRANIAL STIMULATION

Intracerebral stimulation. At the Seattle symposium in 1973, Hosobuchi, Adams, and Fields reported on their first experiences of stimulating the sensory thalamus as treatment of neuropathic pain (Bonica 1974). Studies of "analgesia from focal brain stimulation" were also reviewed by Liebeskind et al. (1974), and reference was given to the first clinical trials with stimulation applied in the central gray. At the subsequent 1st World Congress, Mazars et al. (1976) reported that their group in Paris had been experimenting with such stimulation since 1962, at first using short-term stimulation via temporary connection to an external stimulator, and then introducing an implanted stimulation device in 1972. At the same meeting, Gybels et al. (1976) reported on the effect of stimulation in various brain regions, including the sensory thalamus, on experimentally induced pain. At the second meeting in Montreal in 1978, no less than six papers were presented on stimulation of the periventricular and periaqueductal gray, applied mostly for cancer-related pain. Since then, the practice of intracerebral stimulation has successively diminished, the principle reason being that the long-term results appeared to be unsatisfactory. From the late 1990s there have been few publications on this topic, although a thorough long-term follow-up of patients subjected to periventricular gray stimulation demonstrated a surprisingly favorable outcome (Kumar et al. 1997b). It appears that perhaps we have been too quick to abandon that treatment mode for the management of conditions such as chronic pain in the low back, which is otherwise difficult to control with stimulation. Low back pain is generally mixed, with one dominating component either confined to the low back (mainly nociceptive) or irradiating in the leg (neuropathic or referred). Moreover, medicolegal regulations in the United States, where most of these therapies were practiced, now preclude the use of intracerebral stimulation, i.e., deep brain stimulation (DBS), for pain. This state of affairs is even more regrettable considering that the hardware is now much improved due to the extensive use of DBS for movement disorders. However, in recent years some attempts to re-evaluate the former pain targets have been made.

Recently, therapy-resistant cluster headache has emerged as a new indication for DBS. On the basis of positron emission tomography (PET) findings that cluster attacks are associated with focal activation of the posterior hypothalamus, stimulation was applied in the same region (Franzini et al. 2003). The results, as yet only obtained from a small number of patients, have been very promising, with almost complete suppression of the headache attacks. Considering that cluster headache is one of the most dreadful pain conditions, perhaps DBS will emerge as the therapy of last resort.

Motor cortex stimulation. At the 6th IASP Congress in Adelaide in 1990, much attention was paid to the report by Tsubokawa et al. (1990) that central post-stroke pain could be effectively alleviated by stimulation applied to the *motor* cortex. There seemed, and still seems, to be little rationale for the selection of that target structure, although it was documented, in cats, that deafferented, hyperexcitable thalamic neurons could be inhibited by selective motor cortex stimulation (MCS). In the following year we successfully applied MCS to a therapy-resistant case of trigeminal neuropathy that had also failed to respond to sensory thalamic stimulation (Meyerson et al. 1993) (Fig. 2). Subsequently, MCS has been adopted as a treatment of central and various forms of peripheral, mostly trigeminal, neuropathic pain. The majority of the ensuing studies related to MCS have been reported at the regular IASP meetings and published in *PAIN*. It appears that in most reports the outcome tends to be somewhat more favorable in cases of trigeminal neuropathy (60–80% with pain relief >50%) than in cases of central pain (40–70%). To the best of our knowledge, no controlled studies have been performed. It should be emphasized, however, that MCS, unlike other electrical stimulation modalities, does not evoke any subjective sensations. This unique feature makes it possible for studies to incorporate a double-blind stimulation control.

The practice of MCS requires a great deal of expertise and experience. The epidural placement of the stimulating electrode is critical. Precise identification of the motor cortex strip and the portion corresponding to the site of pain requires both electrophysiological and neuronavigation methods, ideally combined with functional magnetic resonance imaging.

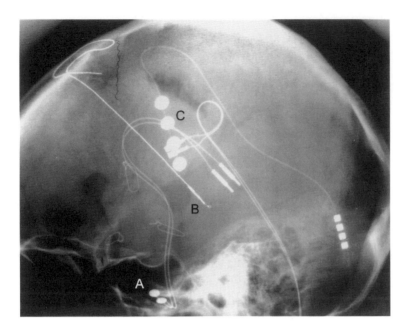

Fig 2. Radiograph of a patient suffering from severe painful trigeminal neuropathy. This case illustrates that such pain may be extremely difficult to manage and that various invasive stimulation procedures may fail. The patient had been subjected first to stimulation of the Gasserian ganglion (A) and then of the sensory thalamus (B), as well as to stimulation of the spinal trigeminal tract (not illustrated). For the past 12 years she has had good, but not complete, pain relief with motor cortex stimulation (C). This stimulation does not evoke any subjective sensations.

The mode of action of MCS is still poorly understood. There are few directly relevant experimental data, although it is known that stimulation applied to the motor cortex can induce presynaptic afferent inhibition in the spinal dorsal horn (Andersen et al. 1962). Tsubokawa et al. (1993) hypothesized that pain following a cerebral lesion is the result of deficient inhibitory control and advanced the notion that MCS acts via activation of large-fiber reciprocal interconnections between the sensory and motor cortices. However, PET studies have demonstrated that MCS is associated with signs of significant activation of the ipsilateral thalamus, cingulate gyrus, and areas in the brainstem (Garcia-Larrea et 1999). At variance with Tsubokawa's theory, it has been argued that the integrity of the sensory cortex and lemniscal system is not a prerequisite for MCS functioning (Nguyen et al. 1999).

Despite having been in use for a decade, and although the number of patients treated with it probably exceeds 350–400, MSC is still a treatment modality under development and cannot be recommended for routine use. However, it has proven to be effective in some cases of otherwise therapy-resistant pain conditions, and therefore a systematic exploration of its potential in managing difficult pains is warranted.

CONCLUDING REMARKS

The various electrical stimulation techniques described in this chapter offer minimally invasive and reversible therapeutic options in cases of both neuropathic and ischemic pain conditions where conventional therapies have failed. TENS and SCS should be regarded as routine therapies in selected neuropathic and ischemic pain conditions. These techniques have far fewer long-term side effects than the pharmaceutical strategies now available for chronic use. Invasive peripheral nerve stimulation remains an option practiced in certain centers, and this treatment modality deserves to be explored more in the future. The more invasive strategies involving supraspinal electrical stimulation for pain should at present be restricted to centers with special experience and interest and with extensive knowledge of pain analysis and patient selection.

No doubt, the further development of microcomputer techniques will enable more sophisticated stimulation regimens and miniaturization of the equipment. During the last decade, better control of paresthesia distribution during SCS has been accomplished by using more complicated electrode designs, devices with many stimulating poles and multiple leads, and dual channel systems. Future testing and programming after initial implantation will probably be automated via a computer, the patients giving just simple dichotomous responses to the various stimulation patterns offered by the system (North et al. 2003).

The history of neurostimulation techniques clearly demonstrates the drawbacks of applying therapies without solid knowledge of their physiological basis. Electrical activation of neuronal circuits may be regarded as comparable to in situ drug administration because the activated neurons deliver neurotransmitters and modulators in physiological amounts to the very site where they will activate their receptors. Some recent neurostimulation research has been conducted along these lines, and new data about transmitters involved in effects of the stimulation have provided some novel therapeutic tools. A spin-off from animal research has thus been the possibility of enhancing the SCS effect by concomitant administration of baclofen and adenosine (Lind et al. 2004). Further, it has been demonstrated that gabapentin, pregabalin and clonidine, when administered intrathecally or intravenously in normally inactive doses can potentiate the SCS-suppressing effect on behavioral signs of tactile allodynia in mononeuropathic rats (Wallin et al. 2002; Schechtmann et al. 2004). There is reason to believe that a more diversified adjuvant pharmacological treatment in the future may help to enhance the efficacy of various stimulation therapies.

From general clinical experience, we know that patients who present with seemingly almost identical symptoms of neuropathy following peripheral nerve injury may respond differently to stimulation therapy. One patient may enjoy almost complete alleviation of both spontaneous and evoked pain, whereas another may not respond at all to stimulation that is technically adequate (which for SCS involves paresthesias covering the entire painful region). It is a salient finding that the same situation seems to occur in nerve-lesioned rats exhibiting marked signs of neuropathy. In some rats these signs are completely suppressed by SCS, whereas in others the treatment has no effect whatsoever. It would be clinically relevant to explore the possible biochemical background to the differential effect of SCS in such animals.

SCS in ischemic syndromes is especially promising because it implies not only symptomatic pain therapy but also—as the primary effect—resolution of the tissue ischemia. Here, increased efforts to explore the relevant mechanisms are called for. SCS is offered to patients with ischemic pain where there are no adequate therapeutic alternatives, and the long-term follow-ups have demonstrated sustained benefit, especially for refractory angina pectoris.

Intracranial stimulation will be restricted to the most severe cases of neuropathic pain and mixed forms of pain in the future. Many of these cases are otherwise candidates for long-term intraspinal morphine administration. However, opioid therapy may involve serious side effects and tolerance, and therefore there is perhaps reason to re-evaluate the old DBS targets. Moreover, modern research in the biology of pain provides indications of brain regions that could serve as novel and more efficient targets, such as the posterior hypothalamus.

Electrical modulation of central pain circuitry, and of central control mechanisms for tissue blood perfusion, will no doubt remain an indispensable part of the therapeutic armamentarium.

REFERENCES

Andersen P, Eccles JC, Sears TA. Presynaptic inhibitory action of cerebral cortex on the spinal cord. *Nature* 1962; 194:740–741.

Basbaum AI, Marley N, O'Keefe J. Spinal cord pathways involved in the production of analgesia by brain stimulation. In: Bonica JJ, Albe-Fessard DG (Eds). *Proceedings of the First World Congress on Pain,* Advances in Pain Research and Therapy, Vol. 1. New York: Raven Press, 1976, pp 511–516.

Bonica JJ. *International Symposium on Pain,* Advances in Neurology, Vol. 4. New York: Raven Press, 1974.

Carroll D, Tramer M, McQuay H, Nye B, Moore A. Randomization is important in studies with pain outcome: systematic review of transcutaneous electrical nerve stimulation in acute postoperative pain. *Br J Anaesth* 1996; 77:798–803.

Chung JM, Fang ZR, Hori Y, Lee KH, Willis WD. Prolonged inhibition of primate spinothalamic tract cells by peripheral nerve stimulation. *Pain* 1984; 19:259–275.

Dickenson AH. Gate control theory of pain stands the test of time. *Br J Anaesth* 2002; 88:755–757.

El-Khoury C, Hawwa N, Baliki M, et al. Attenuation of neuropathic pain by segmental and supraspinal activation of the dorsal column system in awake rats. *Neuroscience* 2002; 112:541–553.

Foreman RD, Beall JE, Applebaum AE, Coulter CJ, Willis WD. Inhibition of primate spinothalamic tract neurons by electrical stimulation of dorsal column or peripheral nerve. In: Bonica JJ, Albe-Fessard DG (Eds). *Proceedings of the First World Congress on Pain,* Advances in Pain Research and Therapy, Vol. 1. New York: Raven Press, 1976, pp 405–410.

Foreman RD, DeJongste MJL, Linderoth B. Integrative control of cardiac function by cervical and thoracic spinal neurons. In: Armour JA, Ardell JL (Eds). *Basic and Clinical Neurocardiology.* Oxford: Oxford University Press, 2004, pp 153–186.

Franzini A, Ferroli P, Leone M, Broggi G. Stimulation of the posterior hypothalamus for treatment of chronic intractable cluster headaches: first reported series. *Neurosurgery* 2003; 52:1095–1099.

Gadsby JG, Flowerdew MW. Transcutaneous electrical nerve stimulation and acupuncture-like transcutaneous electrical nerve stimulation for chronic low back pain. *Cochrane Database Syst Rev* 2000; 2.

Garcia-Larrea L, Peyron R, Mertens P, et al. Electrical stimulation of motor cortex for pain control: a combined PET-scan and electrophysiological study. *Pain* 1999; 83:259–273.

Gybels JM, Nuttin BJ. Peripheral nerve stimulation. In: Loeser JD (Ed). *Bonica's Management of Pain.* Philadelphia: Lippincott Williams & Wilkins, 2001, pp 1851–1856.

Gybels J, Van Hees J, Peluso F. Modulation of experimentally induced pain in man by electrical stimulation of some cortical, thalamic and basal ganglia structures. In: Bonica JJ, Albe-Fessard D (Eds). *Proceedings of the First World Congress on Pain,* Advances in Pain Research and Therapy, Vol. 1. Raven Press, New York, 1976, pp 475–478.

Handwerker HO, Iggo A, Zimmermann M. Segmental and supraspinal actions on dorsal horn neurons responding to noxious and non-noxious skin stimuli. *Pain* 1975; 1:147–165.

Holsheimer J, Wesselink WA. Effect of anode-cathode configuration on paresthesia coverage in spinal cord stimulation, *Neurosurgery* 1997; 41:654–659.

Ignelzi RJ, Nyquist JK. Direct effect of electrical stimulation on peripheral nerve evoked activity: implications in pain relief. *J Neurosurg* 1976; 45:159–165.

Jabbur SJ, Harris FA, Biedenbach MA, Morse RW, Towe AL. Cerebral modulation of neuronal excitability in the cuneate nucleus of the macaque monkey. In: Bonica JJ, Albe-Fessard DG (Eds). *Proceedings of the First World Congress on Pain,* Advances in Pain Research and Therapy, Vol. 1, New York: Raven Press, 1976, pp 461–468.

Johnson MD, Burchiel KJ. Peripheral stimulation for treatment of trigeminal postherpetic neuralgia and trigeminal posttraumatic neuropathic pain: a pilot study. *Neurosurgery* 2004; 55:135–141.

Kemler MA, De Vet HC, Barendse GA, et al. The effect of spinal cord stimulation in patients with chronic reflex sympathetic dystrophy: two years' follow-up of the randomized controlled trial. *Ann Neurol* 2004; 55:13–18.

Kumar K, Nath RK, Toth C. Spinal cord stimulation is effective in the management of reflex sympathetic dystrophy, *Neurosurgery* 1997a; 40:503–508.

Kumar K, Toth C, Nath R. Deep brain stimulation for intractable pain: a 15-year experience, *Neurosurgery* 1997b; 40:736–747.

Liebeskind JC. Pain modulation by central nervous system stimulation. In: Bonica JJ, Albe-Fessard DG (Eds). *Proceedings of the First World Congress on Pain,* Advances in Pain Research and Therapy, Vol. 1. New York: Raven Press, 1976, pp 445–454.

Liebeskind JC, Mayer DJ, Akil H. Central mechanisms by pain inhibition: studies of analgesia from focal brain stimulation. In: Bonica JJ (Ed). *International Symposium on Pain,* Advances in Neurology, Vol. 4. New York: Raven Press, 1974, pp 261–268.

Lind G, Meyerson BA, Linderoth B. Intrathecal baclofen as adjuvant therapy to enhance the effect of spinal cord stimulation in neuropathic pain: a pilot study. *Eur J Pain* 2004; 8:377–383.

Lindblom U, Meyerson BA. Influence on touch, vibration and cutaneous pain of dorsal column stimulation in man. *Pain* 1975; 1:257–270.

Linderoth B, Foreman RD. Physiology of spinal cord stimulation: review and update. *Neuromodulation* 1999; 2:150–164.

Long DM. Use of peripheral and spinal cord stimulation in the relief of chronic pain. In: Bonica JJ, Albe-Fessard DG (Eds). *Proceedings of the First World Congress on Pain,* Advances in Pain Research and Therapy, Vol. 1. New York: Raven Press, 1976, pp 395–404.

Mannheimer C, Carlsson CA, Emanuelsson H, et al. The effects of transcutaneous electrical nerve stimulation in patients with severe angina pectoris. *Circulation* 1985; 71:308–316.

Mazars GJ, Merienne L, Cioloca C. Contribution of thalamic stimulation to the physiology of pain. In: Bonica JJ, Albe-Fessard DG (Eds). *Proceedings of the First World Congress on Pain,* Advances in Pain Research and Therapy, Vol. 1. New York: Raven Press, 1976, pp 483–486.

Meyerson BA. Electrostimulation procedures: effects, presumed rationale, and possible mechanisms. In: Bonica JJ, Lindblom U (Eds). *Proceedings of the Third World Congress on Pain,* Advances in Pain Research and Therapy, Vol. 5. New York: Raven Press, 1983, pp 495–534.

Meyerson B, Håkanson S. Suppression of pain in trigeminal neuropathy by electric stimulation of the Gasserian ganglion. *Neurosurgery* 1986; 18:59–66.

Meyerson BA, Linderoth B. Spinal cord stimulation: mechanisms of action in neuropathic and ischemic pain. In: Simpson BA (Ed). *Electrical Stimulation and the Relief of Pain,* Pain Research and Clinical Management, Vol. 15. Amsterdam: Elsevier Science, 2003, pp 161–182.

Meyerson BA, Lindblom U, Linderoth B, Lind G, Herregodts P. Motor cortex stimulation as treatment of trigeminal neuropathic pain. In: Meyerson BA, Ostertag C (Eds). *Advances in Stereotactic and Functional Neurosurgery,* Vol. 11. Vienna: Springer-Verlag, 1993, pp 150–153.

Nashold BS, Friedman H. Dorsal column stimulation for control of pain. *J Neurosurg* 1972; 36:590–597.

Nguyen JP, Lefaucheur JP, Decq P. Chronic motor cortex stimulation in the treatment central and neuropathic pain. Correlations between clinical, electrophysiological and anatomical data. *Pain* 1999; 82:245–251.

North RB, Kidd DH, Zahurak M, James CS, Long DM. Spinal cord stimulation for chronic, intractable pain: experience over two decades. *Neurosurgery* 1993; 32:384–395.

North RB, Calkins SK, Campbell DS, et al. Automated, patient-interactive, spinal cord stimulator adjustment: a randomized controlled trial. *Neurosurgery* 2003; 52:572–580.

Shealy CM. Six years' experience with electrical stimulation for control of pain. In: Bonica JJ (Ed). *International Symposium on Pain,* Advances in Neurology, Vol. 4. New York: Raven Press, 1974, pp 775–782.

Schechtmann G, Wallin J, Meyerson BA, Linderoth B. Intrathecal clonidine suppresses tactile allodynia and potentiate spinal cord stimulation in neuropathic rats. *Anesth Analg* 2004; 99:135–139.

Sjölund B, Eriksson M. Electro-acupuncture and endogenous morphines. *Lancet* 1976; 2:1085.

Sjölund BH, Eriksson M. Endorphins and analgesia produced by peripheral conditioning stimulation. In: Bonica JJ, Liebeskind JC, Albe-Fessard DG (Eds). *Proceedings of the Second World Congress on Pain,* Advances in Pain Research and Therapy, Vol. 3. New York: Raven Press, 1979, pp 587–592.

Sweet W. Control of pain by direct electrical stimulation of peripheral nerves. *Clin Neurosurg* 1976; 19:103–111.

Sweet WH, Wepsic JG. Stimulation of pain suppressor mechanisms: a critique of some current methods. In: Bonica JJ (Ed). *International Symposium on Pain,* Advances in Neurology, Vol. 4. New York: Raven Press, 1974, pp 737–748.

Taub A, Campbell JN. Percutaneous local electrical analgesia: peripheral mechanisms. In: Bonica JJ (Ed). *International Symposium on Pain,* Advances in Neurology, Vol. 4. New York: Raven Press, 1974, pp 727–732.

Torebjörk HE, Hallin RG. Excitation failure in thin nerve fiber structures and accompanying hypalgesia during repetitive electric skin stimulation. In: Bonica JJ (Ed). *International Symposium on Pain,* Advances in Neurology, Vol. 4. New York: Raven Press, 1974, pp 733–736.

Tsubokawa T, Katayama Y, Yamamoto T. Motor cortex stimulation for control of thalamic pain. *Abstracts: 6th World Congress on Pain.* Seattle: IASP Press, 1990.

Tsubokawa T, Katayama Y, Yamamoto T, et al. Chronic motor cortex stimulation in patients with thalamic pain. *J Neurosurg* 1993; 78:393–401.

Wall PD, Gutnik M. Properties of peripheral nerve impulses originating from a neuroma. *Nature* 1974; 248:740–743.

Wall PD, Sweet WH. Temporary abolition of pain in man. *Science* 1967; 155:108–109.

Weiner RL, Alo KM, Fuller ML. Peripheral neurostimulation to control intractable occipital neuralgia. *Abstracts: 9th World Congress on Pain.* Seattle: IASP Press, 1999, p 61.

White JC, Sweet WH. *Pain and the Neurosurgeon.* Springfield, IL: Charles C Thomas, 1969, pp 888–904.

Wallin J, Cui J-G, Yahknitsa V, et al. Gabapentin and pregabalin suppress tactile allodynia and potentiate spinal cord stimulation in a model of neuropathy. *Eur J Pain* 2002; 6:261–272.

Correspondence to: Björn A. Meyerson, MD, PhD, Department of Neurosurgery, Karolinska University Hospital, SE-17176 Stockholm, Sweden. Email: bjorn.meyerson@karolinska.se.

The Paths of Pain 1975–2005, edited by
Harold Merskey, John D. Loeser, and Ronald
Dubner, IASP Press, Seattle, © 2005.

22

Terms and Taxonomy: Paper Tools at the Cutting Edge of Study

Harold Merskey

*Professor Emeritus of Psychiatry, University of Western Ontario,
London, Ontario, Canada*

When basic or clinical scientists seek to find ways forward in their subjects, classification often seems forced upon us or dull. We may grant that it is essential, but not that it is entrancing. However, there is an encouraging history in the story of pain and classification. It begins with the vision of John Bonica:

"Many people have considered the definition of pain and a uniform list of terms and classification of pain syndromes impossible because of differences of opinion among scientists and clinicians of different disciplines, and also because of differences in national usage. Consequently, we have been markedly impaired in our communication pertaining to pain research and therapy. This became impressively clear to me during the time I wrote my book, *Management of Pain*, when I expended an immense amount of time and effort to analyze and synthesize the results reported by numerous writers who obviously were describing the same condition under a large variety of quite different names." (Bonica 1979)

Undaunted, Bonica developed an impressive classification of pain syndromes in his book, and the experience gave him some firm convictions:

"(a) it is possible to define terms and develop a classification ... acceptable to many, albeit *not all* [emphasis added], readers and workers in the field; (b) even if the definitions and classification are not perfect they are better than "the Tower of Babel" conditions that currently exist; (c) such classification [is] not ... "fixed" for all time ...; and (d) the adoption of such taxonomy with the condition that it can be modified will encourage its use

widely by those who may disagree with some part of the classification. ...
This in fact has been the experience and chronology of [other disorders]."
(Bonica 1979)

When drafting the constitution of the IASP, John Bonica created a Committee on Standards, which had a subcommittee on taxonomy. As a psychiatrist, I was surprised when he suggested that I become chair of this subcommittee and recommended me to Dr. Albe-Fessard, first president of IASP, in 1975. I had thought that the problem would be to bring together individuals concerned with the classification of somatic syndromes, neurologists, rheumatologists, internists, and perhaps anesthetists, rather than psychiatrists, who would have the least to offer in defining pain syndromes. He explained that he wanted someone who had a native command of English and who was not an American, because he was extremely anxious that this most important committee—as he saw it—should not seem to be dominated by his fellow citizens of the United States.

FINDING TERMS

A taxonomy subcommittee was formed, and I agreed to see what could be done. The first members were Madame Albe-Fessard (France), John J. Bonica (USA), Amiram Carmon (Israel), Ronald Dubner (USA), Howard L. Fields (USA), Frederick W.L. Kerr (USA), Ulf Lindlom (Sweden), James M. Mumford (UK), William Noordenbos (Netherlands), Carlo Pagni (Italy), Marcel J. Renaer (Belgium), Richard A. Sternbach (USA), and Sir Sydney Sunderland (Australia). Innocently, I asked around and was told that it would be "impossible" to create an agreed taxonomy. Contemporaneously, an effort at the National Institute of Dental Research (NIDR) in the United States failed to achieve even an agreed classification of oral facial pain—or at least one that was much favored. However, there was an interest in the subcommittee in definitions of pain terms. Ulf Lindblom (a neurologist), James Mumford (a dental surgeon), William Noordenbos (a neurosurgeon), and Peter Nathan (a neurologist and neurophysiologist who was consulted as well) prepared a series of definitions of terms. Lindblom prepared the first draft of pain terms, which after much consideration and minor modification was adopted by the subcommittee and published in 1979 (IASP Subcommittee on Taxonomy 1979).

The neurologists on the subcommittee wanted to establish adequate terms for clinical use in the examination of patients with pain. Their concern was with defining hyperesthesia, hyperalgesia, neuralgia, neuropathy, and similar basic "tools of the trade" needed for comparison of their work with that of others. Agreement was obtained through correspondence and through discussion at the triennial committee meetings at the time of the 2nd and 3rd Congresses in particular.

One term in particular scored an exceptional success: *allodynia.* This word was coined at the request of Noordenbos, Professor of Neurosurgery at the University of Amsterdam, who wanted a term to describe pain arising as a result of the application of non-noxious stimuli to otherwise normal tissue. The tissue might have abnormal innervation or might be a referral site for other loci but was giving rise to pain on stimulation by non-noxious means. The subcommittee could not think of a satisfactory word, and I was commissioned to seek help from a classical scholar with knowledge of medicine. Paul Potter, MD, a translator of Hippocrates and Hannah Professor of the History of Medicine at the University of Western Ontario, recommended the word *allodynia, allo* (meaning "other" in Greek) and *dynia,* derived from *odynia, odune,* or *odyne*—a suffix found already in a number of words meaning pain, such as pleurodynia and coccygodynia. This word had a striking success, even more so with physiologists, for whom it was not primarily intended, but who adopted it enthusiastically so that the literature of neurophysiology often refers to allodynia. A search of the on-line database of the National Library of Medicine of the United States (PubMed) on 27 November 2003 turned up 1365 references to allodynia in articles, among which of the first 100, 20 included allodynia in their title and another two referred to anti-allodynia. A "Google" search found 12,500 occurrences.

The second success of the new terminology was the provision of a definition of pain as "an unpleasant sensory and emotional experience associated with actual or potential tissue damage or described in terms of such damage." This definition was based upon an earlier one (Merskey and Spear 1967) that had achieved some recognition over a period of 12 years. The authority of the IASP gave power to the new version, which is now widely accepted. Like the other terms, the definition of pain was accompanied by a note to explain why we thought it would be useful. The note emphasized that pain is always subjective. Each individual learns the application of the word "pain" through experiences related to injury in early life. These were the types of experience that biologists recognized as causes of tissue damage. Many patients who appeared to have pain did not have tissue damage but described their condition in identical terms to those used when we expected or recognized tissue damage.

One commentator observed:

"It is fascinating how much matter for controversy has been packed into the brief IASP definition of pain. The definition and its supporting annotations gently but surely dissolve any necessary connection between pain and tissue damage. That became a key to the definition. It depended upon the usage of the word pain whether a physical change was apparent. ... Most important, with a daring that merits repetition, the IASP definition recognizes that pain is always a subjective, psychological state. ... At the same time, the Task Force authors also state in the annotation what is surely true: that pain, despite its psychological and subjective nature, "most often has a proximate physical cause." (Morris 2003)

The IASP definition has been adopted fairly broadly and helps to minimize the idea that there is some sort of pain that patients imagine and that is not the same as the pain of "real injury or disease."

The success of the definitions as a whole owes most to Lindblom, Mumford, Nathan, and Noordenbos. The other major task of the subcommittee, which is much further from perfection, was the production of an ideal classification of chronic pain syndromes.

CLASSIFICATION

Once a core of success had been established within the taxonomy subcommittee, members felt that a useful contribution had been made with definitions of terms, and it became possible to float the idea that we should tackle the issue of sorting out chronic pain syndromes into an adequate classification. Here, there was much uncertainty. The subcommittee realized that it would be inappropriate to try to describe all pain syndromes—that would have meant rewriting medicine. Instead, the members agreed that we would describe all chronic pain syndromes that lasted more than 3 months, and we would also include one or two acute syndromes that demonstrated classical patterns that frequently became chronic, such as postherpetic neuralgia.

As chair, I put forward a draft of the scheme for orofacial pain prepared by Aaron Ganz at the NIDR. It was felt and expressed with some turbulence in the subcommittee that this classification of only one region of the body raised considerable difficulties by attempting to determine the causes of the syndromes as a starting point for classification. However, the group did come to an agreement, suggested particularly by Dick Sternbach, that we should commence with the region of the body as a defining starting point and only put causes into the descriptions at the end. He pointed out from the viewpoint of a psychologist that this was how doctors most often commonly made their diagnoses and reports, such as "low back pain" or "left leg pain."

We then drew up a possible arrangement of syndromes by site, including a number of relatively generalized syndromes, and a modal pattern for the description of each syndrome that was to be classified. This pattern normally ran through site, system, main features, associated features, means of obtaining relief (while with proper caution eschewing any detailed advice at all on treatment), signs, pathology, differential diagnoses, and a five- or six-digit code. In the end, not all syndromes were fully described, and perhaps the majority were not fully described, but a separate account was given of each discrete syndrome recognized. A description of this approach was published after having been presented in 1981 to the 3rd World Congress in Edinburgh (Merskey 1983).

The definitions appear to have been generally well received, and the Council of the IASP in particular was encouraging. The effort then continued to establish descriptions of major conditions. Known specialists were contacted throughout the world and asked to provide descriptions of the conditions in question. We were greatly helped in this by the fact that, in organizing the meeting that led to the foundation of the IASP, Bonica had identified 100 individuals who had published significant contributions on pain. Once a description was obtained from an established clinician in the field, it was reviewed by colleagues, and an agreed version was developed by the overall editor of the taxonomy and the colleagues providing the expert information. In this way, many descriptions were assembled, but by no means enough to complete a representative group. As editor, I next met with Bonica, who, from his extensive knowledge, was able to provide basic descriptions for some conditions that had not been fully dealt with otherwise and to suggest other colleagues to recruit. He was also able to give an adequate and experienced critical review of the descriptions themselves. We were helped significantly in developing some descriptions by the existing work of the American Medical Association Ad Hoc Committee on the Classification of Headache (Friedman et al. 1962).

Once sufficient descriptions had been completed to the reasonable satisfaction of the members of the Subcommittee on Classification, comprising Michael Bond, David Boyd, and myself, they were presented in turn to the taxonomy subcommittee and then to the IASP Council. All three members of the small subgroup were psychiatrists, but Bond had trained as well as a neurosurgeon, and Boyd was trained in internal medicine and was practicing in that discipline. Thus, the 1986 version of the *Classification of Chronic Pain Syndromes* emerged and was published in *Pain* (IASP Subcommittee on Taxonomy 1986).

The basis for the taxonomy was conceptually simple. A satisfactory classification should be comprehensive and exhaustive. There should be a place for every item in the field, and no items should overlap. The periodic table and Darwinian classifications of flora and fauna largely achieve those aims. Medical classification cannot do so. When the classification system was planned, we had found in the ninth revision (1978) of the World Health Organization's *International Classification of Disease* (ICD-9) that conditions were classified by causal agent, e.g., infectious diseases or neuroplasms; by systems of the body, e.g., gastrointestinal or genitourinary; or by symptom pattern and type of symptom, as in psychiatric illnesses. Some illnesses were grouped by time of occurrence, e.g., congenital anomalies, or conditions originating in the perinatal period, and even as Symptoms, Signs and Ill-defined Conditions—a group on their own. There was a code in the ICD-9 (ICD-650) for delivery in a completely normal case of pregnancy. Within neurology there are subdivisions by symptom patterns, e.g., epilepsy or migraine; by heredity or by degenerative disease, e.g., degenerations usually manifest in childhood or Parkinson's disease; by location, for example, spinal cerebellar disease; and by infectious causes, e.g., meningitis.

When we come to diagnoses for pain, overlap is the rule rather than the exception. At the time the IASP classification was introduced, the ICD-9 included codes for migraine (346), ankylosing spondylitis (720), and rheumatoid arthritis (714); in the group of Symptoms, Signs and Ill-defined conditions we could find headache (784.0), but atypical face pain (350.2), migraine (346), and tension headache (307.8) were all found elsewhere.

The IASP sets of descriptions, organized largely by region and then by system, were both popular and neglected. Many individuals undertaking work with chronic pain are still appropriately disposed to use the simple and brief arrangements of the *International Classification of Disease* in its 9th and 10th revisions (World Health Organization 1978, 1992). However, IASP's *Classification of Chronic Pain* built up a following in some particular respects. First, where a condition was not well described elsewhere and some consensus was needed, the description tended to be noticed, as in the case of cervical sprain injuries (whiplash). Second, the *Classification* was appreciated when a condition was rare and not well known, but where one or two cases had been seen by colleagues over periods of years. Having a description available tended to help diagnosis of rare conditions such as the syndrome of painful legs and moving toes, which was recognized by a number of pain physicians through the descriptions in the *Classification*. Rare, but remediable forms of headache also were better recognized in this way, e.g., chronic paroxysmal hemicrania. Further, when there was a need to review a controversial category, such as reflex sympathetic dystrophy, help was solicited from the subcommittee in finding a descriptive solution to controversial problems.

The name reflex sympathetic dystrophy, while widely recognized, had been felt to be unsatisfactory because the syndrome in question was not always, or even not often, reflex by origin, and was not always dependent upon sympathetic malfunction. The boundaries of the disorder varied from worker to worker, and the basis for experimental study varied accordingly. Michael Stanton-Hicks of Cleveland, Ohio, and colleagues organized a series of special meetings of interested research workers and clinicians. At the second meeting, held in Orlando, Florida, in 1993, the effort was made to produce a description in a pattern that could be incorporated in the second edition of the *Classification of Chronic Pain Syndromes* (Merskey and Bogduk 1994) that would improve on the description of the disorder as it existed in the first edition. There was unanimous agreement that two changes must be made. The name of the disorder should be changed, for the reasons given, and the notion of a sympathetic disorder should be carefully separated from the common clinical pattern that was of interest, because while the pattern was sometimes poorly understood, it was not necessarily dependent upon sympathetic activity or underactivity. The IASP Task Force on Taxonomy, which replaced the Subcommittee on Taxonomy and was responsible for the creation of the second edition of the *Classification,* addressed these aims by creating the category of complex regional pain syndrome type I to describe what was formerly called reflex sympathetic dystrophy and then by indicating in the overall description, separate from the classification coding, that the disorder could be described as either sympathetically dependent or sympathetically independent (Stanton-Hicks et al. 1996). This category worked well for some 10 years from 1993 to 2003, but studies by Harden et al. (1999) suggested that the criteria were not sufficiently tight to cover those cases that most clinicians thought were characteristic and typical, while excluding other more doubtful cases. This situation was tackled by providing descriptions of narrow criteria and more broad criteria. Four clinically and statistically distinct subgroups within the existing IASP criteria have been proposed by Wilson et al. (2005). It is likely that the next meeting of the Task Force on Taxonomy will recommend identification of patients and cases according to these new criteria.

The most logical reduction in medical classification, but not necessarily a desirable one, is provided by the *International Classification of Primary Care* (Lamberts and Wood 1987). This classification simply registers every reason for content as the patient's records. Thus it describes the work of the doctor, not the world of disease. However, it is a useful classification for physicians who wish to know how much attention they have been giving to different topics and also how to bill for their services. All classification systems are liable to be used for billing purposes, which makes them popular even when they are still dull.

The IASP classification has been used for billing services, particularly in the United States. Such advantages are only part of the reason for classification. In the long run the best reason is for the comparison of cases between different physicians and different sources of clinical information so that uniformity of understanding can be achieved even if advances in understanding are less frequent. In any case, uniformity of understanding is vital for scientific progress whether or not our understanding is incomplete.

THE FUTURE

As this chapter suggests, it is likely that the future of classification will be shaped by its own needs. Further descriptions will evolve, but changes are likely to be introduced piecemeal in a system accessed by computer. There is interest in a system of classifying pain on a mechanistic basis, which, if it develops, will be likely to apply first to neuropathic pain and then perhaps later to other conditions. Clinical disorders will of course be further subdivided and refined, and their descriptions will evolve accordingly. The IASP Task Force on Taxonomy, chaired by John D. Loeser, will remain integral to the ongoing classification of pain through its work on preparation of a new edition of the *Classification of Chronic Pain* and related activities.

REFERENCES

Bonica JJ. The need of a taxonomy. *Pain* 1979; 6:247–252.

Friedman AP, Finley KH, Graham JR, et al. Classification of Headache. Special report of the Ad Hoc Committee. *Arch Neurol* 1962; 6:173–176.

Harden RN, Bruehl S, Galer BS, et al. Complex Regional Pain Syndrome. Are the IASP diagnostic criteria valid and sufficiently comprehensive? *Pain* 1999; 83:211–221.

International Association for the Study of Pain Subcommittee on Taxonomy. Pain terms: a list with definitions and notes on usage, recommended by the IASP Subcommittee on Taxonomy. *Pain* 1979; 6:249–252.

International Association for the Study of Pain Subcommittee on Taxonomy. Classification of chronic pain: descriptions of chronic pain syndromes and definitions of pain terms. *Pain* 1986 (Suppl 3).

Lamberts H, Wood M. *ICPC International Classification of Primary Care.* Oxford: Oxford University Press, 1987.

Merskey H. Development of a universal language of pain syndrome. In: Bonica JJ, Lindblom U, Iggo A (Eds). *Proceedings of the Third World Congress on Pain*, Advances in Pain Research and Therapy, Vol. 5. New York: Raven Press, 1983, pp 37–52.

Merskey H, Bogduk N. *Classification of Chronic Pain: Descriptions of Chronic Pain Syndromes and Definitions of Pain Terms,* 2nd ed. Seattle: IASP Press, 1994.

Merskey H, Spear FG. *Pain: Psychological and Psychiatric Aspects.* London: Baillière, Tindall and Cassell, 1967.

Morris DB. The challenges of pain and suffering. In: Jensen TS, Wilson PR, Rice ASC (Eds). *Chronic Pain.* London: Arnold, 2003, pp 3–13.

Stanton-Hicks M, Jänig W, Hassenbusch S, et al. Reflex sympathic dystrophy. Changing concepts and taxonomy. *Pain* 1996; 63:127–133.

Sub-committee on Taxonomy. International Association for the Study of Pain. *Classification of Chronic Pain, Descriptions of Chronic Pain Syndromes and Definitions of Pain Terms.* In: Merskey H (Ed). *Pain* 1986; (Suppl 3):1–226.

Wilson PR, Stanton-Hicks M, Harden RN. *CRPS: Current Diagnosis and Therapy,* Progress in Pain Research and Management, Vol. 32. Seattle: IASP Press, 2005.

World Health Organization. *Manual of the International Statistical Classification of Diseases, Injuries, and Causes of Death,* 9th rev. Geneva: World Health Organization, 1978. World Health Organization. *International Statistical Classification of Diseases and Related Health Problems,* 10th rev. Geneva: World Health Organization, 1992.

Correspondence to: Harold Merskey, DM, FRCP, FRCP(C), FRCPsych, 71 Logan Avenue, London, ON, Canada N5Y 2P9. Tel: 519-672-2298; Fax: 519-679-6849; email: harold.merskey@sympatico.ca.

The Paths of Pain 1975–2005, edited by
Harold Merskey, John D. Loeser, and Ronald
Dubner, IASP Press, Seattle, © 2005.

23

Epidemiology of Pain

Michael Von Korff[a] and Linda LeResche[b]

*[a]Center for Health Studies, Group Health Cooperative,
Seattle, Washington, USA; [b]Department of Oral Medicine,
University of Washington, Seattle, Washington, USA*

Epidemiology is the study of the distribution, determinants, and control of disease and disability in populations (Lilienfeld and Lilienfeld 1980). The study of pain is an orphan in the field of epidemiology. Despite the substantial social and personal costs of pain, and scientific progress in understanding pain assessment and mechanisms, the importance of epidemiologic studies of pain is not widely appreciated by practicing epidemiologists. The large majority of epidemiologists devote their efforts to three areas: cancer, cardiovascular disease, and infectious disease. Many epidemiologists hesitate to study pain. Pain is a subjective phenomenon, not a well-defined disease state that can be ascertained by objective diagnostic tests. Funding for epidemiologic studies of pain can be difficult to obtain—there is no National Institute of Pain in the United States or other countries. Departments of epidemiology in leading schools of public health do not prepare their graduates to use epidemiologic methods to study pain conditions. As a result, there is not a critical mass of epidemiologists devoted to studying pain.

Despite these limitations, the application of epidemiologic methods to the study of pain over the last 30 years has yielded important information relevant to understanding the distribution, determinants and burden of pain conditions in human populations. Upon the occasion of the 30th anniversary of the 1st World Congress of the IASP, the purpose of this chapter is to review the accumulation of knowledge about the distribution, determinants, and prevention of pain that has developed through application of epidemiologic methods. In fact, the IASP has played a significant role in synthesizing the results of existing epidemiologic research on pain through its role in the organization of a comprehensive review of epidemiologic evidence regarding the distribution and determinants of pain conditions (Crombie et al. 1999). Moreover, the multidisciplinary traditions of the IASP have fostered a biopsychosocial perspective on pain that is consistent with the perspectives of epidemiology (Dworkin et al. 1992).

This brief review is necessarily selective. However, a cursory examination of progress in this field is sufficient to convey a sense of excitement about what has been learned, and about the potential for epidemiologic methods to make fundamental contributions to the study of pain in the next 30 years. This chapter is organized by the uses of epidemiology identified by Morris (1975). In each of the six areas of epidemiologic investigation, significant progress has been made, and important new opportunities for scientific discovery are at hand.

INDIVIDUAL CHANCES AND RISKS

Pain epidemiology has been preoccupied with developing reliable estimates of the prevalence of chronic pain conditions. This focus stands in contrast to epidemiologic investigations of most chronic and infectious diseases, which predominantly concentrate on identifying causes and evaluating methods of prevention and control. Despite the large and growing number of epidemiologic surveys that have estimated the prevalence of common chronic pain conditions, there is an abiding perception that understanding of the frequency and distribution of chronic pain in populations is inadequate. This sense of inadequate knowledge stems from: (1) the perceived need for an overall prevalence estimate across the diverse types of chronic pain; (2) the widely varying prevalence rate estimates produced by different surveys of the same pain condition; (3) the lack of national survey data for some chronic pain conditions; and (4) the lack of consensus on methods of determining whether particular pain conditions are present or absent. Given the large variety of chronic pain conditions, it is probably not realistic to attempt to estimate the prevalence of all forms of chronic pain, just as reliable estimates of the prevalence of all forms of cancer or all forms of neurological disorder are not readily available.

Recent reviews of prevalence surveys of specific chronic pain conditions, in particular the reviews of epidemiologic evidence published in the IASP's volume *The Epidemiology of Pain* (Crombie et al. 1999), suggest that there is more information on the extent of common chronic pain conditions than is generally perceived. As shown in Table I, significant numbers of prevalence surveys have been carried out for many different chronic pain conditions, including headache and migraine (Scher et al. 1999), back pain

Table I
Period prevalence rates (1 year or less) of common chronic pain conditions in adults,
showing median and range of prevalence estimates and pattern of sex differences

Pain Condition	Median Prevalence Estimate (%)	Range of Prevalence Estimates (No. Studies)	Sex Differences in Prevalence Rates
Headache	69% females 46% males	3–99% (F) 3–93% (M) (33 studies)	More common among women
Low back pain	37%	10–63% (11 studies)	Prevalence rates do not differ by sex in most studies
Knee pain	18%	10–29% (11 studies)	More common among women, but sex difference reduced at older ages
Neck pain	16% females 12% males	10–40% (F) 3–29% (M) (4 studies)	More common among women
Migraine	15% females 6% males	2–48% (F) 0–46% (M) (32 studies)	More common among women
Chronic wide-spread pain (fibromyalgia)	8%	0.66–10.7% (8 studies)	More common among women
Temporo-mandibular pain	9% females 5% males	5–14% (F) 3–10% (M) (10 studies)	More common among women
Shoulder pain	7%	2–61% (5 studies)	Sex differences are inconsistent

(Dionne 1999), knee pain (McCartney and Croft 1999), neck pain (Ariens et al. 1999), chronic widespread pain (Macfarlane 1999), temporomandibular pain (Drangsholt and LeResche 1999), and shoulder pain (van der Windt and Croft 1999). While the range of prevalence rate estimates emerging from these surveys is often large, it is typical for survey estimates to cluster around the median estimate. The large range of these estimates is most likely due to the sensitivity of case ascertainment to differences in the questions asked, and to the differences in severity or duration criteria applied. When consensus diagnostic criteria and standardized questions have been applied in epidemiologic surveys, as is the case for headache and temporomandibular pain disorders, there has been increased convergence in prevalence rate estimates.

Interest is now growing in estimating incidence rates (the number of new onsets of a pain condition in a year per unit population). There are likely to be significant difficulties in estimating incidence rates. These difficulties include ascertaining whether a subject is at risk (i.e., has no prior history of the pain condition); developing reliable and valid methods for defining and determining the point of onset of a new pain condition; and implementing surveillance of an at-risk population to ascertain new onsets. If cohorts were established to estimate incidence rates of specific pain conditions, it would probably be necessary to re-interview participants every 3 to 6 months, due to decay of memory for pain with time. While there will be difficulties in estimating incidence rates, such a cohort study could make an important contribution by permitting assessment of mutable risk factors, psychological state, and functional status before, during, and after significant pain episodes have occurred. Given the tendency of multiple pain conditions to occur in the same individuals (Dworkin et al. 1990), it may make sense for cohort studies on pain onset to focus on more than just a single pain condition. This broader focus would permit differentiation of condition-specific risk factors for pain onset from generalized risk factors.

COMMUNITY DIAGNOSIS

Epidemiologic methods have been used to describe the impact of pain conditions in the community. For chronic diseases such as cancer and cardiovascular disease, condition-specific mortality rates have long been used to assess population trends in community impact. For most pain conditions, data concerning work disability, activity limitations, and health care utilization and costs are important for assessing community impact, while mortality data are of limited value. In a recent population survey of almost 29,000 working age adults, Stewart et al. (2003) estimated that 13% of the U.S. population had experienced a loss of productive time in the prior 3 months due to a common pain condition. Headache, back pain, and arthritis pain were the most common types of pain accounting for lost productive time. Over three-quarters of the lost productive time was due to reduced performance while at work, rather then work absence. Hashemi et al. (1998) examined the duration and cost of worker's compensation claims for back pain for a U.S. private insurer. Prior research had shown a dramatic increase in the occurrence of disability claims, followed by a reduction in the number of disability claims for back pain from the late 1980s to the mid-1990s. The authors found that, depending on year, 5–9% of the claimants accounted for 65–85% of total costs and for 78–90% of disability days. From 1988 to 1996, the average duration of disability claims decreased from 156 days to 61 days, resulting in a 41% decrease in the average claim cost, although the median claim cost increased by 20% in the same time period. Comparing the results of these two studies is informative. The total impact of pain on lost productivity appears to be greatest among persons who continue to work, due to their large numbers, but a small proportion of disability claimants account for the large majority of disability insurance costs. These contrasting results indicate the importance of understanding how the societal impact differs depending on what part of the chronic pain population is studied. This consideration highlights the limitations of studying chronic pain only among unrepresentative patients seen in pain clinics, because they account for a small and atypical part of the total spectrum of persons with chronic pain in the population at large.

Progress has also been made in estimating the total economic burden of selected chronic pain conditions on a population basis. Maniadakis and Gray (2000) developed estimates of the societal costs of back pain in the United Kingdom. They found that 37% of the costs of care were for physical therapists, 31% for hospital care, 14% for primary care, 7% for medications, 6% for community care, and 5% for imaging services. However, the costs of productivity losses and informal care were estimated to be over six times greater than the direct costs of health care. Similarly, van Tulder ct al. (1995) estimated that the costs of back pain in the Netherlands amounted to 1.7% of the gross domestic product in 1991, with 93% of the costs due to disability and absenteeism, and medical care costs accounting for only 7% of the total societal costs. In this study, two-thirds of the disability costs were due to absenteeism and one-third was due to disablement.

Given the substantial differences in organization of health care and disability systems across countries, cross-national studies of common chronic pain conditions that compared disability insurance costs, absenteeism, impaired productivity, health care costs and their components, and informal care giving could be highly informative. As health care systems in developed countries implement automated medical records, the feasibility of efficiently identifying large numbers of persons with treated pain conditions may dramatically increase. Differences in functional outcomes after adjustment for case-mix would be of particular interest. With the development of standardized scales that have been validated in diverse languages, international comparative studies of common pain conditions are now highly feasible.

IDENTIFICATION OF SYNDROMES

The application of epidemiologic principles and methods has made important contributions to defining pain syndromes. A fundamental principle of epidemiology is that case definitions should employ standardized diagnostic criteria and reproducible diagnostic methods. As a result of the increased emphasis on operational diagnostic criteria and reproducible diagnostic methods, standardized diagnostic criteria have been developed for a number of prevalent pain conditions, including headache disorders (International Headache Society 2004), temporomandibular disorders (Dworkin and LeResche 1992), fibromyalgia (Wolfe et al. 1990), and irritable bowel syndrome (Drossman et al. 2000). These diagnostic criteria have been applied in prevalence surveys, risk factor studies, clinical studies, and randomized clinical trials. The use of reliable, standardized diagnostic criteria can reduce variation in prevalence rate estimates in population surveys. It can also increase the homogeneity and comparability of cases in risk factor studies, clinical studies, and controlled trials. While considerable progress has been made in developing standardized and reliable diagnostic criteria for many prevalent pain conditions, establishing the validity and the utility of these classifications is more difficult. Establishing the validity of diagnostic criteria is based on showing that they predict meaningful differences in causal processes, risk factors, response to treatment, and/or clinical course. Research on the validity of research diagnostic criteria for pain conditions is an important area for future research.

COMPLETING THE CLINICAL PICTURE

The application of epidemiologic methods can complete the clinical picture by studying cases that would not normally be seen in clinical settings, and by systematically following up cases over time to establish the long-term outcomes among typical cases.

Over the last decade, the conduct of well-designed epidemiologic follow-up studies has changed the understanding of the prognosis of nonspecific back pain. Until the early 1990s, the consensus view was that the prognosis for back pain among persons seeking treatment in primary care settings was excellent; only a small percentage of patients were thought to develop chronic pain (Deyo 1987). During the following decade, numerous follow-up studies of persons seeking general medical care for back pain were conducted. Pengel et al. (2003) reviewed 15 studies of persons seeking treatment for low back pain or sciatica whose back pain had lasted less than 3 weeks and who were followed up for at least 3 months. Among these acute back pain patients, pain and disability ratings improved by an average of 58% over the first month, which is consistent with the traditional view that back pain improves rapidly for most back pain patients seen in primary care. The authors also reported that the large majority of patients initially off work returned to work within 1 month (pooled estimate of 82%). However, from 1 month to 3 months, there was only gradual improvement, and limited improvement thereafter. This review also found that pain and disability typically persist at low levels from 3 months to 12 months, and that about three-quarters of back pain patients had at least one recurrence of back pain within a year. In a review of studies that included a broader spectrum of patients than those with pain of less than 3 weeks' duration, Von Korff and Saunders (1996) concluded that about two-thirds to three-quarters of back pain patients seen in primary care continue to have at least mild pain 1 month after seeking care, whereas one-third report moderate to severe pain and about one-quarter report substantial activity limitations at 1 month. At 1 year, about one-half report pain at the time of the follow-up interview, although pain is often mild. At 1 year, one-third report intermittent or persistent pain of at least moderate intensity, and one in five report substantial activity limitations. About one patient in four has persistent back pain at 1 year, defined as pain present on more than half the days during an extended period of time (6 months to 1 year). Hestback et al. (2003) reviewed 36 studies and concluded that back pain is usually not a self-limiting condition in the traditional meaning of that term.

These studies of back pain outcomes point to conceptual difficulties in how acute pain and chronic pain are differentiated. If most patients experience rapid improvement, but many continue to experience mild to moderate pain over long periods of time, often with an intermittent pattern, then how should acute and chronic pain be distinguished? The IASP defines chronic pain by a duration of 6 months or more (Merskey and Bogduk 1994), but allows that chronic episodes may be intermittent. A definition of chronic pain based on episode duration encounters problems when representative cases are observed over extended periods. Episode duration does not adequately differentiate individuals who have long-lasting pain at low levels of intensity and interference from those with severe and persistent pain. Empirical studies suggest that pain severity and interference with activities may be more important in differentiating pain dysfunction than persistence of pain per se (Von Korff et al. 1992). Developing operational criteria for chronic pain based on episode duration alone is difficult when there is a recurrent pattern of flare-ups of severe pain interspersed with pain-free intervals. Prospective epidemiologic studies can enrich our understanding of the complex patterns of pain outcomes that are common in the population at large. Research to date suggests that widely used criteria for differentiating acute and chronic pain may need to be reconsidered and reconceptualized based on empirical analysis of long-term outcomes among representative cases with various pain conditions.

IN SEARCH OF CAUSES

The predominant focus of epidemiologic research in cancer, cardiovascular disease, and infectious disease is identification of causes and development of methods of disease prevention and control. While survey research has been used to study sociodemographic correlates of various pain conditions, the application of epidemiologic methods to investigate causes of specific pain syndromes is in its infancy. The use of epidemiology to understand gender differences in the occurrence of temporomandibular pain disorders illustrates how epidemiologic methods can complement clinical and basic research on pain mechanisms.

Numerous adult population surveys of temporomandibular disorder (TMD) pain had reported that its prevalence was almost twice as common among females as among males (LeResche et al. 1997). In contrast, the prevalence of TMD pain prior to adolescence was found to be low (2–4%) relative to adult prevalence rates, and it did not seem to differ for boys and girls (LeResche et al. 1997). Moreover, among adult females, the prevalence of TMD pain was lower for women in the postmenopausal years than for those of reproductive age (Von Korff et al. 1988; Carlsson and LeResche 1995). This pattern of decreasing prevalence with age stands in contrast to the prevalence rates of arthritis and other forms of degenerative joint disease, which increase dramatically with age (Corti and Rigon 2003). If TMD pain were typically the result of degenerative processes affecting the temporomandibular joint, an increasing prevalence with age would be expected as observed for other forms of arthritis. The prevalence pattern of TMD pain is similar to that of migraine headache, where hormonal factors have long been known to play a role in a subset of cases (Silberstein and Merriam 1991). Thus, the prevalence pattern suggests the possibility that reproductive hormones might also play an etiologic role in the occurrence of TMD pain. But, how could this hypothesis be tested using epidemiologic methods?

A case-control study design employing health care records was used to evaluate the association of use of exogenous hormones with risk of having treated TMD pain in a large health care organization (LeResche et al. 1997). Among postmenopausal women, those using hormone replacement therapy (HRT) were compared to women not using HRT. In this study, women who were treated for TMD pain were found to be more likely to be using HRT than controls, with an odds ratio of 1.8. More specifically, risk of TMD was related to use of estrogen, with a clear dose-response relationship between amount of estrogen prescribed in the prior year and risk of being treated for TMD pain.

This line of research was then extended in an observational study in which women with TMD pain completed daily diaries over three menstrual cycles (LeResche et al. 2003). In this study, levels of TMD pain were found to vary systematically across the menstrual cycle. Pain was highest when estrogen was at its lowest level and when estrogen level was rapidly changing. The finding that exogenous estrogen use increased risk of developing TMD pain and the finding that the highest pain levels occur at times of low or fluctuating endogenous estrogen initially seems contradictory. However, a common HRT protocol in perimenopausal women involves stopping use of estrogen for 1 week of the cycle to allow a "menstrual" bleed (similar to the protocol for many oral contraceptives). If estrogen serves as a pain modulator in humans, as appears to be the case in animals (Bodnar et al. 1988; Mogil et al. 1993; Sternberg et al. 1995), it may be the *withdrawal* of estrogen that is associated with increased pain (Marcus 1995).

The association of migraine headache with phase of the menstrual cycle is well documented (Schipper 1986; Silberstein and Merriam 1991; Marcus 1995). Although evidence is less clear than for migraine, a number of prospective diary studies have found indications that estrogen fluctuations may be associated with the onset or severity of non-migraine headache. Studies assessing both migraine and non-migraine headaches (Waters and O'Connor 1971; Johannes et al. 1995) have found the risk of all headaches to be significantly higher during the menstrual period than during the remainder of the cycle, although the relationship is stronger for migraine than for non-migraine headaches.

This research suggests that epidemiologic methods, if used in tandem with basic and clinical research on pain mechanisms, have the potential to advance understanding of the causes of pain in human populations. This potential will not be realized, however, if epidemiologic studies of pain are limited to prevalence surveys focused on estimating the frequency and burden of pain in populations, and if there is not increased exchange between persons using epidemiologic methods to study the causes of pain conditions and scientists doing basic or clinical research on pain.

WORKING OF THE HEALTH SERVICES

Epidemiologic methods can also be used to assess whether health services are effectively meeting the needs of particular clinical populations. In the case of common chronic pain disorders, epidemiologic methods are needed to provide guidance because these conditions affect large numbers of people, contact with health services is common, the spectrum of severity is great, and the evidence base for effective and safe care is often inadequate.

An example of how epidemiologic studies can inform debates about appropriate health care for chronic pain is provided by consideration of the use of opioids for management of chronic musculoskeletal pain. Starting in the latter part of the 1980s, there was increased advocacy for using potent opioids to manage chronic benign pain (Portenoy and Foley 1986; Tennant et al. 1988). The reasoning behind this advocacy was as follows. Randomized clinical trials suggested that opioids were effective relative to placebo in controlling pain among persons with chronic musculoskeletal pain (Ballantyne and Mao 2003). Clinical experience of some practitioners suggested that it was possible to manage selected patients, who should be followed closely, with long-term opioid therapy (Portenoy 1996). A letter to the *New England Journal of Medicine* was sometimes cited in support of the low risk of addiction, even though this brief report did not differentiate brief use of opioids from long-term use, and ascertainment of addiction was based on hospital records data unlikely to capture most episodes of substance abuse or dependence (Porter and Jick 1980). Based on these kinds of observations and data, consensus recommendations were promulgated by the American Pain Society and American Academy of Pain Medicine in 1996 recommending that selected patients who were closely monitored could be managed with long-term opioid therapy contingent on documented progress towards agreed-upon clinical goals.

The value of using epidemiologic methods to evaluate health care is that it broadens the policy perspective to consider not only what happens to selected patients treated under ideal circumstances, but also the consequences of changes in care in the entire population, including the majority of patients that may not be closely monitored. Epidemiologic research suggests the need for caution in advocacy for use of potent opioids in management of chronic musculoskeletal pain. Caudill-Slosberg et al. (2004), using United States health survey data from 1980 and 2000, found that among patients seen for chronic musculoskeletal pain, 2% received potent opioids in 1980 whereas 9% received such medications in 2000, with the large majority of these prescriptions occurring in general medical settings where close follow-up and monitoring of treatment progress and adverse effects are difficult. Since the numbers of patients seen for chronic musculoskeletal pain in a year is vast, this change meant that potent opioids were prescribed at almost 5 million additional encounters in 2000 relative to 1980 prescribing patterns (although it is likely that many of these prescriptions were for short-term treatment). The potential risks of increased prescribing of opioids for chronic musculoskeletal pain on a population basis were suggested by a systematic review of studies of the occurrence of substance abuse by Fishbain et al. (1992). The authors found that drug abuse or dependence was observed among 3–19% of chronic pain patients, suggesting that a significant minority of chronic pain patients are at risk. On a population basis, the risks of increased distribution of potent opioids may affect persons other than the individuals filling the prescriptions. The College on Problems of Drug Dependence task force of prescription opioid non-medical use and abuse (Zacny et al. 2003) drew on epidemiologic data to assess the consequences of increased availability of opioids. Based on U.S. national survey data, the report stated that in the year 2000 approximately 2 million persons aged 12 or older reported using a prescription opioid for a nonmedical reason for the first time, a number that had quintupled since the mid-1980s. Survey data from the Monitoring the Future project, an ongoing survey of representative samples of 8th, 10th, and 12th grade high school students in the United States, found that the use of prescription opioids among 12th graders increased from 1.1% in 1991 to 3% in 2001, a 173% increase in one decade. The Drug Abuse Warning Network, a surveillance program for a representative sample of emergency departments, found that the number of mentions of opioid analgesics in emergency department episodes increased by 123% from 1994 to 2001, with a 21% increase between 2000 and 2001 alone. Among the 40 U.S. states that report data on drug abuse treatment episodes, 33 states reported a 20% or greater increase in the number of episodes for non-heroin opioid problems between 1999 and 2001. These population surveillance data indicate that the use of prescription opioids for chronic musculoskeletal pain has increased markedly in the prior two decades, and that during the past decade, there has also been a large increase in the extent of abuse of these medications.

The epidemiologic perspective suggests that it is not sufficient to consider only the safety of prescribing opioids to carefully selected patients monitored closely under optimal conditions. Recommendations for care of chronic pain patients must also consider the effects of guidelines when they are implemented on a mass basis under real-world conditions. Increased application of the epidemiologic perspective and epidemiologic methods to the significant problems in caring for large numbers of persons with chronic pain could provide guidance that would help improve the effectiveness, cost-effectiveness, and safety of health care services for pain.

CONCLUSIONS

The field of epidemiology has already made significant contributions to our understanding of the distribution, burdens, determinants, and management of pain. This chapter was intended to highlight a few examples of the contributions of epidemiology to the field of pain. While the contributions of epidemiologic research to the study of pain over the last 30 years have been substantial, the future potential is even greater. The field of pain would benefit from concerted efforts to recruit trained epidemiologists to study pain. The increased application of epidemiologic methods to etiologic studies of pain and the evaluation of ways to effectively and safely manage and control pain conditions on a population basis are two of the most promising areas for future epidemiologic studies of pain.

REFERENCES

American Pain Society and American Academy of Pain Medicine. *Consensus Statement: The Use of Opioids for the Treatment of Chronic Pain.* American Pain Society and American Academy of Pain Medicine, 1996. Available at: www.ampainsoc.org/advocacy/opioids.htm.

Ariens GAM, Bourghouts JAJ, Koes BW. Neck pain. In: Crombie IK, et al. (Eds). *Epidemiology of Pain.* Seattle: IASP Press, 1999, pp 235–256.

Ballantyne JC, Mao J. Opioid therapy for chronic pain. *New Engl J Med* 2003; 349:1943–1953.

Bodnar RJ, Romero M, Kramer E. Organismic variables and pain inhibition: roles of gender and aging. *Brain Res Bull* 1988; 21:947–953.

Carlsson G, LeResche L. Epidemiology of temporomandibular disorders. In: Sessle B, Bryant P, Dionne R, (Eds). *Temporomandibular Disorders and Related Pain Conditions,* Progress in Pain Research and Management, Vol. 4. Seattle: IASP Press, 1995, pp 211–226.

Caudill-Slosberg MA, Schwartz LM, Woloshin S. Office visits and analgesic prescriptions for musculoskeletal pain in the U.S.: 1980 vs. 2000. *Pain* 2004;109(3):514–519.

Corti MC, Rigon C. Epidemiology of osteoarthritis: prevalence, risk factors and functional impact. *Aging Clin Exp Res* 2003; 15:359–363.

Crombie IK, Croft PR, Linton SJ, LeResche L, Von Korff M (Eds). *Epidemiology of Pain.* Seattle: IASP Press, 1999.

Deyo RA. The role of the primary care physician in reducing work absenteeism and costs due to back pain. In: Deyo RA (Ed). *Spine, State of the Art Review: Occupational Back Pain.* Philadelphia: Hanley and Belfus, 1987, pp 17–30.

Dionne CE. Low back pain. In: Crombie IK, et al. (Eds). *Epidemiology of Pain.* Seattle: IASP Press, 1999, pp 283–298.

Drangsholt M, LeResche L. Temporomandibular disorder pain. In: Crombie IK, et al. (Eds). *Epidemiology of Pain.* Seattle: IASP Press, 1999, pp 203–234.

Drossman DA, Corazziari E, Talley NJ, et al. *The Functional Gastrointestinal Disorders. Diagnosis, Pathophysiology and Treatment: A Multinational Consensus,* 2nd ed. McLean, VA: Degnon Associates, 2000.

Dworkin SF, LeResche L. Research diagnostic criteria for temporomandibular disorders: review, criteria, examinations and specifications, critique. *J Craniomandib Disord* 1992; 6:301–355.

Dworkin SF, Von Korff M, LeResche L. Multiple pains and psychiatric disturbance. An epidemiologic investigation. *Arch Gen Psychiatry* 1990; 47:239–244.

Dworkin SF, Von Korff M, LeResche L. Epidemiologic studies of chronic pain: a dynamic-ecologic perspective. *Ann Behav Med* 1992; 14:3–11.

Fishbain DA, Rosomoff HL, Rosomoff RS. Drug abuse, dependence, and addiction in chronic pain patients. *Clin J Pain* 1992; 8:77–85.

Hashemi L, Webster BS, Clancey EA. Trends in disability duration and cost of workers' compensation low back claims (1988–1996). *J Occup Environ Med* 1998; 40:1110–1119.

Hestback L, Leboeuf-Yde C, Manniche C. Low back pain: what is the long-term course? A review of studies in general patient populations. *Eur Spine J* 2003; 12:149–165.

International Headache Society. International Classification of Headache Disorders, 2nd ed. *Cephalagia* 2004; Suppl 1:1–150.

Johannes CB, Linet MS, Stewart WF, et al. Relationship of headache to phase of the menstrual cycle among young women: a daily diary study. *Neurology* 1995; 45:1076–1082.

LeResche L, Saunders K, Von Korff M, Barlow W, Dworkin SF. Use of exogenous hormones and risk of temporomandibular disorder pain. *Pain* 1997; 69:153–160.

LeResche L, Mancl L, Sherman JJ, Gandara B, Dworkin SF. Changes in temporomandibular pain and other symptoms across the menstrual cycle. *Pain* 2003; 106:253–261.

Lilienfeld AM, Lilienfeld DE. *Foundations of Epidemiology,* 2nd ed. New York: Oxford University Press, 1980.

Macfarlane GJ. Fibromyalgia and chronic widespread pain. In: Crombie IK, et al. (Eds). *Epidemiology of Pain.* Seattle: IASP Press, 1999, pp 113–124.

Maniadakis N, Gray A. The economic burden of back pain in the UK. *Pain* 2000; 84:95–103.

Marcus DA. Clinical review: interrelationships of neurochemicals, estrogen, and recurring headache. *Pain* 1995; 62:129–139.

McCartney R, Croft PR. Knee pain. In: Crombie IK, et al. (Eds). *Epidemiology of Pain.* Seattle: IASP Press, 1999, pp 299–314.

Merskey H, Bogduk N (Eds). *Classification of Chronic Pain: Descriptions of Chronic Pain Syndromes and Definitions of Pain Terms,* 2nd ed. Seattle: IASP Press, 1994.

Mogil JS, Sternberg WF, Kest B, Marek P, Liebeskind JC. Sex differences in the antagonism of swim stress-induced analgesia: effects of gonadectomy and estrogen replacement. *Pain* 1993; 53:17–25.

Morris JN. *Uses of Epidemiology.* Edinburgh: Churchill Livingstone, 1975.

Pengel LH, Herbert RD, Maher CG, Refshauge KM. Acute low back pain: systematic review of its prognosis. *BMJ* 2003; 327:323.

Portenoy RK. Opioid therapy for chronic nonmalignant pain: a review of the critical issues. *J Pain Symptom Manage* 1996; 11(4):203–217.

Portenoy RK, Foley KM. Chronic use of opioid analgesics in non-malignant pain: report of 38 cases. *Pain* 1986; 25(2):171–186.

Porter J, Jick H. Addiction rare in patients treated with narcotics. *N Engl J Med* 1980; 302(2):123.

Scher AI, Stewart WF, Lipton RB. Migraine and headache: a meta-analytic approach. In: Crombie IK, et al. (Eds). *Epidemiology of Pain.* Seattle: IASP Press, 1999, pp 159–170.

Schipper HM. Neurology of sex steroids and oral contraceptives. *Neurol Clin* 1986; 4:721–751.

Silberstein SD, Merriam GR. Estrogens, progestins, and headache. *Neurology* 1991; 41:786–793.

Sternberg WF, Mogil JS, Kest B, et al. Neonatal testosterone exposure influences neurochemistry of non-opioid swim stress-induced analgesia in adult mice. *Pain* 1995; 63:321–326.

Stewart WF, Ricci JA, Chee E, Morganstein D, Lipton R. Lost productive time and cost due to common pain conditions in the US workforce. *JAMA* 2003; 290:2443–2454.

Tennant F Jr, Robinson D, Sagherian A, Seecof R. Chronic opioid treatment of intractable, non-malignant pain. *NIDA Res Monogr* 1988; 81:174–180.

van der Windt DAWM, Croft PR. Shoulder pain. In: Crombie IK, et al. (Eds). *Epidemiology of Pain.* Seattle: IASP Press, 1999, pp 203–234. pp 257–282.

van Tulder MW, Koes BW, Bouter LM. A cost-of-illness study of back pain in the Netherlands. *Pain* 1995; 62:233–240.

Von Korff M, Saunders K. The course of back pain in primary care. *Spine* 1996; 21:2833–2837.

Von Korff M, Dworkin SF, LeResche L, Kruger A. An epidemiologic comparison of pain complaints. *Pain* 1988; 32:173–183.

Von Korff M, Ormel J, Keefe F, Dworkin SF. Grading the severity of chronic pain. *Pain* 1992; 50:133–149.

Waters WE, O'Connor PJ. Epidemiology of headache and migraine in women. *J Neurol Neurosurg Psychiatry* 1971; 34:148–153.

Wolfe F, Smythe HA, Yunus MB, et al. The American College of Rheumatology 1990 Criteria for the Classification of Fibromyalgia. Report of the Multicenter Criteria Committee. *Arthritis Rheum* 1990; 33:160–172.

Zacny J, Bigelow G, Compton P, et al. College on Problems of Drug Dependence taskforce on prescription opioid non-medical use and abuse: position statement. *Drug Alcohol Depend* 2003; 69:215–232.

Correspondence to: Michael Von Korff, ScD, Center for Health Studies, Group Health Cooperative, 1730 Minor Ave, Suite 1600, Seattle WA, 98101, USA. Email: vonkorff.m@ghc.org.

The Paths of Pain 1975–2005, edited by
Harold Merskey, John D. Loeser, and Ronald
Dubner, IASP Press, Seattle, © 2005.

24

Musculoskeletal Pain

James P. Robinson,[a] Dean Ricketts,[b] and David Hanscom[c]

[a]*Department of Rehabilitation Medicine, University of Washington Medical Center, Seattle, Washington, USA;* [b]*Private Practice in Orthopedics, Bellevue, Washington, USA;* [c]*Private Practice in Orthopedics, Seattle, Washington, USA*

Musculoskeletal pain is important to pain medicine because of its high prevalence (Praemer et al. 1999; National Research Council and Institute of Medicine 2001). However, the fact that musculoskeletal disorders are common and often painful does not automatically mean that they should be construed as pain problems, or as problems of interest to physicians who specialize in pain medicine. For example, chest pain is a cardinal symptom of cardiac ischemia, but a patient with angina is almost invariably treated by a cardiologist or a thoracic surgeon rather than by a pain specialist. More generally, traditional medical teaching holds that pain is a symptom of various disorders, and, like other symptoms and signs, is important primarily as a guide to diagnosing the underlying disorder. In this traditional model, treatment is directed toward the abnormal anatomy and physiology that comprise a disorder, rather than toward the symptoms of the disorder. The assumption is that once the underlying biological abnormality has been corrected, the symptoms—including pain—will resolve.

The assumption that diagnosis and treatment should be directed toward pathophysiology rather than toward direct treatment of symptoms is central to the orthopedic approach to musculoskeletal disorders. Orthopedists implicitly assume what might be called the "structural model" of musculoskeletal disorders. They assume that the symptoms and signs of musculoskeletal dysfunction can be explained by anatomical or functional abnormalities in specific musculoskeletal structures and that the most effective way to relieve these symptoms and signs is to correct the underlying structural abnormality.

To the extent that musculoskeletal pain is strongly correlated with evidence of structural lesions and can be eliminated by the diagnosis and treatment of these lesions, musculoskeletal medicine has no need for physicians who specialize in pain management. However, pain specialists become important in musculoskeletal medicine when the most feasible treatment strategy is to manage pain directly rather than to attempt to fix a structural abnormality presumed to be causing pain. Such a strategy is generally appropriate when the structural model fails, either because a patient's pain complaints are dissociated from an identifiable structural lesion, or because the structural lesion thought to be causing the patient's pain cannot be effectively corrected. One or the other of these circumstances holds frequently enough that musculoskeletal pain is appropriately an area of great concern for pain specialists.

This chapter is organized around the structural model of musculoskeletal pain, including its strengths, weaknesses, and changing status over the past 30 years. There are several reasons for this organization. First, the structural model trumps all other approaches when it applies, for example in the treatment of a comminuted fracture of the femur from a skiing accident. This point is so obvious that it may escape reflection. Second, in our opinion, the structural model articulated in orthopedic literature is the only reasonably comprehensive model of musculoskeletal disorders. Third, the orthopedic approach to musculoskeletal disorders is that only one that can fairly easily traced over time, because it is the only one for which multiple editions of basic texts can be compared (Crenshaw 1971; Canale 2003).

As we will see below, pain specialists and pain researchers have greatly added to our understanding of musculoskeletal disorders. But it is important to acknowledge at the outset that the pain medicine perspective on musculoskeletal disorders is only one of many perspectives, and that pain specialists participate very selectively in the treatment of patients with such disorders.

CAVEATS

A history of musculoskeletal medicine from the 1970s to the present is fraught with ambiguities. These include the failure of practitioners of musculoskeletal medicine to describe their conceptual models clearly either in the 1970s or at present, as well as the marked heterogeneity of opinion among different practitioners in both time periods. In addition, musculoskeletal medicine is such a broad field that almost any general statement about it will have numerous exceptions.

We will address this diversity by limiting the scope of our analysis to the following disorders in which mechanical stresses are thought to play a crucial role: (1) *Overt injuries,* such as a fracture of the lower extremity in a skiing accident. (2) *Covert "injuries,"* in which an individual is exposed repeatedly to low-grade mechanical stresses, rather than to a single overwhelming mechanical stress. Examples include lateral epicondylitis and carpal tunnel syndrome. (3) *Degenerative joint disease.* (4) *Nonradicular low back pain (LBP).* This condition is included because of its high prevalence among patients who are seen by pain specialists, and because it highlights difficulties in the application of the structural model. We will also discuss (5) *fibromyalgia (FMS).* FMS patients report pain that appears to involve the musculoskeletal system, but for which no underlying structural abnormality can be identified. It thus represents the ultimate challenge to the structural model.

MAJOR TRENDS DURING THE PAST 30 YEARS

ADVANCES IN THE STRUCTURAL MODEL FOR SERIOUS, OVERT INJURIES

Orthopedic management of overt injuries has advanced dramatically in the past 30 years. The advances have occurred in multiple arenas, including materials science, surgical techniques, and diagnostic testing. Specific examples include the introduction of arthroscopic surgery and marked improvements in the management of fractures. It is beyond the scope of this chapter to attempt to summarize these advances (see Canale 2003).

A striking feature of the improvements in orthopedic management of overt injuries is that most of them are "invisible" to pain specialists. This reflects the basic reality that pain specialists are unlikely to see patients with musculoskeletal disorders from overt injuries unless the patients have failed to benefit from orthopedic management. Thus, for example, pain specialists are unlikely to be familiar with improvements in the orthopedic management of acute meniscal tears or full-thickness rotator cuff tears because they rarely see patients with these conditions.

LIMITATIONS IN THE STRUCTURAL MODEL

As noted above, the most dramatic advances in orthopedics in the past 30 years have come in the management of overt, serious musculoskeletal injuries. The structural model can also claim significant advances in the treatment of degenerative joint disease. In particular, major advances have occurred in joint arthroplasty during the past 30 years. In contrast, the structural model appears less plausible now than it did in the early 1970s as an adequate model for covert injuries, LBP, and FMS, for reasons that are discussed below.

THE EMERGENCE OF NEW VOICES

Pain medicine. In 1975, the IASP was in its infancy, and other organizations of pain medicine physicians had not yet come into existence. Some physicians may have called themselves pain specialists, but they would not be able to pursue specialty training in pain medicine or take any kind of certifying examination. In contrast, the specialty of pain medicine is currently flourishing.

It is significant that aside from epidural injections, virtually none of the interventional treatments currently used by pain specialists were available in the early 1970s. Diskography dates back to the 1940s, but it was used primarily as a means of improving surgical decision making until the late 1990s, when intradiskal electrothermal disk decompression and annuloplasty (IDET) was introduced (Kennedy 1999). Facet joint injections (Mooney and Robertson 1976), facet or medial branch neurotomies (Pawl 1974; Bogduk and Long 1980), spinal cord stimulation (Shealy et al. 1967; Simpson 1999), and intrathecal opiate therapy (Onofrio 1983) were either nonexistent or in their infancy in the early 1970s.

Similarly, many of the rehabilitative and pharmacological approaches currently used by pain specialists were not available in the early 1970s. Intensive multidisciplinary pain rehabilitation was first described in 1973 (Fordyce et al. 1973). Options for pharmacological therapy have expanded with the easing of regulations regarding the use of opiates in chronic nonmalignant pain during the 1990s (Gilson et al. 2003), and with our increased understanding of the role of anticonvulsants and antidepressants in the treatment of chronic pain (Staiger et al. 2003; Backonja 2004).

The increasing role of physical medicine and rehabilitation physicians in musculoskeletal disorders. Physiatrists have played an increasingly prominent role in the management of musculoskeletal pain during the past 30 years. In 1993, the Physiatric Association of Spine, Sports and Occupational Rehabilitation (PASSOR) was formed as a special interest group within the American Academy of Physical Medicine and Rehabilitation. The existence of PASSOR reflects the fact that during the past 20 years physiatrists have been prominent as musculoskeletal medicine specialists, and their specialty uses many of the injection procedures that interventional pain specialists perform.

It is interesting to note that whereas interventional pain specialists are typically trained in anesthesiology and view their role as one of pain management, physiatrists who specialize in musculoskeletal medicine are more likely to accept the basic structural model of musculoskeletal disorders, and to view their role as one of diagnosing and providing nonsurgical treatment within that model.

Rheumatology and FMS. Since the 1970s, rheumatologists have played a prominent role in the development of the fibrositis/fibromyalgia construct. Because FMS is by definition a widespread pain condition, rheumatologists and other researchers have looked assiduously for systemic abnormalities that are specific to it and might explain it. The essentially negative outcome of these investigations has added new dimensions to the dialogue about musculoskeletal pain. In particular, some investigators have concluded that the fundamental abnormality in FMS does not reside in the musculoskeletal system, but in the manner in which the central nervous system (CNS) processes sensory input (Bennett 1999; Banic et al. 2004; Staud 2004; see Moldofsky and Merskey, this volume). This perspective represents a radical break with the structural model of musculoskeletal pain because it asserts that in some settings, pain that is described in terms of musculoskeletal dysfunction may not be a product of any abnormality in the musculoskeletal system.

Complementary and alternative medicine. Practitioners of complementary and alternative medicine (CAM) existed in the early 1970s, but their role in treating musculoskeletal conditions has increased enormously in the past 30 years (Eisenberg et al. 1998; Ni et al. 2002). Although practitioners of different forms of CAM have widely diverse conceptual models of musculoskeletal pain, they are united in their rejection of the structural model as understood in orthopedics. The growing influence of CAM approaches such as massage, acupuncture, and naturopathy highlights the fact that many practitioners and consumers of musculoskeletal medicine reject the orthopedic model.

Patient support groups. The past 30 years have witnessed the emergence of advocacy groups comprising patients with chronic pain (Shorter 1992; Leong and Euller-Ziegler 2004). It is now common for patients with chronic pain conditions to communicate with a network of similar sufferers. These interactions tend to empower patients, who then become more assertive regarding the physicians they are willing to see and the treatments they prefer (Leong and Euller-Ziegler 2004). The effects of patient advocacy groups are difficult to assess, but there is no doubt that such groups create new voices in the dialogue about chronic musculoskeletal pain.

INCREASED RELIANCE ON EMPIRICAL EVIDENCE

A striking feature of orthopedic texts from the early 1970s is that they make only minimal references to empirical studies. The texts are generally silent about the epidemiology of various musculoskeletal disorders, and recommendations about treatment are virtually never buttressed by data.

One reason for the absence of empirical data is that extensive research on most musculoskeletal conditions simply did not exist in the early 1970s. But authors of orthopedic texts did not decry the dearth of data, and it appears that they assumed that experts in musculoskeletal medicine could be trusted to provide valid information about the appropriate management of various disorders. In sharp contrast, the 10th edition of *Campbell's Operative Orthopaedics* (Canale 2003) contains numerous references to published studies on the outcomes of various treatments.

THE RECOGNITION OF UNCERTAINTY

Discussions of nonradicular LBP in texts of the 1970s often provided detailed differential diagnoses and described in detail methods of evaluating the low back. The implicit message was that if a clinician developed the requisite level of clinical acumen, he or she would be able to make a reasonably firm diagnosis in most patients with LBP.

More recent research and opinions challenge the confidence exuded by texts from the early 1970s. As indicated by the book *Symposium on Idiopathic Low Back Pain* (White and Gordon 1982), spine specialists began questioning the specificity of diagnosis for patients with LBP more than 20 years ago. This skepticism continues (Deyo 2002).

Ironically, while some orthopedists and numerous other researchers have argued against the notion of an identifiable structural lesion or pain generator in most nonradicular LBP, the physiatrists and interventional pain specialists who perform spinal injections are moving in the opposite direction (Saal 2002). A major thrust of injection therapy for axial lumbar spine conditions is to make a precise anatomic diagnosis that accounts for a patient's pain, and to provide targeted treatment based on the diagnosis. The growth of this approach can be appreciated when we consider the robust growth of PASSOR and the International Spinal Injection Society (ISIS).

IMPROVEMENTS IN IMAGING

In the early 1970s, imaging studies for musculoskeletal disorders were limited to X-rays, arthrography, myelography, and bone scans. Computer-assisted tomography (CT), introduced during the 1970s, has greatly enhanced the ability of physicians to visualize bony structures. The 1980s saw the introduction of magnetic resonance imaging (MRI) scanning. MRI scans quickly became the studies of choice for virtually all soft tissue lesions, including disk abnormalities in the spine, meniscus cartilage injuries in the knee, and ligament or tendon injuries in virtually all areas of the body. Witte

(2003, p. 123) describes the significance of MRI scans to musculoskeletal medicine as follows:

"Aside from routine roentgenography, no imaging method has as great an effect on the current practice of orthopaedics as magnetic resonance imaging (MRI). MRI provides unsurpassed soft tissue contrast and multiplanar capability with spatial resolution that approaches that of computed tomography (CT). Consequently, MRI has superseded older imaging methods such as myelography, arthrography, and even angiography. In some areas, such as the knee and shoulder, MRI has become a powerful diagnostic tool, helping the surgeon to evaluate structures that are otherwise invisible to noninvasive techniques."

These improvements in imaging technology have produced the paradox of mismatches between symptoms and anatomic findings. Advanced imaging of the lumbar spine, for example, is sometimes entirely normal even in patients who complain bitterly of LBP. At the opposite extreme, studies on both CT scans and MRI scans of the lumbar spine have found high false-positive rates—significant structural abnormalities in individuals who are completely free of symptoms (Jackson et al. 1989; Boos et al. 2000; Jarvik et al. 2001). The studies on false-positive findings clearly indicate that when physicians explain the symptoms of LBP patients on the basis of imaging abnormalities, they are often making their inferences on the basis of incidental structural abnormalities that have little or no relevance to the patients' pain.

The issue of mismatches between patients' musculoskeletal symptoms and the findings on advanced imaging tests is more than just a caution to surgeons not to over-interpret the tests. It potentially goes to the core of the structural model of musculoskeletal pain. In the 1970s, an orthopedist could confidently state that musculoskeletal symptoms following injury were almost always related in systematic ways to structural lesions (except in patients with "psychogenic" pain), but that the lesions were often impossible to find because of limitations in diagnostic tools. This assessment is much less credible today. The difficulties physicians have encountered in "finding pain" on advanced imaging studies have highlighted limitations in the scope of the structural model of musculoskeletal disorders. A reasonable conclusion based on our current knowledge is that musculoskeletal pain is *sometimes* reducible to structural lesions, and that the likelihood of a close correspondence between symptoms and structural abnormalities is greatest for acute injuries from violent mechanical forces. In contrast, relations between structural abnormalities and symptoms are likely to be tenuous in patients with chronic musculoskeletal pain, or those who have developed symptoms in the absence of any clear injury.

PSYCHOLOGY OF CHRONIC PAIN

A major change during the past 30 years has been the development of behavioral medicine as a field within psychology, and the greatly expanded role of psychologists with behavioral medicine training in the evaluation and management of chronic pain. The significance of these developments is discussed by Keefe et al. and by Merskey in other chapters of this book.

THE IMPORTANCE OF ACTIVE REHABILITATION

A striking feature of discussions in the early 1970s is that bedrest is given a prominent role in the treatment of musculoskeletal problems. For example, Salter (1970, p. 214) stated:

> "All patients with degenerative joint disease in the lumbar spine are helped, at least to some degree, by adequate local rest of the spine. Patients with segmental instability, segmental narrowing and intervertebral disc herniation should rest in bed on a firm mattress which is supported by rigid boards. For acute attacks of either lumbago or sciatica, complete bed rest should be continued until at least two or three days after the pain has been relieved."

Prevailing views regarding exercise are entirely different now. For example, research has demonstrated that for nonradicular LBP, bedrest does nothing to facilitate recovery, and may well impede it (Hilde et al. 2002). This research has led experts in LBP to recommend early mobilization of patients with LBP, and specifically to recommend against prolonged bedrest (Atlas and Deyo 2001).

Sports medicine has also advanced greatly during the past 30 years, and concepts developed for athletes have been applied to all patients with musculoskeletal injuries. The message from sports medicine is simple and consistent: regardless of what specific curative procedure is undertaken to help an athlete recover from a significant injury, vigorous rehabilitation on the part of the athlete is almost always required if he or she is to return to competitive sports.

Multidisciplinary pain management programs and functional restoration programs represent the ultimate attempts to rehabilitate patients with chronic pain via physical reactivation in combination with psychosocial support.

PROGRESS IN THE SCIENCE OF MUSCLE PAIN

Muscular pain has been largely ignored by orthopedists. For example, the terms "fibromyalgia," "myofascial pain," and "muscle pain" are not included in the index for the 10th edition of *Campbell's Operative Ortho-paedics* (Canale 2003). In contrast, muscle pain has been an area of particular interest for many pain specialists and for neurobiologists interested in pain mechanisms. Pain described as muscular is frequently found in patients with chronic musculoskeletal disorders. Some of these patients start with injuries to muscles, but a striking feature of muscle pain is that it is often reported by patients whose initial injuries involved structures other than muscles. Pain that appears to be muscular in origin is important not only because of its high prevalence, but also because it can be induced easily and safely in experimental studies, and thus has been used as a prototype of deep somatic pain. Moreover, as discussed below, research on muscle pain has provided insights into the role of the CNS in musculoskeletal pain.

Any discussion of muscle pain can founder at the outset on the problems of defining the term. For example, many writers casually equate muscle pain and myofascial pain. We propose a simple, descriptive definition of muscle pain based on two criteria: (1) a patient's description of his/her pain as being muscular, and of being aching or cramping in quality; (2) hyperalgesia in the symptomatic area when pressure is applied to it (i.e., reduced pressure pain threshold). These criteria almost certainly lack specificity. However, as discussed below, we view the low specificity not as a problem with our definition, but rather as an indicator of the complex factors underlying pain that is described as muscular.

Empirical research on muscle pain was virtually nonexistent in the early 1970s. In the preface to their seminal book *Muscle Pain,* Mense and Simons (2001, p. vii) described the situation as follows:

> "The history of this book reaches back to the year 1978, when the authors met for the first time in Montreal on the occasion of the Second World Congress on Pain, organized by the ... IASP. Contact between the authors was maintained and intensified in ensuing years. The contacts were used for long and vivid discussions of all aspects of muscle pain. In 1978, the mechanisms of muscle pain were largely unknown. ... Very often, [our] discussions started with an effort to account for a clinical observation and ended with the frustrating conclusion that it could not be solved because too little was known about the neurobiology and pathophysiology of muscle pain. In the late 1970s, pain research in general was a relatively new discipline, and the bulk of the available knowledge was obtained in experiments on cutaneous pain. Even though many mechanisms controlling cutaneous pain could be assumed to be functioning also in muscle pain, it became increasingly clear that muscle pain differed from cutaneous pain in many aspects." (Mense and Simons 2001)

Fortunately, research on muscle pain has advanced enormously since 1978. Of the many questions that have been addressed in this research, the ones of greatest relevance to the present chapter include the following: (1) What are the parameters and the physiological basis of the referred pain that is often seen in patients with muscle pain? (2) Is it possible for injuries to nonmuscular structures to cause pain that appears to be muscular in nature? (3) What role does CNS sensitization play in muscle pain? (4) What are the relations between muscle pain and chronic musculoskeletal pain? Research related to these questions is briefly and selectively discussed below. For more complete discussions, the reader should consult the book by Mense and Simons (2001), as well as several recent reviews (Graven-Nielsen and Arendt-Nielsen 2002; Arendt-Nielsen and Graven-Nielsen 2003; Staud 2004).

REFERRED PAIN

Research dating back to Kellgren's work in the 1930s demonstrates that irritation of muscles can produce pain both locally and at distant sites (Kellgren 1938). Other research suggests that noxious stimulation of musculoskeletal structures other than muscles—such as intervertebral disks (Ohnmeiss et al. 1999) or facet joints (Dwyer et al. 1990)—can provoke referred pain in patterns that have some similarity to those postulated for myofascial trigger points (Travell and Simons 1992). More recently, studies have demonstrated that noxious stimulation of various visceral structures can provoke pain referral and hyperalgesia in patterns that mimic pain of muscular origin (Giamberardino et al. 2002; Drewes et al. 2003; Giamberardino 2003).

CENTRAL SENSITIZATION AND MUSCLE PAIN

Several investigators have proposed that the basis for referral of pain following noxious stimulation of muscles, joints, or viscera is sensitization of the CNS (Graven-Nielsen and Arendt-Nielsen 2002; Arendt-Nielsen and Graven-Nielsen 2003). This hypothesis provides a plausible explanation for why noxious stimulation of a musculoskeletal structure can produce pain and hyperalgesia in a remote site, and is consistent with animal studies in which sensitization of the dorsal horn of the spinal cord can be demonstrated following noxious stimulation of muscles (Hoheisel et al. 1994; Mense and Simons 2001). Central sensitization is associated with a reduction in the firing threshold for dorsal horn neurons and expansion of their receptive fields, with the result that the neurons fire in response to gentle tactile stimulation of sites far removed from the site of experimental injury (Hoheisel and Mense 1989).

MUSCLE PAIN IN PATIENTS WITH CHRONIC MUSCULOSKELETAL DISORDERS

Recent research has demonstrated that normal volunteers and patients with chronic musculoskeletal pain respond differently to experimentally in-duced muscular pain, even when the site of experimental pain is far removed from the area where patients have their clinical pain. For example, one study demonstrated that chronic whiplash patients had lower pressure pain thresh-olds than normal controls, both over a muscle in the patients' symptomatic area (the infraspinatus) and over a muscle in a remote site (the tibialis anterior). Moreover, the whiplash patients reported more severe and pro-longed pain following hypertonic saline injections to either muscle (Koelbaek Johansen et al. 1999). The results of this and several other studies (Curatolo et al. 2001; Graven-Nielsen and Arendt-Nielsen 2002) have led at least some investigators to conclude that chronic musculoskeletal pain (whether due to irritation of muscles or other musculoskeletal structures) causes long-term CNS changes that influence individuals' pain experiences to new noxious stimuli.

IMPLICATIONS FOR THE STRUCTURAL MODEL OF MUSCULOSKELETAL PAIN

The above research has significant implications for our understanding of muscle pain in particular and musculoskeletal pain in general. First, it high-lights the difficulty of determining when "muscle pain" truly indicates an abnormality in the muscle where the pain is experienced, as opposed to centrally mediated referred pain or hyperalgesia from other musculoskeletal structures, or from structures that have nothing to do with the musculoskel-etal system. Second, the research strongly suggests that central processing of nociceptive inputs can cause dissociations between the injury or nociceptive event and the pain experience, thereby making it extremely difficult to relate patients' pain reports to a structural lesion.

In a very broad way, research on muscle pain has contributed to a conceptual model of musculoskeletal pain that can be viewed as a "third path" that supplements the structural model and the "psychogenic" model that dominated orthopedic thinking in the early 1970s. This new model has been termed the neurophysiological model (Waddell 2004). Proponents of the model assert that nociceptive inputs from essentially any part of the body can provoke disturbances in the CNS that lead to dissociation between ongoing tissue injury and pain. Moreover, because these disturbances can be demonstrated in infrahuman organisms, as well as in the spinal cord of an organism even after the spinal cord has been functionally isolated from the brain, they cannot be described as "psychological" abnormalities in the usual sense of that term.

CONCLUSIONS AND A TENTATIVE LOOK AHEAD

The structural model has been the dominant model of musculoskeletal disorders during the past 30 years. However, despite the effectiveness of the structural model for overt injuries, research and clinical experience during that period have demonstrated numerous conditions to which it applies imperfectly, if at all. These include nonradicular LBP, repetitive motion disorders, muscular pain, and FMS.

Pain research during the past 30 years has drawn at least the outlines of an alternative model, which has been called the neurophysiological model. It explains chronic musculoskeletal pain on the basis of the physiology of the nervous system, rather than on the basis of structural lesions in peripheral tissues such as bones, joints, ligaments, or muscles.

This new model by no means solves the problem of persistent musculoskeletal pain. In fact, its implications for the treatment of musculoskeletal disorders have thus far been only modest. But there is room for optimism that during the next 30 years, effective pharmacological therapies and perhaps other kinds of treatment based on the neurophysiological model will emerge.

Philosophically, the neurophysiological model occupies an ambiguous middle ground. It rejects the structural model's assumption of a simple relationship between pain and pathology in musculoskeletal tissues, asserting instead that the CNS profoundly influences this relationship and that an individual's experiences following injury must be understood in part on the basis of principles of memory and learning. But because both ongoing tissue injury and altered CNS functioning probably contribute to chronic pain, the boundary between the structural model and the neurophysiological model is likely to remain hazy for the foreseeable future. Also, the boundary between the neurophysiological model and psychological models of chronic pain is currently vague, and is likely to remain so. Neuroscientists, psychologists, and philosophers will be challenged to articulate what differences (if any) exist between physiological processes in the CNS and psychological processes.

REFERENCES

Arendt-Nielsen L, Graven-Nielsen T. Central sensitization in fibromyalgia and other muscu-loskeletal disorders. *Curr Pain Headache Rep* 2003; 7(5):355–361.

Atlas SJ, Deyo RA. Evaluating and managing acute low back pain in the primary care setting. *J Gen Intern Med* 2001; 16(2):120–131.

Backonja M. Neuromodulating drugs for the symptomatic treatment of neuropathic pain. *Curr Pain Headache Rep* 2004; 8(3):212–216.

Banic B, Petersen-Felix S, Andersen OK, et al. Evidence for spinal cord hypersensitivity in chronic pain after whiplash injury and in fibromyalgia. *Pain* 2004; 107(1–2):7–15.

Bennett RM. Fibromyalgia. In: Wall PD, Melzack R (Ed). *Textbook of Pain,* 4th ed. New York: Churchill Livingstone, 1999.

Bogduk N, Long DM. Percutaneous lumbar medial branch neurotomy: a modification of facet denervation. *Spine* 1980; 5:193–200.

Bonica JJ, Albe-Fessard D. *Proceedings of the First World Congress on Pain,* Advances in Pain Research and Therapy, Vol. 1. New York: Raven Press, 1976.

Boos N, Semmer N, Elfering A, et al. Natural history of individuals with asymptomatic disc abnormalities in magnetic resonance imaging: predictors of low back pain-related medical consultation and work incapacity. *Spine* 2000; 25(12):1484–1492.

Canale ST (Ed). *Campbell's Operative Orthopaedics,* 10th ed. St. Louis: Mosby, 2003.

Crenshaw AH (Ed). *Campbell's Operative Orthopaedics,* 5th ed. St. Louis: Mosby, 1971.

Curatolo M, Petersen-Felix S, Arendt-Nielsen L, et al. Central hypersensitivity in chronic pain after whiplash injury. *Clin J Pain* 2001; 17:306–315.

Deyo RA. Diagnostic evaluation of LBP: reaching a specific diagnosis is often impossible. *Arch Intern Med* 2002; 162(13):1444–1447.

Drewes AM, Schipper KP, Dimcevski G, et al. Multi-modal induction and assessment of allodynia and hyperalgesia in the human oesophagus. *Eur J Pain* 2003; 7(6):539–549.

Dwyer A, Aprill C, Bogduk N. Cervical zygapophyseal joint pain patterns. I: A study in normal volunteers. *Spine* 1990; 15(6):453–457.

Eisenberg D, Davis R, Ettner S, et al. Trends in alternative medicine use in the United States, 1990–1997. *JAMA* 1998; 280:1569–1575

Fordyce WE, Fowler RS Jr, Lehmann JF, et al. Operant conditioning in the treatment of chronic pain. *Arch Phys Med Rehabil* 1973; 54(9):399–408.

Giamberardino MA. Referred muscle pain/hyperalgesia and central sensitisation. *J Rehabil Med* 2003; (41 Suppl):85–88.

Giamberardino MA, Berkley KJ, Affaitati G, et al. Influence of endometriosis on pain behav-iors and muscle hyperalgesia induced by a ureteral calculosis in female rats. *Pain* 2002; 95(3):247–257.

Gilson AM, Joranson DE, Maurer MA. Improving state medical board policies: influence of a model. *J Law Med Ethics* 2003; 31(1):119–129.

Graven-Nielsen T, Arendt-Nielsen L. Peripheral and central sensitization in musculoskeletal pain disorders: an experimental approach. *Curr Rheumatol Rep* 2002; 4(4):313–321.

Hilde G, Hagen KB, Jamtvedt G, Winnem M. Advice to stay active as a single treatment for low back pain and sciatica. *Cochrane Database Syst Rev* 2002; (2):CD003632.

Hoheisel U, Mense S. Long-term changes in discharge behaviour of cat dorsal horn neurons following noxious stimulation of deep tissues. *Pain* 1989; 36:239–247.

Hoheisel U, Koch K, Mense S. Functional reorganization in the rat dorsal horn during an experimental myositis. *Pain* 1994; 59:111–118.

Jackson RP, Becker GJ, Jacobs RR, et al. The neuroradiographic diagnosis of lumbar herniated nucleus pulposus: I. A comparison of computed tomography (CT), myelography, CT-myelography, discography, and CT-discography. *Spine* 1989; 14(12):1356–13561.

Jarvik JJ, Hollingworth W, Heagerty P, Haynor DR, Deyo RA. The Longitudinal Assessment
    of Imaging and Disability of the Back (LAIDBack) Study: baseline data. *Spine* 2001;
    26(10):1158–1166.
Kellgren JH. Observations on referred pain arising from muscle. *Clin Sci* 1938; 3:175–190.
Kennedy M. IDET: a new approach to treating lower back pain. *WMJ* 1999; 98:18–20.
Koelbaek Johansen M, Graven-Nielsen T, Schou Olesen A, Arendt-Nielsen L. Generalised
    muscular hyperalgesia in chronic whiplash syndrome. *Pain* 1999; 83(2):229–234.
Leong AL, Euller-Ziegler L. Patient advocacy and arthritis: moving forward. *Bull World
    Health Organ* 2004; 82(2):115–120.
Mense S, Simons DG, Russell IJ. *Muscle Pain.* New York: Lippincott Williams & Wilkins,
    2001.
Mooney V, Robertson J. The facet syndrome. *Clin Orthop* 1976; 115:149–156.
National Research Council and Institute of Medicine. *Musculoskeletal Disorders and the
    Workplace: Low Back and Upper Extremities.* Washington, DC: National Academy Press,
    2001.
Ni H, Simile C, Hardy AM. Utilization of complementary and alternative medicine by United
    States adults: results from the 1999 national health interview survey. *Med Care* 2002;
    140(4):353–358.
Ohnmeiss DD, Vanharanta H, Ekholm J. Relation between pain location and disc pathology: a
    study of pain drawings and CT/discography. *Clin J Pain* 1999; 15(3):210–217.
Onofrio BM. Treatment of chronic pain of malignant origin with intrathecal opiates. *Clin
    Neurosurg* 1983; 31:304–315.
Pawl RP. Results in the treatment of low back syndrome from sensory neurolysis of the lumbar
    facets (facet rhizotomy) by thermal coagulation. *Proc Inst Med Chic* 1974; 30:151–152.
Praemer A, Furner S, Rice DP. *Musculoskeletal Conditions in the United States.* Rosemont, IL:
    American Academy of Orthopaedic Surgeons, 1999.
Saal JS. General principles of diagnostic testing as related to painful lumbar spine disorders: a
    critical appraisal of current diagnostic techniques. *Spine* 2002; 27(22):2538–2545.
Salter RB. *Textbook of Disorders and Injuries of the Musculoskeletal System.* Baltimore:
    Williams & Wilkins, 1970.
Shealy CN, Mortimer JT, Reswick JB. Electrical inhibition of pain by stimulation of the dorsal
    columns: preliminary clinical report. *Anesth Analg* 1967; 46:489–491.
Shorter E. *From Paralysis to Fatigue.* New York: Free Press, 1992.
Simpson BA. Spinal cord and brain stimulation. In: Wall PD, Melzack R (Eds). *Textbook of
    Pain,* 4th ed. New York: Churchill Livingstone, 1999.
Staiger TO, Gaster B, Sullivan MD, Deyo RA. Systematic review of antidepressants in the
    treatment of chronic low back pain. *Spine* 2003; 28(22):2540–2545.
Staud R. Fibromyalgia pain: do we know the source? *Curr Opin Rheumatol* 2004; 16(2):157–
    163.
Travell JG, Simons DG. *Myofascial Pain and Dysfunction: The Trigger Point Manual.* Balti-
    more: Williams & Wilkins, 1992.
Waddell G. *Compensation for Chronic Pain.* London: The Stationery Office, 2004.
White AA, Gordon SL (Eds). *Symposium on Idiopathic Low Back Pain.* St. Louis: Mosby,
    1982.
Witte DH. Magnetic resonance imaging in orthopaedics. In: Canale ST (Ed). *Campbell's
    Operative Orthopaedics,* 10th ed. St. Louis: Mosby, 2003.

Correspondence to: James P. Robinson, MD, PhD, Department of Rehabilitation Medicine, University of Washington Medical Center, Box 356044, Seattle,
WA 98195-6044, USA. Email: jimrob@u.washington.edu.

The Paths of Pain 1975–2005, edited by
Harold Merskey, John D. Loeser, and Ronald
Dubner, IASP Press, Seattle, © 2005.

25

Neck Pain

Nikolai Bogduk

*Department of Clinical Research, Royal Newcastle Hospital,
University of Newcastle, Newcastle, New South Wales, Australia*

In 1978, I treated a 50-year-old gentleman with persistent neck pain. I prescribed for him what was then the conventional treatment: aspirin, traction, and a collar (Jequier and Adams 1974). In 1985, I was asked to provide a medicolegal report on this gentleman. I remember remarking at that time that if only we knew then what we know now, how much more we could have done. This reaction signaled that progress had been made and foreshadowed progress still to come.

CONCEPTS OF NECK PAIN

In the 1970s, medicine had a peculiar attitude to neck pain. It recognized that tumors, infections, and fractures could produce neck pain, but these conditions were not common. For most patients, entities such as cervical spondylosis or osteoarthrosis were invoked as the basis for neck pain (Jequier and Adams 1974). Meanwhile, cervical radiculopathy was recognized as having a cervical cause, but its features were in the upper limb. Nevertheless, it was regarded as a cause of neck pain. The resulting confusion has persisted to this day (Bogduk 2002c, 2003).

In order to resolve the problem of neck pain, I commenced a systematic series of studies (see below) designed to satisfy the following postulates applicable to pain of unknown origin: (1) Whatever the source of pain, it must have a nerve supply. Therefore, the innervation must be established. (2) When stimulated in normal volunteers, the putative source must produce pain like that seen in patients. (3) In patients with pain, anesthetizing the source should relieve their pain. (4) The source should be affected by a condition understood to be capable of producing pain, by initiating nociception. Ultimately, that pain should be terminated by treating the cause, or at least by affecting its source.

ANATOMY

In the 1970s, textbooks of anatomy did not describe the nerve supply of the cervical spine. They still do not. A search of the literature revealed that the distribution of the cervical dorsal rami to the cervical zygapophyseal joints was known to the French for some 20 years (Bogduk 1982). The first English-language study, confirming these features, appeared in 1982 (Bogduk 1982). At typical cervical levels, the zygapophyseal joints were innervated by the medial branches of the cervical dorsal rami with the same segmental numbers as the joints. The C2–3 joint was innervated by the third occipital nerve.

French textbooks had, from the 1920s, recorded that cervical intervertebral disks were innervated by the cervical sinuvertebral nerves (Bogduk et al. 1988), but this knowledge had not transferred to the English-language literature. A formal study, published in 1988, showed that the outer third of the annulus fibrosus of the cervical disk was innervated by branches of the sinuvertebral nerves and the vertebral nerve (Bogduk et al. 1988). Later studies confirmed these findings, and another extended them to include an innervation from the sympathetic trunks (Groen et al. 1990; Mendel et al. 1992). These studies promoted the intervertebral disk to a legitimate potential source of neck pain.

DIAGNOSTIC TECHNIQUES

Two techniques arose by which the proposition could be tested that neck pain arose from the cervical zygapophyseal joints. One was to inject local anesthetic into the joint under fluoroscopic control (Bogduk et al. 1995). The other was to anesthetize the medial branches that innervated the target joint (Bogduk and Marsland 1986, 1988). For the cervical disks, diskography was pioneered by Cloward (1959), but received little attention in the literature until Kikuchi et al. (1981) reported that cervical diskography greatly improved their success rate with anterior cervical fusion for idiopathic neck pain.

STUDIES IN NORMAL VOLUNTEERS

Kellgren (1939) and Feinstein et al. (1954) had demonstrated that noxious stimulation of interspinous structures in the neck could produce local pain and pain referred into the upper limb. These studies showed that nerve root irritation was not the only mechanism by which pain could be referred from the neck to the upper limb. Disorders of the interspinous muscles, however, were not a compelling explanation of neck pain. Therefore, studies were undertaken to demonstrate the capacity of more likely sources to produce neck pain and somatic referred pain.

Dwyer et al. (1990) showed that noxious stimulation of the cervical zygapophyseal joints produced distinct patterns of referred pain (Fig. 1). These patterns were later confirmed by studies using both mechanical stimulation of the joints and electrical stimulation of their nerves (Fukui et al. 1996). Cloward (1960) had shown that mechanical and electrical stimulation of the cervical intervertebral disks would refer pain to the interscapular region. Later studies showed that the patterns of referred pain from the cervical disks were essentially similar to those from the zygapophyscal joints (Schellhas et al. 1996; Grubb and Kelly 2000) (Fig. 1).

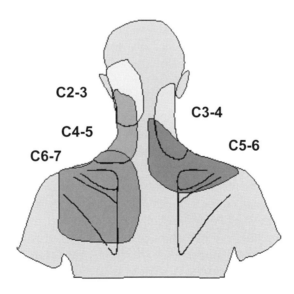

Fig. 1. A map of the referred pain patterns from the zygapophyseal joints and the intervertebral disks at the segments indicated.

PREVALENCE APPROXIMATIONS

Having established the principle that the cervical zygapophyseal joints and the cervical intervertebral disks could be a source of neck pain, investigators sought to estimate how commonly these structures might be the source of pain in patients presenting with neck pain. Small studies reported that about 70% of patients with neck pain or headache could be relieved of their pain by diagnostic blocks of the cervical zygapophyseal joints, most commonly at C2–3 and C5–6 (Bogduk and Marsland 1986, 1988). A larger study involving 318 patients with neck pain found that the prevalence of zygapophyseal joint pain was at least 25% across all patients and as high as 63% in those patients receiving diagnostic blocks (Aprill and Bogduk 1992). Although sentinel, these studies were compromised. They used single diagnostic blocks, which had not been validated, and which could have been affected by false-positive responses.

VALIDATION STUDIES

The validation of a diagnostic test requires several steps. Blocks must be shown to anesthetize the target structure selectively, without implicating other structures that might alternatively be the source of pain; this constitutes face validity. Blocks must faithfully distinguish patients with and without pain from the target source; this constitutes construct validity. Blocks must lead to successful treatment; this constitutes predictive validity, or therapeutic utility.

For cervical zygapophyseal joint blocks, these criteria were all satisfied. Face validity was established by a study that showed that medial branch blocks consistently infiltrated the target nerve but did not spread to any other structure so as to confound the effect (Barnsley and Bogduk 1993). A series of studies established the construct validity of medial branch blocks. One, using comparative local anesthetic blocks, showed that the positive response rate was statistically incompatible with patients having guessed which agent was administered (Barnsley et al. 1993a). Another, using placebo controls, showed that responses to comparative local anesthetic blocks were robust (Lord et al. 1995a). A third study, which showed that single diagnostic blocks were susceptible to a false-positive rate of 30%, mandated that all blocks should be performed under controlled conditions if the response was to be valid (Barnsley et al. 1993b). Predictive validity had to await the development of a successful treatment, but this came in time.

This series of studies made cervical medial branch blocks the most extensively studied and most validated test in the history of pain medicine (Bogduk 2002a). No other test has been so rigorously tested before being applied to clinical practice. In comparison, studies of cervical diskography have lagged behind, but validation data have emerged. An early study showed that some patients in whom diskography appears to be positive have their pain relieved by blocks of the zygapophyseal joints at the same segment (Bogduk and Aprill 1993). This finding implies that diskography is not selective for diskogenic pain in the neck, but might stress painful zygapophyseal joints. A later study showed that to distinguish a symptomatic disk from an asymptomatic one, the evoked pain must exceed 7 on a 10-point numerical pain rating scale (Schellhas et al. 1996). Another study showed that the results of diskography are different if all cervical levels are tested, rather than just the lower three (Grubb and Kelly 2000). Multiple disks are far more often painful than just a single disk. Collectively, these studies warned that, for cervical diskography to be valid, it should be performed after zygapophyseal joint blocks, with close attention to the intensity of pain evoked, and indicated that all segmental levels should be tested.

EPIDEMIOLOGY

Once cervical zygapophyseal joint blocks had been validated, they were applied in epidemiological studies to determine the prevalence of zygapophyseal joint pain. A series of studies from one center found that, in patients with chronic neck pain after whiplash, the prevalence of zygapophyseal joint pain was 54% (95% CI: 40–68%; Barnsley et al. 1995) and 49% (95% CI: 33–64%; Lord et al. 1996a). In patients with headache after whiplash, the prevalence of C2–3 zygapophyseal joint pain was 53% (95% CI: 37–68%; Lord et al. 1994). Among drivers involved in high-speed collisions, the prevalence was as high as 74% (95% CI: 65–83%; Gibson et al. 2000). Studies from other centers have confirmed this pattern. In a rehabilitation practice, the prevalence was at least 36% (27–45%; Speldewinde et al. 2001), and in a pain clinic it was 60% (95% CI: 50–70%; Manchikanti et al. 2002).

Collectively, these studies showed that cervical zygapophyseal joint pain was the single most common basis for chronic neck pain after whiplash. Using diagnostic blocks, under controlled conditions, a source of pain could be verified, and its segmental location specified. Comparable studies to establish the prevalence of zygapophyseal joint pain in patients with idiopathic neck pain have not been conducted, nor has any study yet ventured to determine how often the cervical disks are the source of pain.

TREATMENT

Having found a common, but hitherto unknown, source of neck pain, investigators explored methods of relieving this pain. Intra-articular injection of corticosteroids for cervical zygapophyseal joint pain was found to be no more effective, and even less effective, than injections of local anesthetic (Barnsley et al. 1994). No other form of conservative therapy has been tested for this condition, but a surgical option has been evaluated.

During the late 1970s and the 1980s, several investigators had proposed that cervical zygapophyseal joint pain could be treated by percutaneous denervation of the painful joint, using radiofrequency neurotomy (Lord et al. 1995b, 1998). The techniques used, however, had not been validated for anatomical accuracy, and patients had not been selected using controlled diagnostic blocks (Lord et al. 1995a, 1998).

Lord et al. (1995b) tested a modified technique of cervical medial branch radiofrequency neurotomy. The technique involved placing the electrodes parallel to the target nerve, rather than perpendicular to it, as had been the fashion (Bogduk et al. 1987). Their preliminary study announced that medial branch neurotomy could provide complete relief of neck pain when performed at typical cervical levels. For neurotomy at C2–3, for the treatment of headache, the study warned that technical problems made it difficult to relieve pain consistently.

A subsequent randomized, double-blind, and placebo-controlled study (Lord et al. 1996b) showed that radiofrequency neurotomy was significantly more effective than sham therapy, providing complete relief of neck pain in some 70% of patients treated. Complete relief lasted for a median period of some 280 days, but pain did recur. Nevertheless, relief could be reinstated by repeating the procedure. Subsequent follow-up studies confirmed these outcomes and showed that litigation did not affect outcome (Lord et al. 1998; McDonald et al. 1999; Sapir and Gorup 2001).

For the treatment of headache by third occipital neurotomy, the technical problems identified by Lord et al. (1995b) were addressed and overcome. A study using a revised technique showed that complete relief of headache could be achieved in 86% of patients treated (Govind et al. 2003). If and when pain recurred, relief could be reinstated by repeating the neurotomy.

The success of radiofrequency neurotomy was unprecedented in the history of neck pain. No other intervention had ever been shown to produce complete relief of pain so consistently. Concerned about its implications for the insurance industry, skeptical individuals commissioned an independent inquiry. The agency that conducted this inquiry found no fault in the concept of zygapophyseal joint pain and its treatment by radiofrequency neurotomy (Centre for Health Services and Policy Branch 2001). The agency remarked that the studies constituted a benchmark for studies of treatment of chronic neck pain, but was concerned that the skills to achieve the reported outcomes seemed restricted to one group, and the ability of others to reproduce those skills had not been demonstrated. That problem remains critical in the dissemination of this proven treatment.

For cervical diskogenic pain, treatment has typically been anterior cervical arthrodesis, by various means. The literature on this treatment, however, is meager and unconvincing (Whitecloud and Seago 1987; Garvey et al. 2002). No controlled studies have validated cervical fusion as a treatment for neck pain, and no long-term outcome studies have measured the durability of its effects.

PARALLEL DEVELOPMENTS

While some investigators have pursued a reductionist approach, attempting to isolate the sources of neck pain and treat them, others have used different approaches to address the same problem. Their contributions have been less positive, but have nevertheless served to dispel myths prevalent in the 1970s, some of which persist, despite the evidence against them.

Population studies have shown that plain radiographs are of no value for the diagnosis of neck pain (Bogduk 1999, 2003). Almost universally, radiographs demonstrate either a normal cervical spine or simply age-related changes (Heller et al. 1983). Multiple studies have dispelled the notion that cervical spondylosis might be a cause of pain (Bogduk 1999, 2003). The radiographic changes of spondylosis are equally prevalent in patients with pain and asymptomatic individuals.

Radiography is most often undertaken for fear of missing a lesion, but population studies are reassuring in this regard (Bogduk 1999, 2003). Serious causes of neck pain are evident in the history and are suspected before radiography is undertaken. Reciprocally, no serious diseases would be missed if radiography was not undertaken (Bogduk 1999, 2003). Fractures are an uncommon cause of neck pain (Bogduk 1999, 2003). In trauma patients, the use of radiography can be substantially reduced, without compromising the safety of patients, by following the Canadian C-spine rule (Stiell et al. 2001).

No studies have shown any diagnostic utility for computed tomography in the pursuit of the etiology of neck pain. Several studies have shown that magnetic resonance imaging reveals nothing more than age-related changes, with the same prevalence as in asymptomatic individuals (Bogduk 1999, 2003).

Ergonomic factors are only weak risk factors for neck pain, and standard occupational and demographic features have little influence on prognosis (Bogduk 1999, 2003). What stand out as risk factors are lack of control over workload and an unsupportive work environment (Bogduk 1999, 2003). In contrast with factors that seem to apply to low back pain, personal psychological factors account for no more than 2% of the variance between patients who do and do not develop chronic neck pain (Bogduk 1999, 2003).

In the 1970s the understanding of the mechanics of whiplash as a cause of neck pain was crude, superficial, and wrong. Modern studies have dispelled the notion that it is a flexion-extension injury. During whiplash, the neck does not exceed physiological range of motion (Bogduk and Yoganandan 2001). The critical insult in whiplash is a compression stress in which the neck is compressed from below by a rising trunk. The cervical spine undergoes a sigmoid deformation, during which individual segments exhibit aberrant motion. At C5–6 the anterior vertebral bodies are separated, and the zygapophyseal joints are impacted, as the segment rotates about an abnormally high axis of rotation. This pattern of motion predicts avulsion injuries to the anterior disk and compression injuries to the zygapophyseal joints. These predicted injuries are evident in post-mortem studies (Bogduk and Yoganandan 2001; Uhrenholt et al. 2002). The predicted injury to the zygapophyseal joints correlates with the high prevalence of zygapophyseal joint pain in clinical studies (Bogduk 2002b).

Commonly used interventions for neck pain include analgesics, nonsteroidal anti-inflammatory drugs (NSAIDs), muscle relaxants, collars, acupuncture, traction, physical therapy, exercises, manual therapy, behavioral therapy, and injections. Systematic and pragmatic reviews of the literature on these interventions have been largely disappointing for their advocates. The first such review, by the Quebec Task Force, found very little literature to support commonly practiced interventions for neck pain (Spitzer et al. 1995), and subsequent studies and reviews have done little to change this situation (Bogduk 1999, 2000, 2003; Harms-Ringdahl and Nachemson 2000).

For the treatment of acute neck pain, the most recent evidence-based guidelines (Australian Musculoskeletal Pain Guidelines Group 2003) found no support for most interventions. They could endorse only assurance and activation, exercises, and multimodal therapy involving passive mobilization and exercises. For the treatment of chronic neck pain, the literature is essentially barren (Bogduk 1999, 2003). It attests to a moderate benefit from exercises, but no other intervention has been shown to be effective.

DIFFERENCES BETWEEN NECK PAIN AND BACK PAIN

Studies analogous to those that have been conducted on the causes of neck pain have focused on the causes of back pain. Controlled diagnostic blocks and stringently controlled provocation diskography have been used to determine the various anatomical sources of back pain. The resultant data, however, differ considerably, almost diametrically, with those that apply to chronic neck pain.

For chronic neck pain, as discussed above, the source can be traced to the zygapophyseal joints in about 60% of cases, whereas the prevalence of pain stemming from the cervical intervertebral disks or other structures is unknown. In contrast, chronic low back pain can be traced to internal disk disruption in about 40% of cases (Schwarzer et al. 1995b), to the sacroiliac joints in some 20% of cases (Schwarzer et al. 1995a; Maigne et al. 1996), and to the zygapophyseal joints in only about 15% of cases (Schwarzer et al. 1994). Furthermore, this latter figure may be inflated, because the criterion standard for a positive response was only 50% relief of pain, rather than complete relief, after diagnostic blocks.

The contrast is that whereas low back pain most often stems from the intervertebral disks, with the zygapophyseal joints being an uncommon source, neck pain most often stems from the zygapophyseal joints. These differences can be related to the different structure and mechanics of the disks and zygapophyseal joints of the lumbar and cervical spines. In the neck, the zygapophyseal joints are susceptible to compression injury and extension injury, whereas in the lumbar spine they are relatively spared from injury in the axial and sagittal planes because the disks bear the brunt of compression loading.

SYNOPSIS

In the 1970s, neck pain was attributed to cervical spondylosis. Its treatment was aspirin and physical therapy. These beliefs and practices have been refuted by subsequent research. Yet, ironically, they still persist. Whereas aspirin was replaced by NSAIDs and other agents, none has been shown to be effective for neck pain. Whereas traction and collars were replaced by manipulative therapy, the latter has been found to be ineffective. Of the conventional therapies, exercise is the only one that has attracted evidence. However, exercise is not curative; it is a nonspecific intervention, in that it is not founded on knowledge or diagnosis of the source of pain or its cause. Whereas it may reduce pain, it does not eliminate it.

In the development of knowledge and new procedures, a classical biomedical, reductionist approach has proved effective for neck pain. The paradigm of cervical zygapophyseal joint pain has satisfied the postulates for establishing a source of pain. The joints have a nerve supply. They can be made to hurt in normal volunteers. Neck pain is relieved when the joints are anesthetized in patients. When treatment targets the painful joint, complete relief can be achieved. Furthermore, cervical zygapophyseal joint pain is not a rare, or peculiar, phenomenon. It is the single most common basis for chronic neck pain. Its treatment is the only method that has been proven to achieve complete relief of pain. This novel approach is not a trivial change from what was known, believed, and practiced in the 1970s.

Zygapophyseal joint pain, however, is not the only or total answer to neck pain. Some 40% of patients have some other source and cause of pain. The intervertebral disks are prominent amongst contenders to fill this vacancy. Unfortunately, for those patients who might have diskogenic pain, research has been limited. We urgently need a validated test to determine whether a patient has diskogenic pain. Thereafter, a dependable treatment is required.

REFERENCES

Aprill C, Bogduk N. The prevalence of cervical zygapophyseal joint pain: a first approximation. *Spine* 1992; 17:744–747.

Australian Acute Musculoskeletal Pain Guidelines Group. *Evidence-Based Management of Acute Musculoskeletal Pain.* Brisbane: Australian Academic Press, 2003. Available at: www.nhmrc.gov.au.

Barnsley L, Bogduk N. Medial branch blocks are specific for the diagnosis of cervical zygapophysial joint pain. *Reg Anesthes* 1993; 18:343–350.

Barnsley L, Lord S, Bogduk N. Comparative local anaesthetic blocks in the diagnosis of cervical zygapophysial joint pain. *Pain* 1993a; 55:99–106.

Barnsley L, Lord S, Wallis B, Bogduk N. False-positive rates of cervical zygapophysial joint blocks. *Clin J Pain* 1993b; 9:124–130.

Barnsley L, Lord SM, Wallis BJ, Bogduk N. Lack of effect of intraarticular corticosteroids for chronic pain in the cervical zygapophyseal joints. *N Engl J Med* 1994; 330:1047–1050.

Barnsley L, Lord SM, Wallis BJ, Bogduk N. The prevalence of chronic cervical zygapophysial joint pain after whiplash. *Spine* 1995; 20:20–26.

Bogduk N. The clinical anatomy of the cervical dorsal rami. *Spine* 1982; 7:319–330.

Bogduk N. The neck. *Bailliere's Clin Rheumatol* 1999; 13:261–285.

Bogduk N. Whiplash: why pay for something that does not work? *J Musculoskel Pain* 2000; 8:29–53.

Bogduk N. Diagnostic nerve blocks in chronic pain. *Best Pract Res Clin Anaesthesiol* 2002a; 16:565–578.

Bogduk N. Point of view. *Spine* 2002b; 27:1940–1941.

Bogduk N. Cervical pain. In: Ashbury AK, McKhann GM, McDonald WI, Goadsby PJ, MacArthur JC (Eds). *Disease of the Nervous System: Clinical Neuroscience and Therapeutic Principles.* Cambridge: Cambridge University Press, 2002c, pp 742–759.

Bogduk N. Neck pain and whiplash. In: Jensen TS, Wilson PR, Rice ASC (Eds). *Clinical Pain Management: Chronic Pain*. London: Arnold, 2003, pp 504–519.

Bogduk N, Aprill C. On the nature of neck pain, discography and cervical zygapophysial joint blocks. *Pain* 1993; 54:213–217.

Bogduk N, Marsland A. On the concept of third occipital headache. *J Neurol Neurosurg Psychiatry* 1986; 49:775–780.

Bogduk N, Marsland A. The cervical zygapophysial joints as a source of neck pain. *Spine* 1988; 13:610–617.

Bogduk N, Yoganandan N. Biomechanics of the cervical spine. Part 3: Minor injuries. *Clin Biomech* 2001; 16:267–275.

Bogduk N, Macintosh J, Marsland A. A technical limitations to efficacy of radiofrequency neurotomy for spinal pain. *Neurosurgery* 1987; 20:529–535.

Bogduk N, Windsor M, Inglis A. The innervation of the cervical intervertebral discs. *Spine* 1988; 13:2–8.

Bogduk N, Aprill C, Derby R. Diagnostic blocks of synovial joints. In: White AH (Ed). *Diagnosis and Conservative Treatment, Spine Care*, Vol. 1. St Louis: Mosby, 1995, pp 298–321

Centre for Health Services and Policy Branch. Percutaneous radio-frequency neurotomy treatment of chronic cervical pain following whiplash injury. Vancouver: University of British Columbia, British Columbia Office of Health Technology Assessment 01:5T, 2001.

Cloward RB. Cervical diskography. A contribution to the aetiology and mechanism of neck, shoulder and arm pain. *Ann Surg* 1959; 130:1052–1064.

Cloward RB. The clinical significance of the sinu-vertebral nerve of the cervical spine in relation to the cervical disk syndrome. *J Neurol Neurosurg Psychiatry* 1960; 23:321–326.

Dwyer A, Aprill C, Bogduk N. Cervical zygapophysial joint pain patterns. I: A study in normal volunteers. *Spine* 1990; 15:453–457.

Feinstein B, Langton JBK, Jameson RM, Schiller F. Experiments on referred pain from deep somatic tissues. *J Bone Joint Surg* 1954; 36A:981–997.

Fukui S, Ohseto K, Shiotani M, et al. Referred pain distribution of the cervical zygapophyseal joints and cervical dorsal rami. *Pain* 1996; 68:79–83.

Garvey TA, Transfeldt EE, Malcolm JR, Kos P. Outcome of anterior cervical diskectomy and fusion as perceived by patients treated for dominant axial-mechanical cervical spine pain. *Spine* 2002; 27:1887–1894.

Gibson T, Bogduk N, Macpherson J, McIntosh A. Crash characteristics of whiplash associated chronic neck pain. *J Musculoskel Pain* 2000; 8:87–95.

Govind J, King W, Bailey B, Bogduk N. Radiofrequency neurotomy for the treatment of third occipital headache. *J Neurol Neurosurg Psychiatry* 2003; 74:88–93.

Groen GJ, Baljet B, Drukker J. Nerves and nerve plexuses of the human vertebral column. *Am J Anat* 1990; 188:282–296.

Grubb SA, Kelly CK. Cervical discography: clinical implications from 12 years of experience. *Spine* 2000; 25:1382–1389.

Harms-Ringdahl K, Nachemson A. Acute and subacute neck pain: nonsurgical treatment. In: Nachemson A, Jonsson E (Eds). *Neck and Back Pain: The Scientific Evidence of Causes, Diagnosis, and Treatment*. Philadelphia: Lippincott Williams and Wilkins, 2000, pp 327–338.

Heller CA, Stanley P, Lewis-Jones B, Heller RF. Value of X-ray examinations of the cervical spine. *BMJ* 1983; 287:1276–1278.

Jequier M, Adams RD. Pain in the back and neck. In: Wintrobe MM, Thorm GW, Adams RD, et al. (Eds). *Harrison's Principles of Internal Medicine*, 7th ed. New York: McGraw-Hill, 1974, pp 34–43.

Kellgren JH. On the distribution of pain arising from deep somatic structures with charts of segmental pain areas. *Clin Sci* 1939; 4:35–46.

Kikuchi S, MacNab I, Moreau P. Localisation of the level of symptomatic cervical disc degeneration. *J Bone Joint Surg* 1981; 63B:272–277.

Lord S, Barnsley L, Wallis B, Bogduk N. Third occipital headache: a prevalence study. *J Neurol Neurosurg Psychiatry* 1994, 57:1187–1190.

Lord SM, Barnsley L, Bogduk N. The utility of comparative local anaesthetic blocks versus placebo-controlled blocks for the diagnosis of cervical zygapophysial joint pain. *Clin J Pain* 1995a; 11:208–213.

Lord SM, Barnsley L, Bogduk N. Percutaneous radiofrequency neurotomy in the treatment of cervical zygapophysial joint pain: a caution. *Neurosurgery* 1995b; 36:732–739.

Lord S, Barnsley L, Wallis BJ, Bogduk N. Chronic cervical zygapophysial joint pain after whiplash: a placebo-controlled prevalence study. *Spine* 1996a; 21:1737–1745.

Lord SM, Barnsley L, Wallis BJ, McDonald GJ, Bogduk N. Percutaneous radio-frequency neurotomy for chronic cervical zygapophysial-joint pain. *N Engl J Med* 1996b; 335:1721–1726.

Lord SM, McDonald GJ, Bogduk N. Percutaneous radiofrequency neurotomy of the cervical medial branches: a validated treatment for cervical zygapophysial joint pain. *Neurosurg Q* 1998; 8:288–308.

Maigne JY, Aivaliklis A, Pfefer F. Results of sacroiliac joint double block and value of sacroiliac pain provocation tests in 54 patients with low-back pain. *Spine* 1996; 21:1889–1892.

McDonald G, Lord SM, Bogduk N. Long-term follow-up of patients treated with cervical radiofrequency neurotomy for chronic neck pain. *Neurosurgery* 1999; 45:61–68.

Manchikanti L, Singh V, Rivera J, Pampati V. Prevalence of cervical facet joint pain in chronic neck pain. *Pain Physician* 2002; 5:243–249.

Mendel T, Wink CS, Zimny ML. Neural elements in human cervical intervertebral discs. *Spine* 1992; 17:132–135.

Sapir DA, Gorup JM. Radiofrequency medial branch neurotomy in litigant and nonlitigant patients with cervical whiplash. *Spine* 2001; 26:E268–E273.

Schellhas KP, Smith MD, Gundry CR, Pollei SR. Cervical discogenic pain: prospective correlation of magnetic resonance imaging and discography in asymptomatic subjects and pain sufferers. *Spine* 1996; 21:300–312.

Schwarzer AC, Aprill CN, Derby R, et al. Clinical features of patients with pain stemming from the lumbar zygapophysial joints. Is the lumbar facet syndrome a clinical entity? *Spine* 1994; 19:1132–1137.

Schwarzer AC, Aprill CN, Bogduk N. The sacroiliac joint in chronic low back pain. *Spine* 1995a; 20:31–37.

Schwarzer AC, Aprill CN, Derby R, et al. The prevalence and clinical features of internal disc disruption in patients with chronic low back pain. *Spine* 1995b; 20:1878–1883.

Speldewinde GC, Bashford GM, Davidson IR. Diagnostic cervical zygapophysial joint blocks for chronic cervical pain. *Med J Aust* 2001; 174:174–176.

Spitzer WO, Skovron ML, Salmi LR, et al. Scientific monograph of the Quebec task force on whiplash-associated disorders: redefining "whiplash" and its management. *Spine* 1995; 20:1S–73S.

Stiell IG, Wells GA, Vandemheen KL, et al. The Canadian C-spine rule for radiography in alert and stable trauma patients. *JAMA* 2001; 286:1841–1848.

Uhrenholt L, Grunnet-Nilsson N, Hartvgsen J. Cervical spine lesions after road traffic accidents. A systematic review. *Spine* 2002; 27:1934–1940.

Whitecloud TS, Seago RA. Cervical discogenic syndrome. Results of operative intervention in patients with positive discography, *Spine* 1987; 12:313–316.

Correspondence to: Nikolai Bogduk, MD, PhD, Department of Clinical Research, David Maddison Building, Royal Newcastle Hospital, Newcastle, NSW 2300, Australia. Fax: 61-2-4923-6103; email: mgillam@mail.newcastle.edu.au.

The Paths of Pain 1975–2005, edited by
Harold Merskey, John D. Loeser, and Ronald
Dubner, IASP Press, Seattle, © 2005.

26

Low Back Pain

Gordon Waddell

*Centre for Psychosocial and Disability Research,
University of Cardiff, Cardiff, United Kingdom*

Low back pain is one of the most common pain conditions, and its treatment accounts for 25–50% of the workload of most pain clinics (Crombie et al. 1999). For more than a century, low back pain has been recognized as one of the most common causes of work disability, and it now accounts for about a quarter of workers' compensation costs (Allan and Waddell 1989). For these reasons, there has been more clinical and social research into low back pain and disability than into any other single pain condition. However, many of the findings do not appear to be unique to back pain, so this condition may serve as a good exemplar for many common pain conditions. The focus of this chapter is nonspecific low back pain, which accounts for about 95% of all back problems.

THE POSITION IN 1975

In 1975, low back pain was generally regarded as a physical injury, which was understood and managed in terms of a biomedical model and according to orthopedic principles. Although the gate control theory of pain (Melzack and Wall 1965) was already 10 years old, routine practice was based on a Cartesian model of pain, in which pain was a warning signal of tissue injury, likely to be aggravated by physical activity and work. The basic strategy of management was rest to allow the "injury" to "heal" (even though there was scant evidence of tissue damage in most nonspecific low back pain and little evidence for the effectiveness of rest). Patients were given sick certification and advised to remain off work until the pain was "cured."

The mid-1970s represented a time of great technological advances in Western medicine, with growing professional confidence and public expectation that, if conservative management failed, some medical or surgical specialist would be able to "fix" the problem (Deyo 1998). This was also a time of major social change, during which most industrialized nations entered a continuing period of changing patterns of employment associated with post-industrial restructuring, rising socioeconomic expectations, and changing attitudes to work, health, sickness, and disability. Although objective measures of health have continued to show gradual improvement, the amount of sick leave and long-term incapacity attributed to low back pain was about to increase exponentially (Fig. 1). Since that time, the single greatest social security problem in all Western countries has been the trend toward earlier retirement, and low back pain is one of the most common health grounds contributing to this trend (Waddell et al. 2002).

ADVANCES IN KNOWLEDGE SINCE 1975

Basic science and clinical understanding of pain have been revolutionized since 1975, as discussed elsewhere in this volume. Here, it is enough to highlight several advances in knowledge that have had a direct impact on clinical thinking regarding the management of low back pain. These advances can be summarized as follows: (1) Modern neurophysiology provides a much better basis for understanding clinical pain (Melzack and Wall 1965; Devor 1996; Doubell et al. 1999; Melzack 1999). (2) Pain signals do not pass unaltered to the cerebral cortex, but are always and constantly

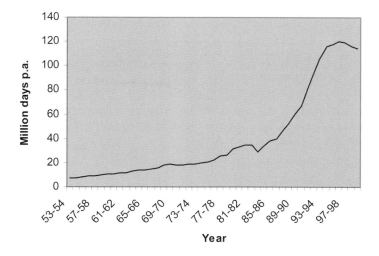

Fig. 1. Trends of social security benefits for back conditions in the United Kingdom; based on statistics from the Department for Work and Pensions (reproduced with permission from Waddell 2004).

modulated at various levels within the central nervous system (CNS).
(3) Pain, emotions, and pain behavior are all integral parts of the pain
experience. (4) The spinal cord and brain are best envisaged as a complex,
integrated neural network or neuromatrix rather than in terms of pain tracts.
(5) The CNS is not like a telephone exchange, but more like a complex
computer network that responds actively to incoming signals. (6) Finally,
there is a return to the holistic view that pain is a response of the whole
human brain.

This new understanding moves clinical thinking beyond the old medical
model. There is now broad agreement that chronic pain can only be understood and managed according to a biopsychosocial model (Fig. 2) that includes biological, psychological *and* social dimensions (Engel 1977; Waddell
2002). In this model, *bio-* refers to the physical or mental health condition;
psycho- recognizes that personal and psychological factors influence functioning; and *social* recognizes the importance of the social context with its
pressures and constraints on behavior and functioning.

Low back pain is not only a cause of great human suffering, but also the
single most common cause of disability during the working years of life.
Pain and disability should be distinguished, both conceptually and in clinical
practice. As a clinical oversimplification, pain is a symptom (which may
have major biopsychosocial ramifications), whereas disability is restricted
functioning. Pain and disability often go together, but the relationship between them is much weaker than many clinicians and patients assume (with
a correlation generally of $< r = 0.40$). Clinical management of low back pain
aims to provide the best possible pain relief or control, but it must also

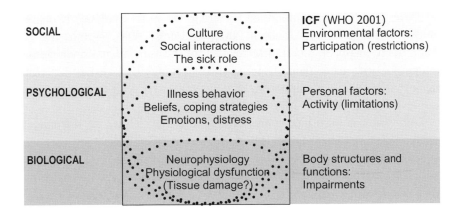

Fig. 2. A biopsychosocial model of chronic pain and disability, with corresponding ICF
components (reproduced with permission from Waddell 2004).

prevent or minimize disability; physicians cannot assume that treating pain will lead to consequent improvement in disability. From this perspective, the biopsychosocial model is not only a model of pain, but a much more comprehensive model of human illness and disability. The *International Classification of Functioning, Disability and Health* (ICF) (World Health Organization 2001), based on the biopsychosocial model, is now a widely accepted framework for disability and rehabilitation (Wade and de Jong 2000; Waddell and Burton 2004). The ICF conceives functioning and disability as a dynamic interaction between the individual, the health problem, and the social context.

TRENDS IN THE MANAGEMENT OF LOW BACK PAIN SINCE 1975

There appear to be several divergent trends in the management of low back pain, which are at best quite separate, and at worst incongruous and running counter to each other.

BASIC CLINICAL MANAGEMENT OF LOW BACK PAIN

Most low back pain is managed in primary care, which is the most appropriate setting for the management for nonspecific symptoms where there is no clear indication for any specialist investigation or intervention (Clinical Standards Advisory Group 1994). It is also where the outcome is largely predetermined.

The advances in knowledge outlined above may seem philosophical, but they have had a very practical impact on the clinical management of low back pain, which is now supported by strong scientific evidence (Cochrane Library; Nachemson and Jonsson 2000; Waddell 2004). Within the past decade, there has been a complete reversal of the fundamental management strategy for low back pain, from a passive strategy of rest to an active strategy of advising and supporting patients to remain active and to continue their ordinary activities as normally as possible (Table I).

This view has been incorporated into clinical guidelines for the management of acute low back pain, which have now been developed in almost every Western country (Royal College of General Practitioners 1999; Koes et al. 2001). These guidelines focus on basic principles of management rather than specific treatments, and all advocate very similar messages (Table II). Randomized controlled trials show that such guidelines can be implemented in clinical practice and can improve clinical outcomes (Rossignol et al. 2000; McGuirk et al. 2001).

Table I
Rest or stay active?

Bed rest:

Is not an effective treatment

May delay recovery

Advice to stay active and continue ordinary activities as normally as possible leads to:

Faster recovery and return to work

Less chronic disability

Fewer recurrent problems

Source: Based on systematic reviews of 28 randomized controlled trials (Hagen et al. 2000, 2002; Waddell 2004).

All clinical guidelines recommend that patients should be given adequate information and advice, and this can be supported by printed material to take home. Most of the older educational material for low back pain, based on traditional ideas about spinal injury and pathology, promotes the need for medical treatment or therapy (Table III), although that approach has never been shown to be effective. More recent, innovative educational material, such as *The Back Book* (Roland et al. 2002), based on the biopsychosocial model and aimed at changing beliefs and behavior (Table III), has proven more effective (Burton et al. 1999; Moore et al. 2000; George et al. 2003). Integrated public and professional education campaigns have been shown to be effective in changing professional advice and public beliefs about how to manage low back pain (Buchbinder et al. 2001a,b; Health Scotland 2005).

Recently published occupational health guidelines have extended clinical management (which too often ignores occupational issues and outcomes) into the occupational context (Carter and Birrell 2000; Kendall 2000; Staal et al. 2003). The basic principles remain the same: providing accurate yet positive information and advice; advising and supporting workers to continue their ordinary activities (including work) as normally as possible; and

Table II
Clinical management of acute low back pain

Exclusion of serious disease

Reassurance

Simple symptomatic measures

Avoidance of over-investigation, labeling, and medicalization

Advice to continue ordinary activities as normally as possible

Early return to work

If patient has not returned to ordinary activities and work within 4–6 weeks, intensive re-activation and rehabilitation

Table III
A comparison of traditional and biopsychosocial information and advice

Traditional Biomedical Education	Modern Biopsychosocial Approach
Focus on pain	Focus on disability *and* pain
Impart "knowledge"	Change patient's beliefs and behavior
Provide "medical" information about anatomy, pathology, diagnosis, indications, and methods of treatment	Provide information about epidemiology, natural history, and prognosis, and about how people react and cope with low back pain
Instruction on ergonomics, technique of lifting, and back-specific exercises	Encourage patient to focus on staying active, continuing ordinary activities as normally as possible, and activities of daily living
Facilitate patient cooperation with treatment; patient remains the passive recipient of professional treatment	Enable patients to share or take over responsibility for their own continued management

Source: Adapted with permission from Waddell (2004).

providing work adjustments or accommodations. However, this requires a major shift in clinical thinking: every doctor and therapist who treats back pain must take an interest in occupational issues and must accept responsibility for helping these patients to remain at work or return to work.

MEDICAL TECHNOLOGIES

During the past two decades, there has been enormous development of medical technology that simply did not exist in 1975. This has led to great advances in the investigation and treatment of serious spinal pathologies such as tumor, infection, and fractures. The problem is that these technologies are not designed for and are largely inappropriate for nonspecific low back pain, yet that is where they are now widely used.

Computerized tomography (CT) and magnetic resonance imaging (MRI) provide detailed information about the anatomy of spinal pathology and neurological compression, which is of enormous value for planning interventions on these specific conditions. The difficulty arises when that approach is transferred to nonspecific low back pain. There, the problem is that most "degenerative changes" are a normal age-related process; most MRI "abnormalities" bear little relationship to clinical symptoms and are equally common in patients with low back pain and normal asymptomatic people (Nachemson and Vingaard 2000). Low back pain is usually due to conditions that cannot be diagnosed on imaging, and most images do not help routine management (Jarvik and Deyo 2000). Yet the pictures are so seductive that they are almost impossible to resist, and too often drive interventions that have little clear clinical indication (Hadler 2003; Jarvik et al. 2003).

The pharmacopeia and the drug industry have expanded greatly since 1975, and there is now very heavy use of analgesics for low back pain, especially in the United States (Schoene 2003). Forty-five percent of American adults take prescription analgesics for some form of pain, and 87% take over-the-counter analgesics. There is particular concern about increasing use of opioids. Hunkele and Vogt (2002) found that 56% of 17,228 patients with back pain received an average of 4.6 analgesic prescriptions: about 33% were for narcotics, 26% for narcotics and nonselective opioids, 9% for narcotics and other analgesics, and 27% for nonsteroidal anti-inflammatory drugs alone. Yet there is limited scientific evidence on effectiveness and continued controversy about the use of strong narcotics for chronic benign pain (Meldrum 2003; Schoene 2004).

The combination of non-invasive investigations, greater biomechanical understanding, safer anesthesia and surgery, and new technology has had the most dramatic impact on spinal surgery. U.S. National Hospital Discharge Surveys show that the number of patients having a low back operation has increased from 150,000 in 1979 to about half a million in 2001, roughly doubling each decade. Back and neck operations are now the third most common form of surgery in the United States, after cesarean section and tubal ligation. There are particularly large increases in rates of spinal fusion, surgery for spinal stenosis, and spinal surgery in older patients. In 1975 there was virtually no use of instrumentation, except for spinal deformity and fractures. Today, there are about 300,000 spinal fusions per annum in the United States, mostly for nonspecific low back pain, and the majority use some form of fusion technology (Mendenhall 2002). Yet there is no good clinical indication for this increase and no evidence that it has improved clinical outcomes (Bono and Lee 2004; Gibson et al. 2004). Perhaps as important as these technological advances has been increasing commercialization and the increasingly sophisticated marketing of medical technologies and products.

COMPLEMENTARY AND ALTERNATIVE MEDICINE

In 1975, there was still strong antipathy between conventional and alternative medicine, and litigation between the American Medical Association and chiropractors was not finally settled till 1987 (Chapman-Smith 2000). Today, osteopathy and chiropractic care are fully established health professions in the United States, the United Kingdom, and many other countries, and it is recognized (in at least some medical quarters) that they have much to offer in the understanding and management of nonspecific low back pain. There are numerous other alternative therapies, of which massage, yoga, relaxation therapies, and energy healing currently appear to be the most popular, while acupuncture seems to have waxed and waned (Eisenberg et al. 1998; Cherkin et al. 2002; Wolsko et al. 2003).

Osteopathic medicine and chiropractic have survived and flourished for more than a century, because many patients have chosen them in preference to conventional medicine. (Fashions for most other alternative therapies have come and gone over the years.) The chiropractic profession, in particular, has become much stronger, and the number of chiropractic visits is doubling roughly every 15 years (Chapman-Smith 2000). In the United States, alternative therapies have now overtaken orthodox medicine in the number of patients they treat for low back pain (Eisenberg et al. 1998). In the United Kingdom, where 97% of all health care is provided by the National Health Service (NHS), more than half of all patients who would be entitled to receive NHS-funded physical therapy for low back pain elect to pay for private physiotherapy, osteopathy, or chiropractic treatment instead (Clinical Standards Advisory Group 1994).

There is growing scientific evidence on the effectiveness of complementary and alternative medicine for low back pain (Chapman-Smith 2003; Cherkin et al. 2003), with particularly good evidence for manipulation (Assendelft et al. 2003). Evidence from four randomized controlled trials and six cohort studies suggests that physiotherapy and chiropractic are equally effective in reducing symptoms and improving function, though overall the evidence is unclear on the relative effectiveness and cost-effectiveness of medical versus chiropractic care for low back pain (Baldwin et al. 2001). Many studies show that chiropractic patients are more satisfied with their care (Chapman-Smith 2003).

Health care for low back pain (particularly in the United States) is a curious mixture of contrasts. It is easy to forget that most people still deal with back pain themselves most of the time, without professional help. Those who go to conventional medical practitioners receive two very different patterns of health care: two-thirds receive essentially conservative treatment in primary care, while one-third are referred to medical specialists who provide high-tech, costly investigations and interventions. But more people with back pain are seeking complementary and alternative health care instead. It used to be thought that patients used *either* conventional *or* alternative health care, but it appears that many patients now visit different professionals at different times, move back and forth, or see more than one health professional at the same time (Cherkin et al. 2002; Wolsko et al. 2003).

DISABILITY TRENDS

Given the advances in knowledge, new investigations and interventions, better professional development and skills, and increasing health care resources devoted to low back pain over the past 30 years, it might be expected that clinical outcomes would be improving and fewer people would be developing chronic pain and disability. Paradoxically, social security statistics show that low back disability has actually increased exponentially (Fig. 1).

It is important to emphasize that these data do not indicate an increase in low back pain. Most of the epidemiological evidence shows that there has not been any significant change in the prevalence of low back pain (Waddell 2004). There is no biological reason to expect any change in the pathology or severity of low back pain. Rather, these data reflect trends of chronic disability, medical certification, social security benefits, and early retirement. Data from the past 30 years show a similar pattern in most Western countries, although these trends do now appear to be changing in some settings in some countries (Waddell et al. 2002). Arguably, this problem is more of a social epidemic, which has little to do with health care. Nevertheless, management of low back pain at the end of the 20th century at best did not solve the problem, and at worst may have contributed to it.

FUTURE DIRECTIONS

It is doubtful if anyone in 1975 could have predicted the state of low back pain today. Given the divergent trends, it is equally impossible to predict what will happen in another 30 years. But it is possible to identify some of the forces that will determine that future, and to envisage some alternative scenarios.

Human beings will certainly continue to have low back pain, just as they always have—today, in 1975, and throughout recorded history. At times, they will continue to seek help, in one form or another. It is almost certain that various groups of health professionals (not necessarily the same ones as today) will continue to make a living from low back pain, and they will probably continue to compete in the health care marketplace. It is more difficult to predict the direction that health care will take. In another 30 years, we will probably have even better knowledge, investigations, and interventions, but will we show any greater wisdom in our handling of an everyday bodily symptom like low back pain? Will we be able to separate health services for serious spinal pathologies from those for nonspecific low back pain? To what extent will health care services and resources be designed to meet the needs of patients with nonspecific low back pain, and to what extent will they serve the vested interests of different groups of health care providers? Would you place your money (perhaps literally) on commercial interests or on scientific evidence about which interventions are effective? The central issue is likely to remain the battle of health care ideologies in the clinic, the health marketplace, and the media: the outcome of that battle is less certain.

But whatever direction health care takes, will that make any difference to disability trends? These trends probably have more to do with social factors and unpredictable shifts in the culture that surrounds back pain, health care, and disability. The future of low back pain, like most human behavior and many health outcomes, will probably depend more on the philosophy of our approach than on further scientific advances.

REFERENCES

Allan DB, Waddell G. An historical perspective on low back pain and disability. *Acta Orthop Scand* 1989; 60(Suppl 234):1–23.

Assendelft WJ, Morton SC, Yu EI, Suttorp MJ, Shekelle PG. Spinal manipulative therapy for low back pain. A meta-analysis of effectiveness relative to other therapies. *Ann Intern Med* 2003; 138:871–881.

Baldwin ML, Cote P, Frank JW, Johnson WG. Cost-effectiveness studies of medical and chiropractic care for occupational low back pain: a critical review of the literature. *Spine J* 2001; 1:138–147.

Bono CM, Lee CK. Critical analysis of trends in fusion for degenerative disc disease over the past 20 years: influence of technique on fusion rate and clinical outcome. *Spine* 2004; 29:455–463.

Buchbinder R, Jolley D, Wyatt M. Population based intervention to change back pain beliefs and disability: three part evaluation. *BMJ* 2001a; 322:1516–1520.

Buchbinder R, Jolley DJ, Wyatt M. Effects of a media campaign on back pain beliefs and its potential influence on the management of low back pain in general practice. *Spine* 2001b; 26:2535–2542.

Burton AK, Waddell G, Tillotson KM, Summerton N. Information and advice to patients with back pain can have a positive effect: a randomized controlled trial of a novel educational booklet in primary care. *Spine* 1999; 24:2484–2491.

Carter JT, Birrell LN (Eds). *Occupational Health Guidelines for the Management of Low Back Pain at Work—Principal Recommendations*. London: Faculty of Occupational Medicine, 2000. Available at: www.facoccmed.ac.uk.

Chapman-Smith DA. *The Chiropractic Profession: Its Education, Practice, Research and Future Directions*. West Des Moines, IA: NCMIC Group, 2000.

Chapman-Smith DA. Chiropractic management of back pain: a treatment that stands up. *Chiropractic Rep* 2003; 17(4):1–8.

Cherkin DC, Deyo RA, Sherman KJ, et al. Characteristics of visits to licensed acupuncturists, chiropractors, massage therapists and physicians. *J Am Board Fam Pract* 2002; 15:463–472.

Cherkin DC, Sherman KJ, Deyo RA, Shekelle PG. A review of the evidence for the effectiveness, safety and cost of acupuncture, massage therapy and spinal manipulation for back pain. *Ann Intern Med* 2003; 138:898–906.

Crombie IK, Croft PR, Linton SJ, LeResche L, Von Korff M (Eds). *Epidemiology of Pain.* Seattle: IASP Press, 1999.

Clinical Standards Advisory Group. *CSAG Report on Back Pain.* London: HMSO, 1994.

Cochrane Library. Oxford: Update Software. *Cochrane Database Syst Rev* 2004; 1:CD000447.

Cochrane Reviews. Toronto: Cochrane Back Review Group. Available at: www. cochrane.iwh. on. ca.

Devor M. Pain mechanisms and pain syndromes. In: Campbell JN (Ed). *Pain 1996—An Updated Review: Refresher Course Syllabus.* Seattle: IASP Press, 1996, pp 103–112.

Deyo RA. Low back pain. *Sci Am* 1998; August:29–33.

Doubell TP, Mannion RJ, Woolf CJ. The dorsal horn: state-dependent sensory processing, plasticity and the generation of pain. In: Wall PD, Melzack R (Eds). *Textbook of Pain,* 4th ed. Edinburgh: Churchill Livingstone, 1999, pp 165–181.

Eisenberg DM, Davis RB, Ettner SL, et al. Trends in alternative medicine use in the United States, 1990–1997: results of a follow-up national survey. *JAMA* 1998; 280:1569–1575.

Engel GL. The need for a new medical model: a challenge for biomedicine. *Science* 1977; 196:129–136.

George SZ, Fritz JM, Biolosky JE, Donald DA. The effect of a fear-avoidance based physical therapy intervention for patients with acute low back pain: results of a randomised clinical trial. *Spine* 2003; 28:2551–2660.

Gibson JNA, Grant IC, Waddell G. The Cochrane review of surgery for lumbar disc prolapse and degenerative lumbar spondylosis. *The Cochrane Library.* Oxford: Update Software, 2004.

Hadler N. MRI for regional back pain: need for less imaging, better understanding. *JAMA* 2003; 289:2863–2865.

Hagen KB, Hilde G, Jamtvedt G, Winnem M. Bed rest for acute low back pain and sciatica (Cochrane Review). *Spine* 2000; 25:2932–2939.

Hagen KB, Hilde G, Jamtvedt G, Winnem M. The Cochrane Review of advice to stay active as a single treatment for acute low back pain and sciatica. *Spine* 2002; 27:1736–1741.

Health Scotland. *Working Backs Scotland.* Edinburgh: Health Scotland. Available at: www.workingbacksscotland.com; accessed 2005.

Hunkele J, Vogt M. Use of narcotics and NSAIDs for low back pain: impact on medication costs. Paper presented at: Annual Meeting of the American College of Rheumatology, New Orleans, 2002.

Jarvik JG, Deyo RA. Imaging of lumbar intervertebral disk degeneration and ageing, excluding disk herniation. *Radiol Clin North Am* 2000; 38:1255–1266.

Jarvik JG, Hollingworth W, Martin B, et al. Rapid magnetic imaging vs. radiographs for patients with low back pain: a randomized controlled trial. *JAMA* 2003; 287:2810–2818.

Kendall NAS. *Active and Working! Managing Acute Low Back Pain in the Workplace: An Employer's Guide.* Wellington, NZ: Accident Rehabilitation & Compensation Insurance Corporation of New Zealand and the National Health Committee, 2000. Available at: www.acc.org.nz.

Koes BW, van Tulder MW, Ostelo R, Burton AK, Waddell G. Clinical guidelines for the management of low back pain in primary care: an international comparison. *Spine* 2001; 26:2504–2513.

McGuirk B, King W, Govind J, Lowry J, Bogduk N. Safety, efficacy, and cost-effectiveness of evidence-based guidelines for the management of acute low-back pain in primary care. *Spine* 2001; 26:2615–2622.

Meldrum ML (Ed). *Opioids and Pain Relief: A Historical Perspective,* Progress in Pain Research and Management, Vol. 25. Seattle: IASP Press, 2003.

Melzack R. From the gate to the neuromatrix. *Pain* 1999; (Suppl)6:S121–S126.

Melzack R, Wall PD. Pain mechanisms: a new theory. *Science* 1965; 150:971–979.

Mendenhall S. Spinal surgery update. *Orthopedic Network News* 2002; 13:1–20.

Moore JE, Von Korff M, Cherkin D, Saunders K, Lorig K. A randomized trial of a cognitive-behavioral program for enhancing back pain self-care in a primary care setting. *Pain* 2000; 88:145–153.

Nachemson AL, Jonsson E (Eds). *Neck and Back Pain: the Scientific Evidence of Causes, Diagnosis, and Treatment.* Philadelphia: Lippincott Williams & Wilkins, 2000.

Nachemson A, Vingard E. Assessment of patients with neck and back pain: a best-evidence synthesis. In: Nachemson AL, Jonsson E (Eds). *Neck and Back Pain: The Scientific Evidence of Causes, Diagnosis, and Treatment.* Philadelphia: Lippincott Williams & Wilkins, 2000, pp 189–235.

Royal College of General Practitioners. *Clinical Guidelines for the Management of Acute Low Back Pain.* London: Royal College of General Practitioners, 1999. Available at: www.rcgp.org.uk.

Roland M, Waddell G, Klaber-Moffett J, Burton K, Main C. *The Back Book,* 2nd ed. London: The Stationery Office, 2002.

Rossignol M, Abenhaim L, Seguin P, et al. Coordination of primary health care for back pain: a randomized controlled trial. *Spine* 2000; 25:251–259.

Schoene M. The treatment of back and neck pain: a new pattern of care? *Back Letter* 2003; 18(3):25–36.

Schoene M. Soaring opioid use. *Back Letter* 2004; 19(1):5.

Staal JB, Hlobil H, van Tulder MW, et al. Occupational health guidelines for the management of low back pain: an international comparison. *Occup Environ Med* 2003; 60:618–626.

Waddell G. *Models of Disability: Using Low Back Pain as an Example.* London: Royal Society of Medicine Press, 2002.

Waddell G. *The Back Pain Revolution,* 2nd ed. Edinburgh: Churchill Livingstone, 2004.

Waddell G, Burton AK. *Concepts of Rehabilitation For the Management of Common Health Problems.* London: The Stationery Office, 2004.

Waddell G, Aylward M, Sawney P. *Back Pain, Incapacity for Work and Social Security Benefits: An International Literature Review and Analysis.* London: Royal Society of Medicine Press, 2002.

Wade DT, de Jong BA. Recent advances in rehabilitation. *BMJ* 2000; 320:1385–1388.

World Health Organization. *International Classification of Functioning, Disability and Health.* Geneva: World Health Organization, 2001. Available at: www.who.int/entity/classifica-tions/icf.en.

Wolsko PM, Eisenberg DM, Davis RB, Kessler R, Phillips RS. Patterns and perceptions of care for treatment of back and neck pain: results of a national survey. *Spine* 2003; 28:292–298.

Correspondence to: Gordon Waddell, CBE, DSc, MD, FRCS, 6 Heatherbrae, Bishopbriggs, Glasgow G64 2TA, United Kingdom. Email: gordon.waddell@virgin.net.

The Paths of Pain 1975–2005, edited by
Harold Merskey, John D. Loeser, and Ronald
Dubner, IASP Press, Seattle, © 2005.

27

From Fibrositis and Psychogenic Rheumatism to Fibromyalgia

Harvey Moldofsky[a] and Harold Merskey[b]

[a]Professor Emeritus, Faculty of Medicine, University of Toronto, Toronto, Ontario, Canada; [b]Professor Emeritus of Psychiatry, University of Western Ontario, London, Ontario, Canada

Striking changes have occurred between 1975 and the present time in our understanding of fibromyalgia, previously known by various names such as fibrositis and psychogenic rheumatism. In 1975, diffuse widespread pain, fatigue, and impaired functional capabilities had more than a 100-year history of diagnostic and etiologic confusion. The older labels of fibrositis and psychogenic rheumatism stemmed from suppositions that pain and fatigue resulted from peripheral pathology that seemingly affected the connective tissue of muscles and joints, or from a malfunction of the nervous system with behavioral and psychosocial disturbances. This chapter summarizes beliefs about the origin and evolution of these differing viewpoints and the subsequent lack of scientific substantiation for the presumed pathogenesis of these clinical diagnoses. However, research over the past 30 years has resulted in the confirmation of diagnostic criteria, while neurobiological research has helped to improve our understanding of the syndrome and comorbid disorders.

CONNECTIVE TISSUE AND MUSCLE PATHOLOGY

Gowers (1904) introduced the term "fibrositis." He speculated that inflammation of fibrous or connective tissue of muscles, joints, and nerve sheaths is the reason for the acute and chronic muscular pain and tenderness of what was then known as lumbago or muscular rheumatism. He claimed that fibrositis might affect the lower and upper limbs (brachial fibrositis), shoulders, neck (stiff neck), and chest (intercostal fibrositis). Rheumatic fibrositis was seldom symmetrical. It could occur as the result of a traumatic injury or faulty habitual posture. Shortly thereafter, Stockman (1904) reported on histological changes indicative of inflammation that were seen in the tender fibrous indurations, known as fibrositic nodules. These nodules, which are felt beneath the skin or in the muscles, were first described by Balfour in 1816 in patients with "muscular rheumatism." The search for a physical condition focused for many years on the possibility of a muscle disorder or a local abnormality of muscle function (Bennett 1999). Some workers examined paraspinal muscles in patients operated on for disk herniation and found an accumulation of acid-mucopolysaccharides in fibrositic nodules identified in the interstitial tissues. Others described "ragged red fibers" identified by light microscopy. Subsequent detailed muscle studies failed to confirm any specific pathology on routine light microscopy and on studies of the morphology of muscle fibers, histochemistry, ultrastructure, and biochemistry (Bennett and Jacobsen 1994). Simms (1996) suggested that abnormal findings in skeletal muscle disclosed by nuclear magnetic resonance spectroscopy were due to chronic deconditioning, which is common among patients with fibromyalgia. Nevertheless, the search persists for local pathology to explain local areas of tenderness or disturbance in muscle function. Studies of muscle biopsies in fibromyalgia have not uncovered abnormalities in the expression of opioid receptors, any specific muscle cytopathology, or any sign of reinnervation to explain peripheral nociceptive mechanisms (Salemi et al. 2003).

BEHAVIORAL AND PSYCHOSOCIAL EXPLANATIONS

Toward the latter part of the 19th and early 20th century, George Miller Beard's concept of "neurasthenia" became a fashionable explanation for bodily aching and exhaustion. Beard saw an analogy between the depletion of electrical power in an electrical circuit by an excessive demand upon Edison's electrical generator and the symptoms of "myelasthenia" (spinal irritation or exhaustion), a variety of neurasthenia. The symptoms supposedly stemmed from exhaustion of the nervous system as the result of the demands of Western industrialized society. However, lack of evidence that the electrical activity of the nervous system was depleted and failure to reveal any disease of the nervous system caused neurological interest to wane and to be replaced by psychological explanations. In the mid-20th century there was a considerable tendency to describe as "psychogenic" various patterns of pain that lacked support from physical diagnostic methods (e.g., Engel 1959), an opinion that was echoed by numerous psychoanalytic writers and others

(Merskey and Spear 1967). The pain was considered to be a musculoskeletal manifestation of a psychoneurosis, called psychogenic rheumatism. The diagnosis was based on an absence of organic disease, the presence of functional disability, and evidence for psychopathology (Boland and Corr 1943). Interest in the relevance of personality to such psychosomatic ailments as rheumatoid arthritis and migraine (Dunbar 1938) spawned the search for specific personality traits contributing to the etiology of psychogenic rheumatism. Currently, these personality traits are held to result from a selection process. The more conditions are examined in the general population, the less likely are the persons who possess them to deviate psychologically from the rest and the less similar they are to typical clinical patients with any disorder.

The lack of any specific explanation for the diffuse pain, tenderness, fatigue, and sleep disturbance seen in patients led Philip Hench in 1976 to introduce the descriptive label "fibromyalgia" to replace such labels as psychogenic rheumatism, tension rheumatism, fibrositis, fibromyositis, interstitial myofibrositis, and myofascial pain syndrome. In subsequent psychological studies conducted in patients with fibromyalgia, three basic considerations apply. First, without evidence of psychological illness, the condition should not be attributed to hidden psychological causes. Second, psychological illness may cause the consultation but not the condition. Third, the psychological illness may follow from having an unpleasant physical disorder.

Kirmayer et al. (1988), using a diagnostic interview schedule, found only seven patients who had ever had a diagnosis of a psychiatric disorder among 20 patients with fibromyalgia and seven among 23 patients with rheumatoid arthritis. Payne et al. (1982) found significant elevations on six scales of the Minnesota Multiphasic Personality Inventory in patients with fibromyalgia compared with a control series of patients with other rheumatic diseases such as rheumatoid arthritis and lupus erythematosus. However, elevated scales in a group can result from a minority of patients being emotionally upset. Studies that employ cut-off criteria will separate those who meet the criteria of a psychiatric illness from others. When these criteria are implemented, between 35% and 72% of patients with fibromyalgia show current or past psychiatric disturbance (e.g., Payne et al. 1982; Clarke et al. 1985). In family practice, and in many medical departments in general hospitals, about 30% of all patients have concomitant psychiatric disorders (Shepherd et al. 1966).

Because fibromyalgia patients are often depressed, and because antidepressants such as amitriptyline may be helpful in easing pain, "affective spectrum disorder" provides a (questionable) theoretical model, rooted in the contemporary interest in the biological origins of primary mood disorder (Hudson and Pope 1990). This mood explanation substitutes for psycho-neurotic or generalized distress explanations about fibromyalgia. The pain, fatigue, and sleep disorder of fibromyalgia are interpreted to be components of an affective spectrum disorder that include cataplexy, migraine, and irritable bowel syndrome. While tricyclic medications may be helpful in curbing cataplexy, improving mood, and easing chronic myalgia, such effects do not imply that their varied neurotransmitter actions have uncovered a common affective disturbance mechanism as the cause of fibromyalgia.

Concerns about growth in insurance compensation claims for disability associated with the diffuse pain and fatigue have led some authors to surmise socioeconomic explanations that initiate and perpetuate these complaints. The symptoms are perceived to provide diagnostic legitimacy for physicians and patients to exploit the insurance industry, or to merely provide credence to overemphasized complaints driven by questions of physicians or ideas that patients developed when going through the medical system (e.g., Hadler 1986).

CONTEMPORARY PERSPECTIVES ON FIBROMYALGIA

DIAGNOSIS

Because of the absence of any definitive inflammatory pathology in the fibrositic nodules and no clear understanding derived from essentially psychiatric assessments of behavior and personality, scientific interest in fibrositis had faded by the early 1970s. Yet rheumatologists continued to apply the term as a "wastebasket" diagnosis to patients with aching in their muscles and joint regions without any evidence for rheumatic or connective disease. As an initial step to a systematic study of such patients, diagnostic criteria were established. Hugh Smythe, influenced by Wallace Graham, was becoming interested in the patterns of tenderness in the body, which were not specific to muscles, tendons, or joints. With Moldofsky, Smythe defined 14 highly reproducible specific areas of localized tenderness, or tender points, where at least 12 were commonly found in patients with persistent diffuse myalgia, fatigue, and unrefreshing sleep (Smythe and Moldofsky 1977). Subsequently, the syndrome of fibrositis/fibromyalgia was validated in a multicenter study commissioned by the American College of Rheumatology (Wolfe et al. 1990). The number of tender points was increased so that in addition to the history of more than 3 months of widespread musculoskeletal pain, tenderness in 11 or more of 18 tender points differentiated the syndrome from other rheumatic diseases. The same criteria appear in IASP's

Classification of Chronic Pain Syndromes (Merskey and Bogduk 1994) and are used internationally, both in clinical practice and in research studies.

Whereas the diagnosis is generally acceptable to rheumatologists as a parsimonious expression of a common clinical phenomenon, fibromyalgia is less likely to be diagnosed in related specialties. Among Canadian physicians, 80% of rheumatologists responding to questions about a case history agreed with the patient's diagnosis with the most contested form of the condition, post-traumatic fibromyalgia, compared to 70.5% of general practitioners, 60.4% of physiatrists, and only 28.8% of orthopedists (White et al. 2000). Skepticism concerning the syndrome is still heard, especially from practitioners who dislike post-traumatic fibromyalgia and its management where there are insurance or compensation claims.

While interest in fibromyalgia is greatest among rheumatologists, similar diagnostic labels have emerged in various medical specialties in order to address unexplained pain and fatigue symptoms in their patients, such as chronic fatigue syndrome (infectious disease specialists); Gulf War syndrome and multiple chemical sensitivity syndrome or sick building syndrome (allergy specialists, clinical immunologists); and chronic pain in somatoform disorder (psychiatrists). Moreover, the disorder is found to occur with other unexplained pain problems such as irritable bowel syndrome, temporomandibular pain syndrome, interstitial cystitis, migraine, chronic headache, and atypical chest pain (Silver and Wallace 2002). Fibromyalgia symptoms may accompany rheumatic or connective tissue disease such as osteoarthritis and rheumatoid arthritis, and they also occur commonly in patients with systemic lupus erythematosus, cancer, and other organic disorders including various infections, myxedema, and hypoparathyroidism (e.g., Bland and Frymoyer 1970; Golding 1970), and in patients experiencing drug reactions.

DISORDER OF THE SLEEPING-WAKING BRAIN WITH NEUROENDOCRINE, NEUROIMMUNE, NEUROTRANSMITTER, AND AUTONOMIC DYSFUNCTIONS

Moldofsky et al. (1975) identified the then-currently accepted clinical criteria for fibrositis/fibromyalgia and attempted to determine the contribution of brain physiology to the syndrome. They aimed to identify clinical features that were common in such patients. In addition to diffuse musculoskeletal pain and specific areas of tenderness, they noted that such patients commonly complained of light unrefreshing sleep. Studying the sleep patterns of fibromyalgia patients, Moldofsky et al. (1975) found alpha rhythms during deep delta-wave sleep (i.e., the alpha-delta sleep pattern) or alpha

EEG frequency in stage 2 non-REM sleep. In order to determine the relationship of sleep patterns to symptoms, the authors studied a group of healthy subjects whose slow-wave (deep) sleep was disrupted by noise over three consecutive nights, after which they were permitted to sleep undisturbed. Over the three days they complained of pain in various muscle groups and showed increased tenderness in the same anatomical areas noted in the patients with fibrositis. Not only did these authors artificially induce the waking symptoms by disturbing deep or restorative sleep, but in a subsequent small study, Moldofsky and Scarisbrick (1976) showed that subjects who took daily exercise and were physically fit did not experience fibromyalgic symptoms following a similar experimental disruption of their sleep. The research implied that physical fitness would benefit patients. This notion was confirmed in a study of cardiovascular fitness training of fibromyalgia patients (McCain et al. 1988).

Approximately 25 years later, experimental studies of sleep fragmentation of slow-wave sleep largely replicated the original findings, confirming the central role of the sleeping and waking cycles of the brain in the etiology of the syndrome. The early research of Moldofsky and Warsh (1978) showing that aspects of serotoninergic neurotransmitter dysfunction relate to the pain provided the basis for the use of tricyclic medications for facilitating sleep and improving pain in fibromyalgia patients (Carrette et al. 1986; Goldenberg et al. 1986; Bennett et al. 1988). These studies provoked interest and confidence in the idea that the fibromyalgia syndrome was a coherent— and intriguing—clinical phenomenon, with a pathophysiological substrate. This renewed interest in the syndrome led to verification of Moldofsky and Smythe's initial clinical criteria by Wolfe et al. (1990), followed by more detailed study of neurophysiological, neurotransmitter, neuroendocrine, neuroimmune, and autonomic disturbances of the syndrome. Later research expanded on alpha EEG sleep disorder, which not only occurs in a phasic relationship to delta sleep (alpha delta sleep), but also may occur tonically in stage 2 non-REM sleep, or in a frequent periodic manner as in K alpha EEG sleep or the cyclical alternating pattern (MacFarlane et al. 1996). In about 20% of cases, sleep may be fragmented because of restless legs and sleep-related periodic involuntary limb movements, and in some cases by sleep apnea (Moldofsky 2001). Disordered nocturnal sleep is not only related to pain, but is also associated with cognitive impairment, variation in fatigue, sleepiness, and depression over the day (Coté and Moldofsky 1997). These findings and subsequent research have led to a neurobiological theory of the etiology of the syndrome that involves a deregulation of underlying sleep/wake-related biological rhythms (Moldofsky 1994; Pillemer et al. 1997).

NEUROTRANSMITTER, CHEMICAL, AND NERVOUS SYSTEM DEREGULATION

Once fibromyalgia was identified as a diffuse disorder with pathophysiological changes in sleep and possibly in aspects of serotonin metabolism (Moldofsky and Warsh 1978), investigations proceeded for other neurotransmitter and chemical changes that might be involved in the pathogenesis of the syndrome. Substance P, which is related to the apparent experience of pain in animals and to the experience of pain in humans (Malmberg and Yaksh 1992), was two to three times higher in the cerebrospinal fluid in patients with fibromyalgia than in normal control subjects (Vaeroy et al. 1988; Russell et al. 1994; Mountz et al. 1995). The elevation in substance P suggests that certain central neurokinin receptor functions may be modulated in the syndrome (Russell 2002). Dynorphin was also found to be raised by about 50% in fibromyalgia (Vaeroy et al. 1991). Increased concentrations of nerve growth factor in the cerebrospinal fluid imply an abnormal central mechanism causing altered levels of this and related neuropeptides (Giovengo et al. 1999). These alterations in neurotransmitter substances that affect pain sensitivity may be responsible for central hypersensitivity (Bennett 1999). While controlling for possible increased general hypervigilance, Lorenz et al. (1996) showed such central hypersensitivity in fibromyalgia with increased brain amplitude of somatosensory potentials N170 and P390.

In addition to such increased nociceptive mechanisms in patients with fibromyalgia, there is circadian sympathetic dysfunction affecting heart rate (Martinez-Lavin 2002). About 65% of patients show evidence of orthostatic intolerance, but it is uncertain whether dysautonomia is a cause or an effect of sedentary behavior (Raj et al. 2000).

Coupled with the recognition of sleep-wake disturbances and changes in somatosensory potentials, it is also clear that light touch and pressure give rise to pain in patients with fibromyalgia, a phenomenon known in general as allodynia (see Chapter 22 by Merskey, this volume). Accordingly, increased temporal summation and "wind-up" from controlled repetitive low-intensity stimulation has been demonstrated from both skin and muscle (Staud et al. 2003), indicating central sensitization. Likewise, functional magnetic resonance imaging has yielded evidence of augmented pain processing in fibromyalgia, thus strengthening the view of the syndrome as a state of central hypersensitivity, with corresponding changes to be expected in neurotransmitters (Gracely et al. 2002).

NEUROENDOCRINE, CYTOKINE, AND NEUROIMMUNE DYSFUNCTIONS

The finding of low concentrations of somatomedin C in fibromyalgia syndrome (Bennett et al. 1992) stimulated studies in deregulation of neuroendocrine functions as playing a role in the etiology and perpetuation of the disorder. Considerable interest has centered on growth hormone, much of which is normally secreted during slow-wave (deep) non-REM sleep. Studies showing that levels of growth hormone tend to be reduced led to the experimental administration of growth hormone to fibromyalgia patients. After 9 months of growth hormone injections, the patients reported an overall improvement and a reduction in the number of tender points (Bennett et al. 1998).

About 5% of fibromyalgia patients have hypothyroidism (Carrette and Lefrancois 1988), and the dynamics of the thyroid axis are of interest. Changes there may be a function of a stress response, but except where there is clear evidence for hypothyroidism, treatment directed to the thyroid is not useful (Geenen et al. 2002).

Whereas there are no consistent abnormalities in prolactin, melatonin, or sex hormone functions, there is evidence for perturbations in cortisol and in the neurohormonal dynamics of the hypothalamic-pituitary-adrenal axis (Demitrack and Crofford 1998). The observed changes may be confounded by the distress induced by pain, sleep disturbances, depression, and physical deconditioning (Geenen et al. 2002). A preliminary study revealed a phase advance in circadian natural killer cell cytotoxicity that accompanied a dampening of the amplitude rhythm of circadian cortisol (Moldofsky et al. 1998).

While no specific neuroendocrine, cytokine, or neuroimmune dysfunctions have been directly related to fibromyalgia, the abnormalities that have been reported provide further evidence for the importance of pursuing brain-related functions in the pathogenesis of the syndrome (Pillemer et al. 1997).

CONCLUSIONS

It seems very likely from the evidence presented in this chapter that disturbance of the sleeping-waking brain, very possibly with aberrations in the development and production of neurotransmitters and the development of central sensitization, serves in the pathogenesis of fibromyalgia, along with perturbations in neuroendocrine, neuroimmune, and autonomic functions. Psychological studies have failed to determine a psychological cause for the syndrome, and psychologically based methods of treatment, such as cognitive-behavioral therapy, have also failed to alter the outcome dramatically.

Unfortunately, even the most successful neuropharmacological treatment has had limited success in providing long-term effective treatment for patients with fibromyalgia.

REFERENCES

Bennett RM. Fibromyalgia. In: Wall PD, Melzack R (Eds). *Textbook of Pain.* Edinburgh: Churchill Livingstone 1999, pp 579–601.

Bennett RM, Jacobsen S. Muscle function and origin of pain in fibromyalgia. *Baillière's Clin Rheum* 1994; 8:721–746.

Bennett RM, Gatter RA, Campbell SM, et al. A comparison of cyclobenzaprine and placebo in the management of fibrositis: a double blind controlled study. *Arthritis Rheum* 1988; 3:1535–1542.

Bennett RM, Clark SC, Campbell SM, et al. Low levels of somatomedin C in patients with the fibromyalgia syndrome. A possible link between sleep and muscle pain. *Arthritis Rheum* 1992; 35:1113–1116.

Bennett RM, Clark SC, Walczyk J. A randomized, double- blind, placebo- controlled study of growth hormone in the treatment of fibromyalgia. *Am J Med* 1998; 104:227–231.

Bland JH, Frymoyer JW. Rheumatic syndromes of myxedema. *N Engl J Med* 1970; 282:1171–1174.

Boland EW, Corr WP. Psychogenic rheumatism. *JAMA* 1943; 123:805–809.

Carrette S, Lefrancois L. Fibrositis and primary hypothyroidism. *J Rheumatol* 1988; 15:1418–1421.

Carrette S, McCain GA, Bell DA, et al. Evaluation of amitriptyline in primary fibrositis: a double blind placebo-controlled study. *Arthritis Rheum* 1986; 29:655–659.

Clarke S, Campbell SM, Forehand ME, et al. Clinical characteristics of fibrositis. II: A "blinded," controlled study using standard psychological tests. *Arthritis Rheum* 1985; 28:132–137.

Coté KA, Moldofsky H. Sleep: daytime symptoms and cognitive performance in patients with fibromyalgia. *J Rheumatol* 1997; 26:2014–2023.

Demitrack MA, Crofford LJ. Evidence for and pathophysiologic implications of the hypothalamic-pituitary-adrenal axis dysregulation in fibromyalgia and chronic fatigue syndrome. *Ann NY Acad Sci* 1998; 840:684–697.

Dunbar HF. *Emotions and Bodily Changes,* 2nd ed. New York: Columbia University Press, 1938.

Engel GL. "Psychogenic" pain and the pain-prone patient. *Am J Med* 1959; 26:899–918.

Geenen R, Jacobs JWG, Bijlsma JWJ. Evaluation and management of endocrine dysfunction in fibromyalgia. *Rheum Dis Clin North Am* 2002; 28:389–404.

Giovengo SL, Russell IJ, Larsen AA. Increased concentrations of nerve growth factor in cerebrospinal fluid of patients with fibromyalgia. *J Rheumatol* 1999; 26:1564–1569.

Goldenberg DL, Felson DT, Dinerman H. A randomized, controlled trial of amitriptyline and naproxen in the treatment of patients with fibromyalgia. *Arthritis Rheum* 1986; 29:1371–1377.

Golding DN. Hypothyroidism presenting with musculoskeletal symptoms. *Ann Rheum Dis* 1970; 29:10–14.

Gowers WR. A lecture on lumbago: lessons and analogues. *BMJ* 1904; 1:117–121.

Gracely RH, Petzke F, Wolf JM, et al. Functional magnetic resonance imaging evidence of augmented pain processing in fibromyalgia. *Arthritis Rheum* 2002; 46, 5:1333–1343.

Hadler NM. A critical reappraisal of the fibrositis concept. *Am J Med* 1986; 81(Suppl.)3A:26–30.

Hudson JI, Pope HG Jr. Affective spectrum disorder: does antidepressant response identify a family of disorders with a common pathophysiology? *Am J Psychiatry* 1990; 147:552–564.

Kirmayer LJ, Robbins MJ, Kapusta MA. Somatization and depression in fibromyalgia syndrome. *Am J Psychiatry* 1988; 145:950–954.

Lorenz J, Grasedyck K, Bromm B. Middle and long latency somatosensory evoked potentials after painful laser stimulation in patients with fibromyalgia syndrome. *Electroencephal Clin Neurophysiol* 1996; 100:165–168.

MacFarlane JG, Shahal B, Moldofsky H. Periodic K-alpha sleep EEG activity and periodic leg movements during sleep: comparisons of clinical features and sleep parameters. *Sleep* 1996; 19:200–204.

Malmberg AB, Yaksh TL. Hyperalgesia mediated by spinal butamate or substance P receptor blocked by spinal cyclo-oxygenase inhibition. *Science* 1992; 257:1276–1279.

Martinez-Lavin M. Management of dysautonomia in fibromyalgia. *Rheum Dis Clin N Am* 2002; 28:379–387.

McCain GA, Bell DA, Mai FM, et al. A controlled study of the effects of a supervised cardiovascular fitness training program on the manifestations of primary fibromyalgia. *Arthritis Rheum* 1988; 31:1135–1141.

Merskey H, Bogduk N. *Classification of Chronic Pain: Descriptions of Chronic Pain Syndromes and Definitions of Pain Terms,* 2nd ed. Seattle: IASP Press, 1994.

Merskey H, Spear FG. *Pain: Psychological and Psychiatric Aspects*. London: Baillière, Tindall and Cassell, 1967.

Moldofsky H. Chronobiological influences on fibromyalgia syndrome: theoretical and therapeutic implications. *Baillière's Clin Rheumatol* 1994; 8:801–810.

Moldofsky H. Sleep and pain. *Sleep Med Rev* 2001; 5:387–398.

Moldofsky H, Scarisbrick P. Induction of neurasthenic musculoskeletal pain syndrome by selective sleep stage deprivation. *Psychosom Med* 1976; 38:35–44.

Moldofsky H, Warsh JJ. Plasma tryptophan and musculoskeletal pain in non-articular rheumatism ("fibrositis syndrome"). *Pain* 1978; 5:65–71.

Moldofsky H, Scarisbrick P, England R, et al. Musculoskeletal symptoms and non-REM sleep disturbance in patients with "fibrositis syndrome" and healthy subjects. *Psychosom Med* 1975; 37:341–351.

Moldofsky H, Lue FA, Dickstein J, et al. Disordered circadian sleep-wake neuroendocrine and immune functions in chronic fatigue/fibromyalgia syndrome. *Arthritis Rheum* 1998; 41(Suppl):S255.

Mountz JM, Bradley JL, Modell JG, et al. Fibromyalgia in women: Abnormalities of regional cerebral blood flow in the thalamus and the caudate nucleus are associated with low pain threshold levels. *Arthritis Rheum* 1995; 38:926–938.

Payne TC, Levitt F, Garron DC, et al. Fibrositis and psychologic disturbance. *Arthritis Rheum* 1982; 25:213–217.

Pillemer SR, Bradley LA, Crofford LJ, et al. The neuroscience and endocrinology of fibromyalgia. *Arthritis Rheum* 1997; 40:1928–1939.

Raj SR, Brouillard D, Simpson CS, et al. Dysautonomia among patients with fibromyalgia: a noninvasive assessment. *J Rheumatol* 2000; 27:2660–2665.

Russell IJ. The promise of substance P inhibitors in fibromyalgia. *Rheum Dis Clin North Am* 2002; 28:329–342.

Russell IJ, Orr MD, Littman B, et al. Elevated cerebrospinal fluid levels of substance P in patients with a fibromyalgia syndrome. *Arthritis Rheum* 1994; 37:1593–1601.

Salemi S, Aeschlimann, Gay RE, et al. Expression and localization of opioid receptors in muscle satellite cells: no difference between fibromyalgia patients and healthy subjects. *Arthritis Rheum* 2003; 48:3291–3294.

Shepherd M, Cooper B, Brown MC, et al. *Psychiatric Illness in General Practice*. London: Oxford University Press, 1966.

Silver DS, Wallace DJ. The management of fibromyalgia-associated syndromes. *Rheum Dis Clin N Am* 2002; 28:405–417.

Simms RW. Is there muscle pathology in fibromyalgia syndrome? *Rheum Dis Clin N Am* 1996; 22:245–266.

Smythe HA, Moldofsky H. Two contributions to understanding of the "fibrositis" syndrome. *Bull Rheum Dis* 1977; 8:928–931.

Staud R, Cannon RC, Mauderli AP, et al. Temporal summation of pain from mechanical stimulation of muscle tissue in normal controls and subjects with fibromyalgia syndrome. *Pain* 2003; 102:87–95.

Stockman R. The causes, pathology and treatment of chronic rheumatism. *Edinburgh Med J* 1904; 15:107–116, 223–235.

Vaeroy H, Helle R, Forre O, et al. Elevated CSF levels of substance P and high incidence of Raynaud phenomenon in patients with fibromyalgia: new features for diagnosis. *Pain* 1988; 32:21–26.

Vaeroy H, Nyberg F, Terenius L. No evidence for endorphin deficiency in fibromyalgia following investigation of cerebrospinal fluid (CSF) dynorphin A and met-enkephalin-Arg6-Phe7. *Pain* 1991; 46:139–143.

White KP, Østbye T, Harth M, et al. Perspectives on post-traumatic fibromyalgia: a random survey of Canadian general practitioners, orthopedists, physiatrists and rheumatologists. *J Rheumatol* 2000; 27:790–796.

Wolfe F, Smythe HA, Yunus MB, et al. The American College of Rheumatology 1990 criteria for the classification of fibromyalgia. Report of the Multicenter Criteria Committee. *Arthritis Rheum* 1990; 33, 2:160–172.

Correspondence to: Harvey Moldofsky, MD, FRCP(C), 3400 College Street, Suite 580, Toronto, ON, Canada M5T 3A9.

The Paths of Pain 1975–2005, edited by
Harold Merskey, John D. Loeser, and Ronald
Dubner, IASP Press, Seattle, © 2005.

28

Psychological Contributions to the Understanding and Treatment of Pain

Francis J. Keefe, Kim E. Dixon, and Rebecca W. Pryor

*Department of Psychiatry and Behavioral Sciences, Duke University
Medical Center, Durham, North Carolina, USA*

The 30 years since IASP's 1st World Congress on Pain have seen major advances in our ability to understand and treat pain. This chapter highlights the specific contributions that psychologists have made to pain theory, research, and practice. The chapter is divided into two sections. In the first, we pinpoint key topics of concern to pain psychologists at the inception of IASP and provide an update describing how these topics have been addressed in the intervening years. In the second section, we identify important new directions for psychological pain research and practice.

KEY TOPICS IN THE PSYCHOLOGY OF PAIN: THEN AND NOW

PAIN THEORY

The IASP's early years were a time of growing dissatisfaction with traditional medical models that viewed pain as a simple sensory event signaling tissue injury or damage. One indication of the thinking of that time was the definition of pain formulated by the IASP: "an unpleasant sensory or emotional experience associated with actual or potential tissue damage or described in terms of such damage" (IASP Subcommittee on Taxonomy 1979). This definition underscores the notion that pain is inherently subjective and complex and that it may occur either in the presence or absence of underlying tissue pathology.

The gate control theory exerted a major early influence on psychological concepts of pain (Melzack and Wall 1965). This theory maintains that pain is a complex experience that involves sensory-discriminative, evaluative-cognitive, and affective-motivational components. A key tenet of the gate control theory is that the brain plays an active role in pain modulation by influencing the transmission of noxious signals at the level of the dorsal horns in the spinal cord. Melzack and Casey (1968) elaborated this notion by discussing central mechanisms responsible for three pain modulation functions: (1) a sensory-discriminative function that selects and modulates sensory input, (2) a motivational-affective function that is responsible for the unpleasant affect and motivational drive associated with pain avoidance, and (3) a central control function that integrates information from past experience and regulates activity in the sensory-discriminative and motivational-affective systems.

The gate control theory had several major influences on the way in which pain specialists viewed the psychology of pain. First, by emphasizing the dynamic role the brain plays in pain processing, it heightened interest in personality, motivation, emotion, cognition, and other psychological factors. Second, by tying psychological processes to physiology, it legitimized, for more biomedically oriented pain specialists, the role of psychological factors in pain management. Finally, it stimulated interest in psychological interventions for pain control such as operant conditioning, relaxation, hypnosis, and cognitive strategies.

The 1980s witnessed the emergence of the cognitive-behavioral model of pain (Turk et al. 1983). This psychological model, strongly influenced by the gate control theory, emphasizes that pain is a complex experience that affects and in turn is affected by cognitions (e.g., thoughts, beliefs, memories, and expectations), emotions (e.g., depression, anger, guilt, and joy), and behaviors (e.g., involvement in distracting or pleasant activities and avoidance of painful activities). A major tenet of the cognitive-behavioral model is that one can enhance patients' ability to cope with pain by systematically training them to alter pain-related cognitions and behavior. Cognitive-behavioral treatment protocols for pain management were developed and refined in the 1980s and 1990s and are now widely used in chronic pain management (Keefe et al. 1992; Turk and Okifuji 2002).

Recently, Melzack (1999) has proposed a neuromatrix model of pain that further highlights the role of psychological processes in pain. According to this model, the brain has a neural network that integrates information from multiple sources to produce the experience that is labeled as pain. Key inputs into the pain neural matrix include: (1) sensory information from somatic receptors, (2) visual and other sensory information that influence how the multiple inputs are interpreted, (3) phasic cognitive and emotional inputs (e.g., attention, anxiety, and expectations), (4) tonic cognitive and emotional inputs (e.g., cultural experiences, memory, and personality traits), (5) intrinsic neural inhibitory inputs, and (6) inputs from the body's stress regulation system. The neuromatrix theory is important because it integrates new findings from brain-imaging studies, studies of the effects of stress on pain, and research on cognitive-behavioral factors and pain. As such, it represents yet another step in the evolution of more complex psychological models of pain.

PAIN MEASUREMENT

In the early 1970s, researchers were just beginning to grasp the complexity of the pain experience. Pain was typically measured using numeric or verbal rating scales that focused on the intensity of pain. Melzack and Torgerson (1971) made a seminal contribution to our understanding of the multidimensional nature of pain when they developed the McGill Pain Questionnaire (MPQ). The MPQ includes a widely used adjective checklist that measures not only an evaluative dimension of pain, but also sensory and affective pain dimensions. It is now widely accepted that a pain measure that focuses solely on pain intensity cannot adequately capture the pain experience and that, in addition to intensity, one needs to measure other important dimensions of pain such as affect and unpleasantness (Jensen and Karoly 2001).

Since the mid-1980s, there has been growing recognition of the need for pain measurement tools that are specific to particular pain syndromes. Examples include the Brief Pain Inventory (Cleeland et al. 1989), developed for use with cancer patients; the Neuropathic Pain Scale (Galer and Jensen 1997); and the Temporomandibular Joint Scale (Levitt et al. 1988). Specific approaches to pain assessment strategies also have been developed for particular patient populations such as older adults (Gagliese 2001) and children and adolescents (McGrath and Gillespie 2001).

Individuals who have pain exhibit certain behaviors (e.g., guarded movement or grimacing) that communicate their pain (Fordyce 1976). Measures of such pain behaviors were in their infancy in the early 1970s and mainly consisted of self-reports of activity level (uptime) or medication intake. In the 1980s, observational protocols for directly recording pain behavior were developed and validated. A protocol developed by Keefe and Block (1982) involves collecting videotaped pain behavior samples of low back pain patients as they engage in a standard set of activities (sitting, standing, walking, and reclining). The videotapes are subsequently viewed by trained observers who code the occurrence of specific pain behaviors (guarded movement, stationary pain-avoidant posturing, grimacing, rubbing the painful area, and sighing). The Keefe and Block (1982) observation protocol has shown strong evidence of reliability and validity, and during the 1980s and 1990s it was adapted for use in patients with a wide range of pain conditions (see Keefe et al. 2001 for a review of this literature).

More recently, research on direct observation of pain behavior has focused on pain-related facial expressions of pain (e.g., Craig et al. 2001;
Hadjistavropoulos et al. 2001). Investigators have begun exploring whether
observations of pain-related facial expressions can be an aid in measuring
pain in persons who are unable to provide valid verbal pain reports, such as
very young children (Gilbert et al. 1999) and older adults with cognitive
deficits or dementia (e.g., Hadjistavropoulos et al. 1998, 2000).

In the 1970s, clinicians often asked patients to reflect on a particular
time period (e.g., the past week or past month) and provide an average
rating of pain. Such cross-sectional measures are subject to recall bias and
fail to capture dynamic day-to-day changes in pain. Over the ensuing years,
there has been growing interest in paper-and-pencil as well as computer-
based diary approaches that involve multiple daily pain assessments collected over long time periods (Affleck et al. 1996, 1999; Keefe et al. 1997).

At the time of the 1st World Congress, there was a strong interest in
psychophysiological measures of pain. In studies involving experimental
pain, the nociceptive flexion reflex threshold, a measure of stimulus-induced
spinal reflexes, was well established as a reliable, valid, and objective pain
assessment technique (Willer 1977). This instrument has remained an important tool of clinical research for more than 30 years (Skljarevski and
Ramadan 2002) and has been used to examine the influence of specific
psychological variables such as catastrophizing (France et al. 2002).

Imaging techniques represent a new development in pain measurement.
Interesting findings regarding the neural correlates of pain affect and pain
intensity have emerged from recent brain-imaging studies. Rainville et al.
(1997) found that a hypnotic intervention designed to manipulate *pain unpleasantness* modulated activity specifically in the anterior cingulate cortex
(ACC), whereas Hofbauer et al. (2001) found that a hypnotic intervention
designed to manipulate *pain intensity* activated the primary somatosensory
cortex. Imaging research has shown unique activation of the contralateral
ACC and ipsilateral lentiform in fibromyalgia patients who scored high on a
measure of pain catastrophizing (Gracely et al. 2004).

PERSONALITY AND PAIN

One of the earliest interests of pain psychologists was the relationship of
personality to pain. A number of early reports attempted to determine whether
the Minnesota Multiphasic Personality Inventory (MMPI; Hathaway and
McKinley 1943) could be used to differentiate chronic pain patients having
organic pain from those with functional pain complaints. Hanvik (1951)
compared the MMPI profiles of 30 chronic back pain patients classified as

experiencing organic pain (based on X-ray and physical examination findings) and 30 patients classified as having functional pain. Only the functional pain patients showed a "Conversion V" profile that consisted of elevations on scales 1 (Hypochondriasis) and 3 (Hysteria) with a substantially lower score on scale 2 (Depression). By the early 1970s, the notion that the Conversion V profile could discriminate organic from functional pain was being called into question. In a study of 50,000 medical patients, Schwartz and Krupp (1971) found that a Conversion V profile was unrelated to a functional pain diagnosis. Beals and Hickman (1972) reported that patients with back injuries (i.e., organically based pain) also displayed a general elevation on the neurotic triad (elevation on scales 1, 2, and 3) as well as a slight Conversion V configuration of scores. Sternbach and Timmermans (1975) were among the first to suggest that the personality variables measured by the MMPI may be a result of pain rather than simply a contributing factor. They reported that patients who received surgery to relieve their pain displayed significant decreases in their scores on MMPI scales 1 and 3.

In the early 1970s, the MMPI was frequently used as a predictor of surgical and medical outcomes. Although positive findings were obtained in some predictive studies (e.g., Wilfling et al. 1973; Wiltse and Rocchio 1975), some findings were negative (Bradley et al. 1992). The mixed findings reported across the predictive studies most likely reflected methodological problems including small sample sizes, variations in the treatment procedures, and lack of consistency in outcome measures (Bradley et al. 1992).

One methodological issue that received considerable attention in the late 1970s to 1980s was that of heterogeneity of patient populations. The basic notion was that, in most studies, data from patients having diverse personality characteristics were being averaged together to produce a composite MMPI profile that gave an illusion of homogeneity. Cluster analysis provides a statistical technique for identifying homogeneous subgroups within a larger, heterogeneous population. Bradley et al. (1978) were the first to use cluster analysis to identify homogeneous MMPI subgroups of low back pain patients. They identified three subgroups for men and four for women. The subgroups for men included those exhibiting a neurotic triad profile, a profile within normal limits, and a profile with elevations on scales F, 1, 2, 3, and 8. The subgroups for women included those exhibiting a neurotic triad profile, a Conversion V profile, a profile within normal limits, and a profile with elevations across all scales. Subsequent cluster analysis studies have identified a variety of MMPI subgroups, several of which were similar to those found by Bradley's team (Prokop et al. 1980; Bernstein and Garbin 1983; Hart 1984). Researchers also have shown that these MMPI subgroups are meaningfully related to measures of adjustment to pain, with patients in the subgroups showing elevations on multiple MMPI scales having the highest levels of pain, disability, and pain behavior. Although this research convincingly demonstrates that one can identify homogeneous MMPI subgroups within heterogeneous chronic pain populations, studies have failed to show that these subgroups are consistently related to the outcome of medical, surgical, or behavioral treatments for chronic pain (Moore et al. 1986; Guck et al. 1988).

The focus of research on personality and pain has shifted significantly from where it was in the 1970s (Keefe et al. 2002a). With the widespread application of the gate control and cognitive-behavioral models of pain, the organic/functional distinction is now seen as overly simplistic and relatively meaningless (Turk 1996). Broadband personality measures such as the MMPI are used less frequently, and measures that focus on more specific personality traits, such as alexithymia, are used more frequently (Keefe et al. 2002a). Patients who are alexithymic (which means that they have difficulty in identifying, communicating, and separating their feelings from other physical sensations) have been found to experience much higher levels of pain and psychological distress compared to non-alexithymic patients (Lumley et al. 1997; Taylor et al. 1997).

PSYCHOLOGICAL TREATMENTS

Behavioral interventions were among the first psychological treatments used in chronic pain management. Derived from operant conditioning, these interventions focused on modifying pain behaviors by altering their relationship to social and environmental contingencies (Fordyce 1976; Gentry 1977). In these interventions, positive reinforcement such as praise or attention was used to increase the frequency of adaptive "well behaviors" such as exercising and spending time up and out of bed. Extinction, or withholding of positive reinforcement (e.g., attention) was used to reduce the frequency of maladaptive "pain behaviors." Evidence for the efficacy of behavioral interventions initially came primarily from studies using single-case experimental designs (Fordyce et al. 1973, 1986). Operant behavioral interventions continue to be used in pain management, and recent randomized clinical trials demonstrate their efficacy (Ersek et al. 2003; Sanders 2003).

By the mid-1980s, there was growing recognition of the role of cognitive factors in the pain experience. Studies showed that cognitive pain-coping strategies, pain beliefs, and self-efficacy could influence pain, psychological distress, and physical disability (Keefe et al. 1988; Keefe and Williams 1989). This was a time of heightened interest in multimodal treatment protocols that combined cognitive interventions (e.g., cognitive restructuring, imagery, and distraction methods) with more traditional behavioral interventions. These cognitive-behavioral protocols were first used successfully in headache treatment and were rapidly adopted in other areas of pain management (Mitchell and White 1977). Turk et al. (1983) were among the first to describe practical strategies for utilizing cognitive-behavioral therapy methods for patients having chronic pain. A number of meta-analyses and systematic reviews are available to support the efficacy of cognitive-behavioral treatment protocols for chronic pain and disease-related pain conditions (Keefe et al. 1992; Compas et al. 1996; Turner 1996; Scheer et al. 1997; Morley et al. 1999).

In the 1970s, biofeedback was a novel intervention. In biofeedback. patients are given accurate, moment-to-moment feedback about physiological responses related to pain (e.g., increased muscle tension) in order to enable them to control these responses. Biofeedback was initially applied in headache management (Stroebel and Glueck 1975; Holroyd and Andrasik 1982), and in recent years, strong empirical support for the efficacy of biofeedback has emerged from randomized clinical trials for both migraine and tension headaches (Arena and Blanchard 2001). Although biofeedback is also used for other chronically painful conditions (e.g., low back pain, Raynaud's disease), controlled studies suggest that it is typically equivalent to other relaxation methods for such conditions.

Hypnosis was also a popular pain management intervention in the 1970s. While it was recognized that hypnosis provided only brief pain relief, it was believed that hypnosis had a role as part of a more comprehensive approach to pain treatment (Barber 1982). Over the years, hypnosis protocols have been developed for a variety of pain conditions including fibromyalgia (Haanen et al. 1991), tension headache (Zitman et al. 1992), and cancer pain (Trijsburg et al. 1992; Redd et al. 2001). A recent meta-review concluded that hypnosis is an efficacious treatment for cancer pain and some acute pain conditions; however, variability in the quality of many of the hypnosis studies reviewed precluded definitive judgments of its efficacy for other pain conditions (Hawkins 2001).

MULTIDISCIPLINARY PAIN PROGRAMS

In the 1970s, pain specialists first developed and refined specialized multidisciplinary treatment programs in which psychological interventions were combined with a wide range of medical, surgical, and other interventions in hopes of improving patient outcome. Many of the early multidisciplinary pain programs were situated on inpatient hospital units. Fordyce and his colleagues (1973), for example, developed an intensive behavioral pain management program in a rehabilitation unit. This program, based on an operant-behavioral model of pain, was designed to decrease maladaptive pain behaviors while increasing more adaptive well behaviors. The staff members on this unit were trained in skills necessary to minimize reinforcement of pain behaviors exhibited by the patients. Conversely, well behaviors such as increasing uptime were reinforced through positive social reinforcement. Patients were switched from an as-needed to time-contingent dosing of pain medications with a goal of decreasing the amount of medication needed. Data collected over the course of treatment showed that patients who participated in this program showed significant increases in their level of uptime and exercise and decreases in medication intake (Fordyce et al. 1973).

Rapid growth in multidisciplinary pain programs continued up through the 1990s to such an extent that by the turn of this century, multidisciplinary pain management was described as "medicine's new growth industry" (Loeser and Turk 2001). Multidisciplinary programs for chronic pain management eventually became available in hospitals and outpatient facilities in many countries around the world (Loeser and Turk 2001; Thomsen et al. 2001). Meta-analyses also provided empirical support for the efficacy of such programs (Flor et al. 1992; Karjalainen et al. 2003). Flor et al. (1992), for example, reported that patients who completed such programs functioned better than 75% of those who were untreated or who had received unimodal treatments.

Despite the popularity and strong empirical support for multidisciplinary approaches to managing chronic pain (Flor et al. 1992; Guzm et al. 2003), there is at least anecdotal evidence that these programs are viewed by many in the insurance industry as costly and inefficient (Thomsen et al. 2001). In the United States and other countries, many well-established programs are now being closed due to problems with reimbursement (Guzm et al. 2003). The loss of these programs is a major concern, particularly given the difficulty of developing them and the fact that they have benefited many patients whose pain had failed to respond to conventional medical or surgical interventions.

FUTURE DIRECTIONS

UNDERSTANDING THE PROCESS OF PAIN COPING

When faced with severe or persistent pain, individuals develop strategies to cope with or minimize their pain. Over the past 15 years, numerous studies have underscored the importance of pain coping strategies in understanding how individuals adjust to persistent pain (Lester and Keefe 1997; Keefe et al. 2002b). Although the literature on this topic is large and varied, the findings obtained support two basic conclusions (Lester and Keefe 1997). First, individuals who are more active in pain coping and who are able to maintain a rational and more positive outlook in the face of pain are better able to adapt to persistent pain. Second, those who are more passive and avoidant in pain coping and who tend to catastrophize (i.e., ruminate about pain, magnify it, and feel helpless) show much poorer adaptations to persistent pain.

Many of the studies on pain coping are limited by the fact that they have relied on cross-sectional measures of coping that may fail to capture important day-to-day changes in the relationships of coping to pain, mood, and other outcomes. Over the past 10 years, psychological researchers have begun to explore daily diary methods for understanding the process of coping (Affleck et al. 1999). In daily diary research, participants may be asked to provide reports of their pain, coping, mood, activity, or other variables at one time or at multiple times during each day. These reports are either entered onto a paper diary form that is mailed in daily, or entered in a database on a handheld computer. Daily diary methods are well tolerated by patients and have several distinct advantages (Affleck et al. 1999). First, they measure rapidly changing processes closer to their real time occurrence. Second, they enable each person to serve as his or her own control, thereby minimizing potential individual difference factors, such as personality or disease severity, that might confound relationships between pain and coping or pain and mood. Finally, they provide repeated measurements that enable the researcher to apply powerful within-person statistical analyses that allow for stronger inferences to be drawn regarding causal sequences between coping and other outcomes.

In our own laboratory, we have conducted a series of studies using daily diary methodology to study pain coping in arthritis patients. In our first study (Keefe et al. 1997), 53 rheumatoid arthritis patients supplied reports of pain coping, positive mood, negative mood, and joint pain for 30 consecutive days. Within-person analyses provided unique information about the relations among coping, pain, and mood. Increases in daily coping efficacy were related not only to decreases in pain, but also to increases in positive mood and decreases in negative mood. Persons who reported frequent use of problem-focused coping efforts—pain reduction efforts and relaxation strategies—also showed a significant improvement in pain the following day and an enhancement in positive mood.

Attempts to understand pain coping processes are likely to continue in the future, particularly since these processes have important implications for pain management. Daily diary records of coping methods provide a promising strategy for studying the pain coping process and are likely to become even more widely used in future research.

ETHNIC/CULTURAL DIFFERENCES

An important new direction in the psychology of pain is the study of how culture and ethnicity influence the experience of pain. Converging lines of evidence gathered in studies conducted in the United States have shown that, when compared to Caucasian Americans, African Americans report higher levels of pain. This pattern has been found in clinical studies of patients having pain due to AIDS (Breitbart et al. 1996), migraine headaches (Stewart et al. 1996), arthritis (Creamer et al. 1999), and chronic pain (Riley et al. 2002). Experimental pain studies also have found that, when compared to Caucasian Americans, African Americans report significantly lower levels of pain tolerance for thermal pain, ischemic pain, and cold pressor pain (Walsh et al. 1989; Edwards and Fillingim 1999; Campbell et al. 2003).

Interestingly, relatively little attention has been given to exploring the underlying biological, psychological, or sociological factors that may be responsible for the differences in pain reports between African Americans and Caucasian Americans. There is some speculation that African Americans may be more prone to hypertension and enhanced cardiovascular reactivity to pain (McNeilly and Zeichner 1989). There is also some evidence that ethnic differences in pain coping styles may influence the pain experience (James et al. 1983; Jordan et al 1998; Clark et al. 1999). Some studies have reported on a link between "John Henryism" (a type of active coping that involves working harder when faced with difficult challenges), hypertension, and pain in African-Americans (James et al. 1983, 1987, 1992). Clark et al. (1999) suggests that the stress experienced by ethnic minorities, such as African Americans, due to social factors such as racism and discrimination, results in higher levels of sympathetic activation and physiological exhaustion, which in turn might contribute to pain. It is also likely that the undertreatment of pain observed in minority populations (Todd et al. 2000; Green et al. 2003) is related to ethnic differences in pain expression, which might affect clinical treatment decisions.

There is a need for additional research examining ethnic differences in pain. Current research also has very little to offer about the interactions that may exist between ethnicity and other subject variables such as sex and age. For example, perhaps ethnic differences are more pronounced in older African Americans who may have developed more marked cultural differences than their younger counterparts. Along these lines, future research must also consider the interaction of ethnic background of the experimenter with that of the subject. At least one study suggests that improved communications between physicians and patients of the same ethnic background may affect the pain experience (Cooper-Patrick et al. 1999). Additionally, Tait and Chibnall (1998) found that higher pain severity was related to more prejudiced stereotyping among clinicians.

In the future, the field of pain research will need to move away from simple comparative studies involving ethnicity and pain toward studies designed to understand the pain experience through ethnic variations. Toward this end, efforts must also be focused on understanding the pain experience within a given ethnicity. Clinical outcome studies should explore ethnic differences in pain-related variables both before and after treatment. Research on pain and ethnicity must begin to include measures of a variety of biopsychosocial factors. In this way, ethnic differences in the experience of pain can serve to contribute much to our knowledge of factors affecting the pain experience in all individuals.

UNDERSTANDING PSYCHOLOGICAL TREATMENT MECHANISMS

As noted above, increasing evidence indicates that cognitive-behavioral therapy and other psychological interventions can be helpful in improving adjustment to persistent pain. What is less clear are the mechanisms through which these interventions influence pain and adjustment. Psychological interventions may exert their influence through several possible pathways. First, these interventions may be beneficial because they produce changes in cognitions—in how patients think about and appraise their pain. Consistent with this view, there is growing evidence that changes in cognitions are related to treatment outcome. For example, patients who show increases in self-efficacy over the course of cognitive-behavioral treatments show much better short- and long-term outcomes (Lorig et al. 1993; Keefe et al. 1996, 1999). Also, individuals who show decreases in maladaptive cognitions, specifically pain catastrophizing, during treatment are more likely to report improvements in pain and psychological distress (Burns et al. 2003).

Second, psychological interventions may benefit people by changing their behavior and social interactions. After completing treatment, participants may be much more active and more likely to re-engage in meaningful social roles and relationships. Although Fordyce (1976) originally emphasized the key role of behavior change in pain management, relatively few studies have examined behavioral and social factors as mediators of the outcome of cognitive-behavioral treatment. Future studies need to examine the influence of changes in behavioral interactions in family, work, health care, and other social settings on treatment outcome. Finally, future research needs to explore whether the benefits of psychosocial pain management interventions can be understood by examining changes in biological pathways such as changes in stress responding, neural inhibition, or immune responses. By incorporating measures designed to capture changes in biological processes, future studies can gain a better understanding of the biological basis of therapeutic improvements in pain and adjustment. By improving insights into the mechanisms underlying psychological treatment effects, we not only can improve our understanding of pain but also can develop new and more effective treatment protocols.

DISSEMINATION OF TREATMENT

Psychological treatments for pain have traditionally been delivered by highly trained, Ph.D.-level psychologists in a series of face-to-face sessions. Dissemination of these interventions to individuals who find it difficult or are unable to participate in such a conventional treatment format is an important challenge for the future. Telephone-based educational interventions have been used in arthritis pain management for a number of years (Weinberger et al. 1989), and a recent study demonstrated the use of an interactive voice response telephone system in enhancing maintenance following pain-coping skills training (Naylor et al. 2002). Another approach to disseminating psychological interventions is the use of lay counselors. Several studies have demonstrated that self-management interventions led by lay persons can improve adjustment to chronically painful conditions such as arthritis (e.g., Lorig and Fries 1995) and low back pain (Von Korff et al. 2002). Lorig et al. (2002) recently conducted a study to test a Web-based format for pain management. In addition to receiving a book and videotape on managing back pain, patients in the treatment arm of this study participated in a closed e-mail listserver facilitated by two moderators and a physician, psychologist, and physical therapist. Compared to a control condition of usual care, this novel format produced significant decreases in pain, disability, distress, and health care visits.

TAILORING PSYCHOLOGICAL TREATMENTS

With recognition of the heterogeneity of chronic pain populations has come increased interest in tailoring treatments so as to better address the needs of individual patients (Keefe et al. 2004). Turk and his colleagues have identified three replicable subgroups of chronic pain patients based on their responses to the West Haven-Yale Multidimensional Pain Inventory (MPI): a dysfunctional group, an interpersonally distressed group, and an adaptive coper group (Kerns et al. 1985; Jamison et al. 1994). In several studies (Rudy et al. 1995; Turk et al. 1998), these patient subgroups have been shown to respond differentially to multidisciplinary pain treatment protocols. In general, patients in the dysfunctional group have shown the best outcomes and those in the adaptive coper and interpersonally distressed groups have shown fewer benefits. On the basis of these findings, Turk and Okifuji (2001) have argued that a standardized treatment protocol may not benefit all patients and that one must tailor treatment so as to address specific needs, such as by involving spouses or family members in treatment protocols for patients who are interpersonally distressed.

Treatment tailoring is only beginning to be explored in the psychological pain management literature. For example, a study by Evers et al. (2002) found that a cognitive-behavioral treatment protocol that was tailored to address specific concerns of patients with early rheumatoid arthritis had significant and positive effects on fatigue, depression, coping, and social support. Another recent study by Dalton et al. (2004) found that a cognitive-behavioral pain management intervention that was tailored based on cancer patients' responses on a biobehavioral pain profile led to better immediate treatment outcomes compared to a standard cognitive-behavioral intervention.

Treatment tailoring is important for two reasons. First, it is responsive to the unique problems and issues that patients present and thus may enhance patient motivation and engagement in treatment. Second, it allows practitioners to streamline treatment, reduce its costs, and make it more readily available to patients who need it.

CONCLUSIONS

Psychological approaches to understanding and treating pain have evolved considerably over the past 30 years. The contributions of psychologists are evident through advances not only in pain theory, but also in pain research and practice. New research initiatives promise to enhance our understanding of how people cope with pain and how psychological treatments influence pain. This research is likely to have important implications for another key future direction: tailoring psychological treatments to fit the needs of particular patients. As the future brings improved dissemination of interventions, the long-standing promise of psychological treatment in pain management is more likely to become a reality.

ACKNOWLEDGMENTS

Supported by several NIH Grants (AR50245, NS46422-01, CA91947, AR047218, MH63429, AR46305) and, in part, by funds provided by the Arthritis Foundation and the Fetzer Institute.

REFERENCES

Affleck G, Urrows S, Tennen H, et al. Sequential daily relations of sleep, pain intensity, and attention to pain among women with fibromyalgia. *Pain* 1996; 68:363–368.

Affleck G, Tennen H, Keefe FJ, et al. Everyday life with osteoarthritis or rheumatoid arthritis: independent effects of disease and gender on daily pain, mood, and coping. *Pain* 1999; 83:601–609.

Arena JG, Blanchard EB. Biofeedback therapy for chronic pain disorders. In: Loeser JP, Butler SD, Chapman CR, Turk DC (Eds). *Bonica's Management of Pain*, 3rd ed. Philadelphia: Lippincott Williams & Wilkins, 2001, pp 1759–1767.

Barber J. Incorporating hypnosis in the management of chronic pain. In: Barber J, Adrian C (Eds). *Psychological Approaches to Management of Pain*. New York: Brunner/Mazel, 1982, pp 40–89.

Beals RK, Hickman NW. Industrial injuries of the back and extremities. *J Bone Joint Surg Am* 1972; 54:1593–1611.

Bernstein IH, Garbin CP. Hierarchical clustering of pain patients' MMPI profiles: a replication note. *J Pers Assess* 1983; 47:171–172.

Bradley LA, Prokop CK, Margolis R, Gentry WD. Multivariate analyses of the MMPI profiles of low back pain patients. *J Behav Med* 1978; 1:253–272.

Bradley LA, Haile JM, Jaworski TM. Assessment of psychological status using interviews and self-report instruments. In: Turk DC, Melzack R (Eds). *Handbook of Pain Assessment*. New York: Guilford Press, 1992, pp 193–213.

Breitbart W, McDonald MV, Rosenfeld B, et al. Pain in ambulatory AIDS patients. I: Pain characteristics and medical correlates. *Pain* 1996; 68:315–321.

Burns J, Glenn B, Bruehl S, Harden R, Lofland K. Cognitive factors influence outcome following multidisciplinary chronic pain treatment: a replication and extension of a cross-lagged panel analysis. *Behav Res Ther* 2003; 41:1163–1182.

Campbell C, Fillingim R, Edwards RR. Ethnic differences in responses to multiple experimental pain stimuli. *J Pain* 2003; 4(Suppl 1):96.

Clark R, Anderson NB, Clark VR, Williams DR. Racism as a stressor for African-Americans: a biopsychosocial model. *Am Psychol* 1999; 54:805–816.

Cleeland CS. Measurement of pain by subjective report. In: Chapman CR, Loeser JD (Eds). *Issues in Pain Measurement*. New York: Raven Press, 1989, pp 391–404.

Compas BE, Haaga DAF, Keefe FJ, et al. Sampling of empirically supported psychological treatments from health psychology: smoking, chronic pain, cancer, and bulimia nervosa. *J Consult Clin Psychol* 1996; 66:89–112.

Cooper-Patrick L, Gallo JJ, Gonzales JJ, et al. Race, gender, and partnership in the patient-physician relationship. *JAMA* 1999; 282:583–589.

Craig KD, Prkachin KM, Grunau RE. The facial expression of pain. In: Turk DC, Melzack R (Eds). *Handbook of Pain Assessment*, 2nd ed. New York: Guilford Press, 2001, pp 153–169.

Creamer P, Lethbridge-Cejku M, Hochberg MC. Determinants of pain severity in knee osteoarthritis: effect of demographic and psychosocial variables using 3 pain measures. *J Rheumatol* 1999; 26:1785–1792.

Dalton J, Keefe FJ, Carlson J, Youngblood R. Tailoring cognitive-behavioral treatment for cancer pain. *Pain Manage Nurs* 2004;5(1):3–18.

Edwards RR, Fillingim RB. Ethnic differences in thermal pain responses. *Psychosom Med* 1999; 61:346–354.

Ersek M, Turner JA, McCurry SM, Gibbons L, Kraybill BM. Efficacy of a self-management group intervention for elderly persons with chronic pain. *Clin J Pain* 2003; 19:156–167.

Evers AWM, Kraaimaat FW, van Riel PLCM, de Jong AJL. Tailored cognitive-behavioral therapy in early rheumatoid arthritis for patients at risk: a randomized controlled trial. *Pain* 2002; 100:141–153.

Flor H, Fydrich T, Turk DC. Efficacy of multidisciplinary pain treatment centers: a meta-analytic review. *Pain* 1992; 49:221–230.

Fordyce WE. *Behavioral Methods for Chronic Pain and Illness*. Saint Louis: Mosby, 1976.

Fordyce WE, Fowler RS, Lehmann JR, et al. Operant conditioning in the treatment of chronic pain. *Arch Phys Med Rehabil* 1973; 54:399–405.

Fordyce WE, Brockway JA, Bergman JA, Spengler D. Acute back pain: a control-group comparison of behavioral vs. traditional management methods. *J Behav Med* 1986; 9:127–140.

France CR, France JL, al'Absi M, Ring C, McIntyre D. Catastrophizing is related to pain ratings, but not nociceptive flexion reflex threshold. *Pain* 2002; 99:459–463.

Gagliese L. Assessment of pain in the elderly. In: Turk DC, Melzack R (Eds). *Handbook of Pain Assessment*, 2nd ed. New York: Guilford Press, 2001, pp 119–133.

Galer BS, Jensen MP. Development and preliminary validation of a pain measure specific to neuropathic pain: the Neuropathic Pain Scale. *Neurology* 1997; 48:332–338.

Gentry WD. Chronic pain. In: Williams RB, Gentry WD (Eds). *Behavioral Approaches to Medical Treatment*. Cambridge, MA: Ballinger, 1977, pp 173–182.

Gilbert CA, Lilley CM, Craig KD, et al. Postoperative pain expression in preschool children: validation of the Child Facial Coding System. *Clin J Pain* 1999; 15:192–200.

Gracely RH, Geisser ME, Giesecke T, et al. Pain catastrophizing and neural responses to pain among persons with fibromyalgia. *Brain* 2004; 127:835–843.

Green CR, Anderson KO, Baker TA, et al. The unequal burden of pain: confronting racial and ethnic disparities in pain. *Pain Med* 2003; 4:277–294.

Guck TP, Meilman PW, Skultety FM, Poloni LD. Pain-patient Minnesota Multiphasic Personality Inventory (MMPI) subgroup: evaluation of long-term treatment outcome. *J Behav Med* 1988; 11:159–169.

Guzm NJ, Esmail R, Karjalainen K, et al. Multidisciplinary bio-psycho-social rehabilitation for chronic low back pain, Cochrane review. *Cochrane Library* 2003; Issue 2.

Haanen HC, Hoenderdos HT, van Romunde, et el. Controlled trial of hypnotherapy in the treatment of fibromyalgia. *J Rheumatol* 1991; 18:72–75.

Hadjistavropoulos T, LaChapelle D, MacLeod F, et al. Cognitive functioning and pain reactions in hospitalized elders. *Pain Res Manage* 1998; 3:145–151.

Hadjistavropoulos T, LaChapelle D, MacLeod F, Snider B, Craig KD. Measuring movement-exacerbated pain in cognitively impaired frail elders. *Clin J Pain* 2000; 16:54–63.

Hadjistavropoulos T, von Baeyer C, Craig K. Pain assessment in persons with limited ability to communicate. In: Turk DC, Melzack R (Eds). *Handbook of Pain Assessment,* 2nd ed. New York: Guilford Press, 2001, pp 134–152.

Hanvik LJ. MMPI profiles in patients with low-back pain. *J Consult Psychol* 1951; 15:350–352.

Hathaway SR, McKinley JC. *The Minnesota Multiphasic Personality Inventory*, 2nd ed. Minneapolis: University of Minnesota Press, 1943.

Hart RR. Chronic pain: replicated multivariate clustering of personality profiles. *J Clin Psychol* 1984; 40:129–133.

Hawkins RMF. A systematic meta-review of hypnosis as an empirically supported treatment for pain. *Pain Rev* 2001; 8:47–73.

Hofbauer RK, Rainville P, Duncan GH, Bushnell MC. Cortical representations of the sensory dimension of pain. *J Neurophysiol* 2001; 86:402–411.

Holroyd KA, Andrasik F. A cognitive-behavioral approach to recurrent tension and migraine headache. In: Kendall PC (Ed). *Advances in Cognitive-Behavioral Research and Therapy*, Vol. 1. New York: Academic Press, 1982, pp 275–320.

IASP Subcommittee on Taxonomy. Pain terms: a list of definitions and notes on usage. *Pain* 1979; 6:249–252.

James SA, Hartnett SA, Kalsbeek WD. John Henryism and blood pressure differences among black men. *J Behav Med* 1983; 6:259–278.

James SA, Strogatz DS, Wing SB, Ramsey DL. Socioeconomic status, John Henryism, and hypertension in blacks and whites. *Am J Epidemiol* 1987; 126:664–673.

James SA, Keenan NL, Strogatz DS, Browning Sr, Garrett JM. Socioeconomic status, John Henryism, and blood pressure in black adults: the Pitt County Study. *Am J Epidemiol* 1992; 135:59–67.

Jamison RN, Rudy TE, Penzien DB, Mosley TH. Cognitive-behavioral classifications of chronic pain: replication and extension of empirically derived patient profiles. *Pain* 1994; 57:277–292.

Jensen MP, Karoly P. Self-report scales and procedures for assessing pain in adults. In: Turk DC, Melzack R (Eds). *Handbook of Pain Assessment,* 2nd ed. New York: Guilford Press, 2001, pp 15–34.

Jordan MS, Lumley MA, Leisen JC. The relationships of cognitive coping and pain control beliefs to pain and adjustment among African-American and Caucasian women with rheumatoid arthritis. *Arthritis Care Res* 1998; 11:80–88.

Karjalainen K, Malmivaara A, van Tulder M, et al. Multidisciplinary biopsychosocial rehabilitation for subacute low back pain among working age adults. *Cochrane Database Syst Rev* 2003, 2:CD002193.

Keefe FJ, Block AR. Development of an observation method for assessing pain behavior in chronic low back pain patients. *Behav Ther* 1982; 13:363–375.

Keefe FJ, Williams DA. New directions in pain assessment and treatment. *Clin Psychol Rev* 1989; 9:549–568.

Keefe FJ, Gil KM, Williams DA. Pain management programs: clinical research perspectives. *NC Med J* 1988; 49:526–529.

Keefe FJ, Dunsmore J, Burnett R. Behavioral and cognitive-behavioral approaches to chronic pain: recent advances and future directions. *J Consult Clin Psychol* 1992; 60:528–536.

Keefe F, Caldwell D, Baucom D, et al. Spouse-assisted coping skills training in the management of osteoarthritis knee pain. *Arthritis Care Res* 1996; 9:279–291.

Keefe FJ, Affleck G, Lefebvre JC, et al. Pain coping strategies and coping efficacy in rheumatoid arthritis: a daily process analysis. *Pain* 1997; 69:35–42.

Keefe F, Caldwell D, Baucom D, et al. Spouse-assisted coping skills training in the management of osteoarthritis knee pain: long-term follow-up results. *Arthritis Care Res* 1999; 12:101–111.

Keefe FJ, Williams DA, Smith SJ, Assessment of pain behaviors. In: Turk DC, Melzack R (Eds). *Handbook of Pain Assessment,* 2nd ed. New York: Guilford Press, 2001, pp 170–187.

Keefe FJ, Lumley MA, Buffington ALH, et al. Changing face of pain: evolution of pain research in psychosomatic medicine. *Psychosom Med* 2002a; 64:921–938.

Keefe FJ, Smith SJ, Buffington ALH, et al. Recent advances and future directions in the biopsychosocial assessment and treatment of arthritis. *J Consult Clin Psychol* 2002b; 70:640–655.

Keefe FJ, Rumble ME, Scipio CD, Giordano L, Perri LM. Psychological aspects of persistent pain: current state of the science. *J Pain* 2004; 5(4):195–211.

Kerns RD, Turk DC, Rudy TE. The West Haven-Yale Multidimensional Pain Inventory (WHYMPI). *Pain* 1985; 23:345–356.

Lester N, Keefe FJ. Coping with chronic pain. In: Baum A, McManus C, Newman S, Weinman J, West R (Eds). *Cambridge Handbook of Psychology, Health and Medicine.* Cambridge: Cambridge University Press, 1997, pp 87–90.

Levitt SR, Lundeen TF, McKinney MW. Initial studies of a new assessment method for temporomandibular joint disorders. *J Prosthet Dent* 1988; 59:490–495.

Loeser JD, Turk DC. Multidisciplinary pain programs. In: Loeser JD, Butler SH, Chapman RC, et al. (Eds). *Bonica's Management of Pain,* 3rd ed. Philadelphia: Lippincott, Williams and Wilkins, pp 2069–2079.

Lorig K, Fries JF. *The Arthritis Helpbook,* 4th ed. Reading, MA: Addison-Wesley, 1995.

Lorig K, Mazonson P, Holman H. Evidence suggesting that health education for self-management in patients with chronic arthritis has sustained health benefits while reducing health care costs. *Arthritis Rheum* 1993; 36:439–446.

Lorig KR, Laurent DD, Deyo RA, et al. Can a back pain e-mail discussion group improve health status and lower health care costs? *Arch Intern Med* 2002; 162:792–796.

Lumley MA, Asselin LA, Norman S. Alexithymia in chronic pain patients. *Compr Psychiatry* 1997; 38:160–165.

McGrath PA, Gillespie J. Pain assessment in children and adolescents. In: Turk DC, Melzack R (Eds). *Handbook of Pain Assessment,* 2nd ed. New York: Guilford Press, 2001, pp 97–118.

McNeilly MD, Zeichner A. Neuropeptide and cardiovascular responses to intravenous catheterization in normotensive and hypertensive blacks and whites. *Health Psychol* 1989; 8:487–501.

Melzack R. From the gate to the neuromatrix. *Pain* 1999; (Suppl 6):121–126.

Melzack R, Casey KL. Sensory, motivation, and central control determinants of pain: a new conceptual model. In: Kenshalo D (Ed). *The Skin Senses.* Springfield, IL: Thomas, 1968, pp 423–239.

Melzack R, Torgerson WS. On the language of pain. *Anesthesiology* 1971; 34:50–59.

Melzack R, Wall PD. Pain mechanisms: a new theory. *Science* 1965; 150:971–979.

Mitchell KR, White RG. Behavioral self-management: an application to the problem of migraine. *Behav Ther* 1977; 8:213–221.

Moore JE, Armentrout DP, Parker JC, Kivlahan DR. Empirically derived pain-patient MMPI subgroups: prediction of treatment outcome. *J Behav Med* 1986; 9:51–63.

Morley S, Eccleston C, Williams A. Systematic review and meta-analysis of randomized controlled trials of cognitive behavioral therapy and behavioral therapy for chronic pain in adults, excluding headaches. *Pain* 1999; 80:1–13.

Naylor MR, Helzer JE, Naud S, Keefe FJ. Automated telephone as an adjunct for the treatment of chronic pain: a pilot study. *J Pain* 2002; 6:429–438.

Prokop CK, Bradley LA, Margolis R, Gentry WD. Multivariate analysis of the MMPI profiles of patients with multiple pain complaints. *J Pers Assess* 1980; 44:246–252.

Rainville P, Duncan GH, Price DD, Carrier B, Bushnell MC. Pain affect encoded in human anterior cingulate but not somatosensory cortex. *Science* 1997; 277:968–971.

Redd WH, Montgomery GH, DuHamel KN. Behavioral intervention for cancer treatment side effects. *J Natl Cancer Inst* 2001; 93:810–823.

Riley JL III, Wade JB, Myers CD, et al. Racial/ethnic differences in the experience of chronic pain. *Pain* 2002; 100:291–298.

Rudy TE, Turk DC, Kubinski JA, Zaki HS. Differential treatment responses of TMD patients as a function of psychological characteristics. *Pain* 1995; 61:103–112.

Sanders SH. Operant therapy with pain patients: evidence for its effectiveness. In: Lebovits AH (Ed). *Seminars in Pain Medicine.* Philadelphia: Saunders, 2003, pp 90–98.

Scheer SJ, Watanabe TK, Radack KL. Randomized controlled trials in industrial low back pain. Part 3. Subacute/chronic pain interventions. *Arch Phys Med Rehabil* 1997; 78:414–423.

Schwartz MS, Krupp NE. The MMPI "conversion V" among 50,000 medical patients: a study of incidence, criteria, and profile elevation. *J Clin Psychol* 1971; 27:89–95.

Skljarevski V, Ramadan NM. The nociceptive flexion reflex in humans. *Pain* 2002; 96:3–8.

Sternbach RA, Timmermans G. Personality changes associated with reduction of pain. *Pain* 1975; 1:177–181.

Stewart WF, Lipton RB, Liberman J. Variation in migraine prevalence by race. *Neurology* 1996; 47:52–59.

Stroebel C F, Glueck BC. Psychophysiological rationale for the application of biofeedback in the alleviation of pain. In: Weisenberg M, Tursky B (Eds). *Pain: New Perspectives in Therapy and Research.* New York: Plenum Press, 1975, pp 75–82.

Tait RC, Chibnall JT. Attitude profiles and clinical status in patients with chronic pain. *Pain* 1998; 78:49–57.

Taylor GJ, Bagby RM, Parker JDA (Eds). *Disorders of Affect Regulation: Alexithymia in Medical and Psychiatric Illness.* New York: Cambridge University Press, 1997.

Thomsen AB, Sorensen J, Sjogren P, Eriksen J. Economic evaluation of multidisciplinary pain management in chronic pain patients: a qualitative systematic review. *J Pain Symptom Manage* 2001; 22:688–698.

Todd KH, Deaton C, D'Adamo AP, Goe L. Ethnicity and analgesic practice. *Ann Emerg Med* 2000; 35:11–16.

Trijsburg RW, van Knippenberg FC, Rijpma SE. Effects of psychological treatment on cancer patients: a critical review. *Psychosom Med* 1992; 54:489–517.

Turk DC. Biopsychosocial perspectives on chronic pain. In: Gatchel RJ, Turk DC (Eds). *Psychological Approaches to Pain Management: A Practitioner's Handbook.* New York: Guilford Press, 1996, pp 33–52.

Turk DC, Okifuji A. Matching treatment to assessment of patients with chronic pain. In: Turk DC, Melzack R (Eds). *Handbook of Pain Assessment*, 2nd ed. New York: Guilford Press, 2001, pp 400–414.

Turk DC, Okifuji A. Psychological factors in chronic pain: evolution and revolution. *J Consult Clin Psychol* 2002; 70:678–690.

Turk DC, Meichenbaum D, Genest M. *Pain and Behavioral Medicine: A Cognitive-Behavioral Perspective.* New York: Guilford Press, 1983.

Turk DC, Okifuji A, Sinclair JD, Starz TW. Differential responses by psychosocial subgroups of fibromyalgia syndrome patients to an interdisciplinary treatment. *Arthritis Care Res* 1998; 11:397–404.

Turner JA. Educational and behavioral interventions for back pain in primary care. *Spine* 1996; 21:2851–2859.

Von Korff, M, Moore JE, Lorig K, et al. A randomized trial of a lay person-led self-management group intervention for back pain patients in primary care. *Spine* 2002; 23:2608–2615.

Walsh NE, Schoenfeld L, Ramamurthy S, Hoffman J. Normative model for cold pressor test. *Am J Phys Med Rehabil* 1989; 68:6–11.

Weinberger M, Tierney WM, Booher P, Katz BP. Can the provision of information to patients with osteoarthritis improve functional status? A randomized, controlled trial. *Arthritis Rheum* 1989; 32:1577–1583.

Wilfling FJ, Klonoff H, Kokan P. Psychological, demographic and orthopaedic factors associated with prediction of outcome of spinal fusion. *Clin Orthop* 1973; 90:153–160.

Willer JC. Comparative study of perceived pain and nociceptive flexion reflex in man. *Pain* 1977; 3:111–119.

Wiltse LL, Rocchio PD. Preoperative psychological tests as predictors of success of chemonucleolysis in the treatment of the low-back syndrome. *J Bone Joint Surg Am* 1975; 57:478–483.

Zitman FG, van Dyck R, Spinhoven P, Linssen AC. Hypnosis and autogenic training in the treatment of tension headaches: a two-phase constructive design study with follow-up. *J Psychosom Res* 1992; 36:219–228.

Correspondence to: Francis J. Keefe, PhD, Box 3159, Duke University Medical Center, Durham, NC 27710, USA. Email: keefe003@mc.duke.edu.

The Paths of Pain 1975–2005, edited by
Harold Merskey, John D. Loeser, and Ronald
Dubner, IASP Press, Seattle, © 2005.

29

Psychiatry and Pain: Causes, Effects, and Complications

Harold Merskey

*Professor Emeritus of Psychiatry, University of Western Ontario,
London, Ontario, Canada*

To explain the coincidental occurrence of pain and psychiatric illness, some clinicians claim that much pain has psychological causes or can be managed behaviorally, while others maintain that the psychogenesis of pain has been overstated so that most patients with pain presenting for treatment in clinical practice suffer from physical disorders that are liable to promote depression and anxiety along with pain (Merskey 1999). The correct mid-point between these opposing views is still a matter for debate.

MID-19TH-CENTURY OPINION

Psychological theory in the 1970s was substantially influenced by Engel (1959), who argued that many patients could adapt themselves to life only by having a traumatic social or personal relationship, such as a bad marriage in which they played a masochistic role, or by suffering from chronic pain. Engel presented an uncontrolled case series together with psychoanalytic ideas from more than 30 individual reports in the literature. He gained support because of the demonstration that pain is often a sign of psychiatric illness (Stengel 1965), a view confirmed by later surveys (Klee et al. 1959; Spear 1967; Delaplaine et al. 1978).

It was believed that Freud had provided a helpful explanation for psychogenic pain in terms of an hysterical conversion disorder. That proposition is now questioned in view of the failure to demonstrate this mechanism satisfactorily even in a case series, and because of the recognition that depression and anxiety follow rather than promote pain in most patients with physical illness. In fact, the whole Freudian theory of repression has been radically undermined by the repressed memory controversy (Ofshe and Watters 1994). Careful studies of experimental repression have also failed to show any evidence for emotional repression as a cause of symptoms (Holmes 1990).

Merskey (1965) and Spear (1967), examining psychiatric patients with and without chronic pain, confirmed Engel's claim that those with pain have had more surgical operations and feel more resentment and irritability than psychiatric patients without pain. However, Spear also demonstrated that psychiatric patients with pain are not more hostile, either covertly or overtly, than those without pain. Adler et al. (1989) provided controlled evidence that in small groups of patients, pain patients reported having experienced more brutality, sexual abuse, punishment, and guilt feelings in childhood than three other types of patients. This evidence, however, could be attributable to social differences, including employment.

Szasz (1957) demonstrated that problems with definition arose repeatedly because of a failure to recognize that pain is a psychological notion and that calling a stimulus or a change in nerve pathways "pain" is a mistake that leads to confusion. Walters (1961) expressed that idea very clearly. I have discussed the question of definition in my chapter on terms and taxonomy in this volume. In making diagnoses of pain disorders, physicians may recognize both physical and psychological etiologies, but in each case the different etiologies or diagnoses must be identified with respect to both organic and psychological causes and effects.

PSYCHOLOGICAL FACTORS IN PAIN

Psychological factors in pain were considered actively at the Florence meeting in 1975 and are dealt with in detail by Keefe et al. in this volume. Brief reference will be made to them here. Notably, Sternbach (1976) recognized that the pattern of responses in acute pain does not persist once the pain resolves, but if the pain is constant and continues for weeks or months, it can cause habituation of the autonomic responses. The systematic and quantitative study of pain and its relationship to personality variables or to emotions was well under way in the mid-1970s, as instanced by articles by Black and Chapman (1976) and Timmermans and Sternbach (1976). A study in the clinic using psychological methods of measurement showed that personality setting or style, as measured by the particular instrument chosen, changed in response to the stress of severe physical illness; in cancer patients, chronic pain appeared to increase emotional responses, which later tended to decrease with the relief of pain (Bond 1976).

Findings with the Minnesota Multiphasic Personality Inventory (MMPI) were discussed at the Florence meeting, especially the "Conversion V profile" in which the Hypochondriasis scale is most elevated, the Depression scale least, and the Hysteria scale some way between the two. Use of this profile became controversial because almost all pain patients, whether their illness originated in physical or psychological problems, show this pattern of illness (Smythe 1984), and using it for a psychological attribution is not justified. An interesting brief report (Blumetti and Modesti 1976) heralded findings in later years, showing that psychological measurements are most helpful in predicting response to surgery and also disability. This may not be so simple in implication as might appear: psychological findings reflect the patient's awareness of both physical and psychological difficulties and therefore are inherently more likely than physical findings to give an indication of what is really going to happen.

Writing on pain management, I observed (Merskey 1976) that psychological factors are not usually responsive to interpretative psychotherapy, but I accepted with reservations that behavioral management may be helpful for patients with chronic low back pain, as demonstrated by Fordyce (1976) and Sternbach (1974). However, the approach in which patients are told that it is within themselves to change their experience of pain is too frequently linked with behavioral techniques. Cognitive psychological treatment is much more promising (see Keefe et al., this volume).

DEPRESSION, SELECTION, AND STRESS

Pain can be associated causally with many psychiatric disorders. Anxiety disorder has various somatic concomitants, such as pain in the chest in those who are worried about their heart, while depression is often associated with headache. Bradley (1963) observed that patients in whom pain preceded depression continued to have pain after the depression subsided. If an episode of depression was marked at onset by the emergence of pain, that pain could be expected to resolve. In the 1970s, hysterical conversion mechanisms, as discussed above, were considered to form part of the pattern of psychiatric illness and to be responsible for many pains. Physicians seemed to want to make the diagnosis of conversion disorder in patients to whom they could not offer any other label. However, they recognized that the following psychological processes might promote complaints of pain: (1) hallucinations (rare either in schizophrenia or depression); (2) muscular tension; (3) hysterical conversion, changed in the third edition of the *Diagnostic and Statistical Manual of the American Psychiatric Association* (DSM-III) to the dubious concept of somatization.

Diagnosing anxiety or depressive disorders as causes for pain is sometimes appropriate in psychiatric practice. Unfortunately, it works less well in the pain clinic, to which patients frequently are referred with some possible, but uncertain, physical cause of chronic pain. The notion was once popular of identifying "chronic pain syndrome" in patients who had some incompletely resolved physical problem that was accompanied by a number of irritating psychological symptoms, but who were not in danger or in need of surgery. The Task Force on Taxonomy of the IASP did not accept that this concept was valid or that the proposed syndrome would make a useful category, holding that psychological phenomena needed to be properly identified and characterized when relevant.

If organic causes were poorly identified and if a specific psychiatric illness was not responsible for the condition, patients were often given a default diagnosis such as "hysteria" or were told mystifyingly that their pain was "psychogenic." Measures of psychotherapy or behavioral management might then be offered. If there was a valid independent psychological problem, this approach worked occasionally, but for the most part, it produced disgruntled patients and troubled clinicians.

Better understanding of the psychiatric complication of physical illness arose from studies of depression in pain clinics, where the frequency of depression ranged from as little as 10% to as much as 100%, depending on the clinic and the type of patients it served (Pilowsky et al. 1977; Romano and Turner 1985). After the publication of such studies, the importance of recognizing selection factors was well established.

Beginning in the 1970s, my colleagues and I undertook a series of studies in patients with chronic pain attending nerve block clinics, an orofacial pain clinic, and my own pain service. We thought that many patients in whom clear examples of causation could not be established might have pain because of muscle tension. Investigations of muscle tension, anxiety, and pain had produced relatively weak correlations among these variables, which were insufficient to account for the great majority of the cases. Relaxation treatments were developed, and they are still properly used, but like many other psychological treatments they generally produced useful relief only in patients whose pain was not severe. Not surprisingly, using quite simple psychological test instruments, we determined that most of our patients did not suffer from psychological disorders (Merskey et al. 1987).

Many patients had depression before or during the course of the painful illness, but it often declined. A subset was shown retrospectively to have developed depression at some point after the onset of their illness. Thus, the psychological illness associated with most pain clinic patients and those seen in medical practice could be accounted for as follows: (1) More patients who have anxiety or depression, for any reason, will consult a doctor concerning non-terminal chronic illnesses than those who do not have anxiety or depression. (2) Painful illness is associated with disability, poor sleep, and the disruption of family relationships. Inevitably patients suffer depression, particularly when the pain is worse and poorly controlled, and when they are faced with financial distress; these factors have an impact on patients' activities of daily living, their quality of life, and their marital and other personal relationships. Unemployment, whether or not it is due to painful illness, will have the same effect.

A supportive psychological attitude is highly desirable, and the treatment of depression and anxiety is appropriate; however, relieving pain is the most effective way to improve depression in chronic pain patients. Chronic pain is not well explained by psychodynamic explanations or by factors attributable to questions of compensation.

ANTIDEPRESSANTS

From the 1950s onward, imipramine and newer antidepressants appeared to have some benefit for patients with pain. First, it was clear that patients whose depression was causing pain benefited by these medications, but subsequently the notion grew that there was an independent effect of some antidepressants on pain (Merskey and Hester 1972). Watson et al. (1982) demonstrated in a double-blind placebo-controlled trial of patients with postherpetic neuralgia, using moderate doses of antidepressants, that amitriptyline had a significant benefit for pain. This benefit occurred not only in patients with depression but also in those who were not depressed, as determined by the Beck Depression Inventory. These findings have been confirmed repeatedly in various types of pain (Sharav et al. 1987; Max et al. 1988; Monks 1999).

THE COMPENSATION ISSUE

The compensation issue is still a chronic sore in medical practice. A turning point occurred with the cogent demonstration by Mendelson in 1982 that pain was not "cured" by the resolution of legal proceedings, as had been alleged. Mendelson rejected the claims of Miller (1961) that headache in particular, and pain in general, was "cured by a verdict." Many practitioners had patients who had not been cured after verdicts, even favorable ones, and Mendelson observed that all of the 10 follow-up studies found in the literature from the end of the Second World War up to 1982 had agreed that at least some patients continued to be ill subsequent to settlement of legal claims.

Cervical sprain injuries received considerable attention. Radanov (a psychiatrist) and colleagues (1991) showed that in a general practice sample of patients, the severity of pain and the extent of emotional or cognitive change after whiplash injury were related to age, to a history of prior injury, and to the intensity of pain immediately following the accident. No later work has refuted these findings. A series of studies by Bogduk and colleagues demonstrated a major organic cause for whiplash and a lack of any adequate psychological explanation (Barnsley et al. 1993; Wallis et al. 1997; see Bogduk, this volume).

The strongest relationship of pain behavior is to be found with physical illness (Keefe et al. 1990), although there is a subgroup of patients who only have moderate complaints of pain but greater evidence of pain behavior. Waddell (1999) has concluded that "nonorganic signs" mainly reflect the severity of pain and *not* etiology.

Physiology also shed light on this field. The theory of conversion pain or somatoform pain was partly based upon the notion that regional pains correspond to an idea in the mind of the patient. Physiological evidence to the contrary had long existed and is well exemplified in studies by McMahon and Wall (1984) and also by Woolf and Thompson (1991), which showed quite clearly that at a physiological level, nociceptive responses from the periphery generalize to regions that do not necessarily correspond to nerve roots or nerve distributions (Merskey 1999).

Traditional methods of diagnosing so-called hysterical pain also proved unreliable (Gould et al. 1986). No current good evidence supports the notion of pain as a sort of conversion disorder, despite its long life in the literature. In fact, this disorder is very rare in developed societies. If pain is a psychological complaint produced for benefit, its production is probably deliberate or conscious. Historically, much pain occurring in conjunction with anxiety and depression was called hysteria (Merskey 1999), and some pain as a consequence of anxiety and depression is understandable. Most so-called somatization pain is wrongly labeled because the term is usually regarded as an indication of unconscious psychological processes, although there is now no good evidence for that explanation.

SOCIAL INFLUENCES ON MEDICAL ATTITUDES

In 1995, a task force appointed by the insurance company of the Province of Quebec, which provides universal no-fault insurance to patients, presented a report based on the literature connected with the treatment of cervical sprain injury (whiplash) and its outcome (Quebec Task Force 1995). Treatment studies were found not to meet requirements for the most satisfactory evidence. The group reported a follow-up study of whiplash and published a consensus statement (thereby undermining the scientific purity of its conclusions about the literature). The task force stated that at the end of one year only 1.9% of individuals making claims of uncomplicated whiplash in 1985 were still disabled and that, including those with both whiplash and other injury, 2.9% of all whiplash claimants were disabled. The literature suggests, however, that as many as 10–30% of individuals with whiplash are still disabled or have symptoms at one year. The comments of the Quebec Task Force are questionable because the determination of disability relied primarily or wholly upon the insurer's view. Teasell and Merskey (1999) further demonstrated that significant data had been neglected in the Quebec Task Force report, which had indicated that there were some "recurrences" not due to further accidents. This information was buried in the middle of a lengthy report without discussion. When the figures for recurrences (cases in which the injured parties had sought to have their claims reopened) were added to those who were acknowledged to still be disabled at one year, it appeared that the percentage who might still be disabled at one year was likely to be 9.5% or more. The original figures have been utilized in legal proceedings well beyond Quebec or North America to argue that patients who complained of symptoms or disability from whiplash injury after one year were seeking compensation on the basis of a condition from which they should have recovered.

Another controversial report (Cassidy et al. 2000) claimed that the elimination of compensation for pain was accompanied by quicker recovery and a reduction in pain and depression under a no-fault system. This report was based on figures collected in Saskatchewan comparing a tort system with its successor, an almost totally no-fault system of motor vehicle insurance. This study, published by the author who had edited the Quebec Task Force report, mentioned still larger numbers of "recurrences," termed "re-openings," which amounted to 28% of subjects. The figures for recurrences were omitted from analysis on the implausible grounds that the insurance company was unable to provide adequate data on patients whose cases had been closed and then re-opened. The report also said they were omitted because of a desire to preserve internal validity. In both studies, the way the data were treated appears to reflect the influence of insurance companies (Merskey et al. 2003).

In Saskatchewan, a vocal movement comprising large numbers of victims who had been cut off from recompense objected to the no-fault regime with evidence of ill-treatment of injured persons and claimed that their reasonable claims had been denied (Terry 2002). Additional problems exist with this study, especially the strong local medical denial of the accuracy of the claims it makes (Russell 2000).

Another insurance company (State Farm), based in the United States and Canada, together with an industrial firm and the Insurance Corporation of British Columbia, founded a charity, the Physical Medicine Research Foundation, which organized meetings and provided some support for research. One of the meetings produced a consensus statement that post-traumatic fibromyalgia should not be diagnosed in the medicolegal situation (Wolfe et al. 1990). Additional comments challenging these conclusions were published by Yunus et al. (1997). That foundation has since changed its name to the Canadian Institute for the Relief of Pain and Disability.

These events are matched by a historical sequence of books and articles demonstrating a consistent tendency for insurers to find medical practitioners who lend their opinions to support the minimizing of pain occurring as a result of accidents (Schmiedebach 1999). We (Merskey and Teasell 2000) have argued that the consequence of these attitudes is to influence doctors' thinking and to obscure the intensity of pain and the suffering of patients, not only with respect to compensable injuries.

OVERVIEW

Numerous studies on pain in the last 30 years reflect an interplay of ideas and facts about mind and body from physiology, psychology, and philosophy. In the case of philosophy, semantics has been an important element (see my chapter, "Terms and Taxonomy," in this volume). Most of the conceptual issues have long been recognized, but we might claim that in the late 20th century some of them became more acute, better identified, and less speculative.

More knowledge in physiology, neurology, and psychiatry has limited what we might call "hysterical" diagnoses and increased our information on the functions of the brain in relation to anxiety, mood, and pain. Where the cerebral cortex was almost an empty continent for pain, we begin to see how some of the conscious phenomena that accompany pain can be expressed in the cerebrum. Note the cautious wording—a change in a cortical area with nociception is not evidence of a "seat of pain." At the same time, we can claim to know a little more about social influences on the evolution and treatment of pain and about doctors' attitudes toward pain.

REFERENCES

Adler RH, Zlot S, Hürny C, Minder C. Engel's psychogenic pain and the pain-prone patient: a retrospective, controlled clinical study. *Psychosom Med* 1989; 51:87–101.

Barnsley L, Lord S, Bogduk N. Comparative local anaesthetic blocks in the diagnosis of cervical zygapophyseal joint pain. *Pain* 1993; 55:99–106.

Black RG, Chapman CR. SAD Index for clinical assessment of pain. In: Bonica JJ, Albe-Fessard DG (Eds). *Recent Advances in Pain Research and Therapy.* New York: Raven Press, 1976, pp 301–305.

Blumetti AE, Modesti LM. Psychological predictors of success or failure of surgical intervention for intractable back pain. In: Bonica JJ, Albe-Fessard DG (Eds). *Recent Advances in Pain Research and Therapy.* New York: Raven Press, 1976, pp 323–325.

Bond MR. Pain in cancer patients. In: Bonica JJ, Albe-Fessard DG (Eds). *Recent Advances in Pain Research and Therapy.* New York: Raven Press, 1976, pp 311–316.

Bradley JJ. Severe localized pain associated with the depressive syndrome. *Br J Psychiatry* 1963; 109:741–745.

Cassidy JD, Carroll LJ, Coté P, et al. Effect of eliminating compensation for pain and suffering on the outcome of insurance claims for whiplash injury. *N Engl J Med* 2000; 342:1179–1186.

Delaplaine R, Ifambuyi O, Merskey H, Zarfas J. Significance of pain in psychiatric hospital patients. *Pain* 1978; 4:361–366.

Engel GL. Psychogenic pain. *Med Clin N Am* 1959; 42:1481–1496.

Fordyce WE. *Behavioral Methods in Chronic Pain and Illness.* St. Louis: Mosby, 1976.

Gould R, Miller BL, Goldberg MA, et al. The validity of hysterical signs and symptoms. *J Nerv Ment Dis* 1986; 174:593–598.

Holmes DS. The evidence for repression: an examination of sixty years of research. In: Singer JL (Ed). *Repression and Dissociation: Implications for Personality Theory, Psychopathology, and Health.* Chicago: University of Chicago Press, 1990, pp 85–102.

Keefe FJ, Bradley LA, Crisson E. Behavioral assessment of low back pain: identification of pain behavior sub-groups. *Pain* 1990; 40:153–160.

Klee GD, Ozelis S, Greenberg I, Gallant LJ. Pain and other somatic complaints in a psychiatric clinic. *Md Med J* 1959; 8:188–191.

Max MB, Schafer SC, Culnane M, et al. Association of pain relief with drug side effects in post-herpetic neuralgia: a single-dose study of clonidine, codeine, ibuprofen and placebo. *Clin Pharmacol Ther* 1988; 43:363–371.

McMahon SB, Wall PD. Receptive fields of rat lamina 1 projection cells move to incorporate a nearby region of injury. *Pain* 1984; 19:235–247.

Mendelson G. Not "cured by a verdict." Effect of legal settlement on compensation claimants. *Med J Aust* 1982; ii:219–230.

Merskey H. Psychiatric patients with persistent pain. *J Psychosom Res* 1965; 9:299–309.

Merskey H. Psychiatric aspects of the control of pain. In: Bonica JJ, Albe-Fessard DG (Eds). *Recent Advances in Pain Research and Therapy.* New York: Raven Press, 1976, pp 711–716 and 929–949.

Merskey H. Pain and psychological medicine. In: Wall PD, Melzack R (Eds). *Textbook of Pain,* 4th ed. Edinburgh: Churchill Livingstone, 1999, pp 929–949.

Merskey H, Hester RN. The treatment of chronic pain with psychotropic drugs. *Postgrad Med J* 1972; 16:594–598.

Merskey H, Teasell RW. The disparagement of pain: social influences on medical thinking. *Pain Res Manage* 2000; 5,4:259–270.

Merskey H, Lau CL, Russell ES, et al. Screening for psychiatric morbidity. The pattern of psychological illness and premorbid characteristics in four chronic pain populations. *Pain* 1987; 30:141–157.

Merskey H, Teasell RW, Nussbaum D. Science, insurance, whiplash and minimizing pain. *J Whiplash Related Disorders* 2003; 2:5–13.

Miller HG. Accident neurosis. *BMJ* 1961; i:919–925, 992–998.

Monks R. Psychotropic drugs. In: Wall PD, Melzack R (Eds). *Textbook of Pain,* 4th ed. Edinburgh: Churchill Livingstone 1999; pp 963–989.

Ofshe R, Watters E. *Making Monsters, False memories, Psychotherapy, and Sexual Hysteria.* New York: Charles Scribner's Sons, 1994.

Pilowsky I, Chapman CR, Bonica JJ. Pain, depression and illness behavior in a pain clinic population. *Pain* 1977; 4:183–192.

Quebec Task Force. *Whiplash-Associated Disorders (WAD). Redefining 'Whiplash' and its Management.* Quebec: Société de l'Assurance Automobile du Québec, 1995.

Radanov BP, Stafano GD, Schnidrig A, Ballinari P. Role of psychosocial stress in recovery from common whiplash. *Lancet* 1991; 338:712–715.

Romano JM, Turner JA. Chronic pain and depression, does the evidence support a relationship? *Psychol Bull* 1985; 97:18–34.

Russell RS. *Oral Testimony to the Personal Injury Protection Plan [PIPP] Review Committee, Saskatoon, SK, 15th June 2000.* Available via the Internet: www.againstno-fault.com; accessed August 31, 2000.

Schmiedebach H-P. Post-traumatic neurosis in 19th century Germany: a disease in political juridical and professional context. *Hist Psychiatry* 1999; 10:27–57.

Sharav Y, Singer E, Schmidt E, et al. The analgesic effect of amitriptyline on chronic facial pain. *Pain* 1987; 31:199–209.

Smythe H. Problems with the MMPI. *J Rheumatol* 1984; 11:417–418.

Spear FG. Pain in psychiatric patients. *J Psychosom Res* 1967; 11:187–193.

Stengel E. Pain and the psychiatrist. The 39th Maudsley Lecture. *Br J Psychiatry* 1965; 111:795–802.

Sternbach RA. *Pain Patients: Traits and Treatment.* New York: Academic Press, 1974.

Sternbach RA. Psychological factors in pain. In: Bonica JJ, Albe-Fessard DG (Eds). *Recent Advances in Pain Research and Therapy.* New York: Raven Press 1976, pp 293–299.

Szasz TS. *Pain and Pleasure. A Study of Bodily Feelings.* London: Tavistock, 1957.

Teasell RW, Merskey H. The Quebec Task Force on whiplash-associated disorders and the British Columbia Whiplash Initiative. A study of insurance company initiatives. *Pain Res Manage* 1999; 4:141–149.

Terry L. Commentary: Insurance, research and medical ethics. *Pain Res Manage* 2002; 7:101–106.

Timmermans G, Sternbach RA. Human chronic pain and personality: a conical correlation analysis. In: Bonica JJ, Albe-Fessard DG (Eds). *Recent Advances in Pain Research and Therapy.* New York: Raven Press, 1976, pp 307–310.

Waddell G. *The Back Pain Revolution.* London: Harcourt Press, 1999.

Wallis BJ, Lord SM, Bogduk N. Resolution of psychological distress of whiplash patients following treatment by radiofrequency neurotomy: a randomized, double-blind, placebo controlled trial. *Pain* 1997; 73:15–22.

Walters A. Psychogenic regional pain alias hysterical pain. *Brain* 1961; 84:1–18.

Watson CPN, Evans RJ, Reed K, et al. Amitriptyline versus placebo in postherpetic neuralgia. *Neurology* 1982; 32:671–673.

Wolfe F, Smythe HA, Yunus MB, et al. The American College of Rheumatology 1990 criteria for the classification of fibromyalgia: report of the Multicenter Criteria Committee. *Arthritis Rheum* 1990; 33:160–172.

Woolf CJ, Thompson SWN. The induction and maintenance of central sensitization is dependent on *N*-methyl-D-aspartic acid receptor activation: implications for the treatment of post-injury pain hypersensitivity states. *Pain* 1991; 44:293–299.

Yunus MB, Bennett RM, Romano TJ, et al. Fibromyalgia: an alternative consensus report. *J Clin Rheumatol* 1997; 3:324–327.

Correspondence to: Harold Merskey, DM, FRCP, FRCP(C), FRCPsych, 71 Logan Avenue, London, ON, Canada N5Y 2P9. Tel: 519-672-2298; Fax: 519-679-6849; email: harold.merskey@sympatico.ca.

The Paths of Pain 1975–2005, edited by
Harold Merskey, John D. Loeser, and Ronald
Dubner, IASP Press, Seattle, © 2005.

30

Children—Not Simply "Little Adults"

Patricia A. McGrath

*Department of Anesthesia, Divisional Centre of Pain Management and
Research, The Hospital for Sick Children; Brain and Behavior Program,
Research Institute, at The Hospital for Sick Children; and the Department of
Anesthesia, The University of Toronto, Toronto, Ontario, Canada*

Before IASP was founded, our knowledge of children's pain was severely limited. Clinical decisions about whether children were experiencing pain and, if so, about the particular pain therapies required, were based primarily on physicians' personal beliefs rather than on scientific evidence. Regrettably, common misbeliefs that children did not feel pain in the same manner as adults and consequently did not require similar analgesics, along with pervasive fears that children were at heightened risk for opioid addiction and should receive minimal analgesic doses, caused many children to suffer needlessly.

Two studies highlight how children's pain problems were undertreated during this period. In 1968, Swafford and Allan surveyed analgesic use for all children treated in an intensive care unit during a 4-month period. Only 14% of children (26 of 180) had received any opioids for pain relief. Moreover, only 3% of children received analgesics after general surgery, presumably because "pediatric patients seldom need relief of pain after general surgery. They tolerate discomfort well" (Swafford and Allan 1968).

Subsequently, Eland (1974) compared medication use for 18 adults and 25 children with similar medical conditions during their hospitalization. While 372 opioid doses and 299 non-opioid doses were administered to adults, only 24 analgesic doses were administered to children. In fact, more than half of the children did not receive any analgesics, despite undergoing major trauma including amputation of the foot, excision of neck mass, and heminephrectomy.

Since Eland's thesis, extensive research has refuted the erroneous beliefs that once guided pediatric practice. Through innumerable personal and professional efforts, children's pain has emerged as an important research and clinical specialty. The last 30 years comprise an unparalleled period of critical advances in this enormous field, encompassing a "bench to bedside to community health research" perspective, covering a population "from in utero through adolescence," and including all types of acute and persistent pain. This chapter provides a historical review of our field, highlighting pivotal discoveries and the challenges encountered to make children's pain control a higher priority throughout the world.

AN EMERGING FIELD

Clinicians and scientists who were interested in children's pain had worked in relative isolation from one another in many different centers around the world until the founding of IASP. The journal *Pain* and the triennial world congresses created a unique opportunity for these interdisciplinary "children's pain people" to connect with one another in a dynamic manner. By 1985, IASP had become a home base for many pediatric specialists. The next few years were an exceptional period, marked by an exhilarating whirlwind of sharing ideas, forming friendships, and laying the foundation for an interdisciplinary and international scientific network devoted to children's pain. Significant historical moments include the first International Conference on Pediatric Pain, convened by Dr. Donald Tyler (July 1988; Seattle, Washington); the first Consensus Conference on the Management of Pain in Childhood Cancer, convened by Dr. Neil Schechter (October 1988; Chester, Connecticut); and the first European Conference on Pediatric Pain, convened by Dr. Huda Abu Saad (June 1989; Maastricht, the Netherlands). These three meetings linked experienced clinicians and scientists to obtain the first "evidence base by consensus" for understanding and treating children's pain.

At that time, the first books to cover all aspects of childhood pain were written: three were authored (McGrath and Unruh 1987; Ross and Ross 1988; McGrath 1990) and three were edited texts (Pichard-Léandri and Gauvain-Piquard 1989; Bush and Harkins 1991; Tyler and Krane 1990). These books, heralding the beginning of the field, continue to provide valuable insights about a child's perception, versatile assessment techniques, and the management of common pain problems from a practical hands-on perspective. Today, thousands of articles and almost a hundred books on children's pain have been published. During the period 2001–2003, 14 books and 1728 articles were published, averaging 575 articles per year in a broad spectrum of pain, medical, dental, nursing, psychology, and health journals.

Yet, in striking contrast, in the 3-year period near the founding of IASP (1973–1975), only one book, *The Child with Abdominal Pains* (Apley 1975) and only 61 articles, an average of 20 articles per year, were published.

Thirty years ago, medical texts contained almost no information about the general topic of children's pain, nor any reference to specific pain conditions. Only 26 pages referred to pain across five major pediatric texts (Forfar 1973; Hutchison 1975; Nelson 1975; Silver et al. 1975; Ziai et al. 1975), whereas 270 pages refer to children's pain in recent texts (Behrman et al. 2002, 2004; Rudolph et al. 2002; Robinson and Roberton 2003; Rudolph and Rudolph 2003). The 1973–1975 medical texts devoted less than 1% of their pages to children's pain, while recent textbooks devoted 4% of pages to the topic.

Today, most texts on pain include at least one chapter devoted to children's issues. Moreover, the pediatric field is enriched by recent comprehensive texts (Olsson and Jylli 2001; Schechter et al. 2003) and by specialized texts on neonates (Anand et al. 2000), children's headache (McGrath and Hillier 2001), procedure-related pain (Finley and McGrath 2001; Liossi 2002), and biological-social factors (McGrath and Finley 2003). The IASP's *Core Curriculum on Pain* has recently been revised with expanded sections to encompass new findings in the fields of developmental neurobiology, pain assessment, and evidence-based pain management (www.iasp-pain.org).

Dynamic growth is noted for almost all scientific and clinical activities related to pediatric pain—the number of scientific presentations on pediatric pain at international and national pain meetings; the formation of special interest groups on pain in children to address common scientific, clinical, and advocacy issues; the establishment of interdisciplinary pain clinics for children; and the organization of interdisciplinary meetings focused exclusively on children's pain.

THE DEVELOPING NOCICEPTIVE SYSTEM: INCREASED SENSITIVITY AND PLASTICITY

Ethical concerns and increasing publicity about the lack of analgesia for infants led to a dramatic upsurge in clinical research to document objectively how infants respond to surgical trauma and how analgesic administration affects postsurgical outcome. At the same time, basic scientific research focused on the development of the nociceptive system in animals. Fitzgerald and colleagues initiated a series of elegant anatomical and physiological investigations to detail the development of the nociceptive system (for review, see Andrews 2003; Fitzgerald and Howard 2003). The basic nociceptive connections are formed before birth, but systems at birth are immature and exhibit increased responsivity in comparison to the adult animal.

Considerable neuronal plasticity is evident throughout the developing system from the periphery to the brain. For example, the conduction velocity of afferent fibers, action potential shape, receptor transduction, firing frequencies, and receptive field properties change substantially over the postnatal period (Fitzgerald 1987; Koltzenburg and Lewin 1997; Fitzgerald and Jennings 1999; Woodbury and Koerber 2003). Both high-threshold Aδ and low-threshold Aβ mechanoreceptors respond with lower firing frequencies at birth compared to those in the adult animal. Aβ afferents extend dorsally into laminae II and I along with C fibers, rather than into only laminae III and IV as in the adult animal. Activation of these Aβ afferents evokes excitatory responses more typical of those evoked by Aδ and C fibers in the adult animal. In addition, the receptive fields of dorsal horn cells and somatosensory cortical cells are larger in the newborn. With these larger receptive fields and the dominant A-fiber input, there is an increased likelihood that central cells will be excited by peripheral sensory stimulation, thereby increasing the sensitivity of infant sensory reflexes to stimulation. Moreover, descending inhibitory mechanisms are not functional at birth (Boucher et al. 1998), so that an important endogenous analgesic system is lacking, which means that noxious input may affect neonates more than adults.

Nerve injury, which can evoke persistent neuropathic pain, has dramatically different effects in neonates and adults. During a critical neonatal period, peripheral nerve injury causes rapid and extensive death of axotomized dorsal root ganglion cells, producing major changes within the spinal cord. The central terminals of damaged axons withdraw while adjacent, intact axon collaterals sprout into the denervated region, disrupting the somatotopic organization of central terminals within the dorsal horn and also at higher levels of the nervous system including the cortex (Kaas et al. 1983). Although this process may be a potentially useful compensatory device to restore sensory input from an area of the body surface in which it has been lost, its effects may be detrimental and may trigger chronic pain (Fitzgerald and Howard 2003).

Most studies in developmental neurobiology have been conducted on rat pups because they have comparable developmental timetables with respect to the anatomy, chemistry, and physiology of maturing human pain pathways. To study neural function in human infants, investigators have monitored behavioral and neurophysiological responses, revealing extensive plasticity and increased excitability in the developing nervous system (for review, see Andrews 2003; Johnston et al. 2003). In comparison to adults, young infants have exaggerated reflex responses (i.e., lower thresholds and longer-lasting muscle contractions) in response to certain types of trauma, such as needle insertion (Andrews and Fitzgerald 1999). Repeated mechanical stimulation at strong (but not pain-inducing) intensities can cause sensitization in very young infants, while repeated painful procedures such as those required during intensive care can profoundly affect sensory processing in infants. Infants after surgery can develop a striking hypersensitivity to touch, as well as to pain.

While we do not know specifically how such injuries may affect the mature human pain system or influence adult pain perception, increasing attention is focused on the possible consequences of untreated pain, particularly in infants (Grunau 2000). For example, circumcised newborn infants display a stronger pain response to subsequent routine immunizations at 4 and 6 months compared to uncircumcised infants, but application of lidocaine-prilocaine anesthetic cream at circumcision attenuates the pain response to subsequent immunizations (Taddio et al. 1997). The results of behavioral studies in humans, like those from neurobiological studies in animals, indicate increased responsivity to pain. Clinicians should appreciate that if an injury or medical procedure is noxious to adults, it will be noxious to infants (Porter et al. 1999).

A CHILD'S PAIN PERCEPTION: PLASTICITY AND COMPLEXITY

A child's pain perception can be regarded as plastic from a psychological, as well as biological, perspective. Tissue damage initiates a sequence of neural events that may lead to pain, but many developmental, social, and psychological factors can intervene to alter the sequence of nociceptive transmission and thereby modify a child's pain. Child characteristics, such as cognitive level, sex, gender, temperament, previous pain experience, family, and cultural background generally shape how children interpret and cope with pain (Katz et al. 1980; Blount et al. 1991; Bennett-Branson and Craig 1993; Schanberg et al. 1998; Peterson et al. 1999; Chen et al. 2000; Chambers et al. 2002).

Other factors vary dynamically, depending on the specific circumstances in which a child experiences pain. These situation-specific factors can be shortened to "what children and parents understand, what they (and health care staff) do, and how children and parents feel." Certain situational factors can intensify pain and distress, while others can eventually trigger pain episodes, prolong pain-related disability, or maintain the cycle of repeated pain episodes in recurrent pain syndrome (McGrath and Hillier 2001). Parents and health care providers can dramatically improve children's pain experience and minimize their disability by modifying children's understanding of a situation, their focus of attention, their perceived control over the pain, their expectations for obtaining eventual recovery and pain relief, and the meaning or relevance of the pain (McGrath and Dade 2004).

Situational factors may affect children even more than adults. Adults typically have experienced a wide variety of pains of diverse etiology, intensity, and quality, providing them with a broad base of knowledge and coping behaviors. When adults encounter new pains, they evaluate them primarily from the context of their cumulative life experience. In contrast, children with more limited pain experience must evaluate new pains primarily from the context of the immediate circumstances.

Children's understanding of pain, pain-coping strategies, and the impact of pain increase with age (Gaffney and Dunne 1987), but many questions remain about the interplay of maturation, cognitive development, and experience in mediating a child's pain. Children's procedural pain generally decreases with age (Jay et al. 1983; Lander and Fowler-Kerry 1991; Goodenough et al. 1999), but the effect of age probably varies depending on the type of pain and the nature of the child's previous pain experiences—that is, positive experiences with similar painful situations (Dahlquist et al. 1986; Bijttebier and Vertommen 1998). For example, some studies show increasing postoperative pain with age (Bennett-Branson and Craig 1993), while others show decreasing pain or no age differences (Palermo and Drotar 1996).

Age, sex, and psychosocial factors are now recognized as important factors in the development of persistent pain and pain-related disability. Although the overall prevalence of pain increases with age, girls may be at greater risk than boys for developing certain types of persistent pain (Unruh and Campbell 1999). We do not yet know the specific prevalence of most types of chronic pain in children, but recent research is focusing on the epidemiology of childhood persistent pain to obtain age- and sex-related prevalence estimates, identify vulnerability and prognostic factors, and determine the long-term impact for children and their families.

PAIN ASSESSMENT: A MULTITUDE OF PAIN MEASURES FOR INFANTS AND CHILDREN

Pain assessment is an intrinsic component of pain management in infants and children. Clinicians need an objective measure of pain intensity and an understanding of the factors that cause or exacerbate pain for an individual child. Thus, extensive research has focused on designing pain measures that are convenient to administer and whose resulting scores provide meaningful information about children's pain experiences. More than 60 pain measures are now available for infants, children, and adolescents (for review, see Champion et al. 1998; McGrath 1998; McGrath and Gillespie 2001; Stevens and Franck 2001). While no single pain measure is appropriate for all children and for all situations in which they experience pain, we should be able to evaluate pain for almost every child.

Physiological parameters including heart rate, respiration rate, blood pressure, palmar sweating, cortisol and cortisone levels, oxygen levels, vagal tone, and endorphin concentrations have been studied as potential pain measures. However, they reflect a complex and generalized stress response, rather than correlating with a particular pain level. As such, they may have more relevance as distress indices within a broader behavioral pain scale. Behavioral scales record the type and amount of pain-related behaviors children exhibit. Since a child's specific pain behaviors depend on the type of pain experienced, different scales are usually required for acute and persistent pain. Clinicians monitor children for a specified time period and then complete a checklist noting distress behaviors such as crying, grimacing, and guarding. Behavioral scales must be used for infants and children who are unable to communicate verbally. Recently, investigators are validating pain scales for children who are developmentally disabled (Breau et al. 2002; Terstegen et al. 2003). However, the resulting pain scores are indirect estimates of pain and do not always correlate with children's own pain ratings (Beyer et al. 1990). Even though clinicians may use diaries rather than formal scales, prospective evaluation of a child's behavior is an essential component of pain management, providing information about medication use, compliance with treatment recommendations, and the extent of pain-related disability (missed school attendance, physical activities, and social activities with peers).

Psychological or self-report measures include a broad spectrum of projective techniques, interviews, questionnaires, qualitative descriptive scales, and quantitative rating scales designed to capture the subjective experience of a child's pain. Since children's understanding and language depends on their cognitive level and previous pain experience, clinicians should communicate with children about pain using their own simple words. Most toddlers (approximately 2 years of age) can communicate the presence of pain, using concrete analogies and words learned from their parents to describe the sensations they feel when they hurt themselves. Gradually children learn to differentiate three basic levels of pain intensity—"a little," "some or medium," and "a lot."

By the age of five, most children can differentiate a wide range of pain intensities, and many can use simple ratio and interval pain scales (e.g., visual analogue scales, numerical scales, faces scales, and verbal descriptor scales) to rate their pain intensity. Many scales have excellent psychometric properties, are convenient to administer, are easy for children to understand, are adaptable to many clinical situations, and help parents to monitor their children's pain at home. Interviews, usually conducted independently with a child and his or her parents, are the cornerstone of assessment for children with persistent pain, enabling clinicians to identify relevant child, family, and situational factors that contribute to children's pain and disability problems (Varni et al. 1987; Savedra et al. 1993; McGrath and Hillier 2001).

CHILD-CENTERED CLINICAL MANAGEMENT: INTEGRATING DRUG AND NONDRUG THERAPIES

Anand and colleagues (1987) dramatically highlighted the adverse impact of untreated postoperative pain in 1987, when they revealed that premature infants undergoing surgery without adequate analgesic medication had significantly increased postsurgical morbidity and mortality in comparison to a group that had received fentanyl. The ensuing publicity as people learned that minimal anesthesia and analgesia represented "the norm in pediatric postoperative management," rather than the exception, sparked a revolution (for review, see Schechter et al. 2003). Amidst increased pressure from health care providers, public advocates, and distressed parents, clinical practice started to change so that children began to receive more appropriate analgesics in adequate doses and at regular dosing intervals. New interest was directed toward the pharmacokinetics and pharmacodynamics of conventional analgesics in infants and children, the development of pain-free transdermal and transmucosal drug delivery methods, the design of improved sedation regimens for children undergoing painful or aversive therapies, the feasibility of "child- and parent-controlled" analgesia, the use of adjunct analgesics for neuropathic pain, and a broader use of regional anesthetic techniques in pediatric medicine.

At the same time, increasing attention was focusing on the problem of undertreated procedural pain for children with cancer. Many children were incredibly anxious and distressed about scheduled lumbar punctures and bone marrow aspirations; despite receiving sedatives and local infiltrations, they experienced intense pain during these procedures. Clinicians designed versatile cognitive-behavioral programs, incorporating hypnosis, attention and distraction, and relaxation training, to help these children (Zeltzer and

LeBaron 1982; Hilgard and LeBaron 1984). Such child-centered programs incorporated proven psychological methods to target the specific child, family, and situational factors that were intensifying children's pain, anxiety, and distress, specifically helping children to understand the procedure and its significance and increasing their ability to control what would happen (McGrath 1990). Generally, as children received age-appropriate accurate information, gained realistic expectations, had more choices and control, and used independent pain control strategies, they had decreased pain and distress.

Today, counseling, distraction, guided imagery, hypnosis, relaxation training, biofeedback, and behavioral management are used routinely to treat a child's pain. Children seem more adept than adults at using psychological therapies, presumably because they are generally less biased than adults about their potential efficacy. Health care providers should teach children a few basic attention and distraction methods to reduce pain and guide families to recognize the particular circumstances that exacerbate pain and distress.

Pain control is not merely "drug versus nondrug therapy," but rather an integrated approach to reduce or block nociceptive activity by attenuating responses in peripheral afferents and central pathways, activating endogenous pain inhibitory systems, and modifying situational factors that exacerbate pain. As reviewed in other chapters, analgesics include acetaminophen, non-steroidal anti-inflammatory drugs, opioids, and adjuvant analgesics such as various anticonvulsants and tricyclic antidepressants. Adjuvant analgesics are the cornerstone of pain control for children with chronic pain, especially when the pain has a neuropathic component. Children with severe pain may require progressively higher and more frequent opioid doses due to drug tolerance and should receive the doses they need to relieve their pain (Collins and Weisman 2003). The fear of opioid addiction in children has been greatly exaggerated. Neonates and infants require the same three categories of analgesic drugs as older children. However, premature and full-term newborns show reduced clearance of most opioids. The differences in pharmacokinetics and pharmacodynamics among neonates, preterm infants, and full-term infants warrant special dosing considerations for infants and close monitoring when they receive opioids

Pre-emptive analgesia is the key for managing acute pain from invasive medical procedures. Depending on the procedure, health care providers may choose psychological methods, anesthetic techniques, sedation, and analgesics (Kazak et al. 1998). Children's postoperative pain should be managed from a similar comprehensive perspective aimed to attenuate nociceptive responses from the surgical trauma (when possible) and to prevent pain throughout the recovery period. Children should receive adequate analgesic prescriptions based on the severity of pain, and drugs should be administered at regular dosing intervals based on their duration of action so as to provide consistent pain relief and prevent breakthrough pain.

As in adults, children's chronic pain often has nociceptive and neuropathic components and requires a multimodal therapeutic regimen comprising pharmacological, physical, and psychological therapies. Most of the pharmacological management of neuropathic pain in children and adolescents is based on extrapolation from adult studies. While tricyclic antidepressants and gabapentin are well-established analgesics for neuropathic conditions in adults, evidence for their efficacy in children is very limited (Rusy et al. 2001). A child's chronic pain is influenced by environmental, family, and psychological factors, necessitating the integration of cognitive-behavioral therapies to mitigate some of the factors that intensify pain, distress, and disability. Strong and consistent evidence supports the efficacy of cognitive-behavioral interventions for relieving children's headache. However, the evidence base supporting use of such interventions for relieving other types of chronic pain is weak, as assessed by the number of controlled trials that have been conducted in children and by the few types of chronic pain that have been formally studied. Pediatric research is just beginning on many of the therapies regarded as complementary to traditional medical approaches, such as acupuncture (Zeltzer et al. 2002).

FUTURE CHALLENGES

As a result of extensive research during the past 30 years, we have gained better insights about how the developing nociceptive system responds to tissue injury, how children perceive pain, how we should assess pain in infants and children, and which drug and nondrug therapies will alleviate their pain. The emphasis has shifted gradually from an almost exclusively disease-centered focus—detecting and treating the putative source of tissue damage—to a more child-centered perspective, assessing the child with pain, identifying contributing psychological and contextual factors, and then targeting interventions accordingly. However, serious challenges remain.

We have discovered much about the plasticity of the developing nociceptive system, but we still have much to learn about how signals from painful stimuli are processed, especially at higher levels. Although we need further developmental research in neurobiology, neurophysiology, and pharmacology, we now know that infants seem particularly vulnerable because of their heightened responsivity to tissue injury and that we must devote particular attention to their pain management.

We need to apply the existing knowledge about pain assessment and pain management more consistently within our clinical practice. Regrettably, many hospitals still do not require consistent documentation of children's pain, preventing us from ensuring that children's pain is adequately controlled. Hospital administrators or accreditation organizations should establish children's pain control as a priority, as recently mandated by the Joint Commission on Accreditation of Healthcare Organizations for the United States. In spite of established analgesic dosing guidelines for infants and children, the undertreatment of postoperative and chronic pain is a continuing problem in many centers.

Moreover, increasing responsibility for evidence-based practice dictates that health care providers adopt clear guidelines for determining when treatments are effective and for identifying children for whom they are most effective. We lack data from well-designed cohort studies and randomized controlled trials to support the efficacy of many interventions (both drug and nondrug therapies) used extensively in clinical practice. Although cognitive-behavioral interventions are critical components of pain management programs for chronic pain, most of the data supporting their efficacy is derived from studies of childhood headache. As Eccleston and colleagues (2002) concluded, we urgently need well-designed studies of non-headache chronic pain in children and adolescents.

We critically need data on child-centered treatment efficacy—that is, when interventions are selected for individual children with pain, based on an assessment of the specific cognitive, behavioral, and emotional factors contributing to their pain and disability. We need longitudinal studies to identify key risk factors that influence a child's vulnerability to chronic pain, in particular the apparent increased vulnerability in females. Future studies should use brain-imaging technology and psychophysical measurement to evaluate the neural mechanisms underlying chronic pain and cognitive function in children. Our ultimate and continuing challenges are to better understand the experience of children's pain and to improve clinical practice, so that health care providers use the existing state-of-the-art pain scales, interpret children's pain scores to guide therapeutic decisions, and document treatment effectiveness.

ACKNOWLEDGMENTS

My thanks to Laura Abbott for her expert assistance in appraising the nature of publications on pediatric pain in 1973–1975 and 2000–2003.

REFERENCES

Anand KJ, Sippell WG, Aynsley-Green A. Randomised trial of fentanyl anaesthesia in preterm babies undergoing surgery: effects on the stress response. *Lancet* 1987; 1:62–66.

Anand KJS, Stevens BJ, McGrath PJ (Eds). *Pain in Neonates.* Amsterdam: Elsevier, 2000.

Andrews KA. The human developmental neurophysiology of pain. In: Schechter NL, Berde CB, Yaster M (Eds). *Pain in Infants, Children, and Adolescents,* 2nd ed. Baltimore: Lippincott Williams & Wilkins, 2003, pp 43–57.

Andrews K, Fitzgerald M. Cutaneous flexion reflex in human neonates: a quantitative study of threshold and stimulus-response characteristics after single and repeated stimuli. *Dev Med Child Neurol* 1999; 41:696–703.

Apley J. *The Child with Abdominal Pains.* Oxford: Blackwell Scientific, 1975.

Behrman RE, Kliegman RM, Nelson WE (Eds). *Nelson Essentials of Pediatrics.* Philadelphia: Saunders, 2002.

Behrman RE, Kliegman R, Jenson HB (Eds). *Nelson Textbook of Pediatrics.* Philadelphia: Saunders, 2004.

Bennett-Branson SM, Craig KD. Post-operative pain in children: developmental and family influences on spontaneous coping strategies. *Can J Behav Sci* 1993; 25:355–383.

Beyer JE, McGrath PJ, Berde CB. Discordance between self-report and behavioral pain measures in children aged 3–7 years after surgery. *Pain Symptom Manage* 1990; 5:350–356.

Bijttebier P, Vertommen H. The impact of previous experience on children's reactions to venepunctures. *J Health Psychol* 1998; 3:39–46.

Blount RL, Davis N, Powers SW, Roberts MC. The influence of environmental factors and coping style on children's coping and distress. *Clin Psychol Rev* 1991; 11:93–116.

Boucher T, Jennings E, Fitzgerald M. The onset of diffuse noxious inhibitory controls in postnatal rat pups: a C-Fos study. *Neurosci Lett* 1998; 257:9–12.

Breau LM, McGrath PJ, Camfield CS, et al. Psychometric properties of the non-communicating children's pain checklist–revised. *Pain* 2002; 99:349–357.

Bush JP, Harkins SW (Eds). *Children in Pain: Clinical and Research Issues from a Developmental Perspective.* New York: Springer-Verlag, 1991.

Chambers CT, Craig KD, Bennett SM. The impact of maternal behavior on children's pain experiences: an experimental analysis. *J Pediatr Psychol* 2002; 27:293–301.

Champion GD, Goodenough B, von Baeyer CL, et al. Measurement of pain by self-report. In: Finley GA, McGrath PA (Eds). *Measurement of Pain in Infants and Children,* Progress in Pain Research and Management, Vol. 10. Seattle: IASP Press, 1998, pp 123–160.

Chen E, Craske MG, Katz ER, et al. Pain-sensitive temperament: does it predict procedural distress and response to psychological treatment among children with cancer? *J Pediatr Psychol* 2000; 25:269–278.

Collins J, Weisman SJ. Management of pain in childhood cancer. In: Schechter NL, Berde CB, Yaster M (Eds). *Pain in Infants, Children, and Adolescents,* 2nd ed. Baltimore: Lippincott Williams & Wilkins, 2003, pp 517–538.

Dahlquist CM, Gil KM, Armstrong FD, et al. Preparing children for medical examinations: the importance of previous medical expense. *Health Psychol* 1986; 5:249–259.

Eccleston C, Morley S, Williams A, et al. Systematic review of randomised controlled trials of psychological therapy for chronic pain in children and adolescents, with a subset meta-analysis of pain relief. *Pain* 2002; 99:157–165.

Eland JM. *Children's Communication of Pain.* Master's Thesis. Iowa City: University of Iowa, 1974.

Finley GA, McGrath PJ (Eds). *Measurement of Pain in Infants and Children,* Progress in Pain Research and Management, Vol. 10. Seattle: IASP Press, 1998.

Finley GA, McGrath PJ (Eds). *Acute and Procedure Pain in Infants and Children,* Progress in Pain Research and Management, Vol. 20. Seattle: IASP Press, 2001.

Fitzgerald M. Cutaneous primary afferent properties in the hind limb of the neonatal rat. *J Physiol* 1987; 383:79–92.

Fitzgerald M, Howard RF. The neurobiologic basis of pediatric pain. In: Schechter NL, Berde CB, Yaster M (Eds). *Pain in Infants, Children, and Adolescents*, 2nd ed. Baltimore: Lippincott Williams & Wilkins, 2003, pp 19–42.

Fitzgerald M, Jennings E. The postnatal development of spinal sensory processing. *Proc Natl Acad Sci USA* 1999; 96:7719–7722.

Forfar JO. *Textbook of Paediatrics*. Edinburgh: Churchill Livingstone, 1973.

Gaffney A, Dunne EA. Children's understanding of the causality of pain. *Pain* 1987; 29:91–104.

Goodenough B, Thomas W, Champion GD, et al. Unravelling age effects and sex differences in needle pain: ratings of sensory intensity and unpleasantness of venipuncture pain by children and their parents. *Pain* 1999; 80:179–190.

Grunau RE. Long-term consequences of pain in human neonates. In: Anand KLS, Stevens BJ, McGrath PJ (Eds). *Pain in Neonates,* 2nd ed. Amsterdam: Elsevier, 2000, pp 55–76.

Hilgard JR, LeBaron S. *Hypnotherapy of Pain in Children with Cancer*. Los Altos: Kaufmann, 1984.

Hutchison JH. *Practical Paediatric Problems*. London: Lloyd-Luke, 1975.

Jay SM, Ozolins M, Elliott CH, et al. Assessment of children's distress during painful medical procedures. *Health Psychol* 1983; 2:133–147.

Johnston C, Stevens B, Boyer K, et al. Development of psychologic responses to pain and assessment of pain in infants and toddlers. In: Schechter NL, Berde CB, Yaster M (Eds). *Pain in Infants, Children, and Adolescents,* 2nd ed. Baltimore: Lippincott Williams & Wilkins, 2003, pp 105–127.

Kaas JH, Merzenich MM, Killackey HP. The reorganization of somatosensory cortex following peripheral nerve damage in adult and developing mammals. *Annu Rev Neurosci* 1983; 6:325–356.

Katz ER, Kellerman J, Siegel SE. Behavioral distress in children with cancer undergoing medical procedures: developmental considerations. *J Consult Clin Psychol* 1980; 48:356–365.

Kazak AE, Penati B, Brophy P, et al. Pharmacologic and psychologic interventions for procedural pain. *Pediatrics* 1998; 102:59–66.

Koltzenburg M, Lewin GR. Receptive properties of embryonic chick sensory neurons innervating skin. *J Neurophysiol* 1997; 78:2560–2568.

Lander J, Fowler-Kerry S. Age differences in children's pain. *Percept Mot Skills* 1991; 73:415–418.

Liossi C. *Procedure-Related Cancer Pain in Children*. Oxford: Radcliffe Medical Press, 2002.

McGrath PA. *Pain in Children: Nature, Assessment and Treatment*. New York: Guilford Press, 1990.

McGrath PA, Dade LA. Effective strategies to decrease pain and minimize disability. In: Price DD, Bushnell MC (Eds). *Psychological Methods of Pain Control: Basic Science and Clinical Perspectives,* Progress in Pain Research and Management, Vol. 29. Seattle: IASP Press, 2004, pp 73–96.

McGrath PA, Gillespie JM. Pain assessment in children and adolescents. In: Turk DC, Melzack R (Eds). *Handbook of Pain Assessment*, 2nd ed. New York: Guilford Press, 2001, pp 97–118.

McGrath PA, Hillier LM (Eds). *The Child with Headache: Diagnosis and Treatment,* Progress in Pain Research and Management, Vol. 19. Seattle: IASP Press, 2001.

McGrath PJ. Behavioral measures of pain. In: Finley GA, McGrath PJ. (Eds). *Measurement of Pain in Infants and Children,* Progress in Pain Research and Management, Vol. 10. Seattle: IASP Press, 1998, pp 83–102.

McGrath PJ, Finley GA (Eds). *Pediatric Pain: Biological and Social Context,* Progress in Pain Research and Management, Vol. 26. Seattle: IASP Press, 2003.

McGrath PJ, Unruh AM. *Pain in Children and Adolescents*. Amsterdam: Elsevier, 1987.

Nelson WE. *Nelson Textbook of Pediatrics,* 10th ed. Philadelphia: Saunders, 1975.

Olsson GL, Jylli L (Eds). *Barn och Smärta*. Lund, Sweden: Studentlitteratur, 2001.

Palermo TM, Drotar D. Prediction of children's postoperative pain: the role of presurgical expectations and anticipatory emotions. *J Pediatr Psychol* 1996; 21:683–698.

Peterson L, Crowson J, Saldana L, et al. Of needles and skinned knees: children's coping with medical procedures and minor injuries for self and other. *Health Psychol* 1999; 18:197–200.

Pichard-Léandri E, Gauvain-Piquard A (Eds). *La douleur chez l'enfant.* Paris: Medsi/McGraw Hill, 1989.

Porter FL, Grunau RE, Anand KJ. Long-term effects of pain in infants. *J Dev Behav Pediatr* 1999; 20:253–261.

Robinson MJ, Roberton DM (Eds). *Practical Paediatrics.* Edinburgh: Churchill Livingstone, 2003.

Ross DM, Ross SA. *Childhood Pain: Current Issues, Research, and Management.* Baltimore: Urban & Schwarzenberg, 1988.

Rudolph CD, Rudolph AM (Eds). *Rudolph's Pediatrics.* New York: McGraw-Hill, 2003.

Rudolph AM, Kamei RK, Overby KJ (Eds). *Rudolph's Fundamentals of Pediatrics.* New York: McGraw-Hill, 2002.

Rusy LM, Troshynski TJ, Weisman SJ. Gabapentin in phantom limb pain management in children and young adults: report of seven cases. *J Pain Symptom Manage* 2001; 21:78–82.

Savedra MC, Holzemer WL, Tesler MD, et al. Assessment of postoperation pain in children and adolescents using the adolescent pediatric pain tool. *Nurs Res* 1993; 42:5–9.

Schanberg LE, Keefe FJ, Lefebvre JC, et al. Social context of pain in children with Juvenile Primary Fibromyalgia Syndrome: parental pain history and family environment. *Clin J Pain* 1998; 14:107–115.

Schechter NL, Berde CB, Yaster M (Eds). *Pain in Infants, Children, and Adolescents.* Baltimore: Lippincott Williams & Wilkins, 2003.

Silver HK, Bruyn HB, Kempe CH (Eds). *Handbook of Pediatrics.* Los Altos: Lange Medical Publications, 1975.

Stevens BJ, Franck LS. Assessment and management of pain in neonates. *Paediatr Drugs* 2001; 3:539–558

Swafford LI, Allan D. Pain relief in the pediatric patient. *Med Clin N Am* 1968; 52:131–136.

Taddio A, Katz J, Ilersich AL, et al. Effect of neonatal circumcision on pain response during subsequent routine vaccination. *Lancet* 1997; 349:599–603.

Terstegen C, Koot HM, de Boer JB, et al. Measuring pain in children with cognitive impairment: pain response to surgical procedures. *Pain* 2003; 103:187–198.

Tyler DC, Krane EJ (Eds). *Pain in Children,* Advances in Pain Research and Therapy, Vol. 15. New York: Raven Press, 1990.

Unruh AM, Campbell MA. Gender variations in children's pain experiences. In: Finley GA, McGrath PJ (Eds). *Chronic and Recurrent Pain in Children and Adolescents*, Progress in Pain Research and Management, Vol. 13. Seattle: IASP Press, 1999, pp 199–241.

Varni JW, Thompson KL, Hanson V. The Varni/Thompson Pediatric Pain Questionnaire: I. Chronic musculoskeletal pain in juvenile rheumatoid arthritis. *Pain* 1987; 28:27–38.

Woodbury CJ, Koerber HR. Widespread projections from myelinated nociceptors throughout the substantia gelatinosa provide novel insights into neonatal hypersensitivity. *J Neurosci* 2003; 23:601–610.

Zeltzer L, LeBaron S. Hypnosis and nonhypnotic techniques for reduction of pain and anxiety during painful procedures in children and adolescents with cancer. *J Pediatr* 1982; 101:1032–1035.

Zeltzer LK, Tsao JC, Stelling C, et al. A phase I study on the feasibility and acceptability of an acupuncture/hypnosis intervention for chronic pediatric pain. *J Pain Symptom Manage* 2002; 24:437–446.

Ziai M, Cooke RE, Janeway CA (Eds). *Pediatrics.* Boston: Little, Brown, 1975.

Correspondence to: Patricia A. McGrath, PhD, Divisional Centre of Pain Management and Pain Research, Department of Anesthesiology, The Hospital for Sick Children, 555 University Avenue, Toronto, Ontario, MSG 1XB, Canada. Email: patricia.mcgrath@sickkids.ca

The Paths of Pain 1975–2005, edited by
Harold Merskey, John D. Loeser, and Ronald
Dubner, IASP Press, Seattle, © 2005.

31

Neural Blockade and Neuromodulation in Persistent Pain Management

Paul M. Murphy and Michael J. Cousins

*Pain Management Research Institute, University of Sydney,
Royal North Shore Hospital, St Leonards, New South Wales, Australia*

Prior to 1975, neural blockade by local anesthetic or neurolytic agent seemed a very logical therapeutic accompaniment to a "hard-wired tele-phone cable" concept of pain. Thus, many anesthesiologists and pain spe-cialists carried out temporary or permanent neural blockade procedures at many levels of the neuroaxis in almost every cancer patient referred to them and in many noncancer patients. The results were often disappointing, or else pain relief that initially seemed promising was not sustained. Such results paralleled the outcomes of neuroablative neurosurgical techniques, with the exception of procedures used to treat trigeminal neuralgia, neuro-lytic/neuroablative procedures for certain types of cancer pain, and neuro-lytic lumbar sympathetic blockade for lower limb ischemia (Cousins and Bridenbaugh 1998).

Increasing awareness among clinicians of the gate control theory (Melzack and Wall 1965), particularly after 1975, ushered in a new era in which modulation became a major aim, rather than temporary or permanent neuroablation (Fig. 1). The use of neurolytic and neurodestructive proce-dures became less common for chronic noncancer pain, with a few excep-tions that are discussed below. While neurolytic procedures were retained for important indications such as celiac plexus blockade for pancreatic carci-noma, neuromodulation became a very acceptable and effective additional modality of cancer pain treatment (Cousins and Bridenbaugh 1998). Inter-estingly, the first application of neuromodulation was transcutaneous electri-cal nerve stimulation (TENS), but shortly afterwards neurosurgeon Norman Shealy reported on direct spinal cord stimulation (SCS) via an electrode placed in the subarachnoid space on the dorsum of the spinal cord. Although SCS proliferated in the 1970s and 1980s, poor patient selection and

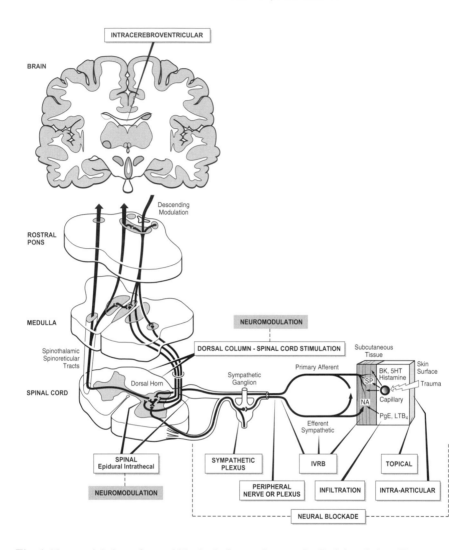

Fig. 1. Neuroaxial sites of neural blockade for persistent pain. Peripheral sites: Temporary neural blockade can be achieved by a variety of topical agents including local anesthetics, capsaicin, guanethidine, corticosteroids, and clonidine (see Watson, this volume, for a discussion of topical agents). Peripheral nerves: Previous neurolytic techniques have been largely replaced by more precise radiofrequency lesioning using anatomical landmarks under image intensifier control and other techniques to control needle placement. Sympathetic ganglia: Neurolytic blocks maintain a valuable role in vascular ischemia and upper abdominal cancer. Temporary blockade with local anesthetics may be of benefit in CRPS and acute-on-chronic or chronic vascular ischemia. Nerve roots: Local anesthetics, corticosteroids, and nonsteroidal anti-inflammatory drugs (experimental) may be used. Spinal cord dorsal horn: Neuromodulation is performed using an increasing array of novel agents. Spinal cord dorsal columns: Neuromodulation is performed by spinal cord stimulation. BK = bradykinin; IVRB = intravenous regional block; LTB_4 = leukotriene B_4; NA = norepinephrine; PgE = prostaglandin E; SP = substance P.

suboptimal technology hampered its development until the mid-1990s. Although spinal modulation by opioid and non-opioid drugs did not develop until 1979, intrathecal (i.t.) and epidural drug administration for acute, chronic and cancer pain was well established by 1984 with a firm scientific foundation and adequate methods of delivery (Cousins and Mather 1984).

Running in parallel with these groundbreaking changes in the use of neural blockade were fundamental shifts in the way that patients with persistent pain were assessed and treated. Although first proposed in the 1940s, the multidisciplinary approach to pain management had not gained widespread application until after the formation of the IASP in 1973, and particularly not until the late 1970s when the biopsychosocial concept of pain management gained momentum. Neuromodulation lent itself much better to a multifaceted approach using drug, nondrug, psychological, and environmental manipulation in a concerted effort to restore mental and physical function. In the early 1980s this approach required the solo-practitioner nerve-block specialist to gain a vast array of new knowledge and to change his or her mode of practice substantially to become part of a team. Some individuals still have not addressed such challenges more than 20 years later.

SPINAL MODULATION BY INTRATHECAL/EPIDURAL DRUG ADMINISTRATION

Although epidural infusions of local anesthetics were widely used for the management of acute obstetrical pain in the late 1960s, application to postoperative and post-trauma pain evolved only gradually during the 1970s as a result of concerns regarding local anesthetic toxicity and cardiovascular side effects (Cousins 2003). Thus the papers of Duggan et al. (1976) and Yaksh and Rudy (1976a,b, 1977) generated great interest among clinicians because of the demonstration of a new potential target in the spinal cord—the opioid receptor.

DEVELOPMENTS SINCE 1975

Electrophysiological studies demonstrated that electrophoretic administration of morphine into the substantia gelatinosa resulted in reduced activity in dorsal horn neurons following noxious skin heating, an effect that was reversible by naloxone (Duggan et al. 1976). The question of clinical applicability began to be resolved in 1976 when it was demonstrated that intrathecal (i.t.) administration of morphine produced dose-dependent, naloxone-reversible analgesia initially in a rat model and subsequently in other animals including primates (Yaksh and Rudy 1976a,b, 1977). The development of a method for implanting a permanent indwelling catheter in rats by this group facilitated additional studies on efficacy, dose response, and neurotoxicity of opioid and non-opioid medications.

Paralleling the initial animal work, the first human studies performed on spinal injury patients demonstrated a naloxone-reversible reduction of spinal polysynaptic reflexes by systemic opioid administration (Willer et al. 1979). Pharmacokinetic and pharmacodynamic studies led to the development of the concept of "selective spinal analgesia," which at the time was considered somewhat controversial (Cousins et al. 1979; Cousins and Mather 1984). Initial concerns arising from anecdotal reports of delayed respiratory depression were allayed with evidence that administration of appropriate minimally effective doses of morphine by the spinal route did not have a significantly different effect on respiratory depression compared to intramuscular administration (Rawal et al. 1987).

SPINAL OPIOID MONOTHERAPY

The spinal cord became recognized during the 1980s as a key target for modulating both acute pain processes and the interlinked mechanisms underlying persistent nociception, including oncogene expression and spinal neuronal reorganization (plasticity) (Basbaum 1999). Spinal (both epidural and i.t.) administration of opioids is now the most frequent method of controlling severe pain due to cancer or advanced disease. Morphine is the most commonly utilized and most widely studied opioid, although hydromorphone and fentanyl are also frequently used. Despite widespread acceptance of long-term administration of i.t. morphine, there are few data on efficacy or safety from controlled clinical trials. There are multiple case reports and retrospective analyses and a small number of prospective studies comprising a database of over 2000 patients. In patients with severe cancer pain, a large, multicenter, international study with a randomized prospective design compared i.t. opioids (in some cases combined with other agents) to "maximal medical therapy." Intrathecal opioids provided clearly superior analgesia and fewer side effects with a trend toward increased survival (Smith et al. 2002, 2004). An important outcome was a significant advantage for i.t. therapy in quality of life measures for both cancer patients and their caregivers. Somewhat dampening the positive results of this study has been evidence of a potential for development of fibrous tissue masses at the tip of i.t. catheters in association with i.t. morphine (particularly following administration of high doses and concentrated solutions) (Yaksh et al. 2003). Recommendations for early diagnosis and treatment have been provided (Yaksh et al. 2002). Intrathecal morphine is approximately 10 times as potent as morphine administered by the epidural route due to high cerebrospinal fluid (CSF) levels, low volume of distribution (approximately 70 mL) and relatively slow elimination kinetics. Animal data suggest that the morphine metabolite morphine-6-glucuronide (M6G) is over 10 times as potent as morphine given by the i.t. route. In chronic morphine infusion, M6G enters the CSF from the plasma and may play an important role in the analgesic effect. A recent evidence-based review suggests that, despite a lack of level 1 and 2 data (from meta-analyses and controlled randomized trials) for long-term i.t. morphine administration, there is significant evidence from cohort studies and nonrandomized trials to support its use (Bennett et al. 2000a). The authors point out that although long-term dose stability is good, dose escalation is not uncommon and may indicate the development of tolerance or disease progression. Initial consensus guidelines considered morphine to be the sole first-line agent for intraspinal infusion in pain management (Bennett et al. 2000b). Hydromorphone was previously considered a second-line agent, suitable for use in the clinical setting when i.t. morphine infusion provides adequate analgesia but with morphine-related toxicity. The algorithm for selection of long-term i.t. drug administration has recently been updated by the Polyanalgesic Consensus Conference, and hydromorphone is now listed as a first-line agent (Hassenbusch et al. 2004). Hydromorphone is five times more potent than morphine when administered by the i.t. route and has gained popularity because it allows for longer intervals between pump refills. An additional benefit is its relatively favorable side-effect profile (Anderson and Burchiel 1999). If adequate analgesia is not achieved with the maximum dosage of first-line agents, addition of an adjuvant agent (bupivacaine or clonidine) should be considered. In instances where neuropathic pain predominates, it may be appropriate to commence with combination therapy (Hassenbusch et al. 2004).

Fentanyl and sufentanil may be utilized as fourth-line agents if an adequate response is not obtained with the addition of adjuvant agents to morphine or hydromorphone. It is also appropriate to commence fentanyl if inadequate analgesia or excessive side effects occur with both first-line opioids (Hassenbusch et al. 2004).

COMBINATION SPINAL ANALGESIC THERAPY

The rapidly evolving knowledge base of neurotransmitters, membrane receptors, and intracellular messenger systems involved in dorsal horn nociception has resulted in the utilization of spinal drug combinations targeting multiple analgesic mechanisms. This approach, paralleling multi-agent therapies in other medical disciplines, has been termed "combination spinal analgesic chemotherapy" (Carr and Cousins 1998).

Opioid-opioid combination.   Spinal administration of two or more opioids with different pharmacological profiles may improve the quality of the analgesic response and reduce potential side effects (Walker et al. 2002). Animal data demonstrate that combining opioids with different receptor kinetics has a dose-sparing effect (Yaksh and Malmberg 1994). A number of human studies have suggested that epidural co-administration of a rapid-onset opioid with morphine improves early analgesia; however, evidence relating to optimal dosing and side effect profile is inconclusive (Sinatra et al. 1991; Tanaka et al. 1997).

Opioid-local anesthetic combination.   Combining drugs with different modalities of action can produce synergy, reducing opioid requirements and thus associated side effects (Prager 2002). Potential combinations include the addition of local anesthetic agents such as bupivacaine, the α_2-adrenoceptor agonist clonidine, NMDA-receptor agonists including ketamine, and midazolam. Despite the growing popularity of such admixtures, it is important to recognize the limited evidence base for the efficacy of many such combination therapies (Walker et al. 2002).

Spinal co-administration of local anesthetic and opioid agents has been extensively reported for the management of acute and chronic pain (Bennett et al. 2000a,b; Walker et al. 2002). Neurotoxicity studies indicate that use of bupivacaine is safe at clinically relevant dosages via both the epidural and i.t. routes, a finding supported by animal data at concentrations well above those in clinical use. Evidence from two prospective studies supports the efficacy and safety of this combination therapy in both cancer (van Dongen et al. 1999) and noncancer pain (Nitescu et al. 1998). Both studies, however, suffer from randomization deficiencies, and in addition, van Dongen et al. use a reduction in progression of i.t. morphine dose in progressive disease as the clinical end point. Case series data support the use of this combination therapy with i.t. bupivacaine/morphine or bupivacaine/hydromorphone combination therapy resulting in a 50% response rate (visual analogue scale, McGill Pain Questionnaire, and Chronic Illness Problem Inventory) in a noncancer pain population (Anderson and Burchiel 1999).

Opioid-clonidine combination.   The analgesic effect of clonidine is mediated via its action on α_2 adrenoceptors located on the superficial layers of the dorsal horn. This action modulates a number of local processes including release of norepinephrine (Yaksh and Malmberg 1994; Goudas et al. 1998) and reduction in spinal nitric oxide release (Lin et al. 2002a). Recently it has been reported that this effect may also be partly mediated via an action on spinal muscarinic receptors (Kang and Eisenach 2003). Studies on healthy human volunteers have demonstrated that the analgesic effect of clonidine administered via the epidural route correlates closely with CSF rather than serum levels, suggesting a direct action at the spinal level (Eisenach et al. 1996). The Epidural Study Group compared the efficacy of epidural morphine plus clonidine versus epidural morphine plus saline in 85 patients with intractable cancer (Eisenach et al. 1995). This randomized, double-blind study demonstrated superior efficacy with the co-administration of clonidine, especially in the setting of neuropathic descriptors. A randomized, controlled, within-patient crossover study of i.t. clonidine and morphine administration in patients suffering neuropathic pain secondary to spinal cord injury demonstrated that co-administration was superior to either agent or placebo; however, the authors could not elucidate whether the effects were additive or synergistic (Siddall et al. 2000). Clonidine has also been utilized in isolation as an effective therapy for chronic neuropathic pain, with a recent phase I/II study indicating its tolerability and efficacy as a long-term therapy (Hassenbusch and Portenoy 2000; Hassenbusch et al. 2002).

Opioid-NMDA antagonist combination. Dorsal horn *N*-methyl-D-aspartate (NMDA) receptors occupy a central role in the process of central sensitization and associated alterations in synaptic plasticity pivotal to the generation of persistent pain. A number of studies have demonstrated potent analgesic effect in neuropathic pain states following neuroaxial administration of racemic ketamine as a co-analgesic with an opioid (Yaksh 1996). Potential neurotoxicity with chronic i.t. administration has been demonstrated in a number of animal models (Hassenbusch et al. 1999), and there has been one case report of leptomeningeal lymphocytic vasculitis following long-term i.t. ketamine infusion (Stotz et al. 1999). A recent report has suggested that preservative-free S (+)-ketamine may be associated with lower risk of neurotoxicity (Vranken et al. 2004); however, no preclinical safety data are available to support the theory. Studies to date do not adequately dissociate the spinal action from possible systemic effects of i.t. ketamine, and it is difficult to determine what role the local anesthetic effect plays. In addition, redistribution may result in supraspinal side effects at therapeutic doses (Bennett et al. 2000a). A recent evidence-based review suggests that due to concerns regarding potential neurotoxicity, currently available NMDA-receptor antagonists must be considered as having a suspect safety profile. It is advocated that use of these agents should be considered only when severe and disabling pain is refractory to more conventional therapies (Hassenbusch et al. 2004).

Opioid-GABA agonist combination. Recent interest has focused on the potential use of i.t. midazolam as an adjuvant analgesic. This benzodiazepine has been used since 1978 for its sedative, anxiolytic, and amnesic properties. The benzodiazepine subunit of the γ-aminobutyric acid (GABA)-A receptor has been demonstrated in the dorsal root ganglion (DRG) and on spinal neurons, correlating with the observation that benzodiazepines suppress afferent evoked excitation in the substantia gelatinosa. Initial animal data demonstrated spinal effects including reduction of spasticity, suppression of afferent evoked somatosympathetic reflexes, and alterations in pain behavior (Yaksh and Allen 2004a,b). Analgesic effects are mediated via the benzodiazepine subunit of the receptor, as co-administration of flumazenil attenuates the response while that of naloxone does not. Sedation and degradation of motor function were identified as the most common side effects; however, all side effects displayed reversibility consistent with the time course of the drug. Maximal analgesic efficacy following i.t. delivery may only be observed at dosages that impair motor function (Walker et al. 2002). Despite its potential analgesic effects, there remains a deficit in safety data regarding spinal administration of this agent. Preclinical studies have concentrated on behavioral indices of toxicity, which, although important, must be correlated with histopathological studies. Despite this lack of histological evidence regarding the safety of midazolam as an i.t. agent, there have been numerous human studies assessing safety. Recently, a cohort study assessed 18 symptoms suggestive of neurological dysfunction in 1100 patients who received i.t. anesthesia with or without midazolam (2 mg) co-administration (Tucker et al. 2004). Follow-up during the first postoperative week and at 1 month suggested that midazolam administration was not associated with an increased risk of neurotoxicity. Recent preclinical data in a sheep model appear to alleviate concerns regarding long-term i.t. midazolam infusion (Johansen et al. 2004). Behavioral and neurological function remained unchanged during a 43-day i.t. infusion of midazolam (5 mg/day or 15 mg/day). Subsequent histological examination of spinal tissue revealed mild inflammation surrounding the catheter in both the midazolam and saline control groups. It now appears that i.t. delivery of midazolam offers potential benefits; however, further preclinical and subsequent clinical studies are required looking at issues including long-term safety and co-administration with other agents (Cousins and Miller 2004). A linked series of editorials and articles in the same volume of *Anesthesia and Analgesia* explore issues in i.t. use of midazolam (Cousins and Miller 2004; Johansen et al. 2004; Tucker et al. 2004; Yaksh and Allen 2004a,b).

Intrathecal baclofen is a recognized treatment for severe spasticity associated with spinal cord injury and multiple sclerosis. Evidence from animal studies and case series suggests that spinal administration of baclofen is associated with an antinociceptive effect at doses that do not produce significant motor blockade. There are several case reports identifying an antinociceptive action in central pain states associated with spasticity, but much less information is available in pain states not associated with spasticity (Slonimski et al. 2004). One case series demonstrates efficacy as a sole agent in the management of diverse conditions including phantom limb pain, failed back surgery syndrome, and peripheral nerve injury (Zuniga et al. 2000). The same authors subsequently report long-term control of pain, allodynia, and autonomic dysfunction by i.t. baclofen administration (with or without clonidine) in two cases of type I complex regional pain syndrome (CRPS-I) (Zuniga et al. 2002). Recent evidence suggests that SCS may mediate its effect in part via an action on spinal GABA$_B$ receptors. A recent study has demonstrated that co-administration of i.t. baclofen may be an important adjuvant therapy with SCS (Lind et al. 2004).

SPINAL PROSTAGLANDIN INHIBITION

Spinal prostaglandins adversely modulate endogenous pain control mechanisms by inhibiting the bulbospinal noradrenergic component of the descending antinociceptive system. Intrathecal administration of aspirin may provide dose-dependent hypoalgesia by inhibiting local prostaglandin synthesis. Two retrospective studies have been carried out to date on 72 patients (5 with cancer pain, 67 with nonmalignant pain). Moderate to excellent analgesia was obtained for a range of 1–30 days following single bolus administration. Mild side effects included generalized fatigue and hallucinations. There are no animal or human data to support the safety or efficacy of chronic i.t. aspirin administration (Bennett et al. 2002a).

NOVEL AGENTS FOR SPINAL MODULATION

As understanding of the complex processes involved in spinal modulation of nociception continues to increase, novel agents directed more specifically to the pathophysiological processes underpinning persistent pain will continue to be added to the armamentarium of i.t. therapies. Potential agents include conopeptides such as ziconotide and antibodies directed against nerve growth factors intimately involved in the spinal processing of nociceptive information.

Conopeptides. Ziconotide, derived from the marine snail *Conus magnus,* is an ω-conopeptide containing 25 amino acids. It is a potent antagonist at the N-type voltage-sensitive calcium channels (VSCCs) that are located on presynaptic terminals in the dorsal horn. It is reported to mediate its antinociceptive effects via an inhibition of neurotransmitter release. There is now some evidence to suggest that dorsal horn opioid receptors may mediate their action in part via a G-protein linkage with N-type VSCCs. Ziconotide has been demonstrated to be effective in animal models of acute and neuro-pathic pain and has not been associated with the development of tolerance. Emerging evidence from human trials supports its efficacy and safety. A recent multicenter randomized, controlled trial (RCT) of 111 patients suffer-ing pain related to intractable AIDS or cancer reported that 52.9% of pa-tients treated with i.t. ziconotide reported moderate to complete relief of pain as compared to 17.5% in the placebo group (Staats et al. 2004). Similar results were obtained in a group of 108 patients who had previously failed to benefit from i.t. opioid therapy. A significantly greater incidence of side effects including ataxia, dysmetria, sedation, and agitation was reported in the ziconotide group (31%) relative to the placebo group (10%) (Doggrell et al. 2004). The place of ziconotide in i.t. therapy is still evolving (Hassenbusch et al. 2004).

Antibodies against growth factors. Neurotrophic factors such as nerve growth factor (NGF) and brain-derived neurotrophic factor (BDNF) play an important role in nociceptive processes (Walker et al. 2002). C fibers that produce substance P and calcitonin gene-related peptide (CGRP) express the NGF receptor tyrosine kinase A (trkA). Inflammatory processes are associ-ated with increased NGF levels, which increase C-fiber discharge and en-hance expression of both the vanilloid receptor (TRPV1) and the purinergic receptor ($P2X_3$). TrkA/immunoglobulin A has been demonstrated to attenu-ate inflammatory hyperalgesia. BDNF is upregulated in DRG neurons in the presence of NGF and acts to modulate the NMDA receptor and potentiate C-fiber-mediated spinal reflexes. Upregulation is seen following nerve injury and is associated with increased expression of BDNF in deeper lamina of the dorsal horn. Animal studies demonstrate that blockade of brain-derived growth factor with trkB/immunoglobulin G attenuates allodynia and hyperalgesia. Neurotrophin-3 (NT-3) mediates neural outgrowth following nerve injury, and the i.t. administration of NT-3 antisense oligonucleotides attenuates post-nerve-injury sprouting and associated allodynia. Intrathecal administra-tion of glial-derived neurotrophic factor (GDNF) has been demonstrated to attenuate spontaneous ectopic neuronal discharge and mechanical allodynia and thermal hyperalgesia associated with sciatic nerve ligation (Walker et al. 2002).

GENE THERAPY

Advances in gene therapy are further expanding the therapeutic options in this field. Interleukin-2 (IL-2) has a potent antinociceptive action, but in vivo its utility is limited by a short duration of action. Recently, a cytomega-lovirus promoter was utilized to clone human IL-2 cDNA into pcDNA (Yao et al. 2002a). Administration of pcDNA-IL-2 resulted in an analgesic action lasting approximately 6 days in a rodent neuropathic pain model as opposed to 10–25 minutes for recombinant human IL-2 administration. Following administration of the pcDNA, IL-2 mRNA was detectable in the DRG, pia mater, sciatic nerve, and dorsal horn (Yao et al. 2003). The same group reported that i.t. delivery of the IL-2 gene resulted in a more potent and prolonged action than other routes of administration (Yao et al. 2002b). Animal models have also identified that i.t. administration of a pro-opiomelanocortin gene vector is associated with modulation of neuropathic pain behavior and correlates with an elevated spinal expression of β-endorphin (Lin et al. 2002b).

The field of combination analgesic chemotherapy has dramatically expanded over the lifespan of the IASP. With ongoing advances in the understanding of nociceptive processes, the possibility of targeting the specific dysfunctional molecular cascades underpinning chronic pain may become a reality, with a circumscribed period of i.t. treatment aiming to be curative—thus fulfilling the concept of spinal analgesic chemotherapy.

SPINAL CORD STIMULATION AND CHRONIC PAIN

DEVELOPMENTS PRIOR TO 1975

Spinal cord stimulation (SCS) developed as a clinical outgrowth of the gate control theory (Melzack and Wall 1965). The application of electrical stimulation to the large fibers in the dorsal columns was proposed to inhibit transmission of nociceptive information in the smaller Aδ and C fibers at the segmental level. This theory predicted that all types of pain would be suppressed equally. Shealy first described the clinical application in 1967 via a subarachnoid route.

DEVELOPMENTS SINCE 1975

Early results published by the European study group indicated the large range of chronic pain conditions for which SCS was being utilized (Krainick and Thoden 1989). These conditions included the common failed back surgery syndrome, phantom limb pain, segmental pain following spinal cord injury, and peripheral nerve and plexus injuries. These early studies reported an initial response greater than 50% in 38% of patients across this diverse range of conditions. Long-term follow-up revealed that only 22.5% of treated patients obtained ongoing pain relief.

NEUROCHEMICAL EFFECTS

No relationship has been demonstrated between SCS and spinal opioid release. Animal data demonstrate an increase in dorsal horn GABA expression in responding rats, but not in animals that fail to respond to SCS. Inhibition of spinothalamic tract transmission by SCS can be antagonized by co-administration of the GABA antagonist bicuculline. This finding has led to the suggestion that co-administration of the GABA agonist baclofen may enhance the efficacy of SCS. This response is abolished by the application of $GABA_B$ antagonists. Spinal levels of substance P and serotonin are also elevated by SCS. Intravenous and i.t. adenosine can alleviate neuropathic pain in the short term, and it has been demonstrated that adenosine may also potentiate the efficacy of SCS. Excitatory amino acid release is suppressed by SCS via an action on $GABA_B$ receptors. The net effect of these neurochemical effects is to reduce dorsal horn neuronal excitability (Oakley and Prager 2002).

NEUROPHYSIOLOGICAL EFFECTS

Application of SCS also induces a number of neurophysiological effects. The antinociceptive effect appears to be mediated via an action on abnormal pain-mediating Aβ-fiber function. The response of wide-dynamic-range neurons in response to thermal, mechanical, and chemical stimuli in animal neuropathic models is suppressed by the application of SCS. Lesions of the dorsal columns in these animals partly attenuate this response. Transection of the cord above the level of SCS also attenuates the response, suggesting that both segmental and supraspinal mechanisms are involved. The partial preservation of the effect following cord transection suggests that the segmental effect is more important. Remote nervous system effects may also play a role because SCS has been demonstrated to activate the descending pain-inhibitory pathways via an action on the anterior pretectal nucleus (Oakley and Prager 2002).

CARDIAC/VASCULAR EFFECTS

In angina pectoris, SCS reduces noxious input to the pain pathway and also stabilizes intracardiac neuronal activity. In ischemic pain models, SCS is associated with peripheral vasodilatation, mediated via pain inhibition and afferent inhibition of the sympathetic nervous system. This effect appears to be mediated via the release of CGRP and is abolished by transection of the dorsal columns.

CLINICAL APPLICATIONS

A wide range of neuropathic pain conditions respond well to SCS in carefully selected patients refractory to other therapies. Pain relief in the order of 50% has been demonstrated in a range of conditions including failed back surgery syndrome (FBSS), CRPS, peripheral nerve and plexus injuries, segmental pain following spinal cord injury, and post-amputation pain (North and Wetzel 2002). Case-control studies suggest response rates of 12–88% for FBSS. In a review of 39 case control studies over a 28-year period, an average of 59% of patients (range: 15–100%) reported 50% or greater pain relief (Turner et al. 1995). Complications were reported in 42% of patients, mostly due to problems with early SCS systems. The authors reported that the evidence was insufficient to draw conclusions about the efficacy of SCS relative to other therapies. Nevertheless, there is evidence to suggest that the majority of patients treated with SCS for FBSS are satisfied with the procedure and would recommend it to others suffering from the same condition (Ohnmeiss and Rashbaum 2001). It has been suggested that SCS may be superior to re-operation in FBSS, but the evidence is limited (North and Wetzel 2002). A recent systematic review of SCS in FBSS and CRPS type I suggested only mild to moderate improvement of pain with SCS (Turner et al. 2004). Only one randomized study was identified, which demonstrated moderately superior efficacy with SCS and physical therapy compared to physical therapy alone in CRPS at 6 months (Kemler et al. 2000) and at 1 year (Kemler and Furnee 2002). On average, 34% of patients in the population studies suffered a stimulator-related adverse occurrence. The authors conclude that further studies are required to fully assess the efficacy of SCS relative to other therapies in chronic pain states. Nevertheless, the consensus of pain clinicians is that SCS has a valuable role in properly selected patients as part of a multimodal approach.

SCS was first utilized in the management of peripheral vascular disease in 1976 and was demonstrated to facilitate the healing of chronic leg ulcers. Multiple retrospective studies have demonstrated efficacy in terms of improved exercise tolerance, reduced pain, and limb salvage (Tiede and Huntoon 2004). The prospective evidence available to date displays a trends toward limb salvage but does not reach statistical significance. The authors suggest that this modality offers significant potential benefit to patients with peripheral vascular disease; however, further studies are warranted to clarify the role of SCS in pain relief and functional improvement.

Since 1985, SCS has emerged as an effective modality for the treatment of refractory angina pectoris. SCS has been demonstrated to significantly reduce the frequency of angina episodes, nitroglycerin consumption, and

Canadian Cardiovascular Society angina class (Yu et al. 2004). It has also been shown to reduce the duration of hospitalization and cost of hospital care. The total cost of SCS implantation was recoverable within 16 months.

A recent 20-year literature review of 68 studies totalling 3679 patients suggests that SCS is a safe and effective therapeutic modality for a range of chronic neuropathic conditions (Cameron 2004). Despite the positive findings, the author concludes that there is an urgent need for randomized, controlled, long-term studies on the efficacy of SCS in large patient populations.

RADIOFREQUENCY LUMBAR FACET DENERVATION

In 1933, Ghormley first proposed facet joint arthropathy as a potential source of back pain. Lumbar zygapophyseal joints are considered to be responsible for 15–40% of chronic back pain (Bogduk 2004). Since the technique of percutaneous radiofrequency (RF) current for denervation of the zygapophyseal joint was first utilized (Shealy 1976), it has been modified and used with varying results. Initial RCTs demonstrated only moderate benefit; however, subsequent studies have reported significant benefit in both analgesia and disability scores (van Kleef et al. 1999). In a recent systematic review of RCTs, only six studies were considered acceptable for inclusion, and as a result of both the small number and a degree of clinical and technical heterogeneity between studies, statistical analysis was precluded (Geurts et al. 2001). All studies analyzed reported positive results, and the authors concluded that there is moderate evidence that RF lumbar facet denervation is more effective than placebo. Appropriate patient selection is of paramount importance; with controlled diagnostic blockade as a diagnostic tool, 60% of patients can reasonably expect 80% pain relief, and 80% can expect in excess of 60% relief at 12 months (Dreyfuss et al. 2000; Bogduk 2004); these figures are derived from one RCT of 31 patients and one observational study. A more recent critical review found only level 3–4 evidence for short-term benefit of intrafacet joint injection of local anesthetic and a steroid. Conflicting evidence for the benefit of RF denervation in chronic lumbar pain has been reported (Niemisto et al. 2003). Certainly, there is a need for large prospective, randomized trials with uniformity in inclusion and exclusion criteria, therapy, outcome measures, and duration of follow-up to allow appropriate recommendations for the management of lumbar zygapophyseal pain to be made. However, chronic low back pain almost invariably is associated with factors in all three of the physical, psychological, and environmental areas. Thus, lumbar RF should be utilized as part of a multimodal approach, aiming to take advantage of the inevitably circumscribed duration of pain relief to implement other measures.

EPIDURAL STEROID INJECTION

Controversy continues to reign over the role of epidural steroid injection (ESI) in chronic low back pain. A number of questions remain unresolved, including: Who to inject? The appropriate volume and content of injectate? The site for injection? The potential benefit of fluoroscopic guidance? The optimal number of injections? Despite a continued growth in the number of case series and retrospective reviews, prospective controlled data are limited. A systematic review of RCTs of the most common interventions suggested that ESI is moderately more effective than placebo in the short-term management of chronic back pain (van Tulder et al. 1997). McQuay and Moore (1998) estimated the number needed to treat (NNT) as 7 for 75% short-term pain relief and 13 for 50% benefit in the long term. Epidural administration of methylprednisolone in 158 patients with radiologically proven disk herniation demonstrated an improvement in function at 3 weeks and a reduction in leg pain at 6 weeks, but ultimately no long-term benefit (Carette et al. 1997). A recent RCT of 85 patients with presumed disk herniation failed to demonstrate any difference in outcome (pain and function) between epidural prednisolone and epidural isotonic saline (Valat et al. 2003). A potential role for epidural administration of nonsteroidal anti-inflammatory drugs (NSAIDs) has been suggested. An RCT comparing the effects of epidural methylprednisolone with indomethacin suggests that a 2-mg dose of indomethacin is equianalgesic to 80 mg of methylprednisolone in failed back surgery syndrome (Aldrete 2003). The prevailing wisdom suggests that ESI may be of benefit in the setting of painful radiculopathy; however, no study has focused only on such patients. Evidence for ESI in the management of lumbar spinal stenosis remains weak. A retrospective review suggested that ESI provides a reasonable option in refractory patients, quoting an analgesic response lasting more than 2 months in 32% of patients (Delport et al. 2004). In an attempt to identify possible indicators of response, Schiff and Eisenberg (2003) recently identified a correlation between response to ESI and evidence of Aδ-fiber dysfunction in quantitative sensory testing. Much work remains to be done in delineating the exact role of ESI in the chronic back pain patient.

SELECTIVE NERVE ROOT INJECTION

Current literature suggests a favorable role for corticosteroid selective nerve root injection (SNRI) in the nonsurgical management of radiculopathy (Slipman and Chow 2002). Improvements in imaging have facilitated precise placement of the injectate close to the disk-nerve interface and the DRG, apparently maximizing potential efficacy. Outcomes appear better for radicular pain secondary to focal disk herniation than for epidural/intraneural fibrosis, a finding consistent with the biochemical construct of radicular pain. The results of SNRI for the management of cervical or lumbar stenosis are intermediate, perhaps indicating the multifactorial pathology of this condition. The complication rate associated with SNRI was assessed in a cohort study of 207 patients over a 4-month period (Botwin et al. 2000). This study identified a number of complications including transient non-postural headache (3.1%), increased back pain (2.4%), facial flushing (1.2%), increased leg pain (0.6%), vasovagal reaction (0.3%), and intra-procedural hypotension (0.3%); dural puncture was not identified. Recently Rozin and colleagues (2003) reported death secondary to vertebral artery penetration in a C7 transforaminal steroid injection. Since inadvertent needle trauma to a nerve root could cause further neuropathic pain, a key question is whether transforaminal needle insertion has any benefit over periforaminal injection at the appropriate site.

CELIAC PLEXUS BLOCK

Recent studies offer conflicting results on the potential benefit of celiac plexus blockade in terms of survival and quality of life in unresectable pancreatic carcinoma. A key meta-analysis of celiac plexus block (CPB) for the treatment of cancer pain retrieved only 24 papers containing data on two or more patients, of which only two studies were RCTs (Eisenberg et al. 1995). From this database of 989 patients, the majority of cases involved pancreatic carcinoma, with 36% being non-pancreatic. Fluoroscopy and radiographic guidance was only utilized in 39% of patients, while 28% of procedures used CT guidance, 1% were guided by ultrasound, and 32% were non-radiologically guided. During the initial 2-week period following CPB, 89% of patients reported good to excellent pain relief, with partial to complete relief continuing in 90% at 3 months and in 70–90% until death. Significant complications were only identified in 2% of patients; however, local pain (96%), diarrhea (44%), and hypotension 38% were common short-term sequelae. The authors concluded that neurolytic CPB has long-lasting efficacy and is complicated by mild and transient adverse effects. Conflicting data exist on the potential beneficial effect on survival of neurolytic CPB in cancer patients. An RCT comparing alcohol neurolytic CPB with placebo reported an elevation in mood, reduced interference in activity, and increased survival in the CPB group (Staats et al. 2001). A recent RCT comparing neurolytic CPB with sham injection plus systemic opioid analgesia demonstrated improved pain control at 6 weeks with CPB, but no difference in opioid consumption, quality of life, or survival (Wong et al. 2004). Neurolytic CPB has an established role in managing severe pain due to pancreatic carcinoma and other intra-abdominal malignancies; however, its effect on survival remains controversial.

EPIDUROSCOPY

Epiduroscopy has been proposed as both a potential diagnostic tool and a useful interventional modality. In a recent prospective study of 58 elderly patients suffering from degenerative spinal stenosis who underwent epiduroscopy, saline adhesion lysis and application of local anesthetic and steroids were associated with significant reduction of leg pain at 12 months (Igarashi et al. 2004). As an investigative tool, epiduroscopy can identify adhesions not visible on magnetic resonance imaging (Geurts et al. 2002). These authors further reported that targeted epidural injection resulted in significant pain relief that was maintained in 35% of patients at 12 months. The technique currently suffers from a lack of controlled studies.

INTRADISKAL ELECTROTHERMAL THERAPY

It has been suggested that over 40% of chronic back pain may be secondary to internal disk disruption (Bogduk 2004). Intradiskal electrothermal therapy (IDET) offers a minimally invasive alternative to arthrodesis in the management of pain due to internal disk disruption. Initial lack of evidence for this modality led to a degree of reluctance in its utilization among clinicians, but the evidence base is continuing to expand.

IDET has been demonstrated to produce superior results compared to physical rehabilitation programs (Bogduk and Karasek 2002). However, a retrospective study of 60 patients with diskogenic back pain reported persistence of pain in 97% of patients, with 29% reporting an increase in pain after IDET (Davis et al. 2004). A recent placebo-controlled RCT of 64 patients with diskogenic pain offers more optimistic results, reporting that 50% of patients sustained pain reduction in excess of 50%. This study derived an NNT of 5 patients to achieve 75% relief (Pauza et al. 2004). This novel therapy appears to offer potential benefit to a subset of patients suffering from diskogenic pain. Further data are required to delineate specific factors that may be predictive of successful therapy.

CONCLUSION

Neural blockade techniques have evolved in an exciting new direction since 1975. While local anesthetic agents continue to be valuable, they are increasingly being used in new ways—at lower doses and in combination with other drugs. There are real prospects of developing more selective sodium-channel-blocking drugs that target only nociceptive fibers, and highly selective calcium-channel-blocking drugs are already in use spinally. The GABA receptor has emerged as a potent option for spinal administration. Antibodies against growth factors, gene therapy, and other strategies to directly treat neuroplasticity changes are opening up a new era in treatment of persistent pain. An indication of the continued high level of interest in the spinal cord as a target for pain control is the placement of a 1984 review on spinal opioids (Cousins and Mather 1984) as the most cited paper in the anesthesiology literature over the last 60 years (Baltussen and Kindler 2004).

REFERENCES

Aldrete JA. Epidural injections of indomethacin for postlaminectomy syndrome: a preliminary report. *Anesth Analg* 2003; 96:463–468.

Anderson VC, Burchiel KJ. A prospective study of long-term intrathecal morphine in the management of chronic non-malignant pain. *Neurosurgery* 1999; 44:289–300.

Baltussen A, Kindler CH. Citation classics in anesthetic journals. *Anesth Analg* 2004; 98:443–451.

Basbaum AI. Spinal mechanisms of acute and persistent pain. *Reg Anesth Pain Med* 1999; 24:59–67.

Bennett G, Serafini M, Burchiel K, et al. Evidence-based review of the literature on intrathecal delivery of pain medication. *J Pain Symptom Manage* 2000a; 20:S19–S36.

Bennett G, Burchiel K, Buscher E, et al. Clinical guidelines for intraspinal infusion: report of an expert panel. *J Pain Symptom Manage* 2000b; 20:S37–S43.

Bogduk N. Management of chronic low back pain. *Med J Aust* 2004; 180:79–83.

Bogduk N, Karasek M. Two-year follow-up of a controlled trial of intradiscal electrothermal anuloplasty for chronic low back pain results from internal disc disruption. *Spine J* 2002; 2:343–350.

Botwin KP, Gruber RD, Bouchlas CG, et al. Complications of fluoroscopically guided transforaminal lumbar epidural injections. *Arch Phys Med Rehabil* 2000; 81:1045–1050.

Cameron T. Safety and efficacy of spinal cord stimulation for the treatment of chronic pain: 20-year literature review. *J Neurosurg* 2004; 100:254–267.

Carette S, Leclaire R, Marcoux S, et al. Epidural corticosteroid injections for sciatica due to herniated nucleus pulposus. *N Engl J Med* 1997; 336:1634–1640.

Carr DB, Cousins MJ. Spinal route of analgesia: opioids and future options. In: Cousins MJ, Bridenbaugh PO (Eds). *Neural Blockade in Clinical Anesthesia and Management of Pain.* Philadelphia: Lippincott-Raven, 1998, pp 915–983.

Cousins MJ. History of the development of pain management with spinal opioid and non-opioid drugs. *Opioids and Pain Relief: A Historical Perspective,* Progress in Pain Research and Management, Vol. 25. Seattle: IASP Press, 2003, pp 141–155.

Cousins MJ, Bridenbaugh PO (Eds). *Neural Blockade in Clinical Anesthesia and Management of Pain.* Philadelphia: Lippincott-Raven, 1998.

Cousins MJ, Mather LE. Intrathecal and epidural administration of opioids. *Anesthesiology* 1984; 61:276–310.

Cousins MJ, Miller RD. Intrathecal midazolam: an ethical editorial dilemma. *Anesth Analg* 2004; 98:1507–1508.

Cousins MJ, Reeve TS, Glynn CJ, Walsh JA, Cherry DA. Neurolytic lumbar sympathetic blockade: duration denervation and relief of rest pain. *Anaesth Intensive Care* 1979; 7:121–135.

Davis TT, Delamarter RB, Sra P, Goldstein TB. The IDET procedure for chronic discogenic low back pain. *Spine* 2004; 29:752–756.

Delport EG, Cucuzzella AR, Marley JK, Pruitt CM, Fisher JR. Treatment of lumbar spinal stenosis with epidural steroid injections: a retrospective outcome study. *Arch Phys Med Rehabil* 2004; 85:479–484.

Doggrell SA. Intrathecal ziconotide for refractory pain. *Expert Opin Investig Drugs* 2004; 13:875–877.

Dreyfuss P, Halbrook B, Pauza K, et al. Efficacy and validity of radiofrequency neurotomy for chronic lumbar zygapophyseal joint pain. *Spine* 2000; 25:1270–1277.

Duggan AW, Hall JG, Headley PM. Morphine, enkephalin and the substantia gelatinosa. *Nature* 1976; 264:456–458.

Eisenach JC, DuPen S, Dubois M, Miguel R, Allin D. Epidural clonidine analgesia for intractable cancer pain. The epidural clonidine study group. *Pain* 1995; 61:391–399.

Eisenach JC, De Kock M, Klimscha W. Alpha-2-adrenergic agonists for regional anesthesia: a clinical review of clonidine (1984–1995). *Anesthesiology* 1996; 85:655–674.

Eisenberg E, Carr DB, Chalmers TC. Neurolytic celiac plexus blockade for treatment of cancer pain: a meta-analysis. *Anesth Analg* 1995; 80:290–295.

Geurts JW, van Wijk RM, Stolker RJ, Groen GJ. Efficacy of radiofrequency procedures for the treatment of spinal pain: a systematic review of randomized clinical trials. *Reg Anesth Pain Med* 2001; 26:394–400.

Geurts JW, Kallewaard JW, Richardson J, Groen GJ. Targeted methylprednisolone acetate/hyaluronidase/clonidine injection after diagnostic epiduroscopy for chronic sciatica: a prospective 1-year follow up study. *Reg Anesth Pain Med* 2002; 27:343–352.

Goudas LC, Carr DB, Filos KS. The spinal clonidine-opioid interaction: from laboratory animals to the postoperative ward-a literature review of pre-clinical and clinical evidence. *Analgesia* 1998; 3:277–290.

Hassenbusch SJ, Portenoy RK. Current practices in intraspinal therapy—a survey of clinical trends and decision making. *J Pain Symptom Manage* 2000; 20:S4–S11.

Hassenbusch SJ, Satterfield WC, Gradert TL. A sheep model for continuous intrathecal infusion of test substances. *Hum Exp Toxicol* 1999; 18:82–87.

Hassenbusch SJ, Gunes S, Wachsman S, Willis KD. Intrathecal clonidine in the treatment of intractable pain: a phase I/II study. *Pain Med* 2002; 3:85–91.

Hassenbusch SJ, Portenoy RK, Cousins MJ, et al. Polyanalgesic Consensus Conference 2003: an update on the management of pain by intraspinal drug delivery—report of an expert panel. *J Pain Symptom Manage* 2004; 27:540–563.

Igarashi T, Hirabayashi Y, Seo N, et al. Lysis of adhesions and epidural injection of steroid/local anaesthetic during epiduroscopy potentially alleviate low back and leg pain in elderly patients with lumbar spinal stenosis. *Br J Anaesth* 2004; 93:181–187.

Johansen MJ, Gradert TL, Satterfield WC, et al. Safety of continuous intrathecal midazolam infusion in the sheep model. *Anesth Analg* 2004; 98:1528–1535.

Kang YJ, Eisenach JC. Intrathecal clonidine reduces hypersensitivity after nerve injury by a mechanism involving m4 muscarinic receptors. *Anesth Analg* 2003; 96:1403–1408.

Kemler MA, Furnee CA. Economic evaluation of spinal cord stimulation for chronic reflex sympathetic dystrophy. *Neurology* 2002; 59:1203–1209.

Kemler MA, Barendse GAM, van Kleef M, et al. Spinal cord stimulation in patients with chronic reflex sympathetic dystrophy. *N Engl J Med* 2000; 343:618–624.

Krainick JU, Thoden U. Spinal cord stimulation. In: Wall PD, Melzack R (Eds). *Textbook of Pain,* 2nd ed. New York: Churchill Livingston, 1989, pp 701–705.

Lin CR, Chuang YC, Cheng JT, Wang CJ, Yang LC. Intrathecal clonidine decreases spinal nitric oxide release in a rat model of complete Freund's adjuvant induced inflammatory pain. *Inflammation* 2002a; 26:161–166.

Lin CR, Yang LC, Lee TH, et al. Electroporation-mediated pain-killer gene therapy in mononeuropathic rats. *Gene Ther* 2002b; 9:1247–1253.

Lind G, Meyerson BA, Winter J, Linderoth B. Intrathecal baclofen as adjuvant therapy to enhance the effect of spinal cord stimulation in neuropathic pain: a pilot study. *Eur J Pain* 2004; 8:377–383.

McQuay HJ, Moore RA. Epidural corticosteroids for sciatica. In: McQuay HJ, Moore A. *An Evidence-Based Resource for Pain Relief.* Oxford University Press, 1998, pp 216–218.

Melzack R, Wall PD. Pain mechanisms: a new theory. *Science* 1965; 150:971.

Nitescu P, Dahm P, Appelgren L, Curelaru I. Continuous infusion of opioid and bupivacaine by externalized intrathecal catheters in long-tern treatment of "refractory" non-malignant pain. *Clin J Pain* 1998; 14:17–28.

North RB, Wetzel FT. Spinal cord stimulation for chronic pain of spinal origin: a valuable long term solution. *Spine* 2002; 27:2584–2591.

Oakley JC, Prager JP. Spinal cord stimulation: mechanisms of action. *Spine* 2002; 27:2574–2583.

Ohnmeiss DD, Rashbaum RF. Patient satisfaction with spinal cord stimulation for predominant complaints of chronic, intractable low back pain. *Spine J* 2001; 1:358–363.

Pauza KJ, Howell S, Dreyfuss P, et al. A randomized placebo controlled trial of intradiscal electrothermal therapy for the treatment of intradiscal low back pain. *Spine J* 2004; 4:27–35.

Prager JP. Neuroaxial medication delivery: the development and maturity of a concept for treating chronic pain of spinal origin. *Spine* 2002; 27:2593–2605.

Rawal N, Arner S, Gustafsson LL, Allvin R. Present state of extradural and intrathecal opioid analgesia in Sweden. A nationwide follow-up survey. *Br J Anaesth* 1987; 59:791–799.

Rozin L, Rozin R, Koehler SA, et al. Death during transforaminal epidural steroid nerve root block (C7) due to perforation of the left vertebral artery. *Am J Forensic Med Pathol* 2003; 24:351–355.

Schiff E, Eisenberg E. Can quantitative sensory testing predict the outcome of epidural steroid injections in sciatica? A preliminary study. *Anesth Analg* 2003; 97:828–832.

Shealy CN. Facet denervation in the management of back and sciatic pain. *Clin Orthop* 1976; 115:157–164.

Siddall PJ, Molloy AR, Walker S, et al. The efficacy of intrathecal morphine and clonidine in the treatment of pain after spinal cord injury. *Anesth Analg* 2000; 91:1493–1498.

Sinatra RS, Sevarino FB, Chung JH, et al. Comparison of epidurally administered sufentanil, morphine and sufentanil-morphine combination for post-operative analgesia. *Anesth Analg* 1991; 72:522–527.

Slipman CW, Chow DW. Therapeutic spinal corticosteroid injections for the management of radiculopathies. *Phys Med Rehabil Clin N Am* 2002; 13:697–711.

Slonimski M, Abram SE, Zuniga RE. Intrathecal baclofen in pain management. *Reg Anesth Pain Med* 2004; 29:269–276.

Smith TJ, Staats PS, Deer T, et al. Randomized clinical trial of an implantable drug delivery system compared with comprehensive medical management for refractory cancer pain: impact on pain, drug related toxicity, and survival. *J Clin Oncol* 2002; 20:4040–4049.

Smith TJ, Swainey C, Coyne PJ. Pain management, including intrathecal pumps. *Curr Oncol Rep* 2004; 6:291–296.

Staats PS, Hekmat H, Sauter P, Lillemoe K. The effects of alcohol celiac plexus block, pain, and mood on longevity in patients with unresectable pancreatic cancer: a double blind randomized, placebo-controlled study. *Pain Med* 2001; 2:28–34.

Staats PS, Yearwood T, Charapata SG, et al. Intrathecal ziconotide in the treatment of refractory pain in patients with cancer or AIDS: a randomized controlled trial. *JAMA* 2004; 291:63–70.

Stotz M, Oehen HP, Gerber H. Histological findings after long term infusion of intrathecal ketamine for chronic pain; a case report. *J Pain Symptom Manage* 1999; 18:223–228.

Tanaka M, Watanabe S, Matsumiya N, et al. Enhanced pain management for postgastrectomy patients with combined epidural morphine and fentanyl. *Can J Anaesth* 1997; 44:1047–1052.

Tiede JM, Huntoon MA. Review of spinal cord stimulation in peripheral arterial disease. *Neuromodulation* 2004; 7:168–175.

Tucker AP, Lai C, Nadeson R, Goodchild CS. Intrathecal midazolam I: a cohort study investigating safety. *Anesth Analg* 2004; 98:1512–1520.

Turner JA, Loeser JD, Bell KG. Spinal cord stimulation for chronic low back pain: a systematic literature synthesis. *Neurosurgery* 1995; 37:1088–1096.

Turner JA, Loescer JD, Deyo RA, Sanders SB. Spinal cord stimulation for patients with failed back surgery syndrome or complex regional pain syndrome: a systematic review of effectiveness and complications. *Pain* 2004; 108:137–147.

Valat JP, Giraudeau B, Rozenberg S, et al. Epidural corticosteroid injections for sciatica: a randomized, double-blind, controlled clinical trial. *Ann Rheum Dis* 2003; 62:639–643.

van Dongen RT, Crul BJ, van Egmond J. Intrathecal coadministration of bupivacaine diminishes morphine dose progression during long-term intrathecal infusion in cancer patients. *Clin J Pain* 1999; 15:166–172.

van Kleef M, Barendse GA, Kessels A, et al. Randomized trial of radiofrequency lumbar facet denervation for chronic low back pain. *Spine* 1999; 24:1937–1942.

van Tulder MW, Koes BW, Bouter LM. Conservative treatment of acute and chronic nonspecific low back pain. A systematic review of randomized controlled trials of the most common interventions. *Spine* 1997; 22:2128–2156.

Vranken JH, van der Vegt MH, Kal JE, Kruis MR. Treatment of neuropathic cancer pain with continuous intrathecal administration of S + -ketamine. *Acta Anaesthesiol Scand* 2004; 48:249–252.

Walker SM, Goudas LC, Cousins MJ, Carr DB. Combination spinal analgesic chemotherapy: a systematic review. *Anesth Analg* 2002; 95:674–715.

Willer JC, Boureau F, Albe-Fessard D. Supraspinal influences on nociceptive flexion reflex pain sensation in man. *Brain Res* 1979; 179:61–68.

Wong GY, Schroeder DR, Carns PE, et al. Effect of neurolytic celiac plexus block on pain relief, quality of life and survival in patients with unresectable pancreatic cancer: a randomized controlled trial. *JAMA* 2004; 291:1092–1099.

Yaksh TL. Epidural ketamine: a useful, mechanistically novel adjuvant to epidural morphine? *Reg Anesth* 1996; 21:508–513.

Yaksh TL, Allen JW. Preclinical insights into the implementation of intrathecal midazolam: a cautionary tale. *Anesth Analg* 2004a; 98:1509–1511.

Yaksh TL, Allen JW. The use of intrathecal midazolam in humans: a case study of process. *Anesth Analg* 2004b; 98:1536–1545.

Yaksh TL, Malmberg AB. Interaction of spinal modulatory receptor systems. In: Fields HL, Liebeskind JC (Eds). *Pharmacological Approaches to the Treatment of Chronic Pain, Progress in Pain Research and Management*, Vol. 1. Seattle: IASP Press, 1994, pp 1164–1172.

Yaksh TL, Rudy TA. Analgesia mediated by a direct spinal action of narcotics. *Science* 1976a; 192:1357–1358.

Yaksh TL, Rudy TA. Chronic catheterization of the spinal subarachnoid space. *Physiol Behav* 1976b; 17:1031–1036.

Yaksh TL, Rudy TA. Studies on the direct spinal action of narcotics in the production of analgesia in the rat. *J Pharmacol Exp Ther* 1977; 202:411–428.

Yaksh TL, Hassenbusch S, Burchiel K, et al. Inflammatory masses associated intrathecal drug infusions: a review of preclinical evidence and human data. *Pain Med* 2002; 3:300–312.

Yaksh TL, Horais KA, Tozier NA, et al. Chronically infused intrathecal morphine in dogs. *Anesthesiology* 2003; 99:174–187.

Yao MZ, Wang JH, Gu JF, et al. Interleukin-2 gene has superior antinociceptive effects when delivered intrathecally. *Neuroreport* 2002a; 13:791–794.

Yao MZ, Gu JF, Wang JH, et al. Interleukin-2 gene therapy of chronic neuropathic pain. *Neuroscience* 2002b; 12:409–416.

Yao MZ, Gu JF, Wang JH, et al. Adenovirus-mediated interleukin-2 gene therapy on nociception. *Gene Ther* 2003; 10:1392–1399.

Yu W, Maru F, Edner F, et al. Spinal cord stimulation for refractory angina pectoris: a retrospective analysis of efficacy and cost-benefit. *Coron Artery Dis* 2004; 15:31–37.

Zuniga RE, Schlicht CR, Abram SE. Intrathecal baclofen is analgesic in patients with chronic pain. *Anesthesiology* 2000; 92:876–880.

Zuniga RE, Perera S, Abram SE. Intrathecal baclofen: a useful agent in the treatment of well-established complex regional pain syndrome. *Reg Anesth Pain Med* 2002; 27(1):90–93.

Correspondence to: Professor Michael J. Cousins, MD, Professor of Anaesthesia and Pain Medicine, University of Sydney, Pain Management Research Institute, Royal North Shore Hospital, St Leonards, New South Wales 2065, Australia. Email: mcousins@doh.health.nsw.gov.au.

The Paths of Pain 1975–2005, edited by
Harold Merskey, John D. Loeser, and Ronald
Dubner, IASP Press, Seattle, © 2005.

32

Opioid Treatment for Cancer Pain and Chronic Noncancer Pain

Dwight E. Moulin

*Departments of Oncology and Clinical Neurological Sciences,
University of Western Ontario, and London Regional Cancer Centre,
London, Ontario, Canada*

Opium and its derivative, morphine, have been recognized for millennia as powerful analgesics. In 1680, Sydenham wrote, "Among the remedies which it has pleased Almighty God to give to man to relieve his sufferings, none is so universal and so efficacious as opium." Despite this awareness, Christian teaching saw pain as an expression of vitality and as a means of redemption. In the Victorian era, there was argument about the justification for using analgesia for childbirth and, to a lesser extent, for surgery, but the benefits of anesthesia quickly overwhelmed opposition. Popular use of opium preparations and derivatives was widespread in Victorian England, where the public was prone to self-medication, and concern arose over the indiscriminate and unregulated use of morphine and alcohol-based compounds (Holmes 2003). In the United States, the alarming spread of morphine use to the working class, coupled with a rising concern over iatrogenic addiction, led to the passage of the Harrison Narcotic Control Act in 1914. Opioid use came under such strict regulatory control that physicians were reluctant to prescribe narcotics at all, and, as a result, pain was grossly undertreated (Hill 1996). Even cancer pain did not escape the stigma attached to opioid use. An authoritative pronouncement in the *Journal of the American Medical Association* in 1941 had a major negative impact on a generation of physicians (Lee 1941). The article stated, "The use of narcotics in terminal cancer is to be condemned if it can possibly be avoided. Morphine and terminal cancer are in no way synonymous. Morphine use is an unpleasant experience to the majority of human subjects because of undesirable side effects. Dominant in the list of these unfortunate effects is addiction." Fortunately, by the time of the 1st World Congress of the IASP in 1975, this situation had changed due to advances on both sides of the Atlantic. Under the direction of Cicely Saunders in the United Kingdom in the early 1950s, the hospice movement was born. Saunders asserted that opioids were not addictive for patients with pain from advanced cancer, that opioids did not cause a major problem of tolerance, and that treatment of pain requires consideration of the whole person (Faull and Nicholson 2003). Concurrently, Beecher, Houde, and Rogers in the United States developed analgesic scales and testing methods using double-blind crossover trials to provide guidelines for the rational use of opioids in clinical practice (Meldrum 2003). Through this pioneering work, opioid therapy was re-established as accepted treatment for pain due to cancer and pain caused by any terminal disease. This chapter will outline some of the advances and controversies in opioid pharmacology and treatment over the past 30 years.

OPIOID PHARMACOLOGY

In 1975, clinicians appreciated that there was tremendous interindividual variability in opioid responsiveness, but very little was known about response mechanisms. The discovery of endogenous opioids or enkephalins in that year, coupled with the identification of the opiate receptor 2 years earlier, set the stage for an explosive increase in our knowledge of opioid pharmacology (Gutstein and Akil 2001). These advances explain some of the variability in opioid responsiveness and have provided important guidelines for the clinical use of opioid analgesics.

PHARMACOGENOMICS

Three distinct opioid receptor types have been characterized (mu, delta, and kappa), and splice variants of the µ-opioid receptor have been identified (Pasternak 2001). Polymorphisms in the µ-opioid receptor may explain differential responses to opioids with high µ-opioid affinity such as fentanyl. Polymorphisms also exist in the cytochrome P450 enzyme system that metabolizes many opioids. Codeine serves as a pro-drug for morphine, and about 10% of the Caucasian population lacks the CYP2D6 isoenzyme responsible for this conversion, making codeine ineffective as an analgesic for this subpopulation (Gutstein and Akil 2001).

METABOLISM

Metabolites play an important role in the analgesic and side-effect profiles of several opioids. Meperidine has a toxic metabolite, normeperidine, which accumulates with repetitive dosing and is cleared by the kidneys (Szeto et al. 1977). Normeperidine is a central nervous system (CNS) stimulant that leads to agitation, twitching, and seizures—especially in the setting of renal failure. Morphine-6-glucuronide (M6G) is an active metabolite of morphine that is also cleared by the kidneys. It is even more potent than the parent compound (Portenoy et al. 1992) and may contribute to the analgesic effects of morphine by acting through a splice variant of the morphine receptor (Rossi et al. 1996). M6G plays a significant role in the analgesic and side-effect profile of morphine, making morphine a poor choice in patients with renal failure. Morphine-3-glucuronide (M3G) and hydromorphone-3-glucuronide (H3G) do not have opioid activity, but they have neuroexcitatory effects in animals after direct injection into the CNS (Smith 2000). The role of M3G and H3G in generating agitation, myoclonus, and seizures in humans requires further study.

PHYSIOCHEMICAL PROPERTIES

There is conflicting evidence that protein binding alters opioid pharmacokinetics (Bernards 1999). However, lipid solubility is known to play an important role in opioid potency and bioavailability by different routes of administration (Bernards 1999). Fentanyl is several orders of magnitude more lipid soluble than morphine and allows for transdermal drug delivery. By bypassing the gastrointestinal tract, transdermal fentanyl probably causes a lower incidence of constipation than orally administered opioids (Ahmedzai and Brooks 1997). Rapid absorption via the oral mucosa makes the fentanyl lollipop useful in pediatric patients and makes sublingual fentanyl a good choice in adult patients with incident pain (Gourlay 1999).

ADJUVANT PROPERTIES OF OPIOIDS

Prolonged opioid therapy can lead to opioid-induced neurotoxicity, a state of abnormal pain sensitivity characterized by increased pain from noxious stimuli (hyperalgesia) and pain from previously innocuous stimuli (allodynia) (Ballantyne and Mao 2003). The observation of paradoxical hyperalgesia as an apparent manifestation of increased pain may prompt dose escalation, which would only make matters worse. Animal studies indicate that opioid-induced neurotoxicity and tolerance are linked to N-methyl-D-aspartate (NMDA) receptor activity (Mao et al. 1995) and suggest that NMDA antagonists may reverse both phenomena.

Opioids produce hormonal changes primarily by acting on the hypothalamic-pituitary-gonadal axis to increase prolactin and decrease gonadotrophic hormones. Prolactin elevation may result in amenorrhea and galactorrhea, and testosterone depletion may lead to decreased libido and, over the long term, osteoporosis (Abs et al. 2000).

Animal studies strongly suggest that prolonged opioid exposure can suppress both humoral and cell-mediated immunity (Roy and Loh 1996). The identification of morphine receptors on immune cells makes opioid modulation of the immune system even more convincing (Makman 1994). However, pain can also impair immune function, and the role of long-term opioid exposure remains to be elucidated.

OPIOID EQUIANALGESIC DOSES

Knowledge of relative analgesic potencies allows clinicians to switch from one opioid or one route of administration to another. Opioid rotation is common practice in cancer pain management (see below) and requires guidelines to facilitate proper dosing. Table I shows standard guidelines for equianalgesic doses of some common opioid analgesics based on a review of literature published between 1975 and 2004 (Jaffe and Martin 1975; Houde 1978; Foley 1985; Levy 1996; Bruera and Kim 2003). Clinicians recognized that early equianalgesic dose estimates were based on single-dose studies and served only as a useful reference point for initiation of dose titration (Foley 1985). As indicated in Table I, these guidelines have evolved over the years and reflect the empirical use of these drugs in clinical practice. Much of this evolution is based on the consequences of repetitive

Table I
Oral and parenteral equianalgesic doses of opioid analgesics

Drug	Route	Equianalgesic Dose (mg)	
		1975*	2005†
Morphine	i.m.	10	10
	p.o.	60	30
Codeine	i.m.	130	100
	p.o.	200	200
Hydromorphone	i.m.	1.5	2
	p.o.	7.5	6
Oxycodone	i.m.	15	–
	p.o.	30	15
Levorphanol	i.m.	2	2
	p.o.	4	4
Methadone	i.m.	10	0.75–5
	p.o.	20	1.5–10

* Adapted from Jaffe and Martin (1975) and Houde (1978).
† Adapted from Levy (1996) and Bruera and Kim (2003).

dosing. For instance, repetitive dosing of oral morphine allows for accumulation of M6G as an active metabolite, which may be responsible for the change in relative potency of intramuscular to oral morphine from 1:6 to 1:2 or 1:3 (Mercadante 1999). Although there is no evidence that hydromorphone has active analgesic metabolites, many centers use a 1:2 or 1:3 ratio for intramuscular to oral hydromorphone. The analgesic potency of methadone relative to other opioid analgesics is difficult to characterize because of its unique properties (Fishman et al. 2002). Methadone is lipophilic and has a long and variable elimination half-life due to its accumulation in fat stores. This feature results in prolongation of the duration of analgesia with repetitive dosing (8–12 hours or longer) in a manner that could not be predicted from single-dose studies. In addition, the d-isomer of methadone has NMDA-antagonist properties that may reverse analgesic tolerance to morphine and other opioids. This incomplete cross-tolerance between morphine and methadone is highly variable and is reflected in an oral methadone to morphine potency ratio in the range of 1:3 to 1:20 (Ripamonti et al. 1998; Bruera and Kim 2003).

OPIOID THERAPY FOR CANCER PAIN

Opioid analgesics remain the cornerstone of treatment for cancer patients with moderate to severe pain. Access to effective analgesics is important because more than 80% of patients with advanced cancer develop pain (Foley 2000). Guidelines for managing cancer pain have been developed by the World Health Organization (1990) and by the Agency for Healthcare Policy and Research (Jacox et al. 1994). These guidelines are based on the WHO three-step analgesic ladder and involve a combination of nonsteroidal anti-inflammatory drugs, opioids, and adjuvant analgesics titrated to pain severity and pathophysiology. Fortunately, field testing and clinical experience indicate that pain can be controlled in about 80% of cancer pain patients using these simple guidelines (Zech et al. 1995). Pain management is still challenging because some clinicians have inadequate pain assessment skills and lack knowledge of analgesic drug therapy. A review of cancer pain management in 54 oncology centers in the United States found that over one-third of patients had pain severe enough to impair their ability to function and that almost half were not given adequate analgesic therapy (Cleeland et al. 1994).

OPIOID ROTATION

Opioid rotation has become a valuable technique in managing cancer patients with difficult pain problems. It involves switching to a different opioid analgesic with the goal of improving analgesia and reducing limiting side effects (Noemi et al. 1995; Bruera et al. 1996). The rationale for opioid rotation is multifactorial. It may eliminate the adverse effects produced by the accumulation of toxic metabolites from the previous opioid. It may acknowledge differential opioid receptor affinity—for instance, methadone has greater affinity for the δ-opioid receptor than morphine (Fishman et al. 2002). The NMDA-antagonist properties of the *d*-isomer of methadone may make methadone especially useful for neuropathic pain (Gagnon et al. 2003). Perhaps the most important factor in the success of opioid rotation is interindividual differences in analgesic responsiveness, which may in part be related to pharmacogenomics (Pasternak 2001). In respect of incomplete cross-tolerance between opioids, the new opioid regimen should start at a daily dose at least 50% lower than the equianalgesic recommendation (Bruera and Kim 2003). This caveat is especially important in switching from other opioids to methadone.

ALTERNATE ROUTES OF OPIOID ADMINISTRATION

Although oral opioids are most convenient, most patients require at least two routes of drug administration, and 20% need up to four routes (Cherny et al. 1995). Buccal, sublingual, rectal, and transdermal routes are useful for patients with gastrointestinal tract dysfunction or intractable nausea or vomiting. The same population benefits from subcutaneous or intravenous infusions when intermittent dosing fails or when dose requirements become so high that they are no longer practical by other routes of administration. For patients who do not have intravenous access, subcutaneous infusion provides equivalent analgesia (Moulin et al. 1991).

The role of epidural and intrathecal infusions of opioids for refractory cancer pain remains controversial and requires further study. A randomized, double-blind comparison of the effectiveness of epidural and subcutaneous morphine in a crossover study in cancer patients found that the two modes of administration provided equal pain relief both at rest and during movement; there were no significant differences in adverse effects (Kalso et al. 1996). However, only 10 patients participated in this trial, and each stage of treatment was only 48 hours. A large randomized, controlled trial of intraspinal analgesia involving patients with refractory cancer pain reported benefit, but there was inadequate blinding of patients and investigators, and the findings are probably inconclusive (Smith et al. 2002).

ADVANCES IN THE MANAGEMENT OF CANCER PAIN

Our knowledge of the pharmacology of opioid analgesics has expanded rapidly over the past 20–30 years. These advances have provided some direction in selecting the right drug and the optimal route of administration for each patient. However, most of the factors responsible for interindividual variation in opioid responsiveness remain unexplained, and there is still a lot of trial and error in opioid selection. In addition, the principles guiding opioid management have essentially remained unchanged over the years (Houde 1978; Foley 1985; Levy 1996; Bruera and Kim 2003). Controlled-release opioids were introduced in the early 1980s and were found to be as effective as immediate-release preparations (Warfield 1998). This option provides convenience and perhaps compliance in pain management, but it is unlikely to change the outcome. Non-opioid advances include the use of bisphosphonates for bone pain and newer anticonvulsants such as gabapentin for neuropathic pain (Bruera and Kim 2003). Most clinicians are aware of the increasing gap between bench research and the bedside in pain management. In 1999, several prominent leaders in the pain field were asked whether advances in opioid pharmacology had influenced pain management. Patrick Wall stated, "astonishingly not," and similar sentiments were expressed by Cicely Saunders and Robert Twycross in the same year (Faull and Nicholson 2003). The major advance in cancer pain management over the past 20–30 years has probably been the ongoing education of physicians and allied health care workers in the management of cancer pain and other symptoms, although progress in this area is still woefully inadequate (Meier et al. 1997; Caron et al. 1999).

OPIOID THERAPY FOR CHRONIC NONCANCER PAIN

Management of chronic noncancer pain is an urgent problem. Extensive epidemiologic studies indicate that the prevalence of chronic pain in the developed world is in the range of 20–30% (Blyth et al. 2001; Moulin et al. 2002; Eriksen et al. 2003). Given the magnitude of the problem, a major dilemma for physicians is whether and how to prescribe opioid therapy for chronic pain. Extensive survey data on opioid use in chronic noncancer pain dating back to 1982 (Moulin 1999) suggested benefit without significant adverse events. In contrast, studies originating in multidisciplinary pain management programs suggested that chronic opioid therapy led to greater psychological distress, impaired cognition, and poor outcome (Portenoy 1994). All of these studies suffer from lack of adequate controls and inherent biases.

EVIDENCE FROM RANDOMIZED CONTROLLED TRIALS

Twelve high-quality randomized controlled trials have been published on the use of opioids for chronic noncancer pain using repetitive dosing for up to 9 weeks (Arkinstall et al. 1995; Moulin et al. 1996; Harati et al. 1998; Watson and Babul 1998; Caldwell et al. 1999; Peloso et al. 2000; Roth et al. 2000; Huse et al. 2001; Caldwell et al. 2002; Maier et al. 2002; Raja et al. 2002; Watson et al. 2003). These trials involve chronic musculoskeletal pain, neuropathic pain, and mixed pain syndromes at a maximal morphine dose of 180 mg per day. Fig. 1 shows that the spectrum of reduction of pain intensity relative to placebo in these studies is in the range of 20–40%. This percentage is probably significant given that Farrar et al. (2001) showed that a reduction of 2 points or 30% in a 0–10-point numerical rating scale of pain intensity represents a clinically important difference. However, 11 of these studies also examined disability outcomes; only six showed functional improvement, which was only marginal in two studies (Fig. 2). Evidence of substance abuse was extremely rare in these studies.

Evidence to date strongly suggests that significant pain relief can be achieved with opioid therapy for chronic noncancer pain. However, the outcome regarding functional improvement is less clear, which creates controversy due to lack of consensus as to what constitutes an acceptable outcome. In addition, evidence of efficacy from randomized controlled trials is limited by inherent selection biases in tertiary care centers and by the relatively small size and duration of these studies (Fig. 1). Evidence of effectiveness from data generated in the "real world" would be more meaningful, but such evidence is presently lacking. We need large-scale longitudinal observational studies with uniform well-defined outcome measures to determine the real benefit of opioid therapy for chronic noncancer pain.

RISK OF ADDICTION

Available data suggest that the rates of opioid abuse in chronic pain patients on long-term opioid therapy ranges from 3.2% to 18.9% (Fishbain et al. 1992). Absence of a history of substance abuse decreases the risk, but does not eliminate it. In our enthusiasm to relieve pain and suffering, physicians have dramatically increased the use of opioids for management of chronic pain over the last two decades. A recent survey found that the use of major opioids for chronic musculoskeletal pain increased from 2% of chronic pain visits in 1980 to 9% in 2000 (Caudill-Slosberg et al. 2004). Another survey found a similar increase in opioid prescriptions dispensed between 1994 and 2001 and, strikingly, the ratio of illicit to licit use of opioids

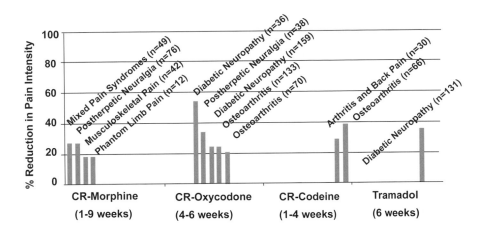

Fig. 1. Percentage reduction in pain intensity relative to placebo in double-blind, placebo-controlled studies of opioids in chronic noncancer pain. CR = controlled-release. Drugs studied, from left to right, were morphine (Maier et al. 2002; Raja et al. 2002; Moulin et al. 1996; Huse et al. 2001), oxycodone (Watson et al. 2003; Watson and Babul 1998; Gimbel et al. 2003; Roth et al. 2000; Caldwell et al. 1999), codeine (Arkinstall et al. 1995; Peloso et al. 2000), and tramadol (Harati et al. 1998).

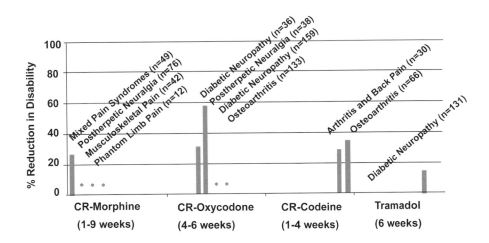

Fig. 2. Percentage reduction in disability in double-blind, placebo-controlled studies of opioids in chronic noncancer pain. Drugs studied, from left to right, were morphine (Maier et al. 2002; Raja et al. 2002; Moulin et al. 1996; Huse et al. 2001), oxycodone (Watson et al. 2003; Watson and Babul 1998; Gimbel et al. 2003; Roth et al. 2000), codeine (Arkinstall et al. 1995; Peloso et al. 2000), and tramadol (Harati et al. 1998). Asterisks (*) denote zero reduction in disability.

increased over 2000–2001—especially for oxycodone (Zacny et al. 2003). However, the problem is not specific to oxycodone. Screening for potential substance abuse and monitoring the risks and benefits of opioid treatment is time consuming. Standard guidelines for opioid management of chronic pain include documentation of the five A's—analgesia, analgesic dose, adverse effects, activity level, and aberrant drug-related behavior (Jovey et al. 2003). In the real world of primary and specialty care clinics, the tendency to bypass these guidelines increases the risk of substance abuse and drug diversion (Von Korff and Deyo 2004). Long-term opioid therapy is best carried out in practice settings where the resources are available to ensure comprehensive assessment and structured follow-up.

FUTURE ADVANCES IN OPIOID ANALGESICS

The holy grail of finding an opioid analgesic that provides good pain relief without significant adverse effects has been sought for over 100 years and is probably unattainable (Rice 2003). However, novel peripheral opioid antagonists have the ability to block the peripheral actions of opioids without affecting centrally mediated analgesia (Bates et al. 2004). Agents such as methylnaltrexone act outside the blood-brain barrier and have the potential to block nausea and vomiting as well as more classical peripheral opioid actions such as constipation. Conversely, opioid receptors are known to reside on peripheral sensory nerve terminals, and there is evidence that intra-articular injection of small doses of morphine during knee surgery can relieve postoperative pain. Peripherally selective opioid agents are being developed that might provide analgesia without central side effects (Schäfer 1999).

Pharmacogenomics is an exciting emerging field. Genetic mapping of the opioid receptor profile of an individual might facilitate the use of the right opioid analgesic for the right patient—perhaps one more step in unraveling the mystery of interindividual variation in opioid responsiveness.

REFERENCES

Abs R, Verhelst J, Maeyaert J, et al. Endocrine consequences of long-term intrathecal administration of opioids. *J Clin Endocrinol Metab* 2000; 85:2215–2222.

Ahmedzai S, Brooks D. Transdermal fentanyl versus sustained-release oral morphine in cancer pain: efficacy and quality of life. *J Pain Symptom Manage* 1997; 13:254–261.

Arkinstall W, Sandler A, Goughnour B, et al. Efficacy of controlled-release codeine in chronic non-malignant pain: a randomized, placebo-controlled clinical trial. *Pain* 1995; 62:169–178.

Ballantyne JC, Mao J. Opioid therapy for chronic pain. *N Engl J Med* 2003; 349:1943–1953.

Bates JJ, Foss JF, Murphy DB. Are peripheral opioid antagonists the solution to opioid side effects? *Anesth Analg* 2004; 98(1):116–122.

Bernards CM. Clinical implications of physicochemical properties of opioids. In: Stein C (Ed). *Opioids in Pain Control: Basic and Clinical Aspects.* New York: Cambridge University Press, 1999, pp 166–187.

Blyth FM, March LM, Brnabic AJM, et al. Chronic pain in Australia: a prevalence study. *Pain* 2001; 89:127–134.

Bruera E, Kim HN. Cancer pain. *JAMA* 2003; 290:2476–2479.

Bruera E, Pereira J, Watanabe S, et al. Opioid rotation in patients with cancer pain: a retrospective comparison of dose ratios between methadone, hydromorphone and morphine. *Cancer* 1996; 78:852–857.

Caldwell JR, Hale ME, Boyd RE, et al. Treatment of osteoarthritis pain with controlled release oxycodone or fixed combination oxycodone plus acetaminophen added to nonsteroidal anti-inflammatory drugs: a double-blind, randomized, multicentre, placebo controlled trial. *J Rheumatol* 1999; 26:862–869.

Caldwell JR, Rapoport RJ, Davis JC, et al. Efficacy and safety of a once-daily morphine formulation in chronic, moderate-to-severe osteoarthritis pain: results from a randomized, placebo-controlled, double-blind trial and an open-label extension trial. *J Pain Symptom Manage* 2002; 23:278–291.

Caron AT, Lynn J, Keaney P. End of life care in medical textbooks. *Ann Intern Med* 1999; 130:82–86.

Caudill-Slosberg MA, Schwartz LM, Woloshin S. Office visits and analgesic prescriptions for musculoskeletal pain in the U.S.: 1980 vs. 2000. *Pain* 2004; 109:514–519.

Cherny NI, Chang V, Frager G, et al. Opioid pharmacology in the management of cancer pain. *Cancer* 1995; 76:1283–1293.

Cleeland CS, Gonin R, Hatfield AK, et al. Pain and its treatment in outpatients with metastatic cancer. *N Engl J Med* 1994; 330:592–596.

Eriksen J, Jensen MK, Sjogren PS, et al. Epidemiology of chronic non-malignant pain in Denmark. *Pain* 2003; 106:221–228.

Farrar JT, Young JP, LaMoreaux L, et al. Clinical importance of changes in chronic pain intensity measured on an 11-point numerical pain rating scale. *Pain* 2001; 94(2):149–158.

Faull C, Nicholson A. Taking the myths out of the magic: establishing the use of opioids in the management of cancer pain. In: Meldrum ML (Ed). *Opioids and Pain Relief: A Historical Perspective,* Progress in Pain Research and Management, Vol. 25. Seattle: IASP Press, 2003, pp 111–129.

Fishbain DA, Rosomoff HL, Rosomoff RS. Drug abuse, dependence and addiction in chronic pain patients. *Clin J Pain* 1992; 8:77–85.

Fishman SM, Wilsey B, Mahajan G, et al. Methadone reincarnated: novel clinical applications with related concerns. *Am Acad Pain Med* 2002; 3:339–348.

Foley KM. The treatment of cancer pain. *N Eng J Med* 1985; 313:84–95.

Foley KM. Controlling cancer pain. *Hosp Pract (Off Ed)* 2000; 35:101–108, 111–112.

Gagnon B, Almahrezi A, Schreier G. Methadone in the treatment of neuropathic pain. *Pain Res Manage* 2003; 8(3):149–154.

Gourlay GK. Different opioids—same actions? In: Kalso E, McQuay HJ Wiesenfeld-Hallin Z (Eds). *Opioid Sensitivity of Chronic Noncancer Pain,* Progress in Pain Research and Management, Vol. 14. Seattle: IASP Press, 1999, pp 97–115.

Gutstein HB, Akil H. Opioid analgesics. In: Hardman JG, Limbird LL (Eds). *Goodman & Gilman's The Pharmacological Basis of Therapeutics,* 10th ed. New York: McGraw-Hill, 2001, pp 569–619.

Harati Y, Gooch C, Swenson M, et al. Double-blind randomized trial of tramadol for the treatment of pain of diabetic neuropathy. *Neurology* 1998; 50(6):1842–1846.

Hill CS Jr. Government regulatory influences on opioid prescribing and their impact on the treatment of pain of nonmalignant origin. *J Pain Symptom Manage* 1996; 11:287–298.

Holmes MS. The grandest badge of his art: three Victorian doctors, pain relief, and the art of medicine. In: Meldrum ML (Ed). *Opioids and Pain Relief: A Historical Perspective,* Progress in Pain Research and Management, Vol. 25. Seattle: IASP Press, 2003, pp 21–34.

Houde RW. Systemic analgesics and related drugs: narcotic analgesics. In: Bonica JJ, Ventafridda V, Fink RB, Jones LE, Loeser JD (Eds). *International Symposium on Pain of Advanced Cancer,* Advances in Pain Research and Therapy, Vol. 2. New York: Raven Press, 1978, pp 263–273.

Huse E, Larbig W, Flor H, et al. The effect of opioids on phantom limb pain and cortical reorganization. *Pain* 2001; 90:47–55.

Jacox A, Carr DB, Payne R, et al. *Management of Cancer Pain.* Clinical Practice Guideline No. 9, AHCPR Publication No. 94–0592. Rockville, MD: Agency for Health Care Policy and Research, 1994.

Jaffe JH, Martin WR. The pharmacological basis of therapeutics. In: Gilman A, Goodman LS (Eds). *Opioid Analgesics and Antagonists.* New York: MacMillan, 1975, pp 245–283.

Jovey RD, Ennis J, Gardner-Nix J, et al. Use of opioid analgesics for the treatment of chronic noncancer pain—a consensus statement and guidelines from the Canadian Pain Society, 2002. *Pain Res Manage* 2003; 8:3A–14A.

Kalso E, Heiskanen T, Rantio M, et al. Epidural and subcutaneous morphine in the management of cancer pain: a double-blind cross-over study. *Pain* 1996; 67:443–449.

Lee LE. Medication in the control of pain in terminal cancer. *JAMA* 1941; 116:216–219.

Levy MH. Pharmacologic treatment of cancer pain. *N Engl J Med* 1996; 335:1124–1132.

Maier C, Hildebrandt J, Klinger R, et al. Morphine responsiveness, efficacy and tolerability in patients with chronic non-tumour associated pain—results of a double-blind placebo-controlled trial (MONTAS). *Pain* 2002; 97:223–233.

Makman MH. Morphine receptors in immunocytes and neurons. *Adv Neuroimmunol* 1994; 4:69–82.

Mao J, Price DD, Mayer DJ. Mechanisms of hyperalgesia and opiate tolerance: a current view of their possible interactions. *Pain* 1995; 62:259–274.

Meier DE, Morrison RS, Cassel CK. Improving palliative care. *Ann Intern Med* 1997; 127;3–25.

Meldrum ML. A capsule history of pain management. *JAMA* 2003; 290:2470–2475.

Mercadante S. The role of morphine glucuronides in cancer pain. *Palliat Med* 1999; 13:95–104.

Moulin DE. Opioids in chronic nonmalignant pain. In: Stein C (Ed). *Opioids in Pain Control: Basic and Clinical Aspects.* New York: Cambridge University Press, 1999, pp 295–308.

Moulin DE, Kreeft JH, Murray-Parsons N, et al. Comparison of continuous subcutaneous and intravenous hydromorphone infusions for management of cancer pain. *Lancet* 1991; 337:465–468.

Moulin DE, Iezzi A, Amireh R, et al. Randomized trial of oral morphine for chronic non-cancer pain. *Lancet* 1996; 347:143–147.

Moulin DE, Clark AJ, Speechly M, et al. Chronic pain in Canada—prevalence, treatment, impact and the role of opioid analgesia. *Pain Res Manage* 2002; 7(4):179–184.

Noemi D, de Stoutz MD, Bruera E, et al. Opioid rotation for toxicity reduction in terminal cancer patients. *J Pain Symptom Manage* 1995; 10:378–384.

Pasternak GW. Incomplete cross-tolerance and multiple mu opioid peptide receptors. *Trends Pharmacol Sci* 2001; 22:67–70.

Peloso PM, Bellamy N, Bensen W, et al. Double-blind randomized placebo control trial of controlled-release codeine in the treatment of osteoarthritis of the hip or knee. *J Rheumatol* 2000; 19:764–771.

Portenoy RK. Opioid therapy for chronic nonmalignant pain: current status. In: Fields HL, Liebeskind JC (Eds). *Pharmacological Approaches to the Treatment of Chronic Pain: New Concepts and Critical Issues,* Progress in Pain Research and Management, Vol. 1. Seattle: IASP Press, 1994, pp 247–287.

Portenoy RK, Thaler HT, Inturrisi CE, et al. The metabolite morphine-6-glucuronide contributes to the analgesia produced by morphine infusion in patients with pain and normal renal function. *Clin Pharmacol Ther* 1992; 51:422–431.

Raja SN, Haythornthwaite JA, Pappagallo, et al. Opioids versus antidepressants in postherpetic neuralgia: a randomized, placebo–controlled trial. *Neurology* 2002; 59:1015–1021.

Rice KC. Analgesic research at the National Institutes of Health: state of the art 1930s to the present. In: Meldrum ML (Ed). *Opioids and Pain Relief: A Historical Perspective,* Progress in Pain Research and Management, Vol. 25. Seattle: IASP Press, 2003, pp 57–83.

Ripamonti C, Groff L, Brunelli C, et al. Switching from morphine to oral methadone in treating cancer pain: what is the equianalgesic dose ratio? *J Clin Oncol* 1998; 16:3216–3221.

Rossi GC, Brown GP, Leventhal L, Yang K, Pasternak GW. Novel receptor mechanisms for heroin and morphine-6 beta-glucuronide analgesia. *Neurosci Lett* 1996; 216:1–4.

Roth SH, Fleischmann RM, Burch RX, et al. Around-the-clock, controlled-release oxycodone therapy for osteoarthritis-related pain: placebo-controlled trial and long-term evaluation. *Arch Intern Med* 2000; 160:853–860.

Roy S, Loh HH. Effects of opioids on the immune system. *Neurochem Res* 1996; 21:1375–1386.

Schäfer M. Efficacy of peripheral opioid analgesia in inflammatory pain: evidence from clinical studies. In: Kalso E, McQuay HJ, Wiesenfeld-Hallin Z (Eds). *Opioid Sensitivity of Chronic Noncancer Pain,* Progress in Pain Research and Management, Vol. 14. Seattle: IASP Press, 1999, pp 327–336.

Smith MT. Neuroexcitatory effects of morphine and hydromorphone: evidence implicating the 3-glucuronide metabolites. *Clin Exp Pharmacol Physiol* 2000; 27:524–528.

Smith TJ, Staats PS, Deer T, et al. Randomized clinical trial of an implantable drug delivery system compared with comprehensive medical management for refractory cancer pain: impact on pain, drug-related toxicity and survival. *J Clin Oncol* 2002; 20:4040–4049.

Szeto HH, Inturrisi CE, Houde R, et al. Accumulation of normeperidine, an active metabolite of meperidine, in patients with renal failure or cancer. *Ann Intern Med* 1977; 86:738–741.

Von Korff M, Deyo RA. Editorial—potent opioids for chronic musculoskeletal pain: flying blind? *Pain* 2004; 109:207–209.

Warfield CA. Controlled-release morphine tablets in patients with chronic cancer pain: a narrative review of controlled clinical trials. *Cancer* 1998; 82(12):2299–2306.

Watson CPN, Babul N. Efficacy of oxycodone in neuropathic pain: a randomized trial in postherpetic neuralgia. *Neurology* 1998; 50:1837–1841.

Watson CPN, Moulin DE, Watt-Watson J, et al. Controlled-release oxycodone relieves neuropathic pain: a randomized, controlled trial in painful diabetic neuropathy. *Pain* 2003; 105:71–78.

World Health Organization. *Cancer Pain Relief and Palliative Care.* Geneva: World Health Organization, 1990.

Zacny J, Bigelow G, Compton P, et al. College on Problems of Drug Dependence taskforce on prescription opioid non-medical use and abuse: position statement. *Drug Alcohol Depend* 2003; 69:215–232.

Zech DFJ, Grond S, Lynch J, et al. Validation of the World Health Organization guidelines for cancer pain relief: a 10-year prospective study. *Pain* 1995; 63:65–76.

Correspondence to: Dwight E. Moulin, MD, London Regional Cancer Centre, 790 Commissioners Road East, London, Ontario N6A 4L6, Canada. Tel: 519-685-8661; Fax: 519-685-8636; email: dwight.moulin@lrcc.on.ca.

The Paths of Pain 1975–2005, edited by
Harold Merskey, John D. Loeser, and Ronald
Dubner, IASP Press, Seattle, © 2005.

33

Topical Agents for Neuropathic Pain: A Systematic Review

C. Peter N. Watson

University of Toronto, Toronto, Ontario, Canada

"about 1550 B.C. ... in Thebes, death befell an architect by the name of Cha. He was laid in his grave with an alabaster pot full of ointment ... chemically and physiologically ... like morphine. What opium would be doing in an ointment I do not know." Guido Majno (1975, p. 111)

The above quotation perhaps provides an example of the use in the ancient world of a topical analgesic for pain. We now know that morphine has a peripheral as well as a central action. Contemporary scientifically proven oral drugs such as antidepressants, anticonvulsants, and opioids are effective in treating some chronic painful conditions. None of these has better than a modest effect, and adverse effects are problematic, particularly in older patients. Furthermore, many patients with chronic pain receive little, if any, benefit from these agents. Simple, effective approaches without significant adverse effects would be an advantage for use alone or as adjunctive therapy. Topical approaches offer the promise of such a treatment.

Topical agents for pain include local anesthetics, capsaicin, and nonsteroidal anti-inflammatories, among others. The most extensively studied are capsaicin and local anesthetics, particularly lidocaine. Capsaicin has had significant limitations because its effect is modest at best, the side effect of burning is problematic, and there may be a large placebo effect. Past clinical trials could not be adequately blinded due to the burning sensation the compound almost always elicits. New research on capsaicin receptors and new compounds have regenerated interest in this area. Local anesthetics appear to be the most practical of the topical agents, and the most extensive research has been done with lidocaine. Interesting new data have emerged about topical antidepressants. This chapter will focus on randomized controlled trials (RCTs) (Table I), particularly in neuropathic pain, but will also

Table I

Published randomized controlled trials of topical agents for neuropathic pain

Condition (Reference)	Agent	N*	Effect	Score†	Comments
Local Anesthetics					
Postherpetic neuralgia (Rowbotham et al. 1995)	5% lidocaine gel	46/39 (16 cranial; 23 torso-limb)	Yes	4	Long-term; 23/31 reported moderate or better relief after 2 months.
Postherpetic neuralgia (Rowbotham et al. 1996)	5% lidocaine patch	36/35	Yes	4	Limb/torso only, cranial not included; 10/35 (28%) had moderate or better relief; "patch effect."
Postherpetic neuralgia (Galer et al. 1999)	5% lidocaine patch	33/32	Yes	5	Enriched enrollment (only patch responders entered into trial); aim to assess the "patch effect." Skin reaction in about 30%.
Focal peripheral pain syndromes (Meier et al. 2003)	5% lidocaine patch	58/40	Yes	5	NNT = 4.0 (overall); 8.4 (allodynia).
Postherpetic neuralgia (Galer et al. 2002)	5% lidocaine patch	96	Yes	4	Used neuropathic pain scale. All non-allodynia qualities benefited.
Capsaicin					
Postherpetic neuralgia (Bernstein et al. 1989)	Capsaicin 0.075% vs. vehicle parallel	33/29	Yes	4	30% of capsaicin had burning. Blinding broken?
Postherpetic neuralgia (Watson et al. 1993)	Capsaicin 0.075% vs. vehicle parallel	143/131	Yes	4	60% burning with capsaicin (vs. 33%). Effectiveness not assessed.
Postmastectomy syndrome (Watson et al. 1993)	0.075% capsaicin vs. vehicle parallel, 6 wk.	25/24	Yes	4	Capsaicin burning a problem. Blinded?
Diabetic neuropathy (Chad et al. 1990)	0.075% capsaicin vs. vehicle parallel, 4 wk.	58/46	Yes	4	Only one outcome measure significant (VAS pain relief). Placebo effect large (50%).
Diabetic neuropathy (Capsaicin Study Group 1991)	0.075% capsaicin vs. vehicle parallel, 8 wk.	277/219	No	4	ITT analysis no difference. Placebo effect = 58%. Burning a problem. Blinded?

		No. patients entered/completed[*]		Score[†]	
Capsaicin					
Painful polyneuropathy (Low et al. 1995)	0.075% capsaicin vs. placebo (methyl nicotinate), other limb control, 12 wk.	40/39	No	4	Large placebo effect (66.7%). Due to active agent? 73% burning with capsaicin. Blinded?
Surgical neuropathic pain in cancer patients (Ellison et al. 1997)	Capsaicin cream 0.075% vs. placebo, 8 wk. cross-over	101/71	Yes	4	Pain reduction = 53% vs. 17%. Adverse effects increased with capsaicin. Blinded? Equal dropouts.
HIV-associated neuropathy (Paice et al. 2000)	Capsaicin cream 0.075% vs. vehicle, 8 wk. parallel	26/14	No	4	Increased dropouts with capsaicin (67% vs. 18%)
Cluster headache (Saper et al. 2002)	Intranasal civamide vs. vehicle, 7 days parallel	28/24	Yes	4	Decreased headache with civamide. Increased burning with civamide. Blinded?
Migraine (Diamond et al. 2000)	Intranasal civamide 20 mg vs. 150 mg, single headache, Rx parallel	37/36	Yes	4	No placebo. "May be effective." Results similar at both doses.
Nonsteroidals					
Postherpetic neuralgia (McQuay et al. 1990)	Benzydamine cream, 6 wk. cross-over	23	No	4	
Antidepressants					
Neuropathic pain (McCleane 2000a)	Topical 5% doxepin vs. placebo, 4 wk.	40/30	Yes	5	Intent-to-treat analysis. Minimal side effects. Statistically significant difference, but clinical meaningfulness unclear.
Neuropathic pain (McCleane 2000b)	Topical doxepin vs. capsaicin vs. doxepin/capsaicin vs. placebo	200/151 (41 dox.; 33 cap.; 36 dox./cap.; 41 plac.)	Yes	4	Intent-to-treat analysis. Blinding may have been threatened by capsaicin-related burning sensation. Clinical meaningfulness unclear, but 40% said they wanted to continue with capsaicin or doxepin. Delay in onset of analgesia of 2 wk. Capsaicin alone reduced sensitivity and shooting pain.

* No. patients entered/completed (no./group). † Score on a 0–5-point rating scale to assess the quality of trials (Jadad et al. 1996).

include uncontrolled data and information on topical agents for non-neuropathic pain. It will also consider the history of topical agents and mention future possible approaches.

METHODS

A systematic review was conducted utilizing the terms "topical agents, "chronic pain," "neuropathic pain," and "randomized controlled trial" to search for RCTs published in English between 1966 and 2004. Specific searches were also conducted for "topical lidocaine," "topical capsaicin," "topical nonsteroidals," and "topical antidepressants" in chronic and neuropathic pain. In order to be as complete as possible, literature searches were carried out with the help of a librarian. Databases used were Medline, EMBASE, CINAHL, PubMed, and the Cochrane Library of Systematic Reviews. I also searched reference lists of previous reviews and sent email inquiries to researchers in this area. Important historical and uncontrolled observations were also sought. For inclusion in the evidence-based group studies (Table I), the study was required to be published in full in English, involve adults, be double blinded and randomized, account for withdrawals, and have a control group. Important historical data and uncontrolled trials were also sought. The specific quality assessment measure used for RCTs was the rating scale described by Jadad et al. (1996). A particular issue was whether the positive results of an RCT are of clinical importance. In order to evaluate clinical importance, number-needed-to-treat (NNT) data (Laupacis et al. 1988; Cook and Sackett 1995) were obtained from previous systematic reviews and, when available, from recent publications (Table II). These numbers were used to compare different topical agents and to provide comparative data for antidepressants, gabapentin, pregabalin, opioids, tramadol, and other drugs shown by RCT to relieve neuropathic pain. Some caution should be taken in using these figures because they compare studies of differing experimental designs (crossover versus parallel), different numbers of study patients, and various methods of data analysis.

LOCAL ANESTHETICS

> " Pure cocaina … leaves upon the tongue a peculiar numbness, followed by a sensation of cold." Albert Niemann (1860)

Table II
Number-needed-to-treat (NNT) data in some neuropathic pain conditions

Drug and Reference	Condition				Comments
	PHN	PDN	PN	CP	
Antidepressants					
McQuay et al. 1996	2.3	3.0		1.7	SR
Sindrup and Jensen 1999	2.3	2.4		1.7	Review
Collins et al. 2000	2.1	3.4			RCT
Venlafaxine					
Sindrup et al. 2003			5.2		RCT
Imipramine					
Sindrup et al. 2003			2.7		RCT
Gabapentin					
Sindrup and Jensen 1999	3.2	3.7			SR
Rice et al. 2001	5.0				RCT
Pregabalin					
Dworkin et al. 2003	3.4				RCT
Oxycodone					
Watson and Babul 1998	2.5				RCT
Watson et al. 2003		2.6			RCT
Tramadol					
Sindrup and Jensen 1999			3.4		SR
Lidocaine patch					
Meier et al. 2003			4.4		RCT
Capsaicin					
Sindrup and Jensen 1999			5.3		SR

Note: Caution should be used in interpreting these figures as they involve studies of differing experimental designs, numbers of patients, and data analyses. CP = central pain; PDN = painful diabetic neuropathy; PHN = postherpetic neuralgia; PN = painful neuropathy; RCT = randomized controlled trial; SR = systematic review.

HISTORICAL ASPECTS

Cocaine, the first local anesthetic, has the topical effect of numbness on the mucous membrane of the tongue, as noted by Albert Niemann in 1860 when he first isolated the drug. Since then, local anesthetics have been given to count-less patients by various routes to control acute and chronic pain.

MECHANISM OF ACTION

Local anesthetics act on cell membranes to prevent the generation and spread of nerve impulses (Catterall and Mackie 1996). They act by blocking voltage-gated sodium channels, which are responsible for the transient increase in the permeability of excitable membranes to Na^+ that is normally produced by depolarization of the membrane. This anesthetic effect elevates the threshold and slows the rate of rise of the action potential and at lower concentrations slows conduction velocity. The Aδ and C fibers that subserve pain are more susceptible to local anesthetics than are large fibers because they are blocked earlier and to greater degree. This greater susceptibility is thought to be related to such factors as the shorter internodal distances of smaller fibers. An important factor in the action of local anesthetics is pH. Because these agents are only slightly soluble as unprotonated amines, they are marketed as water-soluble hydrochlorides, which causes them to be mildly acidic and thus more stable. The unprotonated form is necessary for diffusion across cell membranes, but the cationic (basic) form seems to act preferentially on sodium channels. Both forms, however, have anesthetic activity. The action of topical local anesthetics in neuropathic pain could depend on an effect on peripheral factors such as ectopic discharges from sensitized cutaneous nerves bombarding the dorsal horn of the spinal cord. These damaged or regenerating sensitized fibers undergo changes in the number and location of sodium channels. Ectopic impulses from injured peripheral nerves may be sensitive to lower concentrations of local anesthetic than are required for blocking normal impulse conduction (Chabal et al. 1989). Normal, intact skin is a significant barrier to the action of topical agents. Areas of greater skin thickness, such as the palm of the hand, are subject to a slower onset of analgesia. Highly vascular skin, such as facial skin, is associated with a more rapid onset but a shorter duration of anesthetic effect. The damaged skin in such neuropathic pain conditions as postherpetic neuralgia (PHN) may also influence the action of topical agents, although it is not clear in which direction. The skin is better penetrated by base forms of local anesthetics than by the mildly acidic hydrochloride forms commonly used (Dalili and Adriani 1971). Formulations such as EMLA Cream (Astra Pharmaceuticals; 2.5% lidocaine and 2.5% prilocaine) and Lidoderm (Endo Pharmaceuticals; 5% lidocaine) were developed to improve transdermal delivery.

UNCONTROLLED TRIALS

Uncontrolled trials have reported a benefit of EMLA in PHN (Stow et al. 1989; Attal et al. 1999). Devers and Galer (2000) have shown benefit for the lidocaine patch in several neuropathic pain states, including incisional neuralgia, painful diabetic neuropathy, complex regional pain syndrome, and post-amputation stump pain.

RANDOMIZED CONTROLLED TRIALS

Rowbotham and coworkers (1995) reported an RCT of 5% lidocaine in gel form in PHN. A total of 39 out of 46 patients entering the study completed the three-session crossover study. The 16 patients with facial or upper cervical PHN had gel applied without an occlusive dressing during the 8-hour ses-sions, and the 23 patients with PHN of the torso and limbs had gel applied under Tegaderm dressings for 24 hours. A significant decrease in pain intensity and a significant increase in pain relief scores occurred with lidocaine gel compared to vehicle at 8 and 24 hours in the torso/limb group. In the facial upper cervical group, there were no significant differences between active drug and vehicle in pain scores, but pain relief scores significantly favored the active drug at nearly all time points. Because occlusive dressings used with topical agents are poorly tolerated and are impractical for many PHN sufferers, a gel of 5% lidocaine has been incorporated into adhesive patches with a non-woven, polyethylene adhesive backing that can be used to cover the area of pain. Rowbotham et al. (1996) have demonstrated the benefit of the lidocaine patch in subjects with PHN affecting the torso or extremities who completed a four-session, crossover, random-order, double-blinded, vehicle-controlled study of the patch's analgesic effects. Lidocaine patches were superior to both no-treatment observations and vehicle patches in pain relief scores. Minimal systemic absorption was documented. No systemic side effects occurred, and the patches were well tolerated on allodynic skin for 12 hours. The majority (24 of 35 subjects) reported partial pain relief, with 10 of 35 subjects (28%) noting moderate or better relief. The vehicle patch alone had a significant pain-reducing effect compared with no treatment, presumably by protecting painful, sensitive skin from contact with clothing and gentle touch.

Galer et al. (1999) addressed the contribution of the vehicle patch versus the lidocaine patch in providing relief in PHN. This study had an enriched enrollment design as all 33 subjects had experienced moderate or better relief with topical lidocaine patches on a regular basis for at least a month prior to study enrollment. Twenty-five of 32 subjects (78%) preferred the lidocaine patch as compared with 3/32 (9.4%) for the vehicle patch. The most common untoward effect was "application site reaction" (skin redness or rash), which occurred in about 30% of patients in each group. The authors concluded that the topical lidocaine patch gave significantly better pain relief than did the vehicle patch.

Galer et al. (2002) conducted an RCT that found that the 5% lidocaine patch improved all non-allodynic pain qualities in 96 patients with PHN using a neuropathic pain scale. Meier et al. (2003) carried out an RCT of the

5% lidocaine patch in patients with a variety of peripheral neuropathic pain syndromes. Forty of 58 patients completed this crossover study of the patch as an add-on therapy. The important findings were that the patch was effective over 7 days and that it was useful in neuropathic pain other than PHN. An NNT of 4.4 was obtained, with a higher NNT for allodynia of 8.4.

In conclusion, the topical lidocaine patch holds promise for the treatment of PHN and other neuropathic conditions. The patch itself appears to be an advance over occlusive "food wrap" type dressings because it seems better tolerated, can be cut to fit the area of pain, and may protect against the light tactile stimuli that so often provoke pain in PHN. The patch may have limitations if the pain is in the distribution of the ophthalmic division of the trigeminal nerve (one of the most common sites for intractable PHN) because patients may have severe pain in the scalp areas (to which the patch cannot easily be affixed). Of interest is the lesser effect on allodynia noted and the relief of all the components of non-allodynic pain. One might have expected that allodynia might be better relieved by the patch than other pain types. Skin reactions, reported in 30% of patch users, are one possible limiting adverse effect. The lidocaine patch can be recommended as monotherapy in neuropathic pain or, if a partial effect occurs, as an adjunct to oral agents such as antidepressants, anticonvulsants, or opioids. Further studies of the lidocaine patch are necessary in other neuropathic pain conditions.

TOPICAL CAPSAICIN

"My plan of treatment is to saturate a piece of flannel with concentrated tincture of capsicum and to rub well over the chilblains until a strong tingling and electrical feeling is produced. … The application ought to be continued daily until the disease is removed … relief will be experienced on the very first application … the manner of using it [capsicum] for toothache is by putting a drop … of the tincture on cotton and applying it to the part affected." A. Turnbull (1850)

HISTORICAL ASPECTS

Capsaicin is derived from chili peppers and similar plants of the capsicum plant family. These plants contain about 0.1–2.0% capsaicin. They were used in Mexico in cooking and probably as pharmacological agents as long ago as 7000 BC (Lembeck 1987). Capsaicin seeds and plant stock were brought to Europe and then to Persia, Africa, India, and the Far East by Columbus and subsequent explorers to the New World. It is possible that hot peppers became popular as food additives in hot climates because the gustatory perspiration induced by the effects of capsaicin on thermoregulation could potentially diminish the heat produced by the ingestion of a heavy meal and thereby aid digestion in these warm conditions. The use of these plants' derivatives as pharmacological agents is more difficult to explain because application of capsaicin to the skin or mucous membranes usually increases the severity of a painful condition. It is interesting to speculate that this phenomenon caused ancient physicians to believe that capsaicin was a powerful therapy. Alternatively, they may have recognized that this initial aggravation of symptoms was sometimes followed by pain relief. Perhaps cutaneous vasodilation and the feeling of warmth generated by capsaicin topically led to its use in rheumatic disorders. In 1850, Turnbull reported that hot pepper extract applied on cotton to an aching tooth relieved the pain; he also recommended it for chilblains. In 1878, Hogyes first reported the typical burning caused by capsaicin after mucous membrane application or subcutaneous injection, stating that this sensation was associated with salivation, gastric secretion, and hyperemia, but with no other signs of inflammation. The pain produced by capsaicin is produced by stimulation of unmyelinated fibers sensitized by thermal stimuli. Animals treated with increasing doses of parenteral capsaicin, or given local applications of capsaicin, became desensitized to various chemical stimuli, with a subsequent slow recovery (Jansco 1964). This capsaicin-induced desensitization prevents neurogenic inflammatory responses due to a variety of causes. Later studies demonstrated that neonatal rats given systemic capsaicin developed permanent loss of sensitivity to chemical irritations, which was associated with destruction of small dorsal root ganglion cells and unmyelinated primary afferents, with no damage to the larger-diameter sensory fibers. These findings prompted many laboratories to study the action of capsaicin, yielding an expansion of information about its action as a specific toxin for C fibers. Capsaicin has been found to bind to the vanilloid receptor (Caterina et al. 1997; see the Mechanism of Action section below).

Over-the-counter topical remedies containing capsaicin have been available for years. A recent application of capsaicin has been its addition to bird seed as a squirrel repellant. Birds are less affected by capsaicinoids, perhaps related to their role in disseminating the seeds of these plants. Capsaicin spray is in widespread use as an animal and human repellant. Capsaicin formulations have been recommended for a variety of ailments, chiefly rheumatic. Early clinical trials of topical capsaicin were performed in PHN (Bernstein et al. 1987; Watson et al. 1988). Positive preliminary results led to the use of capsaicin to treat a variety of other neuropathic pain problems, as well as arthritis and disorders of the skin and mucous membranes. To date, it has been difficult to interpret the suggested positive results of these open-label trials by RCT because of the impossibility of maintaining blinding due to the burning sensation induced by the active agent capsaicin and in some trials a large placebo effect.

MECHANISM OF ACTION

Capsaicin causes highly selective excitation of unmyelinated C-fiber afferents (Lynn 1990). In the skin, this mechanism involves nociceptive C fibers of the polymodal (or "mechano-heat") class. Other types of C fibers and larger afferents are unaffected. Levels of the neuropeptide substance P are greatly reduced by capsaicin. Other peptide neurotransmitters are also reduced, including calcitonin gene-related peptide (CGRP), somatostatin, vasoactive intestinal polypeptide (VIP), and probably others. It is of interest that substance P alone is only weakly excitatory to cutaneous afferents and is not painful on application to cutaneous blister bases in humans (Lynn 1990). This finding argues for the initial burning sensation induced by capsaicin being due to more than substance P release. In 1997 a gene was discovered to code for the capsaicin receptor (Caterina et al. 1997). This receptor is the vanilloid receptor (TRPV1) and is expressed only on C fibers. This receptor is thought to mediate the flow of calcium and sodium from the outside to the inside of the neuron and is activated by above-normal temperature, suggesting the transduction of thermal stimuli (Caterina et al. 1997). Chemical activation of this receptor results in desensitization and degeneration of C fibers, thereby blocking afferent input. Degeneration of epidermal fibers has been shown in humans with repeated application of capsaicin (Biro et al. 1997), and this finding might account for some of the analgesia. How significant this effect is with current commercial capsaicin products is unknown. In humans, topical application of capsaicin causes marked hyperalgesia to skin heating and pressure (Carpenter and Lynn 1981), vasodilation, and a burning sensation. After repeated exposures, desensitization occurs with peptide depletion, and the above effects diminish and may disappear. Pain reduction in humans may be due to a block of afferent input (Lynn 1990). The observed delay in onset with some studies may be due to the time required for the relatively low concentrations of capsaicin in the topical preparations to take effect. It is also possible that capsaicin might diminish the increased peripheral and central excitability that may occur in chronic pain statues due to excessive C-fiber input. Selective reduction in afferent input may be more important in pain relief than the more complete interruption that occurs with surgical deafferentation procedures, which are usually unsuccessful and can make the painful state worse. There is some evidence that repeated topical application of 0.075% capsaicin in humans may cause degeneration of epidermal nerve fibers (Nolano et al. 1996). This degeneration may contribute to the analgesic effect, but the eventual clinical importance of this finding is uncertain.

POSTHERPETIC NEURALGIA: RANDOMIZED CONTROLLED TRIALS

An RCT of 33 patients with PHN (Bernstein et al. 1989) was carried out using 0.075% capsaicin. All patients had pain of 12 months' duration or longer (mean = 3 years), and 29 patients completed the trial. An efficacy analysis revealed improvement in favor of capsaicin on scales of pain severity and pain relief. Of capsaicin-related patients, 30% experienced cutaneous burning, making the study impossible to totally blind. An RCT of topical 0.075% capsaicin in PHN indicated an improvement in the pain severity and relief scales in favor of the active agent (Watson et al. 1993). Long-term follow-up suggested a persistent beneficial effect. The burning induced by capsaicin rendered blinding of the trial problematic (60% of the patients utilizing capsaicin experienced burning versus 33% of those treated with placebo, and 18% of the capsaicin group discontinued therapy because of it). Overall, this trial did not adequately assess the clinical meaningfulness of this agent because it did not determine how many patients were satisfied with the amount of pain relief obtained. The pain severity and relief scales suggest that the amount of change with capsaicin was modest (only 20% of patients had nearly complete pain relief). The authors concluded that capsaicin was not a panacea. Both the results of these studies and clinical experience indicate that in PHN the improvement from current capsaicin preparations, if it occurs, is modest, that burning is problematic, and that many patients are dissatisfied with the degree of relief when capsaicin is used as the only therapy. Thus, this agent may work best as an adjuvant to other agents, such as antidepressants, anticonvulsants, and opioids.

PAINFUL DIABETIC NEUROPATHY: RANDOMIZED CONTROLLED TRIALS

There are five published reports of RCTs of 0.075% capsaicin to treat painful diabetic neuropathy (Chad et al. 1990; Capsaicin Study Group 1991). Four of these are smaller studies, and three seem to be part of the largest trial. Chad and colleagues reported the result of an RCT in 58 patients with diabetic polyneuropathy. Patients received topical capsaicin 0.075% four times daily for 4 weeks; 46 patients completed the trial, of whom 24 received

capsaicin. Results reached statistical significance in only one outcome measure—a visual analogue pain relief scale—at 4 weeks. These authors concluded that they could not answer the primary study questions, noting that
their study may have been too small and of too short a duration to show
efficacy, particularly given the large placebo effect (41–50%).The Capsaicin
Study Group reported an 8-week trial of topical capsaicin 0.075% in painful
diabetic neuropathy or radiculopathy. A total of 277 patients entered this
trial, and 219 patients completed it, with 138 receiving capsaicin. Although
significant changes were reported in favor of capsaicin for three rating scales
of pain severity and relief, an intent-to-treat analysis showed no statistical
difference between treatment groups. Pain relief did not always occur immediately or within days, but sometimes after weeks. A large placebo effect
was noted (up to 58.1%). Capsaicin-induced burning and other side effects
were common, occurring in 135 of the 138 active treatment patients, and
posed a threat to the blinding of the trial. Although the authors concluded
that topical capsaicin could be beneficial, either singly or as an adjuvant, in
the treatment of painful diabetic neuropathy or radiculopathy, this study
does not give clear information about how clinically effective this approach
is in terms of patient satisfaction with the degree of pain relief and tolerability of side effects such as burning.

POSTMASTECTOMY PAIN SYNDROME

The postmastectomy pain syndrome affects 4–14% of woman after various surgical procedures on the breast. It usually occurs immediately after
surgery and may be misdiagnosed. It is probably due to intercostal and/or
intercostobrachial nerve injury. The pain can persist and can be very resistant to different therapies. Two uncontrolled trials (Watson et al. 1989; Dini
et al. 1993) and one controlled trial (Watson and Evans 1992) suggest that
topical capsaicin is useful for some patients with this disorder. Watson and
Evans (1992) carried out a randomized, vehicle-controlled, parallel-group
trial of topical capsaicin 0.075% in 25 patients with the syndrome. Reduced
pain was found with capsaicin, and 8 of the 13 patients who responded
favorably had 50% or greater improvement. Five of these 13 patients had a
good or excellent response in that pain was never worse than mild. Only one
of 10 patients responded to placebo. Capsaicin-induced burning was problematic in that it threatened blinding of the trial, but only one patient found
it intolerable and had to stop therapy.

OTHER CONDITIONS: RANDOMIZED CONTROLLED TRIALS

Deal and colleagues (1991) conducted an RCT of capsaicin 0.025% in 101 patients with arthritis; 70 patients had osteoarthritis (OA), and 31 suffered rheumatoid disease (RA) of one or both knees. A total of 93 patients completed the 4-week trial. Capsaicin treatment yielded a statistically significant reduction in pain in both OA (33% less) and RA (57% less). There was a high placebo response rate (up to 48%). Burning occurred in over 40% of capsaicin-treated patients and in only one patient in the placebo group, but only two patients dropped out as a result. The authors concluded that topical capsaicin 0.025% was effective and safe for arthritis pain, although complete relief of pain was rarely observed. McCarthy and McCarty (1992) evaluated topical capsaicin 0.075% in a 4-week, placebo-controlled, double-blind, parallel-group trial of 21 patients with arthritis of the hands (14 with OA and 7 with RA). An effect on pain severity was seen only in OA (on a visual analogue scale of pain severity but not on category scales), but the effects with RA were quite small. OA patients experienced a reduction in pain and tenderness of 40%. All capsaicin-treated patients experienced burning, but only one patient stopped the treatment. Ellison et al. (1997) concluded in an RCT that 0.075% capsaicin decreased surgical neuropathic pain. Topical 0.075% capsaicin had no effect in HIV-associated neuropathy (Paice et al. 2000) or in other distal sensory polyneuropathies (Low et al. 1995). Intranasal civamide, a synthetic isomer of capsaicin and a vanilloid receptor agonist, has been reported as "modestly effective" in migraine (Diamond et al. 2000) and cluster headache (Saper et al. 2002). The burning sensation persists as an issue in these trials.

UNCONTROLLED TRIALS OF MISCELLANEOUS PAINS

Open-label trials suggest improvement in complex regional pain syndrome, notalgia paresthetica, meralgia paresthetica, Guillain Barré syndrome, and multiple sclerosis. A dose-related response of topical capsaicin has been reported by Robbins et al. using single-dose 7.5–10% capsaicin and encouraging compliance with regional anesthesia and morphine (Robbins et al. 1998; Robbins 2000).

In conclusion, the chief limitations of topical capsaicin are its limited clinical effectiveness and the often intense initial burning sensation. Although a number of studies indicate that capsaicin is more effective than placebo, few patients seem to have a very good response when the drug is used as the sole therapy, and others who may have some relief find it is unsatisfactory because of the inadequate pain relief or the burning. This burning sensation has led to a high dropout rate in some studies. Current commercially available topical capsaicin preparations appear safe but are quite expensive. The optimal concentration remains unknown. Future research must look for a way of improving clinical effectiveness, perhaps by exploring similar agents that differ in structure. If higher concentrations are to be used topically, a way must be found of reducing or dealing with the intense burning sensation that so often limits or ends treatment and, as previously mentioned, makes clinical trials impossible to blind. The work of Robbins and colleagues is of interest in this regard with the use of higher doses and regional anesthesia (Robbins et al. 1998; Robbins 2000). Although topical capsaicin appears to have an effect greater than placebo in relieving some chronic pain syndromes, its effect seems to be modest. A number of trials appear to demonstrate statistically significant changes in rating scales of pain severity and relief, but this finding does not necessarily indicate clinical effectiveness.

NONSTEROIDAL ANTI-INFLAMMATORY AGENTS

Thou shalt make him cool applications for drawing out the inflammation from the mouth of the wound ... leaves of willow ... apply to it.
Smith papyrus, 2500 BC, cited by James Breasted (1930)

Three reviews of topical nonsteroidal anti-inflammatory drugs (NSAIDs) in musculoskeletal conditions (Vaile and Davis 1998; Heyneman et al. 2000) and pain (Moore et al. 1998) have concluded that these drugs are effective. There are few specific data in regard to neuropathic pain. The following will review the data with regard to PHN.

The proposed mechanism of action for this approach is still uncertain. For a detailed account the reader is referred elsewhere (Sawynok 2003). Once PHN is well established it is likely that active tissue inflammation is no longer present. In theory, abnormal activity in damaged or sensitized primary afferents may produce neurogenic inflammation by release of substance P and other peptides into the skin. Benzydamine is a pyrazole inhibitor of prostaglandin synthetase. Applied on the skin and mucous membranes in cream form, it is marketed as a topical analgesic and anti-inflammatory agent. Initial uncontrolled studies suggested benefit in PHN patients. This suggestion was not confirmed in a multiple-dose, placebo-controlled, crossover study using 3% benzydamine cream by McQuay et al. (1990). In 1988, King reported his experience with a time-honored remedy he had learned from a local physician. Although King had used the technique for years, his paper recounted the effects in his most recent 12 patients with acute zoster or PHN. The technique consists of crushing two 325-mg aspirin tablets and mixing the powder with 15–30 mL of chloroform. Kassirer (1988) reported good results in a few cases treated with crushed aspirin mixed in an over-the-counter skin cream, indicating that the vehicle may not need to be a powerful solvent such as chloroform. DeBenedittis et al. (1992) reported their uncontrolled experience with 750–1500 mg of crushed aspirin mixed with 20–30 mL of ethyl ether in patients with acute herpetic neuralgia and PHN, and also compared this mixture with two other NSAIDs in 28 patients with acute herpetic neuralgia. Aspirin treatment appeared to accelerate healing and prevent the development of PHN. Patients with PHN also responded. Only aspirin was superior to placebo in the 11-subject comparison of aspirin, indomethacin, and diclofenac in topical form. In summary, topical aspirin and other NSAIDs may have some effect, but work to date does not clarify how clinically meaningful this effect is, and better studies are required. Clinical experience indicates that this method is not very useful. Aspirin in chloroform, ethyl ether, or other vehicles has the advantage of being readily available, but the applications arc difficult to use, and some solvents can be very irritating to mucous membranes.

TOPICAL ANTIDEPRESSANTS

McCleane (2000b) studied topical doxepin (3.3%) versus topical capsaicin (0.025%) versus a combination of the two and against placebo in a 4-week, parallel-design RCT in neuropathic pain. Overall, pain was significantly reduced by all three active treatments to a similar extent. More rapid onset of relief occurred with doxepin/capsaicin. Capsaicin reduced sensitivity and shooting pain. Burning pain was increased by all three active treatments. The authors concluded that all three active treatments produced analgesia of a similar magnitude. If one looks at the details of this study, the diagnostic type of neuropathy was not specified. Forty-nine patients withdrew during the trial. The analysis was, however, intent to treat. Burning pain was increased by treatment, and shooting pain was unchanged by doxepin but reduced by capsaicin. This finding suggests a differential effect of topical agents on the different components of neuropathic pain, something that studies with oral antidepressants and opioids have not demonstrated. Burning was noted by 81% in the capsaicin group, 61% in the doxepin/capsaicin group, and 17% in the doxepin group, and was not stated for placebo. Thus, blinding was threatened by capsaicin as in other studies. No testing of the blinding was reported; blinding may, however, have been secure with doxepin.

A parallel RCT by McCleane (2000a) compared topical 5% doxepin with placebo. Thirty of 40 patients completed the trial. An intent-to-treat analysis favored doxepin. Adverse events were minimal. It was difficult to assess the clinical meaningfulness of these results.

OVERALL CONCLUSIONS AND FUTURE AGENTS

Comparative NNT data are given in Table II; however, as mentioned, these data must be interpreted with some caution because of differing experimental designs, patient numbers, and data analyses. Of the topical agents, the lidocaine patch appears to be the most practical. There is some evidence of a capsaicin effect, and if a way could be found to reduce the burning induced by capsaicinoids it would be easier to study this approach scientifically (maintaining blinding) and to utilize higher concentrations for possibly better relief. Topical NSAIDs and antidepressants require further study. Sawynok (2003) has recently admirably reviewed a number of possible future topical agents, and the reader is referred to that article for details. Included are topical opioids for which there are uncontrolled data for painful skin problems such as burns and ulcers. Glutamate receptor antagonists may prove useful topically. Ketamine, a noncompetitive NMDA antagonist, may have a peripheral site of action, and there are favorable reports of its use in sympathetically maintained pain and in palliative care. Alpha-adrenergic receptor agents such as clonidine have been used in a transdermal patch for diabetic neuropathy, sympathetically maintained pain, and orofacial pain. It is suggested that inhibition of presynaptic norepinephrine release may mediate this effect. Adenosine may act peripherally, and a topical preparation of such an agonist or an adenosine kinase inhibitor may be possible. There has been great interest recently in cannabinoids as a result of the finding of peripheral and central receptors. The anticonvulsant gabapentin may be applicable for topical use. A variety of inflammatory mediators such as prostanoids, bradykinin, adenosine triphosphate, biogenic amines, and nerve growth factor may have useful topical antagonists (Sawynok 2003). The treatment of neuropathic pain with topical agents may always be limited because such pain often has a major central component.

REFERENCES

Attal N, Brasseur L, Chauvin M, et al. Effects of single and repeated applications of a eutectic mixture of local anaesthetics (EMLA) cream on spontaneous and evoked pain in post-herpetic neuralgia. *Pain* 1999; 81(1–2):203–209.

Bernstein JE, Bickers DR, Dahl MV, et al. Treatment of chronic postherpetic neuralgia with topical capsaicin. *J Am Acad Dermatol* 1987; 17:93–96.

Bernstein JE, Korman NJ, Bickers DR, Dahl MV, Millikan LE. Topical capsaicin treatment of chronic postherpetic neuralgia. *J Am Acad Dermatol* 1989; 21:265–270.

Biro T, Acs, G, Acs P, et al. Recent advances in understanding of vanilloid receptors: a therapeutic target for treatment of pain and inflammation in skin. *J Invest Dermatol* 1997; 2:56–60.

Breasted JH. *The Edwin Smith Surgical Papyrus* (2 vols.). University of Chicago Press, 1930.

Capsaicin Study Group. Treatment of painful diabetic neuropathy with topical capsaicin: a multi-centre, double-blind, vehicle-controlled study. *Arch Intern Med* 1991; 151:2225–2229.

Carpenter SE, Lynn B. Vascular and sensory responses of human skin to mild injury after topical treatment with capsaicin. *Br J Pharmacol* 1981; 73:755–758.

Caterina MJ, Schumacher MA, Tominaga M, et al. The capsaicin receptor: a heat-activated ion channel in the pain pathway. *Nature* 1997; 380:816–824.

Catterall W, Mackie K. Local anaesthetics. In: Hardman JG, Limbird LE, Morinoff PB, et al. (Eds). *Goodman and Gilman's The Pharmacological Basis of Therapeutics,* 9th ed. New York: McGraw-Hill, 1996.

Chabal C, Russell LC, Burchiel K. The effect of intravenous lidocaine, tocainide and mexiletine on spontaneously active fibres arising in rat sciatic nerve neuromas. *Pain* 1989; 38:333–338.

Chad DA, Aronin N, Lundstrom R, et al. Does capsaicin relieve the pain of diabetic neuropathy? *Pain* 1990; 42:337–338.

Collins SL, Moore RA, McQuay JH. Antidepressants and anticonvulsants for diabetic neuropathy and postherpetic neuralgia: a quantitative systematic review. *J Pain Symptom Manage* 2000; 20:449–458.

Cook RJ, Sackett DL. The number needed to treat: a clinically useful measure of treatment effect. *BMJ* 1995; 310:452–454.

Dalili H, Adriani J. The efficacy of local anaesthetics in blockading the effects of itch, burning and pain in normal and "sunburned" skin. *Clin Pharmacol Ther* 1971; 12:913–919.

DeBenedittis G, Besana F, Lorenzetti A. A new topical treatment for acute herpetic neuralgia and postherpetic neuralgia: the aspirin/diethyl ether mixture. An open label study plus a double-blind controlled clinical trial. *Pain* 1992; 48:383–390.

Deal CL, Schnitzer TJ, Lipstein E, et al. Treatment of arthritis with topical capsaicin: a double-blind trial. *Clin Ther* 1991; 13:385–395.

Devers A, Galer BS. Topical lidocaine patch relieves a variety of neuropathic pain conditions: an open label study. *Clin J Pain* 2000; 16:205–208.

Diamond S, Freitag F, Phillips SB, et al. Intranasal civamide for the acute treatment of migraine headache. *Cephalalgia* 2000; 20:597–602.

Dini D, Bertelli G, Gozza A, Forno GG. Treatment of the postmastectomy pain syndrome with topical capsaicin. *Pain* 1993; 54:223–226.

Dworkin RH, Corbin AE, Young JP. Pregabalin for the treatment of postherpetic neuralgia. *Neurology* 2003; 60:1274–1283.

Ellison N, Loprinzi CL, Kugler J, et al. Phase III placebo-controlled trial of capsaicin cream in the management of surgical neuropathic pain in cancer patients. *J Clin Oncol* 1997; 15:2974–2980

Galer BS, Rowbotham MC, Perander J, Friedman E. Topical lidocaine patch relieves postherpetic neuralgia more effectively than a vehicle topical patch: results of an enriched enrollment study. *Pain* 1999; 80:533–538.

Galer BS, Jenson MP, Ma T, et al. The lidocaine patch effectively treats all neuropathic pain qualities: results of a randomized double blind, vehicle controlled trial efficacy study with the use of a neuropathic pain scale. *Clin J Pain* 2002; 18:297–301.

Heyneman CA, Lawless-Liday C, Wall GC. Oral versus topical NSAIDs in rheumatic diseases: a comparison. *Drugs* 2000; 60:555–574.

Hogyes A. Beiträge für physiologischen Wirkung der Bestandtheile des *Capsicum annuum*. *Arch Exp Pathol Pharmakol* 1878; 9:117.

Jadad AR, Moore A, Carroll et al. Assessing the quality of reports of randomized clinical trials: is blinding necessary? *Control Clin Trials* 1996; 17:1–12.

Jansco N. Neurogenic inflammatory responses: proceedings of the Hungarian Physiology Society symposium on inflammation, Budapest, 1963. *Acad Sci Hung* 1964; 24(Suppl):3.

Kassirer MR. King and Robert, concerning the management of pain associated with herpes zoster and of post-herpetic neuralgia. *Pain* 1988; 35:368–369.

King RB. Concerning the management of pain associated with herpes zoster and of postherpetic neuralgia. *Pain* 1988; 33:73–78.

Laupacis A, Sackett DL, Roberts RS. An assessment of clinically useful measures of the consequences of treatment. *N Engl J Med* 1988; 318:1728–1733.

Lembeck F. Columbus, capsicum and capsaicin: past, present, and future. *Acta Physiol Hung* 1987; 69:265–273.

Low PA, Opfer-Gehrking TL, Dyck PJ. Double-blind, placebo-controlled study of the application of capsaicin cream in chronic distal painful neuropathy. *Pain* 1995; 62:163–168.

Lynn B. Capsaicin: actions on nociceptive C-fibres and therapeutic potential. *Pain* 1990; 41:61–69.

Majno G. *The Healing Hand, Man and Wound in the Ancient World.* Cambridge, MA: Harvard University Press, 1975.

Meier T, Wasner G, Faust M, et al. Efficacy of lidocaine patch 5% in the treatment of focal peripheral neuropathic pain syndromes. A randomized, double-blind, placebo-controlled trial. *Pain* 2003; 106:151–158.

McCarthy GM, McCarty DJ. Effect of topical capsaicin in the therapy of painful arthritis of the hands. *J Rheumatol* 1992; 19:604–607.

McCleane G. Topical doxepin hydrochloride reduces neuropathic pain: a randomized double-blind placebo-controlled trial. *Pain Clin* 2000a; 12:47–50.

McCleane G. Topical application of doxepin hydrochloride, capsaicin and a combination of both produces analgesia in chronic human neuropathic pain: a randomized double-blind, placebo-controlled trial. *Br J Clin Pharmacol* 2000b; 49:574–579.

McQuay HJ, Carroll D, Moxon A, Glynn CJ, Moore RA. Benzydamine cream for the treatment of post-herpetic neuralgia: minimum duration of treatment periods in a cross-over trial. *Pain* 1990; 40:131–135.

McQuay H, Trainer M, Nye BA, et al. A systematic review of antidepressants in neuropathic pain. *Pain* 1996; 68:217–227.

Meier T, Wasner G, Faust M, et al. Efficacy of lidocaine patch 5% in the treatment of focal neuropathic pain syndromes: a randomized placebo-controlled trial. *Pain* 2003; 106:151–158.

Moore RA, Tramer MR, Carroll D, et al. Quantitative systematic review of non-steroidal anti-inflammatory. *BMJ* 1998; 316:333–338.

Niemann A. On the alkaloid and other constituents of coca leaves. *Am J Pharmacy* 1860; 122–126.

Nolano M, Simone JA, Wendellschafer-Crabb G, et al. Decreased sensation and loss of epidermal nerve fibers following repeated application in humans. *Soc Neurosci Abstr* 1996; 22:1802.

Paice JA, Ferrans CE, Lashley FR, et al. Topical capsaicin in the management of HIV-associated peripheral neuropathy. *J Pain Symptom Manage* 2000; 19:45–52.

Rice ASC, Maton S, Postherpetic Neuralgia Study Group. Gabapentin in postherpetic neuralgia: a randomized, double-blind, placebo-controlled study. *Pain* 2001; 94:215–224.

Robbins W. Clinical application of capsaicinoids. *Clin J Pain* 2000; 16(Suppl):86–89.

Robbins WR, Staats PS, Levine J. Treatment of intractable pain with topical large-dose capsaicin: preliminary report. *Anaesth Analg* 1998; 86(3):579–583.

Rowbotham MC, Davies PS, Fields HL. Topical lidocaine gel relieves postherpetic neuralgia. *Ann Neurol* 1995; 37:246–253.

Rowbotham MC, Davies PS, Verkempinck, C, et al. Lidocaine patch: double-blind Controlled study of a new treatment method for post-herpetic neuralgia. *Pain* 1996; 65:39–44.

Saper JR, Klapper J, Mathew NT. Intranasal civamide for the treatment of episodic cluster headache. *Arch Neurol* 2002; 59:990–994.

Sawynok J. Topical and peripherally acting analgesics. *Pharmacol Rev* 2003; 55:1–20.

Sindrup SH, Jensen TS. Efficacy of pharmacological treatment of neuropathic pain: an update and effect related to mechanism of drug action. *Pain* 1999; 83:389–400.

Sindrup SH, Bach FW, Madsen C, et al. Venlafaxine versus imipramine in painful neuropathy: a randomized controlled trial. *Neurology* 2003; 60:1284–1289.

Stow PJ, Glynn CJ, Minor B. EMLA cream in the treatment of post-herpetic neuralgia: efficacy and pharmacokinetic profile. *Pain* 1989; 39:301–305.

Turnbull A. Tincture of capsaicin as a remedy for chilblains and toothache. *Dublin Free Press* 1850; 1:95–96.

Vaile JH, Davis P. Topical NSAIDs for musculoskeletal conditions. A review. *Drugs* 1998; 56:723–799.

Watson CPN, Babul N. Oxycodone relieves neuropathic pain: a randomized trial in postherpetic neuralgia. *Neurology* 1998; 50:1837–1841.

Watson CPN, Evans RJ. The postmastectomy pain syndrome and topical capsaicin: a randomized trial. *Pain* 1992; 51:375–379.

Watson CP, Evans RJ, Watt VR. Postherpetic neuralgia and topical capsaicin. *Pain* 1988; 33:333–340.

Watson CPN, Evans RJ, Watt VR. The postmastectomy pain syndrome and the effect of topical capsaicin. *Pain* 1989; 88:177–186.

Watson CPN, Tyler K, Bickers DR, et al. A randomized, vehicle-controlled trial of topical capsaicin in the treatment of postherpetic neuralgia. *Clin Ther* 1993; 15:51–520.

Watson CPN, Moulin D, Watt-Watson JH, Gordon A, Eisenhoffer J. Controlled-release oxycodone relieves neuropathic pain: a randomized controlled trial in painful diabetic neuropathy. *Pain* 2003; 105:71–78.

Correspondence to: C. Peter N. Watson, MD, FRCP(C), 1 Sir William's Lane, Toronto, Ontario, Canada M9A 1T8. Tel: 416-239-3494; Fax: 416-239-6365; email: peter.watson@utoronto.ca.

The Paths of Pain 1975–2005, edited by
Harold Merskey, John D. Loeser, and Ronald
Dubner, IASP Press, Seattle, © 2005.

34

Multidisciplinary Pain Management

John D. Loeser

Departments of Neurological Surgery and Anesthesiology,
University of Washington, Seattle, Washington, USA

The multidisciplinary pain clinic, with its complement of physicians, psychologists, nurses, physical therapists, occupational therapists, vocational counselors, and other types of health care providers, is a format for health care delivery with less than 50 years of documented history. The existence of this type of health care activity can be traced to the efforts of one man, John J. Bonica, although others have certainly played a significant role both in setting the stage for Bonica's actions and in further developing the diagnostic and treatment options that have occurred since he initiated this concept of how to treat patients with chronic pain (Bonica and Loeser 2001).

The direct antecedents of the multidisciplinary pain clinic can be found in the second half of the 19th century; prior to that time few, if any, physicians were specialized in the alleviation of pain and suffering. Indeed, few pharmacological or surgical therapies were available then to treat pain, opiates and salicylates being the primary drugs available. Pain was always thought of as the byproduct of a disease; if the disease was successfully treated, the pain could be expected to disappear. Pain was a clue to be pursued in the search for diagnosis. It was commonly thought that a somatic pathological process must be present if a patient reported pain. As the Industrial Age gained momentum, it was recognized that some factory workers and those injured on the railroads could complain of pain and suffer from it in the absence of discernible pathology. Such people were thought either to have a mental illness or to be malingering. This phenomenon was often considered to be outside of the purview of physicians and not amenable to health care. Chronic pain patients were not often discussed in the medical literature.

The beginnings of pain management can be traced to a French surgeon, Jean Joseph Emile Letievant, who was apparently the first to recognize that neurosurgical procedures could be used to alleviate pain in about 1873. The surgical approaches to the treatment of chronic pain were also developed by Robert Waldo Abbe, who first described dorsal rhizotomy in 1889, and by Victor Horsley, who performed the first gasserian ganglionectomy in the same year. Other pioneers included James Leonard Corning, who described the use of cocaine to block nerves in 1884, and Rudolph Schlosser, who used alcohol to destroy nerves in 1900. In the first 20 years of the 20th century, the use of both temporary and lytic blocks of the sympathetic nervous system was the result of studies by Felix Mandl, George Swetlow, and René Leriche (Bonica and Loeser 2001). Subarachnoid alcohol rhizotomy was described by Achille M. Dogliotti in 1931 (Bonica and Loeser 2001). All of these efforts were predicated on the concept that cutting or blocking nerves could turn off pain and thereby offer the patient a more normal life. No other approaches to pain management were discussed in their papers, and none of these early workers had clinics devoted to the treatment of pain. Although narcotics were in widespread, nonprescription use, they were rarely recommended for chronic pain patients.

The first clinic established specifically to treat pain was founded by Emery Rovenstine at New York University in 1936 (Rovenstine and Wertheim 1941). This was a nerve block clinic staffed exclusively by anesthesiologists. Although there may have been other such block clinics elsewhere in the United States or other countries, I cannot find any written references to them, and informal discussions with senior anesthesiologists have not uncovered any earlier treatment programs utilizing nerve blocks. Patients with both acute and chronic pains were treated by local anesthetic nerve blocks.

Bonica started the first recorded multidisciplinary pain clinic in Tacoma, Washington, in 1946. He had provided care to many soldiers with painful injuries during his military career at Madigan Army Hospital and had recognized the advantages of a multidisciplinary approach to care focused upon alleviating pain. When he entered civilian practice after the end of World War II, he enlisted the help of other physicians to provide a broader range of assessment and treatment strategies than one physician could provide. Obviously, the lessons of war injuries were learned by others as well, and similar multidisciplinary clinics were started by F.A. Duncan Alexander in a Veterans Affairs hospital in McKinney, Texas, in 1947 and by William Livingston at the University of Oregon in Portland, Oregon, in 1951(Alexander 1978). Several nerve block clinics were also founded in the United States and in Europe in the 1950s and 1960s, as reviewed by Swerdlow (1992). There were no textbooks or journal articles that described this form of health care delivery and no organizations or meetings that facilitated such activities. These early multidisciplinary pain clinics consisted only of physicians and really focused upon accurate diagnosis and biomedical treatments. Some of them had psychiatrists involved in patient assessment, but there was little understanding of the roles of emotional and environmental factors in the genesis and perpetuation of pain. Traditional ego-based psychiatry did not do well with pain patients, who denied that they had any emotional problems and did not see the need to change their ways of thinking and feeling.

Bonica became the founding Professor of Anesthesiology at the University of Washington in 1960. Shortly after his arrival, with the assistance of a neurosurgeon, Lowell E. White, Jr., and a nurse, Dorothy Crowley, he started the University of Washington Multidisciplinary Pain Clinic. This was a physician multispecialty clinic that evaluated a limited number of patients, presented them at a weekly conference, and recommended treatment. Sometimes one of the Pain Clinic physicians implemented such treatment, and sometimes the patient was referred back to his general practitioner with management recommendations. In the mid-1960s, Wilbert Fordyce, a psychologist who had been hired by the Department of Physical Medicine and Rehabilitation in 1959, became interested in the treatment of chronic pain patients utilizing behavioral strategies, specifically operant conditioning. Fordyce has described, in his interview with John Liebeskind and elsewhere, his fortuitous discovery that pain behaviors could be influenced by environmental contingencies (Fordyce 1976; oral history interview with Wilbert E. Fordyce, 10 July 1993). After some anecdotal patient successes, a formal treatment program of 8 weeks' duration was established with an allocation of three beds in the Department of Physical Medicine and Rehabilitation in 1968. Fordyce also became an active participant in the Multidisciplinary Pain Clinic, participating in patient evaluation and educating all of its physicians about behavioral medicine. However, his operant program was not an integral part of the Pain Clinic; only specific patients were referred to him for treatment. This limitation did not stop Bonica and his protégés from touting the importance of psychologists and behavioral modification in pain management. Psychologists were hired to participate in the Pain Clinic and to work with Dr. Fordyce in 1978.

In this era, Bonica and many of his disciples traveled the world promulgating behaviorally based multidisciplinary pain clinics. The International Association for the Study of Pain played a large role in the dissemination of such clinics by encouraging the formation of national chapters, regional courses, and meetings and by serving as a forum for scientists and clinicians. The ideal that Bonica espoused did not reach fruition at the University of Washington until 1982, when I became the Director of the Multidisciplinary Pain Center and the Fordyce program became the centerpiece of its treatment activities. The fusion of the two programs resulted in a highly structured, 3-week, inpatient program designed to address pain, disuse, depression, and disability that became the model for the burgeoning world of multidisciplinary pain management. Patients were evaluated by a physician, a psychologist, and a vocational counselor and, when appropriate, placed in the Structured Program. The goals of the Structured Program were to: (1) manage inappropriate medications; (2) improve physical conditioning, strength, and flexibility; (3) improve psychological well-being; (4) identify reasonable vocational goals and begin the process of return to gainful employment; (5) educate the patient about human anatomy, physiology, and psychology; (6) educate the patient to be a wise consumer of health care; and (7) treat depression. Other patients who needed procedures or other types of treatment were appropriately managed or referred. Many of these early patients had inappropriate medications—usually opiates, sedative hypnotics, or diazepam—and many such patients had to be admitted for detoxification prior to the attempt to restore well behaviors. The multidisciplinary pain clinic was the last-resort treatment for most of these patients, who, on average, had been off work for over 3 years and had been subjected to multiple operations. Medication management issues, a well as the need to change the patient's environment and contingent reinforcement by family members, mandated an inpatient program. At its zenith, this program treated 18 inpatients every 3 weeks, and the professional staff included five physicians and four psychologists who rotated coverage, as well as physical and occupational therapists, vocational counselors, and nurses (Loeser 2001a,b; Turk and Loeser 2001). This exciting and gratifying but labor-intensive program was a radical departure from traditional medical care (Loeser and Egan 1989). Although there were some issues with payment for services, the program made money for the hospital, and the professionals involved received adequate payment for their time. However, it was the collegial attitude and marvelous cooperation of the entire health care team that made this a wonderful experience for both providers and most patients. Visitors came looking for our operational secrets and were told, "The magic is in the interactions between the providers, not in some hidden skills or treatment strategies."

The apparent success of such treatment programs with the most difficult of chronic pain patients led to the replication of our program at many other institutions. Early multidisciplinary pain clinics included City of Hope in Duarte led by Benjamin Crue, the Denver clinic led by Richard Steig, the San Diego clinic led by Richard Sternbach, the Portland clinic led by Joel Seres and Richard Newman, the Atlanta clinic led by Steven Brena, the Mayo Clinic led by David W. Swanson and Toshihiko Maruta, the Boston clinic led by Gerald M. Aronoff, the Maastricht clinic led by Nico H. Groenman, and the Adelaide clinic led by Issy Pilowsky. When IASP was launched in 1973, multidisciplinary pain clinics encompassing behavioral principles were few, but within a decade they became a growth industry in North America, Australia, New Zealand, and Europe. Behavioral medicine led to the involvement of psychologists in the management of chronic pain. They rapidly built upon Fordyce's ideas and added cognitive treatment strategies to the treatment programs (Rosenstiel and Keefe 1983), which enhanced the efficacy of such treatment programs and broadened the mix of patients who could be successfully treated. The number of articles published on cognitive and behavioral treatment strategies rapidly increased. Case series were reported, as were a few cohort controlled studies. Gradually, a literature evolved that demonstrated the efficacy of this type of treatment program. By 1990, cognitive-behavioral pain management programs were widespread and were becoming the standard of care. Many books were written describing the diagnostic and treatment strategies implemented at different clinics. Other types of treatment for chronic pain did not receive the recognition that multidisciplinary pain clinics gathered in both the professional and lay press. The Commission on Accreditation of Rehabilitation Facilities (CARF), in conjunction with the American Pain Society, established a pain clinic certification process in the United States with criteria that mandated a multidisciplinary diagnostic and treatment program that included physicians, psychologists, physical and occupational therapists, nurses, and other providers (Commission on Accreditation of Rehabilitation Facilities, 1891 E. Grant Road, Tucson, AZ 85712, USA). Outcomes measures were essential for accreditation, and the emphasis was on functional improvement, including return to work.

In the last two decades of the 20th century, many case series were published. Multiple meta-analyses were undertaken, and factors that influenced success were elucidated (Guzman et al. 2001). An excellent compilation of the data is contained in Williams's summary from the IASP's 10th World Congress (Williams 2003). She nicely demonstrated in her literature review that cognitive-behavioral therapy was every bit as effective for a heterogeneous group of chronic pain sufferers (the main complaint being low back pain) as was any published therapy for any specific type of pain. However, the increasing evidence that cognitive-behavioral therapies were more effective than any other form of treatment for chronic pain has not led to the continued expansion of this type of treatment. Economic and political factors seemed to be playing a larger role than evidence for efficacy. Furthermore, the dominance of the biomedical approach to pain has not allowed physicians to broaden their perspectives on how to treat chronic pain patients. Reimbursement schemes often excluded non-physicians from health care. Sociology, not medical science, determined what types of health care would be available to the public.

Pain treatment facilities of all types proliferated during 1980–1995. Brena (1985) documented the early growth of such facilities in 1985 using data from a 1979 survey. There were reportedly 119 multidisciplinary pain centers in the United States and another 43 in the rest of the world. At that time there were 256 other types of pain clinics, usually focusing upon one modality or one diagnosis. The growth in other types of pain clinics was largely due to increased utilization of nerve blocks, epidural steroid injections, and percutaneous approaches to the evaluation and treatment of disk and facet joint diseases. It appeared that the number of pain clinics had quadrupled by 1990 (Loeser 2001b). Some procedurally based pain treatment facilities included psychologists and other providers on their rosters, but needle-based procedures were the most common treatment. Unfortunately, the self-styled appellation "multidisciplinary pain clinic" did not necessarily mean that a biopsychosocial approach to patient care was utilized. Indeed, there is ample evidence of the chaos in the delivery of services for pain management from small area analyses of the prevalence of current procedural terminology (CPT) codes to surveys of treatment facilities and what types of care they offered (Csordas and Clark 1992).

Several forces came into play that changed the status of large, complex multidisciplinary pain programs. The training of large numbers of anesthesiologists who believed that nerve blocks were useful for chronic pain management created a competitive treatment strategy. The reimbursement for operating room anesthesia was no longer so lucrative that those who were interested in pain patients could support themselves with operating room work. Now, procedures were required to fund the time spent with chronic pain patients. Anesthesia department chairs wanted pain clinics to be financially successful, and this could not happen unless procedures were undertaken. The American Board of Anesthesiology required nerve block exposure for an accredited residency and for pain fellowships. Unfortunately, in most institutions, pain management was under the auspices of the anesthesiology department. This situation diverted anesthesia pain specialists away from participating in cognitive-behavioral programs and into offering nerve blocks, stimulators, and pumps. Multidisciplinary pain management programs were severely impacted by this turn toward procedures. Furthermore, the idea that opiates could be useful in the treatment of chronic pain patients undermined pain clinic strategies to eliminate drug usage.

In addition, the rising costs of inpatient treatment programs led to a movement toward outpatient treatment, often in facilities remote from the parent medical center, making multidisciplinary participation more difficult. Outpatient treatment programs often have difficulty dealing with drug-related issues that more readily could be handled with inpatients. Billing issues for outpatient care also created a new problem that adversely affected this form of care.

Particularly in the United States, health care and its funding are separate from disability status. Hence, most health care programs are often not interested in whether or not the insured person goes back to work. This means that health care that has little or no likelihood of returning people to gainful employment may be funded, because the billing codes for physicians exist, whereas multidisciplinary pain management, which is harder to comprehend from the billing perspective, is often not funded, because much of the money goes to non-physicians. In the absence of the requirement for evidence-based medicine, multidisciplinary pain management is not as well funded, even though the published outcomes data show far greater success than for any other type of treatment for chronic pain.

The attempt to quantify changes in the number and types of pain clinics is thwarted by parochial uses of terminology and self-description. However, the CARF accreditation standards in the United States have remained fairly constant, and they only accredit multidisciplinary pain programs. In 1988 they had accredited 90 programs, and in 1998 over 200 programs, but in 2004 there were only 125 programs that maintained accreditation.

By 2004, many of the well-established multidisciplinary pain clinics had shifted their focus and no longer offered a structured rehabilitation program, particularly in the United States. Some have disappeared altogether, as funding for pain management has been curtailed. Instead of being housed in large academic institutions, many of the persisting programs are smaller, private-practice clinics that rely on referring physicians to rule out any treatable anatomical or physiological problem and then address physical, psychological, and pharmacological issues in a rehabilitative mode with an emphasis on return to work. However, even if the specific treatment programs have diminished in number, the influence of the cognitive-behavioral conceptualization of chronic pain has permeated all of the pain treatment world. Health care is a social convention; it is not based upon outcomes data. Multidisciplinary pain management will survive only if the culture of providing care for chronic illness can evolve so that it addresses more than the patient's symptoms and encompasses the treatment of the patient's mind and body as well as his or her environment. The long-standing predominance of the biomedical perspective on disease threatens the existence of cognitive-behavioral programs. Pain and illness belong to patients, not to an outdated conceptualization of the meaning of symptoms. Even as the call for evidence-based medicine spreads throughout the developed world, the existence of cognitive-behavioral diagnostic and therapeutic programs is threatened. Yet published evidence indicates the superiority of these treatment strategies over procedural interventions for low back pain, which is the most common chronic pain seen in pain treatment facilities (Turk and Loeser 2001).

Multidisciplinary pain management identifies all of the relevant factors in the production of pain, suffering, pain behaviors, and disability. Its treatment strategies are aimed at functional restoration as well as symptom control. It recognizes that human behavior is influenced not only by events within the body, but also by environmental and cognitive factors, fears, anticipation, and culture. It works better than any known alternatives, but many patients still fail to get better. Perhaps earlier treatment would improve results. Perhaps better diagnostic strategies and patient selection would improve outcomes. Perhaps more effective treatment programs could be constructed to improve outcomes. However, the real mission of multidisciplinary pain management is to identify the factors that may lead a person into the miseries of being a chronic pain patient. When that happens, programs aimed at prevention could render the need for treatment obsolete. In the interim, multidisciplinary pain management remains the most effective treatment strategy for chronic pain we have at our disposal.

REFERENCES

Alexander FAD. The genesis of the pain clinic. *Pain Abstracts: 2nd World Congress on Pain.* Seattle: International Association for the Study of Pain, 1978, p 250.

Bonica JJ, Loeser JD. Basic consideration of pain: history of pain concepts and therapies. In: Loeser JD (Ed). *Bonica's Management of Pain,* 3rd ed. Philadelphia: Lippincott, 2001, pp 3–16.

Brena SF. Pain control facilities: patterns of operation and problems of organization in the USA. *Clin Anesth* 1985; 3:183–.

Csordas TJ, Clark JA. Ends of the line: diversity among chronic pain centers. *Soc Sci Med* 1992; 34(4):383–393.

Fordyce WE. *Behavioral Methods for Chronic Pain and Illness.* St. Louis: Mosby, 1976.

Guzman J, Esmail R, Karjalainen K, et al. Multidisciplinary rehabilitation for chronic low back pain: systematic review. *BMJ* 2001; 322(7301):1511–1516.

Loeser JD. Multidisciplinary pain assessment. In: Loeser JD (Ed). *Bonica's Management of Pain,* 3rd ed. Philadelphia: Lippincott, 2001a, pp 363–368.

Loeser JD. Basic consideration of pain: multidisciplinary pain programs. In: Loeser JD (Ed). *Bonica's Management of Pain,* 3rd ed. Philadelphia: Lippincott, 2001b, pp 255–264.

Loeser JD, Egan K. *Managing the Chronic Pain Patient: Theory and Practice at the University of Washington Pain Clinic.* New York: Raven Press, 1989.

Oral History Interview with Wilbert E. Fordyce. John C. Liebeskind History of Pain, History & Special Collections Division, Louise M. Darling Biomedical Library. University of California, Los Angeles, July 1993.

Rosenstiel AK, Keefe FJ. The use of coping strategies in chronic low back pain patients: relationship to patient characteristics and current adjustment. *Pain* 1983; 17(1):33–44.

Rovenstine EA, Wertheim HM. Therapeutic nerve block. *JAMA* 1941; 117:1599.

Swerdlow M. The early development of pain relief clinics in the UK. *Anaesthesia* 1992; 48:977–908.

Turk DC, Loeser JD. Methods for symptomatic control: multidisciplinary pain management. In: Loeser JD (Ed). *Bonica's Management of Pain,* 3rd ed. Philadelphia: Lippincott, 2001, pp 2069–2079.

Williams A. Cognitive behavioral treatment. In: Dostrovsky JO, Carr DB, Koltzenburg MD (Eds). *Proceedings of the 10th World Congress on Pain,* Progress in Pain Research and Management, Vol. 24. Seattle: IASP Press, 2003, pp 825–837.

Correspondence to: John D. Loeser, MD, Department of Neurological Surgery, University of Washington, Campus Box 356470, 1959 NE Pacific Street, Seattle, WA 98195, USA. Tel: 206-543-3570; Fax: 206-543-8315; email: jdloeser@u.washington.edu.

The Paths of Pain 1975–2005, edited by
Harold Merskey, John D. Loeser, and Ronald
Dubner, IASP Press, Seattle, © 2005.

35

The Future of Pain Therapy: Something Old, Something New, Something Borrowed, and Something Blue

Allan I. Basbaum

Departments of Anatomy and Physiology and W.M. Keck Foundation Center for Integrative Neuroscience, University of California, San Francisco, California, USA

This is not the first opportunity that I have been given to write an article on the future of pain research and therapy. In 1998, I was charged with a similar task, to commemorate the 25th anniversary of the founding of the IASP (Basbaum 1998). Given the minimal success of my predictions 15 years ago, I do not particularly welcome the opportunity to prognosticate once again. Predictions about the future of pain therapy are as reliable as our most recent New Year's resolutions. Therefore, with a view to being conservative, yet optimistic, I adapted the title of this chapter from a traditional marriage ritual, which encourages a bride to wear to the wedding "something old, something new, something borrowed, and something blue." This recommendation is presumably designed to bring good luck to the marriage. In my opinion, pain therapy in the future will include a mix. Something old—we cannot abandon opiates or nonsteroidal anti-inflammatory drugs (NSAIDs). Something new—what is on the short-term horizon will come, I hope, from a successful transfer of knowledge and technology from the laboratory to the clinic. Something borrowed—more likely we will borrow a lot, including many anticonvulsants and antidepressants. Something blue—the blue could include a pessimistic perspective, but I prefer the more optimistic "blue sky" interpretation. I believe that the future will be strongly influenced by breakthroughs that derive from the molecular revolution, from insights that new imaging techniques will provide about the transmission of injury messages and about the integrative and perceptual aspects of the pain experience, and finally from novel technologies and models. Success in any of these areas will speed up the development of new analgesics with better side-effect profiles, so that the patient can be better served.

SOMETHING OLD

OPIOIDS

On the 25th anniversary of the founding of IASP I recalled a meeting that Jean-Marie Besson and I organized in Berlin in 1989. It was a wonderful and stimulating meeting, but it was most memorable because it began the day that the Berlin Wall came down. One year before the start of the meeting, we were asked to consider the title of the book that was to arise from the deliberations at this conference. We chose: *Towards a New Pharmacotherapy of Pain: Beyond Morphine.* Unfortunately, after a solid week of discussions we concluded that morphine could not yet be replaced, and so we dropped the words "Beyond Morphine" from the title (Basbaum and Besson 1991). Fifteen years has passed since the Berlin meeting, and I am sad to say that morphine and related opioids are still the drugs of choice for most severe pains. Perhaps this pessimistic perspective is an element of the "something blue" part of the title.

I certainly do not wish to denigrate morphine's utility in the management of pain. Morphine is an excellent analgesic, limited of course by an unfortunate side-effect profile that could be entirely predicted from the distribution of opioid receptors (in the gut, leading to constipation; in the medulla, contributing to respiratory depression; and in the limbic system, contributing to its problematic rewarding and potentially addictive properties). The problem of opioid tolerance and dependence also continues to be a significant topic of discussion. Although it is readily demonstrated that animals develop rapid and profound tolerance to morphine and other opioids, the extent to which tolerance to the analgesic properties of opioids develops in patients is still debated. The experiment is not an easy one to perform in humans. Most patients taking high doses of opioids have ongoing disease, which may be progressive, as in the case of cancer. For this reason, it is difficult to determine whether dose escalation results from tolerance or from increased pain. With continued discussions concerning the utility and advisability of long-term morphine for persistent noncancer pain (Gilson et al. 2004), there is a greater likelihood that future studies will be able to rigorously address the magnitude of tolerance in humans.

The other side of the coin concerning long-term opioid use is dependence. Everyone agrees that physical dependence develops in humans. The question is whether psychological dependence (i.e., craving) also occurs, in which patients, and to what extent. One longstanding dogma is that patients who take opioids for pain and who do not have a history of abuse of drugs never develop psychological dependence. Recent news stories (particularly in the United States) of well-known individuals becoming dependent have, however, reopened the discussion. This critical issue must be addressed, particularly if the use of chronic opioids increases in non-terminal patients.

NONSTEROIDAL ANTI-INFLAMMATORY DRUGS

Novel selective inhibitors of cyclooxygenase-2 (COX-2), sometimes called coxibs, have carved a large niche in the analgesic market. Although it was suggested that they had fewer gastrointestinal side effects than non-selective COX-1 and COX-2 inhibitors, concerns about serious cardiovascular side effects have now raised questions about their future in pain therapy. Only time will tell whether these adverse side effects are unique to specific inhibitors or whether there is a COX-2 class effect. Regardless, the concerns point to the need for alternatives. Looking downstream from the COX enzyme in the pathway of arachidonic acid metabolism provides new approaches such as antagonizing the receptors that are targeted by the pronociceptive products of arachidonic metabolism, namely prostaglandins. There are four subtypes of prostaglandin receptors (EP-1 to EP-4), and there is evidence that all four receptors contribute to nociceptive processing (Bar et al. 2004). There is also evidence for the utility of EP antagonists in the clinic (Sarkar et al. 2003). Another interesting approach is to target other enzymes in the pathway of arachidonic acid metabolism. The COX isoenzymes, in fact, catalyze the synthesis of PGH_2, a precursor of key prostaglandins such as PGE_2. Prostaglandin synthase converts PGH_2 to PGE_2, and its deletion (in mutant mice) is associated with profound anti-inflammatory and antinociceptive effects (Trebino et al. 2003). Whether the adverse effects of prostaglandin synthase inhibition will be acceptable remains to be seen, but the approach is promising.

What is perhaps more interesting is the evidence for central as well as peripheral actions of coxibs. Thus, although sensitization of the peripheral terminal of nociceptors by prostaglandins is well established, there is now considerable evidence that prostaglandins also influence the central terminals of the primary afferent. Indeed, intrathecal administration of coxibs, at doses that clearly do not act peripherally, can have profound antinociceptive effects. A plethora of recent studies followed upon an earlier report (Malmberg and Yaksh 1992) that showed an antinociceptive effect of NSAIDs at the spinal level. Of interest, the new studies identified novel and diverse mechanisms through which the COX inhibitors contribute (Ghilardi et al. 2004).

For example, Samad et al. (2001) provided evidence that the COX-2 isoenzyme is induced in the spinal cord when there is peripheral inflammation and that an interleukin-1β-mediated link is involved in its induction. That study illustrated the complex interplay of injury in the periphery with central changes that contribute to, enhance, and prolong nociceptive processing.

A very different interpretation is that the COX inhibitors interfere with a glycinergic regulation of inhibitory tone in the spinal cord (Ahmadi et al. 2002). These authors showed that there is normally a tonic inhibitory control of dorsal horn nociresponsive neurons, via an action at the strychnine-sensitive glycine receptor. When there is injury, noxious input evokes the synthesis and release of prostaglandins in the dorsal horn (via induction of a COX enzyme). The prostaglandins, in turn, target the glycine receptor (indirectly through a complex signaling pathway), resulting in its functional downregulation. The resultant loss of glycinergic inhibition, of course, is equivalent to enhancing central sensitization, but in this case, the problem could be "treated" with a COX enzyme inhibitor. Still unknown is the source of the dorsal horn COX enzyme and thus the source of the pronociceptive prostanoids. Some studies point to glial cells (Marriott et al. 1991), and in this regard the recent papers implicating astroglial and microglial changes in the development of long-term pain conditions is of great interest (see Watkins and Maier, this volume). Clearly, future studies need to pinpoint the origin of this important COX contribution, with a view to selectively targeting it for persistent pain conditions.

SOMETHING NEW

LOTS OF TARGETS, NOT ENOUGH ARROWS

Since my last article that looked to the future pain research and therapy. our understanding of the mechanisms that underlie the generation of pain, particularly tissue- and nerve injury-induced persistent pain, has grown tremendously. But this is both a good and a bad news story. The good news is that the number of possible therapeutic targets has increased significantly (Basbaum and Woolf 1999; Woolf and Salter 2000; Julius and Basbaum 2001; see Dickenson and Besson, this volume). Many of these targets are associated with elements of the "pain" transmission circuitry, and some are expressed selectively in these loci. The bad news is that few new drugs have been developed that target these sites, and more importantly, there is some evidence that targeting a single locus may leave too many routes through which nociceptive messages, and thus pain, can be generated.

Put another way, to some researchers and clinicians, the abundance of signaling molecules that can be targeted in the treatment of pain is the proverbial cup that is half full; to others, the cup is half empty. One must first choose among the many targets, but one cannot ignore the possibility that compensatory changes that overcome the targeting of a single molecule will occur. This is a legitimate clinical concern. As noted below, despite an abundance of targets, the long-sought magic bullet for pain relief has not been found. The cup-half-full contingent also recognizes the likelihood of there being adverse side effects that limit the utility of targeting a single entity, unless the target has a very restricted distribution in the central nervous system (CNS). This concern probably increases proportionately with the diversity of the circuits to which any particular molecular target contributes.

NMDA RECEPTORS: THE HOLY GRAIL IS STILL ILLUSIVE

Despite the presence of multiple pronociceptive molecules/transmitters in primary afferent nociceptors, the key neurotransmitter is still glutamate, and thus understanding the physiology of glutamate's action in the dorsal horn is critical (Carpenter and Dickenson 2001). There are multiple receptors through which glutamate exerts its effects, but not all are candidates for developing novel therapies. Until recently, the simplest view held that acute pain results from glutamate action at α-amino-3-hydroxy-5-methyl-4-isoxazole propionate (AMPA) receptors, which mediate brief depolarization of postsynaptic membrane and action potential generation in postsynaptic neurons (e.g., spinothalamic tract neurons). By contrast, the *N*-methyl-D-aspartate (NMDA) receptor, which at resting membrane potential is inactive, opens when the postsynaptic membrane is slightly depolarized. When glutamate binds to the NMDA receptor, Ca^{2+} enters the postsynaptic neuron. Recent studies have identified many other routes through which glutamate can increase intracellular Ca^{2+}. For example, some subtypes of AMPA receptors gate Ca^{2+}. Moreover, glutamate action at G-protein-linked, metabotropic glutamate receptors can increase intracellular Ca^{2+}, in this case from intracellular stores. The consequences of increased intracellular Ca^{2+} are profound and include activation of a variety of second-messenger systems and enzymes, as well as increased gene transcription, resulting in the synthesis of new proteins. Together these changes contribute to central sensitization, which underlies the hyperexcitability of CNS circuits and contributes to the allodynia and hyperalgesia produced by tissue and nerve injury (Woolf and Salter 2000).

Because the NR1 subunit of the NMDA receptor is ubiquitous, it is not a good target for therapy; the adverse side effects produced by NR1 interference are very high. However, because the NR1 subunit occurs along with a mix of NR2 subunits (A through D), the possibility of developing antagonists directed at the NR2 subunits has been examined. The NR2B subunit is of particular interest. It is concentrated in the superficial dorsal horn, has been implicated in the development of central sensitization and of tissue- and nerve-injury-induced persistent pain, and can be targeted by selective antagonists (Boyce et al. 1999; Chizh et al. 2001; Malmberg et al. 2003; Guo et al. 2004). Also of interest are the many regulatory proteins with which the NMDA-receptor subunits are complexed, for example, the membrane-associated guanylate kinase proteins (Garry and Fleetwood-Walker 2004), notably postsynaptic density 95 protein (PSD-95) and PSD-93 . Mice in which PSD-95 has been deleted do not show mechanical hypersensitivity after nerve injury (Garry et al. 2003), while loss of inflammatory hypersensitivity occurs in PSD-93 mutant mice (Tao et al. 2003; Zhang et al. 2003).

Clearly, the development of highly selective antagonists that can be targeted to the spinal cord has appeal, provided that other contributors to central sensitization and persistent pain do not become predominant. Once again, the critical balance between highly selective drug targeting, which should open therapeutic windows, must be weighed against the need for drugs that eliminate the back doors through which injury inputs sustain long-term, maladaptive plastic changes in the CNS.

OTHER "SOMETHING NEW" TARGETS

The number and diversity of the new targets that have been implicated in the development and maintenance of persistent pain are impressive, yet daunting. I am often reminded of a review that highlighted the number of molecules implicated in the phenomenon of long-term potentiation (LTP), which many researchers believe is a critical basis for learning and memory (Sanes and Lichtman 1999). That article included a table with over 100 molecules, any or all of which could be manipulated in molecular, genetic, or pharmacological studies to enhance or reduce LTP. Many of these molecules have also been implicated in central sensitization, inhibition of which many pain researchers predict will have clinical utility for persistent pain (Ji et al. 2003). Unfortunately, just as the translation of knowledge about LTP to the clinic (e.g., for the treatment of Alzheimer's disease) has been largely unsuccessful, the translation of molecules that interfere with central sensitization to the clinic for pain management has yet to materialize. The most pessimistic view is that an effective drug against central sensitization may have very deleterious side effects because it will also block LTP.

Tetrodotoxin (TTX)-resistant Na⁺ channels. There is little consensus as to what is the best "new" target to attack clinically. In my opinion, the TTX-resistant Na⁺ channel is among the most important targets to consider in the development of novel analgesics (Akopian et al. 1996; Lai et al. 2004). Most importantly, this channel is only expressed by primary afferents. The vast majority of these afferents are unmyelinated, and thus likely to be nociceptors (Djouhri et al. 2003). There is, of course, unequivocal evidence for the utility of local anesthetics in treating complicated persistent pain conditions, such as postherpetic neuralgia, whether applied topically (Rowbotham et al. 1995; see Watson, this volume) or systemically (Rowbotham et al. 1991). The problem is that local anesthetics indiscriminately block Na⁺ channels, resulting in a highly unfavorable therapeutic index, including CNS side effects that are often poorly tolerated. Because the TTX-resistant Na⁺ channel is not expressed in the CNS, its targeting should be associated with a much larger therapeutic window.

Not only is the TTX-resistant Na⁺ channel highly restricted in its distribution, but evidence also indicates that the channel is altered in the setting of tissue and nerve injury (Gold et al. 2003) and contributes to the abnormal spontaneous activity of injured peripheral nerves (Roza et al. 2003). Furthermore, delivery of molecules to target this channel should be simpler because drugs can access the channel in the dorsal root ganglia and peripheral nerves, without having to cross the blood-brain barrier. Unfortunately, development of selective inhibitors has not yet been successful, in part because the molecular structures of TTX-resistant and TTX-sensitive Na⁺ channels do not differ sufficiently. An alternative approach is to use methods that reduce expression of the mRNA that codes for the channel. Antisense studies have proven successful in preclinical animal studies (Lai et al. 2002), but this technology has not proven very successful for clinical practice. Conceivably, newer technologies (see below), including the use of small interfering RNA (siRNA), will permit selective inhibition of the TTX-resistant Na⁺ contribution in patients.

The vanilloid/capsaicin receptor. The difficulty in choosing targets based on molecular characterization of molecules that are enriched in nociceptors is further illustrated by the example of TRPV1, the first member of the transient receptor potential family of channels, also known as the capsaicin receptor. Animals with deletions of this channel show reduced acute pain response to heat and significantly reduced thermal sensitization (Caterina et al. 2000; Davis et al. 2000). On the other hand, tissue- and nerve-injury-induced mechanical hypersensitivity is not altered in these animals. Because mechanical hypersensitivity is a far greater clinical problem than thermal hypersensitivity, the significance of TRPV1 to clinical pain problems is not clear. However, because lowered pH can dramatically lower the temperature threshold for activating TRPV1, it has been suggested that TRPV1 might be relevant in pain conditions where there is inflammation of the viscera. Lowered pH in the setting of visceral inflammation conceivably could activate the normally silent visceral nociceptor, resulting in intense, spontaneous visceral pain. Future studies that use new visceral pain models, followed by clinical trials, should answer this question in a relatively short time period.

Potassium channels. The idea that reduced K^+ channel activity underlies injury-induced increases in neuronal excitability is not new; it has been a mainstay in the epilepsy field (Rogawski and Loscher 2004). Conceivably, therefore, enhancing K^+ channel activity in the setting of hyperexcitability could have equivalent therapeutic value, as would decreasing the activity of TTX-resistant Na^+ channels. For example, Dost et al. (2004) reported that opening the KCNQ potassium channel with the anticonvulsant retigabine is effective in different pain models, even after oral administration. Somewhat paradoxically perhaps, other examples exist in which inhibiting K^+ channel activity is effective. For example, inhibitors of a hyperpolarization-activated cyclic nucleotide-gated potassium channel that is expressed in dorsal root ganglion neurons (Chaplan et al. 2003) not only reduced the hyperactivity of injured peripheral nerves, but also reduced the associated mechanical allodynia. Importantly, there was no effect on normal pain sensitivity. Other approaches to regulating channel activity may be achieved through advances in gene therapy, using viral vectors to increase the expression of the channel of interest. Clearly, a critical factor will be the selectivity of the agents used to regulate the remarkably heterogeneous population of potassium channels, many of which are expressed in primary afferent nociceptors.

Targeting mechanical hypersensitivity. The major clinical problem is not ongoing pain, but mechanical hypersensitivity: "It hurts when I move." Recent research has identified myriad ways that innocuous mechanical inputs can gain access to "pain" transmission circuits in the setting of tissue or nerve injury. Reorganization of spinal cord circuits after injury certainly contributes, including the inappropriate interaction of input carried by $A\beta$ mechanoreceptive afferents with spinal cord circuits that are involved in nociceptive processing. Loss of inhibitory GABAergic tone (Drew et al. 2004), sprouting of large-diameter afferents (Woolf et al. 1995; Bennett et al. 1996), and the de novo synthesis of pronociceptive neurotransmitters by large-diameter afferents have also been implicated (Neumann et al. 1996). A key unanswered question is the nature of the peripheral channel that transduces mechanical stimulation by primary afferents (Lewin and Moshourab

2004). Several families of molecule have been implicated (Price et al. 2000, 2001), notably members of the degenerin/epithelial sodium channel family and most recently, TRPV4, an osmosensor that contributes to mechanical hypersensitivity in the setting of peripheral injury (Alessandri-Haber et al. 2004). Clearly, when the critical channel is identified, the opportunity to develop novel drugs to counter the problem of mechanical hypersensitivity in the setting of injury will be greatly increased.

Targeting the glial cell. Far from being the glue that holds neurons together, glial cells have rapidly become a major focus of research into the pathophysiology of persistent pain conditions (Wieseler-Frank et al. 2004). Although it was traditionally assumed that CNS glial cells only proliferate when there is frank injury to CNS tissue, recent studies demonstrate that glial cells are remarkably responsive to injury to peripheral tissue (including nerves) and that the response is topographic (Honoré et al. 2000). The changes are not mapped as precisely as those of afferents, which may explain why the distribution of pain, such as secondary hyperalgesia, often expands beyond the site of injury. What triggers glial hypertrophy is not known, but studies indicate that neural activity or trophic factors transported by neurons (or not transported, in the case of peripheral nerve injury) are important drivers of the glial response. Another possibility is that humoral factors, including tissue-injury-induced peripheral cytokines, could trigger a spinal cord CNS glial response (Wieseler-Frank et al. 2004). Most importantly, perhaps, there is evidence that the dorsal horn glial cell is the source of many of the CNS mediators, such as prostaglandins, that contribute to central sensitization. To what extent targeting the glial cell could have beneficial effects in the management of pain remains to be determined, but this highly novel approach should clearly be pursued.

Targeting something new (very new). Yet another very novel target for therapy is derived from analysis of the cell's ubiquitination pathway. This pathway is the route through which proteins are trafficked in the cell, either to a different location to specify function, or to the proteosome for degradation (Glickman and Ciechanover 2002). The learning/synaptic plasticity literature has provided a clue to the function of this system and to its possible relevance in persistent pain conditions. Ubiquitination of synaptic proteins has been implicated in long-term plasticity by regulating proteins that interact with the glutamate receptors (Colledge et al. 2003). Studies in the Fleetwood-Walker laboratory (Moss et al. 2002) have shown that intrathecal injection of a selective proteosome inhibitor that prevents ubiquitination significantly reduced nerve-injury-induced hypersensitivity in several pain models.

The complexity of the potential targets is further illustrated by studies that implicated lysophosphatidic acid (LPA; Inoue et al. 2004). LPA is a lipid-derived messenger that acts via a G-protein-coupled receptor. LPA is released in the setting of nerve injury (from platelets), and its inhibition can reduce the allodynia and hyperalgesia produced by nerve injury. For the record, neither the ubiquitination pathway nor LPA are on the Sanes and Lichtman (1999) list of key molecules that contribute to LTP. In other words, the list is getting longer, not shorter, and the route to identifying the best target is less, not more clearly, marked.

MAGIC BULLETS OR COCKTAILS?

Few IASP meetings go by without a heated discussion about the feasibility of developing novel, effective analgesics that only target a single molecule, the so-called "magic bullet" analgesic. The fact that so many mutant mice with single gene deletions show remarkable loss of persistent pain in the setting of tissue or nerve injury suggests that interfering with a single target in patients may be successful in treating difficult pain conditions (Mogil et al. 2000). My colleagues and I have contributed extensively to this literature, implicating neurotransmitters, receptors, and a variety of second-messenger molecules (Malmberg et al. 1997a,b; Cao et al. 1998; Caterina et al. 2000; Zeitz et al. 2002). The hope, of course, is that the phenotype of the mutant mouse translates to the clinical condition, but that hope may not be realized. Rather, the complex array of channels that transduces noxious information and the multiple ways in which hypersensitivity of dorsal horn circuits can be generated raise the unfortunate concern that inhibiting a single mechanism may not be sufficient, or that it will eventually be overcome by redundant circuits. If this is true, then cocktails that target multiple mechanisms should be seriously considered. This is not the first suggestion that polypharmacy may be more common in the future, but the science certainly points that way.

SOMETHING BORROWED

That anticonvulsants have great utility in the management of many pain syndromes has been known for decades. In fact, some of the newest anticonvulsants, notably gabapentin, have proven more effective for pain management than for epilepsy. Although the mechanism of action of gabapentin is still not clear, there is convincing evidence that it binds to the $\alpha_2\delta$ subunit of Ca^{2+} channels (Klugbauer et al. 2003). Whether this is indeed the functional target in humans is not yet established, but research and drug development in the future will clearly focus on this channel, with a view to generating more selective and efficacious analgesics. Identifying the particular neuron or population of neurons where gabapentin acts in different neuropathic pain conditions will also help in this effort and more importantly, should provide new insights into the mechanisms that underlie nerve-injury-induced pain.

Borrowing from other fields is not limited to epilepsy. The same is, of course, true for the development and adaptation of antidepressants for the treatment of neuropathic pain (Max 1994; Dworkin et al. 2003). To this day, however, the mechanisms through which these drugs work for diabetic neuropathic or postherpetic neuralgia are not known. The early ideas that the mechanism involved enhancement of descending controls of "pain" transmission at the level of the spinal cord have largely been abandoned, in part because the most selective serotonin reuptake inhibitors are not particularly effective in the treatment of neuropathic pain. Obviously, the noradrenergic component might predominate, but it is equally likely that an as yet unknown underlying mechanism will be uncovered. Future studies, perhaps with better animal models will home in on the likely target. Is it in the spinal cord, in the brain, or both?

INSIGHTS FROM CANCER CHEMOTHERAPY

More and more I have come to appreciate that there are important similarities between the problems faced by the pain management physician and the oncologist. For example, the oncologist has numerous drugs with which to begin treatment. Most are very effective for in vitro models using tumor cell lines, and prior to their introduction into the clinic, most proved effective in mouse models, typically involving xenografts of tumor cell lines. Indeed, the rule is that if the drug does not work in the mouse, it will not work in the human. Unfortunately, the fact that it works in the mouse in no way ensures success in the humans.

These features have obvious parallels in the development of novel analgesics. Many drugs work in animals, but not all are effective in patients, or they may not provide relief beyond that produced by presently available compounds. As noted above, molecular studies have identified many proteins, deletion of which can have dramatic effects in animal models of persistent pain. Yet translating this information to the clinic has proven difficult. Either designing drugs that interfere selectively with the target has been problematic, or the molecules have failed in the clinic. Just as the preclinical in vivo models for cancer do not necessarily model the human cancer condition, so the extent to which a particular animal model of persistent pain models the clinical persistent pain condition needs further study.

The issue of animal models is particularly important. Recent years have seen an enormous growth in the development of animal models of persistent pain. Neuropathic pain, in particular, is much more readily studied now because of the development of various nerve-injury- and chemotherapy-induced persistent pain models (Bennett and Xie 1988; Seltzer et al. 1990; Kim and Chung 1992; Aley et al. 1996; Malmberg and Basbaum 1998; Decosterd and Woolf 2000). Is it reasonable to assume that one animal neuropathic pain model fits all clinical neuropathic pain conditions? Is a single model, or are three partial nerve injury models, predictive of the pain of postherpetic neuralgia, phantom limb pain, diabetic neuropathy, or post-stroke pain? This surmise is unlikely, not because the models are poor, but because the clinical conditions are diverse and probably do not have a unitary underlying mechanism.

It is of interest that only rarely has a drug been brought to the clinic for neuropathic pain after it proved effective in one or more animal models. As noted above, most analgesics that are effective for neuropathic pain were initially developed as anticonvulsants. They were tested in animal models only after they were evaluated in humans. In effect, this is a retrospective validation of the preclinical neuropathic pain models, supporting the view that these models are predictive of analgesic efficacy in the clinic. A good example in this regard is ziconotide, a cone-snail-derived toxin that targets N-type calcium channels. The efficacy of ziconotide was, in fact, first shown to be effective in animal models of pain (Chaplan 2000; Malmberg and Yaksh 1995). Studies in patients followed these preclinical reports of analgesic efficacy (Atanassoff et al. 2000; Jain 2000).

The other major problem with cancer treatment is that the most effective drugs are often the ones with the worst side-effect profile. Killing tumor cells without killing normal cells is difficult; the window of therapy is generally very small, and the side effects are often so negative that a patient will turn to other approaches, including complementary medicine. Of course, the adverse side effects of opioids are their major limitations, and indeed many patients will turn to alternative therapies, despite the evidence that few are more effective than placebo. Clearly, we need to develop new analgesics with better side-effect profiles, or we need to focus on the management of the side effects so that the therapeutic window of the available analgesics (such as morphine and other opiates) can be significantly increased.

SOMETHING BLUE

TECHNOLOGY, MODELS, AND INSIGHTS

Recent papers have discussed the importance of a genetic contribution to different pain conditions and to drug sensitivity. Gender differences are now well established, in animals as well as in humans (Casey 1999; Craft 2003; Mitrovic et al. 2003; Mogil et al. 2003; Craft et al. 2004; Rustoen et al. 2004). Whether identifying genes will direct therapy in the future of pain therapy, in the way that pharmacogenomics and individual tailoring of drugs is considered the next revolution in cancer chemotherapy, seems unlikely, at least in the near future. On the other hand, improved understanding of the mechanisms underlying different pain conditions and, most importantly, a better grasp of their heterogeneity should come out of such studies. Clinicians and basic scientists regularly use the term "neuropathic pain," but the lack of specificity in the term ignores the complexity and heterogeneity of these pain conditions. Everyone understands the term; it is pain produced by nerve injury, but the term obliterates what are clearly profound differences in the nature of the insult that induces the pain. To what extent a pharmacogenetic analysis of patients with different neuropathic pain conditions will reveal molecular markers of these different conditions remains to be seen. This possibility needs to be evaluated, as it could lead to the development of analgesic drugs that are more effective and have a lower adverse side-effect profile, and most importantly better predictability. Future research should better characterize the clinical syndromes, identifying their commonalities and differences so that drug therapy can be appropriately tailored.

MORE ON MAGIC BULLETS

Because of the explosion of targets that the molecular biologists have identified in different elements of the "pain" transmission system, it is not surprising that therapies based on delivery of genes is seriously considered. The technology to deliver genes is advancing rapidly, as are approaches to selectively reduce the expression of "undesirable" genes. Antisense technology has proven effective in animal models (Lai et al. 2002; Shimoyama et al. 2005), but the technical hurdles to adapt it to patients have not been overcome. For this reason the early enthusiasm for antisense approaches to "knock down" the level of messenger RNA for particular molecules has subsided. The idea that molecular reduction of "bad" genes can have great clinical utility has not, however, been abandoned. On the contrary, the explosion of interest in the utility of RNA interference, which relies on small interfering (siRNA) molecules to reduce or eliminate mRNAs, has revitalized the field (Jones et al. 2004; Novina and Sharp 2004). Using viral vectors to deliver the siRNA molecules, it should be possible not only to target single genes, but also to generate long-term suppression of expression of pronociceptive molecules. Only recently has the technology proven effective in animal models of persistent pain (Dorn et al. 2004; Ganju and Hall 2004). The results are encouraging, and the likelihood of clinical applicability, I believe, is high.

NOVEL ABLATIVE PROCEDURES

Although anterolateral cordotomy has very limited application for the treatment of intractable pain, other, more restricted ablative procedures are being investigated. A molecular-based therapy is receiving considerable attention, although it has not yet been studied in patients. Mantyh and colleagues (1997) adapted a longstanding approach from the cancer field, which takes advantage of surface proteins to define, target, and selectively kill tumor cells, leaving normal cells unaffected. The technology uses a neurotoxic substance P-saporin conjugate, which binds to neurokinin-1 (NK1) receptors on the plasma membrane of a small subset of spinal cord neurons. The substance P component of the toxin conjugate binds to the NK1 receptors, leading to internalization of the entire molecule. The saporin is cleaved in the cytoplasm and then it kills the cell by interfering with protein synthesis. Because the conjugate can only enter cells that express the NK1 receptor, there is hope that the therapeutic window will be large enough to limit side effects. Preliminary results in animals are exciting and encouraging, but the consequence of long-term elimination of subsets of neurons remains to be determined. This is an irreversible ablative procedure, and thus will probably be introduced in a limited number of terminal cancer pain patients before it is evaluated in other persistent pain conditions.

It is, of course, possible that other subsets of spinal cord nociresponsive neurons, or for that matter primary afferents or thalamic neurons, could be targeted with saporin conjugates. If there are indeed labeled lines for different modalities of pain (a controversial topic, to say the least; see Craig 2003), then eliminating one subset may not be sufficient to produce satisfactory, long-term relief of pain. On the other hand, if the NK1 receptor is expressed by all of these subsets of labeled lines, then the problem may be overcome. As more information is gathered about the cell surface markers that characterize the myriad populations of neurons that transmit nociceptive information to the brain, other candidates for selective targeting will almost certainly be identified.

WHAT PROTOCOL SHOULD DIRECT THE SEARCH FOR NEW ANALGESICS?

How then should the scientist and by extension, the pharmaceutical industry proceed? Should their efforts be directed at one or a few of the molecules that are differentially expressed in normal and injured nociceptors? If a subset of these nociceptors is altered by the drug, will that be sufficient to produce adequate pain relief? Or is there too large an escape route, via nociceptors that are injured but do not express the particular molecule, or because there are dozens of other critical molecules that are also dysregulated by injury? The $P2X_3$ subtype of purinergic receptor provides a good illustration of the latter problem. The $P2X_3$ receptor is almost exclusively expressed by a subset of the nonpeptide-containing, IB4-binding population of unmyelinated nociceptors (Snider and McMahon 1998; Vulchanova et al. 1998). Importantly, its elimination, through gene deletion (Cockayne et al. 2000; Souslova et al. 2000), antisense technology (Barclay et al. 2002), or siRNA technology (Dorn et al. 2004), can reduce persistent pain behavior in different animal models. Do these studies provide a sufficient body of evidence to spend the millions of dollars required to test for the effects of antagonizing this receptor in patients? The fact is that the subset of neurons that express the $P2X_3$ receptor is very small. My bias is that targeting of molecules that are more ubiquitously expressed, such as the TTX-resistant Na^+ channel or different Ca^{2+} channel subtypes, has advantages. The downside of that approach is that the adverse side-effect profile is probably directly related to the extent to which the molecule is expressed in a ubiquitous, or a highly distributed fashion.

CONCLUDING THOUGHTS

There is no question that I have concentrated on the nociception component of the pain experience. For this reason it is not surprising that my predictions about future directions in pain therapy emphasize pharmacological targets that regulate nociceptive processing. These are concentrated in the periphery (at the nociceptor) and in the spinal cord, a critical locus for central sensitization. Of course, targets must also be present at higher levels of the neuraxis, but we have much less information about the neurochemical and molecular basis of nociceptive processing at these levels.

This situation could change significantly in the next few years. Imaging techniques are opening a fascinating window into the thalamic and cortical mechanisms that contribute to the experience of pain. Of particular interest are the insights that these studies provide about the sensory-discriminative and emotional components of the pain experience, as discussed by Bushnell in this volume. In this regard, I also recognize that I have not at all discussed nonpharmacological approaches to the management of pain. Clearly, the complexity of the pain experience requires that a multidisciplinary approach should integrate the future of pharmacotherapy with novel nonpharmacological approaches, including psychological approaches, as discussed by Keefe et al. in this volume.

To what extent brain-imaging studies will affect pain therapy is unclear. Imaging cannot yet be used to objectively measure pain. On the other hand, there is a very interesting possibility on the horizon. The ability to perform neurochemical analyses of different brain regions and to evaluate drug action through imaging techniques offers the promise of a new approach to drug assessment (Zubieta et al. 2002). The resolution of imaging techniques is advancing so rapidly that it may soon be possible to localize drug actions at the level of one or several neurons. This technique may, in fact, revolutionize the development of drugs and make it possible to design and evaluate novel analgesics for individual pain conditions.

Finally, let me return to the title of this chapter. The original marriage recommendation was, in fact, to wear: "Something old, something new, something borrowed and something blue, *and a silver sixpence in her shoe.*" The sixpence presumably was a good luck token to ensure the financial security of the marriage. For all the basic scientists and clinicians, as well as the pharmaceutical industry, which spends millions of dollars to develop new drugs for pain therapy, I wish you the "sixpence in your shoe." May funding agencies continue to support pain research, and may the pharmaceutical industry be successful in its efforts to bring safe and effective drugs to the clinic in the shortest time possible.

ACKNOWLEDGMENTS

The author's research is supported by grants from the NIH. The author has consulting relationships with several pharmaceutical companies and specifically has studied NR2B antagonists with support from Cognetix, Inc.

REFERENCES

Ahmadi S, Lippross S, Neuhuber WL, Zeilhofer HU. PGE_2 selectively blocks inhibitory glycinergic neurotransmission onto rat superficial dorsal horn neurons. *Nat Neurosci* 2002; 5:34–40.

Akopian AN, Sivilotti L, Wood JN. A tetrodotoxin-resistant voltage-gated sodium channel expressed by sensory neurons. *Nature* 1996; 379:257–262.

Alessandri-Haber N, Dina OA, Yeh JJ, et al. Transient receptor potential vanilloid 4 is essential in chemotherapy-induced neuropathic pain in the rat. *J Neurosci* 2004; 24:4444–4452.

Aley KO, Reichling DB, Levine JD. Vincristine hyperalgesia in the rat: a model of painful vincristine neuropathy in humans. *Neuroscience* 1996; 73:259–265.

Atanassoff PG, Hartmannsgruber MW, Thrasher J, et al. Ziconotide, a new N-type calcium channel blocker, administered intrathecally for acute postoperative pain. *Reg Anesth Pain Med* 2000; 25:274–278.

Bar KJ, Natura G, Telleria-Diaz A, et al. Changes in the effect of spinal prostaglandin E2 during inflammation: prostaglandin E (EP1–EP4) receptors in spinal nociceptive processing of input from the normal or inflamed knee joint. *J Neurosci* 2004; 24:642–651.

Barclay J, Patel S, Dorn G, et al. Functional downregulation of P2X3 receptor subunit in rat sensory neurons reveals a significant role in chronic neuropathic and inflammatory pain. *J Neurosci* 2002; 22:8139–8147.

Basbaum AI. New techniques, targets and treatments for pain: what promise does the future hold? In: *Celebrating 25 Years, International Association for the Study of Pain, 1973–1998.* Seattle: IASP Press, 1998, pp 16–18.

Basbaum AI, Besson J-M. *Towards a New Pharmacotherapy of Pain,* Life Sciences Research Reports, Vol. 49. London: Wiley, 1991.

Basbaum AI, Woolf CJ. Pain. *Curr Biol* 1999; 9:R429–431.

Bennett GJ, Xie Y-K. A peripheral mononeuropathy in rat that produces disorders of pain sensation like those seen in man. *Pain* 1988; 33:87–107.

Bennett DL, French J, Priestley JV, McMahon SB. NGF but not NT-3 or BDNF prevents the A fiber sprouting into lamina II of the spinal cord that occurs following axotomy. *Mol Cell Neurosci* 1996; 8:211–220.

Boyce S, Wyatt A, Webb JK, et al. Selective NMDA NR2B antagonists induce antinociception without motor dysfunction: correlation with restricted localisation of NR2B subunit in dorsal horn. *Neuropharmacology* 1999; 38:611–623.

Cao YQ, Mantyh PW, Carlson EJ, et al. Primary afferent tachykinins are required to experience moderate to intense pain. *Nature (Lond)* 1998; 392:390–394.

Carpenter KJ, Dickenson AH. Amino acids are still as exciting as ever. *Curr Opin Pharmacol* 2001; 1:57–61.

Casey KL. Forebrain mechanisms of nociception and pain: analysis through imaging. *Proc Natl Acad Sci USA* 1999; 96:7668–7674.

Caterina MJ, Leffler A, Malmberg AB, et al. Impaired nociception and pain sensation in mice lacking the capsaicin receptor. *Science* 2000; 288:306–313.

Chaplan SR. Neuropathic pain: role of voltage-dependent calcium channels. *Reg Anesth Pain Med* 2000; 25:283–285.

Chaplan SR, Guo HQ, Lee DH, et al. Neuronal hyperpolarization-activated pacemaker channels drive neuropathic pain. *J Neurosci* 2003; 23:1169–1178.

Chizh BA, Headley PM, Tzschentke TM. NMDA receptor antagonists as analgesics: focus on the NR2B subtype. *Trends Pharmacol Sci* 2001; 22:636–642.

Cockayne DA, Hamilton SG, Zhu QM, et al. Urinary bladder hyporeflexia and reduced pain-related behaviour in P2X3-deficient mice. *Nature* 2000; 407:1011–1015.

Colledge M, Snyder EM, Crozier RA, et al. Ubiquitination regulates PSD-95 degradation and AMPA receptor surface expression. *Neuron* 2003; 40:595–607.

Craft RM. Sex differences in opioid analgesia: "from mouse to man." *Clin J Pain* 2003; 19:175–186.

Craft RM, Mogil JS, Aloisi MA. Sex differences in pain and analgesia: the role of gonadal hormones. *Eur J Pain* 2004; 8:397–411.

Craig AD. Pain mechanisms: labeled lines versus convergence in central processing. *Annu Rev Neurosci* 2003; 26:1–30.

Davis JB, Gray J, Gunthorpe MJ, et al. Vanilloid receptor-1 is essential for inflammatory thermal hyperalgesia. *Nature* 2000; 405:183–187.

Decosterd I, Woolf CJ. Spared nerve injury: an animal model of persistent peripheral neuropathic pain. *Pain* 2000; 87:149–158.

Djouhri L, Fang X, Okuse K, et al. The TTX-resistant sodium channel Nav1.8 (SNS/PN3): expression and correlation with membrane properties in rat nociceptive primary afferent neurons. *J Physiol* 2003; 550:739–752.

Dorn G, Patel S, Wotherspoon G, et al. siRNA relieves chronic neuropathic pain. *Nucleic Acids Res* 2004; 32:e49.

Dost R, Rostock A, Rundfeldt C. The anti-hyperalgesic activity of retigabine is mediated by KCNQ potassium channel activation. *Naunyn Schmiedebergs Arch Pharmacol* 2004; 369:382–390.

Drew GM, Siddall PJ, Duggan AW. Mechanical allodynia following contusion injury of the rat spinal cord is associated with loss of GABAergic inhibition in the dorsal horn. *Pain* 2004; 109:379–388.

Dworkin RH, Backonja M, Rowbotham MC, et al. Advances in neuropathic pain: diagnosis, mechanisms, and treatment recommendations. *Arch Neurol* 2003; 60:1524–1534.

Ganju P, Hall J. Potential applications of siRNA for pain therapy. *Expert Opin Biol Ther* 2004; 4:531–542.

Garry EM, Fleetwood-Walker SM. Organizing pains. *Trends Neurosci* 2004; 27:292–294.

Garry EM, Moss A, Delaney A, et al. Neuropathic sensitization of behavioral reflexes and spinal NMDA receptor/CaM kinase II interactions are disrupted in PSD-95 mutant mice. *Curr Biol* 2003; 13:321–328.

Ghilardi JR, Svensson CI, Rogers SD, Yaksh TL, Mantyh PW. Constitutive spinal cyclooxygenase-2 participates in the initiation of tissue injury-induced hyperalgesia. *J Neurosci* 2004; 24:2727–2732.

Gilson AM, Ryan KM, Joranson DE, Dahl JL. A reassessment of trends in the medical use and abuse of opioid analgesics and implications for diversion control: 1997–2002. *J Pain Symptom Manage* 2004; 28:176–188.

Glickman MH, Ciechanover A. The ubiquitin-proteasome proteolytic pathway: destruction for the sake of construction. *Physiol Rev* 2002; 82:373–428.

Gold MS, Weinreich D, Kim CS, et al. Redistribution of $Na_V1.8$ in uninjured axons enables neuropathic pain. *J Neurosci* 2003; 23:158–166.

Guo W, Wei F, Zou S, et al. Group I metabotropic glutamate receptor NMDA receptor coupling and signaling cascade mediate spinal dorsal horn NMDA receptor 2B tyrosine phosphorylation associated with inflammatory hyperalgesia. *J Neurosci* 2004; 24:9161–9173.

Honoré P, Rogers SD, Schwei MJ, et al. Murine models of inflammatory, neuropathic and cancer pain each generates a unique set of neurochemical changes in the spinal cord and sensory neurons. *Neuroscience* 2000; 98:585–598.

Inoue M, Rashid MH, Fujita R, et al. Initiation of neuropathic pain requires lysophosphatidic acid receptor signaling. *Nat Med* 2004; 10:712–718.

Jain KK. An evaluation of intrathecal ziconotide for the treatment of chronic pain. *Expert Opin Investig Drugs* 2000; 9:2403–2410.

Ji RR, Kohno T, Moore KA, Woolf CJ. Central sensitization and LTP: do pain and memory share common mechanisms? *Trends Neurosci* 2003; 26:696–705.

Jones SW, Souza PM, Lindsay MA. siRNA for gene silencing: a route to drug target discovery. *Curr Opin Pharmacol* 2004; 4:522–527.

Julius D, Basbaum AI. Molecular mechanisms of nociception. *Nature* 2001; 413:203–210.

Kim SH, Chung JM. An experimental model for peripheral neuropathy produced by segmental spinal nerve ligation in the rat. *Pain* 1992; 50:355–363.

Klugbauer N, Marais E, Hofmann F. Calcium channel alpha-2-delta subunits: differential expression, function, and drug binding. *J Bioenerg Biomembr* 2003; 35:639–647.

Lai J, Gold MS, Kim CS, et al. Inhibition of neuropathic pain by decreased expression of the tetrodotoxin-resistant sodium channel, Na$_V$1.8. *Pain* 2002; 95:143–152.

Lai J, Porreca F, Hunter JC, Gold MS. Voltage-gated sodium channels and hyperalgesia. *Annu Rev Pharmacol Toxicol* 2004; 44:371–397.

Lewin GR, Moshourab R. Mechanosensation and pain. *J Neurobiol* 2004; 61:30–44.

Malmberg AB, Basbaum AI. Partial injury to the sciatic nerve in the mouse: neuropathic pain behavior and dorsal horn plasticity. *Pain* 1998; 76:215–222.

Malmberg AB, Yaksh TL. Hyperalgesia mediated by spinal glutamate or substance P receptor blocked by spinal cyclooxygenase inhibition. *Science* 1992; 257:1276–1279.

Malmberg AB, Yaksh TL. Effect of continuous intrathecal infusion of omega-conopeptides, N-type calcium-channel blockers, on behavior and antinociception in the formalin and hot-plate tests in rats. *Pain* 1995; 60:83–90.

Malmberg AB, Brandon EP, Idzerda RL, et al. Diminished inflammation and nociceptive pain with preservation of neuropathic pain in mice with a targeted mutation of the RIβ subunit of PKA. *J Neurosci* 1997a; 17:7462–7470.

Malmberg AB, Chen C, Tonegawa S, Basbaum AI. Preserved acute pain and reduced neuropathic pain in mice lacking PKCγ. *Science* 1997b; 278:279–283.

Malmberg AB, Gilbert H, McCabe RT, Basbaum AI. Powerful antinociceptive effects of the cone snail venom-derived subtype-selective NMDA receptor antagonists conantokins G and T. *Pain* 2003; 101:109–116.

Mantyh PW, Rogers SD, Honoré P, et al. Inhibition of hyperalgesia by ablation of lamina I spinal neurons expressing the substance P receptor. *Science* 1997; 278:275–279.

Marriott DR, Wilkin GP, Wood JN. Substance P induced release of prostaglandins from astrocytes: regional specialisation and correlation with phosphoinositol metabolism. *J Neurochem* 1991; 56:259–265.

Max MB. Treatment of post-herpetic neuralgia: antidepressants. *Ann Neurol* 1994; 35(Suppl): 50–53.

Mitrovic I, Margeta-Mitrovic M, Bader S, et al. Contribution of GIRK2-mediated postsynaptic signaling to opiate and alpha 2-adrenergic analgesia and analgesic sex differences. *Proc Natl Acad Sci USA* 2003; 100:271–276.

Mogil JS, Yu L, Basbaum AI. Pain genes? natural variation and transgenic mutants. *Annu Rev Neurosci* 2000; 23:777–811.

Mogil JS, Wilson SG, Chesler EJ, et al. The melanocortin-1 receptor gene mediates female-specific mechanisms of analgesia in mice and humans. *Proc Natl Acad Sci USA* 2003; 100:4867–4872.

Moss A, Blackburn-Munro G, Garry EM, et al. A role of the ubiquitin-proteasome system in neuropathic pain. *J Neurosci* 2002; 22:1363–1372.

Neumann S, Doubell TP, Leslie T, Woolf CJ. Inflammatory pain hypersensitivity mediated by phenotypic switch in myelinated primary sensory neurons. *Nature* 1996; 384:360–364.

Novina CD, Sharp PA. The RNAi revolution. *Nature* 2004; 430:161–164.

Price MP, Lewin GR, McIlwrath SL, et al. The mammalian sodium channel BNC1 is required for normal touch sensation. *Nature* 2000; 407:1007–1011.

Price MP, McIlwrath SL, Xie J, et al. The DRASIC cation channel contributes to the detection of cutaneous touch and acid stimuli in mice. *Neuron* 2001; 32:1071–1083.

Rogawski MA, Loscher W. The neurobiology of antiepileptic drugs for the treatment of nonepileptic conditions. *Nat Med* 2004; 10:685–692.

Rowbotham MC, Reisner-Keller LA, Fields HL. Both intravenous lidocaine and morphine reduce the pain of postherpetic neuralgia. *Neurology* 1991; 41(7):1024–1028.

Rowbotham MC, Davies PS, Fields HL. Topical lidocaine gel relieves postherpetic neuralgia. *Ann Neurol* 1995; 37:246–253.

Roza C, Laird JM, Souslova V, Wood JN, Cervero F. The tetrodotoxin-resistant Na$^+$ channel Na$_v$1.8 is essential for the expression of spontaneous activity in damaged sensory axons of mice. *J Physiol* 2003; 550:921–926.

Rustoen T, Wahl AK, Hanestad BR, et al. Gender differences in chronic pain: findings from a population-based study of Norwegian adults. *Pain Manag Nurs* 2004; 5105–5117.

Samad TA, Moore KA, Sapirstein A, Billet S, et al. Interleukin-1-beta-mediated induction of Cox-2 in the CNS contributes to inflammatory pain hypersensitivity. *Nature* 2001; 410:471–475.

Sanes JR, Lichtman JW. Can molecules explain long-term potentiation? *Nat Neurosci* 1999; 2:597–604.

Sarkar S, Hobson AR, Hughes A, et al. The prostaglandin E2 receptor-1 (EP-1) mediates acid-induced visceral pain hypersensitivity in humans. *Gastroenterology* 2003; 124:18–25.

Seltzer Z, Dubner R, Shir Y. A novel behavioral model of neuropathic pain disorders produced in rats by partial sciatic nerve injury. *Pain* 1990; 43:205–218.

Shimoyama N, Shimoyama M, Davis A, Monaghan DT, Inturrisi CE. An antisense oligonucleotide to the *N*-methyl-D-aspartate (NMDA) subunit, NMDAR1, attenuates NMDA-induced nociception, hyperalgesia and morphine tolerance. *J Pharmacol Exp Ther* 2005; 2005; 312:834–840.

Snider WD, McMahon SB. Tackling pain at the source: new ideas about nociceptors. *Neuron* 1998; 20:629–632.

Souslova V, Cesare P, Ding Y, et al. Warm-coding deficits and aberrant inflammatory pain in mice lacking P2X3 receptors. *Nature* 2000; 407:1015–1017.

Tao YX, Rumbaugh G, Wang GD, et al. Impaired NMDA receptor-mediated postsynaptic function and blunted NMDA receptor-dependent persistent pain in mice lacking postsynaptic density-93 protein. *J Neurosci* 2003; 23:6703–6712.

Trebino CE, Stock JL, Gibbons CP, et al. Impaired inflammatory and pain responses in mice lacking an inducible prostaglandin E synthase. *Proc Natl Acad Sci USA* 2003: 100:9044–9049.

Vulchanova L, Riedl MS, Shuster SJ. P2X3 is expressed by DRG neurons that terminate in inner lamina II. *Eur J Neurosci* 1998; 10:3470–3478.

Wieseler-Frank J, Maier SF, Watkins LR. Glial activation and pathological pain. *Neurochem Int* 2004; 45:389–395.

Woolf CJ, Salter MW. Neuronal plasticity: increasing the gain in pain. *Science* 2000; 288:1765–1769.

Woolf CJ, Shortland P, Reynolds M, et al. Reorganization of central terminals of myelinated primary afferents in the rat dorsal horn following peripheral axotomy. *J Comp Neurol* 1995; 360:121–134.

Zeitz KP, Guy N, Malmberg AB, et al. The 5-HT3 subtype of serotonin receptor contributes to nociceptive processing via a novel subset of myelinated and unmyelinated nociceptors. *J Neurosci* 2002; 22:1010–1019.

Zhang B, Tao F, Liaw WJ, et al. Effect of knock down of spinal cord PSD-93/chapsin-110 on persistent pain induced by complete Freund's adjuvant and peripheral nerve injury. *Pain* 2003; 106:187–196.

Zubieta JK, Smith YR, Bueller JA, et al. Mu-opioid receptor-mediated antinociceptive responses differ in men and women. *J Neurosci* 2002; 22:5100–5107.

Correspondence to: Allan I. Basbaum, PhD, Department of Anatomy, University of California, San Francisco, 513 Parnassus Avenue, Box 0452, San Francisco, CA 94143-0452, USA. Tel: 415-476-5270; Fax: 415-476-4845; email: aib@phy.ucsf.edu.

Index